HIV/AIDS Management

HIV/AIDS Management

Edited by **Roger Mostafa**

hayle medical

New York

Published by Hayle Medical,
30 West, 37th Street, Suite 612,
New York, NY 10018, USA
www.haylemedical.com

HIV/AIDS Management
Edited by Roger Mostafa

International Standard Book Number: 978-1-63241-255-3 (Hardback)

Printed in the United States of America.

Contents

Preface

This book encompasses detailed information related to the management of HIV/AIDS. It neither presents an alternative to any book regarding HIV/AIDS nor exhausts the topic in question. The purpose of this book is to complement the content already in circulation and add value to explanation of certain concepts in order to generate more room for reasoning and arrive at solutions against this global pandemic. Further, this book is expected to complement a varied range of studies and analyses conducted in this field, and provide a platform for latest information on this subject. The aim of this book is to serve as a valuable source of reference and equip the readers with knowledge and skills to work towards decreasing HIV transmission and enhance the quality of life of those suffering from this disease as well as those affected by it.

The information contained in this book is the result of intensive hard work done by researchers in this field. All due efforts have been made to make this book serve as a complete guiding source for students and researchers. The topics in this book have been comprehensively explained to help readers understand the growing trends in the field.

I would like to thank the entire group of writers who made sincere efforts in this book and my family who supported me in my efforts of working on this book. I take this opportunity to thank all those who have been a guiding force throughout my life.

Editor

Part 1

Prevention of HIV/AIDS in General

1

HIV Surveillance

Ali Mirzazadeh[1,2] and Saharnaz Nedjat[3]
[1]*Regional Knowledge Hub for HIV/AIDS Surveillance, Kerman University of Medical Sciences, Kerman,*
[2]*HIV/AIDS & Communicable Disease Unit, WHO Representative Office, Tehran,*
[3]*School of Public Health, Knowledge Utilization Research Center, Tehran University of Medical Science, Iran*

1. Introduction

Epidemiological surveillance is defined as the ongoing systematic collection, recording, analysis, interpretation and dissemination of data reflecting the current health status of a community or population. It is essential to planning, implementation and evaluation of public health practice and is closely integrated with the timely dissemination of these data to those who need to know. The definition emphasizes the use of data for public health action, not simply the collection of information as an end in itself.
The objectives of HIV surveillance include the provision of timely and reliable information for:

- advocacy for resources for prevention and care, mobilization of political commitment
- appropriate resource allocation between affected populations and areas
- effective targeting of prevention, care and support programmes
- monitoring and evaluation of the aggregate impact of programmes
- developing new programmes
- informing the public
- tracking the leading edge of the epidemic
- projecting future care and prevention needs
- identifying information gaps and guiding research to fill those gaps
- making health policies to maximize the effectiveness of the above.

So, HIV surveillance is trying to provide qualified evidences for decision makers to better response to HIV epidemic. In order to reach the above objectives, different elements of HIV surveillance has been developed and implemented in different settings. In this chapter we review these elements. Before addressing the different elements of HIV surveillance, we should have a view of HIV infection and its natural phases of infection.

2. The natural history of HIV disease and disease stages

HIV infection results in a chronic condition which is started from *primary HIV infection* with unspecified signs/symptoms (such as fever, muscle aches and swollen glands). Then most affected persons have mild or no symptoms for several years. Gradually, as their immune system weakens, they will experiences HIV-related clinical symptoms and illnesses. Without specific treatment, the HIV infected person will experience all clinical stages ended with the end-stage disease called AIDS (**Figure 1**).

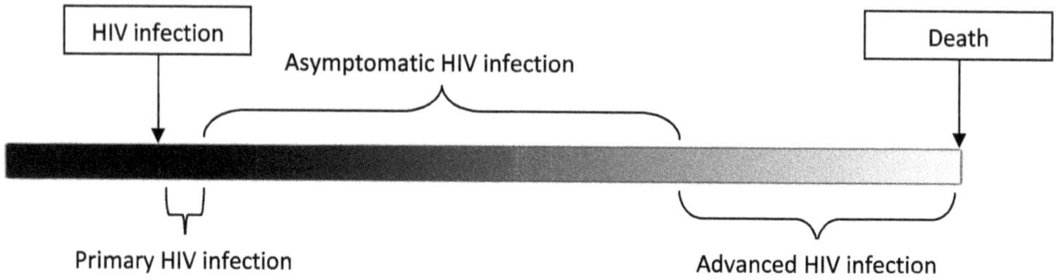

Fig. 1. Key HIV stages which could be reported in HIV case reporting surveillance

HIV transmitted from an infected person to another mainly through:
- Unsafe sexual contact
- Unsafe drug injection
- Delivery of Breast feeding of a child by the affected mother
- Unsafe blood transfusion

As it's obvious, there drivers of the HIV epidemics in a community are risk behaviors. To control the spread of the HIV epidemic, we need to collect information not only on the number of affected people and their previous risky behaviors, but also gather strategic information on the behaviors of the subpopulations especially who are most at risk for acquiring the HIV infection naming female sex workers, injecting drug users, men who have sex with men. Second generation surveillance for HIV/AIDS has been proposed by WHO and UNAIDS to provide such information to response to HIV/AIDS epidemic efficiently.
Second generation surveillance for HIV/AIDS is the regular, systematic collection, analysis and interpretation of information for use in tracking and describing changes in the HIV/AIDS epidemic over time. Second generation surveillance for HIV/AIDS also gathers information on risk behaviors, using them to warn of or explain changes in levels of infection. As such, second generation surveillance includes, in addition to HIV surveillance and AIDS case reporting, STI surveillance to monitor the spread of STI in populations at risk of HIV and behavioral surveillance to monitor trends in risk behaviors over time. These different components achieve greater or lesser significance depending of the surveillance needs of a country, determined by the level of the epidemic it is facing: low level, concentrated or generalized.
The core elements of HIV/AIDS Surveillance included
- HIV/AID Case Reporting
  It's comparable as disease routine reporting system. Persons diagnosed HIV infection (clinical stages 1-4) and/or advanced HIV disease (clinical stages 3 and 4) registered and reported systematically through the health system.
- HIV sentinel sero-prevalence Surveys
  In some health centers, blood is collected routinely for other proposes such as routine antenatal cares for pregnant women. A portion of this blood can be used for HIV testing.
- Behavioral Sero-Surveys (or Bio-Behavioral Surveys)
  Surveys of HIV-related behavior that involve asking a sample of people about their risk behaviors, such as their sexual and drug-injecting behavior. In addition to behavioral questionnaire, blood or saliva also collected to be tested for HIV and/or other sexual

transmitted diseases. In some settings test for tuberculosis is also integrated. Data on behavioral and serological exams are linked and analysis jointly to provide more comprehensive information on the HIV epidemics and its determinants. These Bio-Behavioral surveys could be divided into two categories: (1) facility based surveys (2) community bases surveys. The main differences between these two methods are coming from the sampling schemes that applied for recruiting the subjects into the survey and the definition of the target population.

We elaborate different components of HIV surveillance by the course of HIV infection in Figure 2. Surveillance for HIV infection could be done at four key points: Before, at, after the time of HIV infection and death:

- Surveillance components at the phase before acquiring HIV infection (Behavioural and STI):

  It includes Behavioural and STI surveillance activities. Surveys for estimating the prevalence of risky behaviours and inadequate knowledge on ways to prevent HIV transmission are measures among the general population or high-risk subpopulation (i.e FSWs, IDUs and MSM depend on the context). Sexual Transmitted Infections (STIs) surveillance is also helping the country to track the high-risk populations who are susceptible to get the HIV infection through sexual routes. STIs treatment and care will reduce this susceptibility.
- Surveillance components at the time of acquiring HIV infection (Incidence):

  It's addressing the surveillance activities which could provide an estimated of HIV incidence. HIV incidence is very hard to be estimated and new methods are proposed and implemented. However, many countries did not apply these methods as they are expensive and also laboratories do not have the capacities to do these new tests. As a strategic alternative, it's recommended to include early infant diagnosis surveillance for having a proxy for incidence measures.
- Surveillance components after acquiring the HIV infection (Morbidity):

  These include a verity of surveillance activities such as HIV case reporting, Advanced HIV case reporting, prevalence studies among the general population or high-risk groups, sentinel HIV surveillance among specific groups such as pregnant women at the antenatal clinics. These activities will provide information on the direction of the HIV epidemic in the population and the burden of disease. HIV drug resistance studies also included as the advance component of this phase
- Surveillance components of dead AIDS cases (Mortality):

  This part includes vital registry of all cases died due to AIDS.

The rest of the chapter focuses on HIV case reporting surveillance. If you are interested on the other components such as Sentinel HIV Surveillance and Bio-Behavioral Surveys, more could be found in Guidelines for conducting HIV sentinel serosurveys among pregnant women and other groups (2003) and Guidelines for repeated behavioral surveys in populations at risk of HIV; Durham, North Carolina, Family Health International (2000)

3. HIV case reporting

As one part of the HIV surveillance system, HIV in all clinical stages (including advanced HIV cases and AIDS) is an ongoing reporting system in many countries including the low- and middle-income countries. Since 2006, World Health Organization (WHO) has recommended to replace AIDS case reporting with HIV cases and advanced HIV infection.

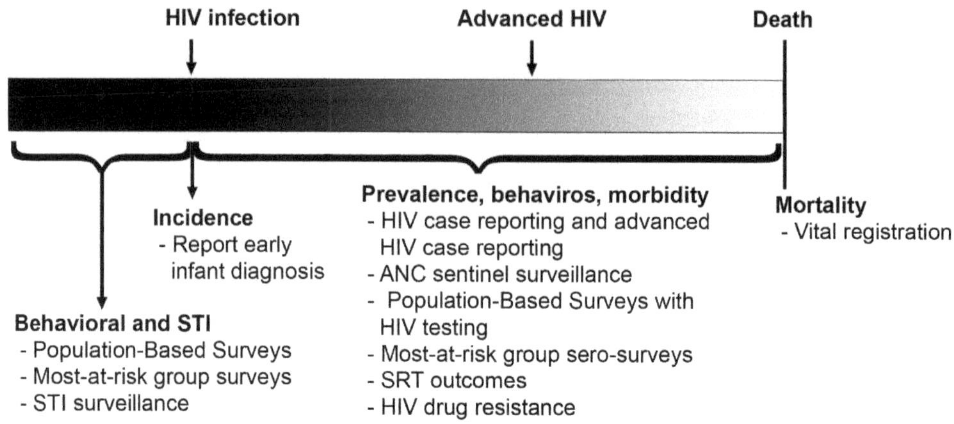

Fig. 2. Key HIV Surveillance Component by phases of HIV infection [Advances and future directions in HIV surveillance Diaz et al. Curr Opin HIV AIDS 4:253-259]

These identified cases are reported confidentially either by names or by anonymous codes. HIV case reporting refers to the methods used to capture individual-level information about persons with HIV infection. Each person with HIV infection is reported using a single case report form which contains information pertaining only to that person. This type of reporting occurs at the level of the health facility and is forwarded to the local level as individual case reports. The local-level surveillance officers combine the data and forward them on to the national surveillance programme where they will be computerized.

WHO refers to reporting all stages of HIV as "HIV infection reporting (all clinical stages)" (Table1) and to reporting of advanced HIV (clinical stages 3 and 4 only) as "advanced HIV infection (disease) reporting." Reporting advanced HIV infection includes AIDS.

Adults and children 18 months or older	HIV infection is diagnosed based on: Positive HIV antibody testing (rapid or laboratory-based enzyme immunoassay). This is confirmed by a second HIV antibody test (rapid or laboratory-based enzyme immunoassay) relying on different antigens or of different operating characteristics; and/or; Positive biological test for HIV or its components (HIV-RNA or HIV-DNA or ultrasensitive HIV p24 antigen) confirmed by a second virological test obtained from a separate determination.
Children younger than 18 months:	HIV infection is diagnosed based on: positive virological test for HIV or its components (HIV-RNA or HIV-DNA or ultrasensitive HIV p24 antigen) confirmed by a second virological test obtained from a separate determination taken more than four weeks after birth. Positive HIV antibody testing is not recommended for definitive or confirmatory diagnosis of HIV infection in children until 18 months of age.

Table 1. WHO case definition for HIV infection

Cases diagnosed with advanced HIV infection (including AIDS) not previously reported should be reported according to a standard case definition. Advanced HIV infection (Table 2) is diagnosed based on clinical and/or immunological (CD4) criteria (Table 3) among people with confirmed HIV infection. AIDS case reporting for surveillance is no longer required if HIV infection or advanced HIV infection is reported.
Advanced HIV infection is diagnosed based on clinical and/or immunological (CD4) criteria among people with confirmed HIV infection:

Criteria for diagnosis of advanced HIV (including AIDS) for reporting
Clinical criteria for diagnosis of advanced HIV in adults and children with confirmed HIV infection: • Presumptive or definitive diagnosis of any stage 3 or stage 4 condition. *and/or;* **Immunological criteria** for diagnosing advanced HIV in adults and children five years or older with confirmed HIV infection: • CD4 count less than 350 per mm3 of blood in an HIV-infected adult or child. *and/or;* **Immunological criteria** for diagnosing advanced HIV in a child younger than five years of age with confirmed HIV infection: • %CD4+ <30 among those younger than 12 months; • %CD4+ <25 among those aged 12–35 months; • %CD4+ <20 among those aged 36–59 months.

Table 2. WHO case definition of advanced HIV (infection or disease) (including AIDS) for reporting[1]

HIV-associated immunodeficiency	Age-related CD4 values			
	<11 months (%CD4+)	12-35 months (%CD4+)	36 -59 months (%CD4+)	>5 years (absolute number per mm3 or %CD4+)
None or not significant	>35	>30	>25	> 500
Mild	30-35	25-30	20–25	350–499
Advanced	25–29	20–24	15–19	200–349
Severe	<25	<20	<15	<200 or <15%

Table 3. WHO immunological classification for established HIV infection

[1]World Health Organization, WHO case definitions of HIV for surveillance and revised clinical staging and immunological classification of HIV-related disease in adults and children. 2007

4. Events which could be reported in HIV case reporting

HIV case reporting, if developed / implemented properly, can provide the health authorities necessary information which are needed for better understanding of the HIV epidemic and monitoring the success of the programmes. The reported cases at any stages of the disease could be used for producing the following indicators:

- HIV incidence (the number or percentage of new HIV infections)
- HIV prevalence (the number or percentage of all persons living with HIV, regardless of how long they have been infected or whether or not they are aware of their infection)
- The incidence of advanced HIV infection
- The prevalence of advanced HIV infection
- Deaths from advanced HIV infection.

5. Elements of a case report form

A comprehensive case report form should include:

- Administrative information
    - Name and address of facility where the report is submitted from (reporting source)
    - Date form completed
    - Report status (new or update)
- Demographic information
    - Patient identifier (name or code)
    - Date of birth
    - Sex
    - Current status (alive, dead, unknown)
    - Country of residence
- Information on the patient's HIV-related risk behaviour
    - Sex with male
    - Sex with female
    - Injected non-prescription drugs
    - Perinatal/MTCT
    - Blood transmission-related variables
    - Occupational exposure
- Diagnosis information
    - Date of HIV diagnosis
    - Facility of diagnosis
- HIV clinical stage
    - Date of first clinical stage
    - Clinical stage
    - Date of first clinical stage 3 diagnosis
    - Date of first clinical stage 4 diagnosis
- Immunologic status
    - Date of first CD4 test
    - Result of first CD4 test (count and/or percentage)
    - Date of first CD4 count <350 cells/mm^3
    - Date of first CD4 count <200 cells/mm^3

- Care and treatment
    - Use of ART
    - Date first used ART
    - Use of prophylaxis against Pneumocystis jirovecii pneumonia
- Vital status
    - Date of death
    - Cause of death.

Countries should carefully consider which elements to include in the case report form. It should include only information that is readily available to the person completing the form and that can be collected from most of the reporting facilities. It should not be a burden to people who complete it.

6. Flow of data

We elaborate this section by presenting an example of health system in a country which medical universities providing health for the people in all areas of the country. Here, the flow of data is divided into four levels (**Figure 3**).

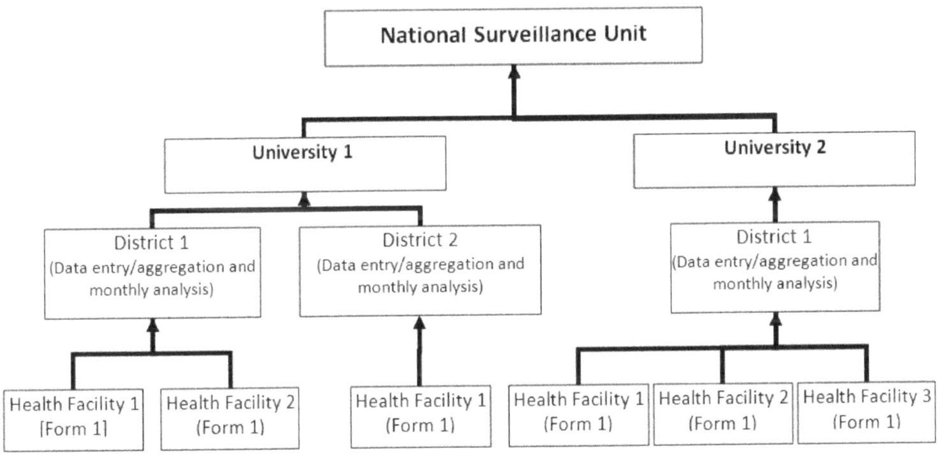

Fig. 3. Flow of data in a country designed in four levels

Level 1 - Health Facilities: all urban and rural health centers, clinics, hospitals, private offices at the time of diagnosis an HIV case in all clinical stages should report the case.

- **Activities**: the responsible staff fill Form 1 for every one who meets the case definition and report the case to level 2

Level 2 - District health centers: these are district health centers which are responsible for providing health to district inhabitants.

- **Activities**: every month, the responsible staff will compile the received data and then fill an aggregated data reporting form and submit it to the Center for Disease Control of the University. By doing sort of data analysis, feedbacks developed and send to the health facilities working in the district.

Level 3 – Center for Disease Control at the University:

- **Activities**: every month, the responsible staff will compile the received data and then fill out an aggregated data reporting form to be sent to the Center for Disease Control of the Ministry (National Surveillance Unit). By doing sort of data analysis, feedbacks developed and send to the district health centers.

Level 4 -Center for District Control at the Ministry (National Surveillance Unit):

- **Activities**: every three months, the responsible staff will compile the received data, make a comprehensive analysis on the received data, and draft the quarterly national surveillance report and distribute it to all the stakeholders to be used.

7. Analysis and feedbacks on cases reporting surveillance

Most of the time, analysis of surveillance data is mainly done only by descriptive analysis to estimate the level of indicators such as the number of affected people by sex, percentage of those cases reported sexual contact as the most probable route of transmission. These estimates should be interpreted according to time to explore the trends and direction of the epidemic. As an example, here we elaborate the analysis and feedback steps of a national HIV case reporting surveillance (in line with the previous section)

Level 2 feedbacks: every three months, HIV surveillance report including the last status of HIV in the district and the trend analysis of the reported data should be sent to all health facilities (even if they did not reported any case of HIV during the period). Such report should have at least the following information:

1. Three months trend
2. Three months trend in compare to the previous three-month period
3. Total number of reported cases by age and sex groups including the main routes of transmission.

Level 3 feedbacks: every three months, HIV surveillance report including the last status of HIV in the province and the trend analysis of the reported data should be sent to all district health centers (even if they did not reported any case of HIV during the period).

Such reports should have at least the following information:

1. Three months trend
2. Three months trend in compare to the previous three-month period
3. Total number of reported cases by age and sex groups including the main routes of transmission.

Level 4 feedbacks: every three months, HIV surveillance report including the last status of HIV in the province and the trend analysis of the reported data should be sent to all district health centers (even if they did not reported any case of HIV during the period).

Such reports should have at least the following information:

1. Three months trend
2. Three months trend in compare to the previous three-month period
3. Total number of reported cases by age and sex groups including the main routes of transmission.

If an increase of 10% has been observed in a university for a period of two sequential months, the feedback should be send to that university and the neighborhood universities at the earliest convenience. It should be done separately from the CDC three-month report.

8. Core indicators according to the phases of the infection

- Surveillance components at the phase before acquiring HIV infection (Behavioural and STI):

  As mentioned before, here the focus is on measuring the risky behaviors which make people susceptible for acquiring the infection. So, samples of people requited in a behavioral survey and complete a questionnaire including sections for sexual behaviors, drug injection and knowledge for HIV prevention, and history of HIV testing and counseling. This data is applied for produce behavioral indicators which used to compare populations, geographic areas and programme impact over time. Examples of these interfamily wide-use indicators are:

• percentage of women and men aged 15–49 who received HIV testing in the previous 12 months and who know their results
• percentage of most-at-risk populations reached by HIV prevention programmes
• percentage of young women and men who have had sexual intercourse before the age of 15
• percentage of female and male sex workers reporting use of a condom with their most recent client
• percentage of injection drug users who reported using sterile injection equipment the most recent time they injected

- Surveillance components after acquiring the HIV infection (Morbidity):

• Percentage of young women and men aged 15 to 24 who are HIV-infected
• Percentage of most-at-risk populations who are HIV-infected.

Although different indicators have been proposed by many international bodies including UNAIDS and WHO, countries should decide from which they will benefit from and is much related to the context and their level of HIV epidemics. They should define the target groups of HIV surveillance and adopt the indicators accordingly.

9. References

[1] World Health Organization and UNAIDS. Second generation surveillance for HIV: compilation of basic materials. CD-ROM. Geneva, World Health Organization (WHO/HIV/2002.07).2002

[2] World Health Organization and UNAIDS. Initiating Second Generation HIV Surveillance Systems: Practical Guidelines. Geneva, World Health Organization (WHO/HIV/2002.17). 2002

[3] World Health Organization and UNAIDS. Guidelines for Second Generation HIV Surveillance for HIV:The Next Decade. Geneva, World Health Organization (WHO/CDS/EDC/2000.05). 2000

[4] Introduction to HIV, AIDS and STI Surveillance: HIV Clinical Staging and Case Reporting, September 2009

[5] Theresa Diaza, Jesus M. Garcia-Callejab, Peter D. Ghysc and Keith Sabina, Advances and future directions in HIV surveillance in low- and middle-income countries, Curr Opin HIV AIDS 4:253–259

[6] World Health Organization, WHO case definitions of HIV for surveillance and revised clinical staging and immunological classification of HIV-related disease in adults and children. 2007

[7] Guidelines for conducting HIV sentinel serosurveys among pregnant women and other groups. Geneva, UNAIDS and WHO, 2003
[8] HIV surveillance in the Middle East and North Africa: a handbook for surveillance planners and implementers / World Health Organization. Regional Office for the Eastern Mediterranean, Joint United Nations Programme on HIV/AIDS, 2010

2

Social Determinants of HIV Health Care: A Tale of Two Cities

Rupali Kotwal Doshi, Carlos del Rio and Vincent C. Marconi
Emory University School of Medicine and Rollins School of Public Health
United States

1. Introduction

Despite unprecedented scale up and advances in the treatment of HIV/AIDS in the last fifteen years, the great majority of individuals around the world who need antiretroviral therapy (ART) are not receiving it. Furthermore, it has now become apparent that even in locations where there is access to treatment, segments of the population do not engage in care because of multiple barriers that prevent them from accessing care, thus losing the potential benefits of ART. A social ecological framework can be applied to understand the multiple layers of factors at the individual, interpersonal and structural levels, that affect HIV clinical outcomes and consequently transmission (Stokols 1996). The institutional barriers include those imposed by the very institutions developed to care for people with HIV. Beyond institutional barriers, factors related to poverty and economics, politics, and the sociocultural and psychological context of the individual all contribute to the challenges faced by people seeking treatment.

Acknowledging the difficulties that HIV-infected individuals confront, the World Health Organization (WHO) has put forth the goal of universal access to HIV/AIDS prevention, treatment, and care (WHO 2010). In addition to improving the individual's personal health, access and treatment with subsequent virologic suppression on a population level may help decrease transmission of HIV (Das et al. 2010). Until a cure for HIV is found, individuals infected with HIV face a lifetime of requiring health care access and antiretroviral drug therapy to control the virus, in addition to the comorbidities associated with chronic HIV infection.

For those able to enter and remain in care, additional obstacles can prevent them from maintaining high levels of adherence to the available therapies. In this chapter, we will explore how the sociocultural context of a particular region can influence health care outcomes for individuals living with HIV. First, we exemplify two epidemics and two health care systems separated geographically and culturally from one another, Atlanta, Georgia, United States, and Durban, KwaZulu-Natal, South Africa, in order to illustrate how these factors can impede a successful response to ART. Following this description, we describe efforts that have been undertaken to address some of these barriers to improve engagement in health care within and beyond these settings. We also review creative approaches that can be used to maximize adherence to treatment. Finally, a course for the ultimate way forward is chartered, detailing steps necessary to address these barriers in a variety of settings around the world.

2. Atlanta, Georgia, USA

2.1 The city too busy to hate

Atlanta is located in the northwest corner of the state of Georgia, which is in the southeastern region of the US. Atlanta was incorporated in 1847 and began as a railroad hub, connecting multiple cities across the US. During the American Civil War (1861-1865), the city was set on fire, destroying a large percentage of its infrastructure. In the years following the Civil War, the city was rebuilt gradually, with the intention to create a modern city that was less reliant on agriculture than previously. For example, the Georgia Institute of Technology, a prominent science and engineering university, was founded in 1885 in order to advance these goals (*The New Georgia Encyclopedia*). In addition, two historically black colleges, Spellman College (for women) and Morehouse College (for men) were established soon after the Civil War.

As the population of Atlanta expanded significantly in the wake of the Civil War, tensions between blacks and whites grew, and Jim Crow laws supporting segregation of the races in housing, school, and socialization began to take effect. In 1906, on the backdrop of Georgia's gubernatorial race which highlighted racial segregation and after newspapers reported 4 incidents of alleged sexual abuse of white women by black men, Atlanta's first documented race riot occurred. The death toll for the event was approximately 25 to 40 African-Americans and 2 whites. After 3 days of fighting, city officials, prominent clergy, and newspapers proposed an end to the violence. White and black community and business leaders came together to support racial reconciliation, in order to protect Atlanta's image as a "thriving New South City." As a result of these efforts, Atlanta did not feature as a major city for civil rights infringement during the riots in the 1960s throughout the south. Furthermore, Atlanta has a strong historical connection with the Civil Rights movement of the mid-twentieth century, because Martin Luther King, Jr., preached at the Ebenezer Baptist Church, located in downtown Atlanta, and the city was seen as a major organizing center for students and other civil rights leaders (*The New Georgia Encyclopedia*).

Atlanta currently has a population of approximately 500,000 within the city limits, and 5 million in the entire metropolitan statistical area (MSA), which includes 31 counties. The racial makeup of the city is approximately 50% African-American, 43% Caucasian, 13% Asian, and 5% Hispanic. In comparison, as of 2009 the state of Georgia's population was estimated to be 9.8 million, consisting of 65% white and 30% black (*United States Census*).

Atlanta's population has grown considerably after the opening of Hartsfield-Jackson International Airport in 1980 (which is one of the busiest in the US) (Yee 2007) and the hosting of the Summer Olympics in 1996. Twenty percent of the population lives below the poverty level. Major industries in Atlanta include professional and administrative services, waste management, education, arts, and food services (*United States Census*). Savannah, located on the Atlantic Ocean, is the second largest port eastern seaboard of the US and serves as a major hub for international shipping. Much of this traffic moves through Atlanta as it passes on to other cities throughout the country. Atlanta has a confluence of racial and ethnic diversity, industry, high-quality colleges and universities, and trade that give it a uniquely metropolitan feel in this region.

2.2 HIV Epidemic in Atlanta and the southeastern U.S.

According to surveillance statistics for HIV/AIDS, the southeast has been among the most significantly affected regions in the US since 2005. Georgia ranked 8th in the nation for its reported prevalence rate of AIDS, and a substantial proportion of HIV cases in this region is diagnosed in Atlanta. The same factors that contribute to high rates of infection and advanced disease in this region also lead to poor entry and retention in care. These factors include poverty (9th most poor state in US), inadequate education (8th worst high school graduation rate in the US), substance abuse, poor access to health care, food insufficiency (Kalichman et al. 2010), and child sex trade (Longerbeam 2010). In Atlanta, crack cocaine use and homelessness impact transmission of HIV, but there is also significant transmission among heterosexuals and men who have sex with men (MSM).

It is important to point out that while 78% of HIV (non-AIDS) cases and 75% of AIDS cases diagnosed in 2008 in Georgia were among Blacks, they make up only 30% of the state population (Mangla and Gant 2008). Among cases of HIV/AIDS diagnosed in Georgia in 2008, about half (53%) occurred between the ages of 30 and 49, one quarter (28%) between ages 20 and 29, and 14% among people 50 years of age of older (Mangla and Gant 2008).

The Atlanta eligible metropolitan area (EMA) is a 20-county region designated by the US Department of Health and Human Services (DHHS) Health Resources and Services Administration (HRSA) to receive federal funding through the Ryan White Comprehensive AIDS Resources Emergency (CARE) Act. As of the end of 2009, a total of 26,546 persons were living with HIV/AIDS in the 20-county Atlanta EMA; of these, 15,548 were AIDS cases and 10,998 are HIV-infected but do not yet have AIDS (eHARS Reporting System 2010). The racial distribution is 68% among blacks and 24% among whites (eHARS Reporting System 2010). The majority of cases are among men, and the main risk factor for transmission is MSM (46%), followed by heterosexual contact (8.4%), injection drug use (7.3%) (eHARS Reporting System 2010).

Within the city of Atlanta, HIV is largely concentrated in one large cluster located in downtown and southwest Atlanta that consists of 157 census tracts and covers about 180 square miles. The cluster contains 60% of prevalent HIV/AIDS cases in the Atlanta MSA, and the HIV prevalence within the cluster is 1.34% compared to 0.32% outside the cluster (Hixson et al. 2011). Thus, as a whole, the city of Atlanta has a "generalized epidemic" with an HIV prevalence of >1% (see Figure 1).

3. Durban, KwaZulu-Natal, South Africa

3.1 The city of gold

Durban (eThekwini), located on the eastern coast of the Republic of South Africa, is the largest city in the province of KwaZulu-Natal (KZN). A well-known tourist destination for South Africans and international travelers, Durban is the third largest city in the Republic and one of the busiest seaports in the southern hemisphere. Durban has a population of nearly 3,500,000 including nearby townships. A very culturally diverse community, Durban's population is 68% black African, 20% Asian (one of the largest Indian populations outside of India and largest Asian community on the African continent), 9% white, and 3% coloured. Manufacturing, tourism, finance and transport are the major industrial sectors in the city. A recent principal host city for the 2010 Fédération Internationale de Football Association World Cup, eThekwini boasts the highest credit rating in Africa for a municipality in September 2004.

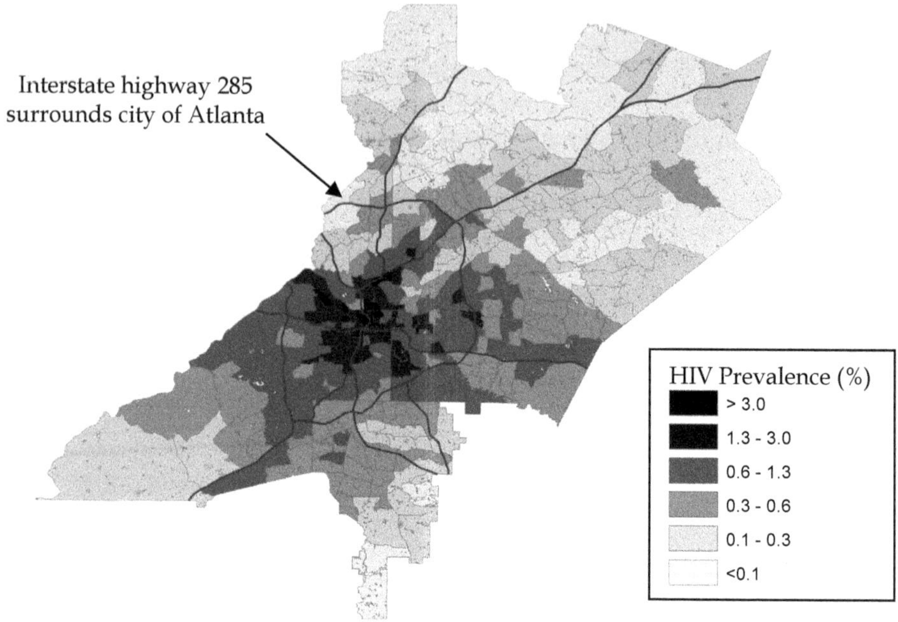

Fig. 1. HIV prevalence estimates for city of Atlanta and Fulton, DeKalb, Gwinnett, and Clayton counties, 2008 (Produced from Georgia Department of Public Health surveillance data)

The aboriginal population of KZN was believed to have settled in the area around 100,000 BC and was eventually overtaken by the Bantu expansion in 300 AD. Early exploration by the Portuguese began in the 15th century (Russell 1899). The Dutch and British later formed more lasting settlements on the coast. The peaceful relationship between the Kingdom of Shaka Zulu and the early British settlers was disrupted after tensions developed between colonists and native Africans (Bulpin 1977). This was followed by major conflicts known as the Anglo-Zulu (1879) and Anglo-Boer Wars (1880-1881 and 1899-1902). The colonizers suppressed and dominated the black South Africans (Shillington 2005).

During this period, a large population of indentured laborers was brought in from India to work in the sugar cane industry, along with black migrant workers from rural areas of KZN. In 1893 Mahatma Gandhi arrived in Durban to serve as a legal adviser for an Indian law firm. The widespread denial of civil liberties and political rights to Indian immigrants inspired his struggle for Indians' rights there and in India. By the end of the 19th century, industry, especially mining, used coercive tactics to maintain inexpensive black labor in the cities. Over time, this severely disrupted traditional family structures and eroded the rural agricultural economy of black South Africans, further increasing the income disparity (Coovadia et al. 2009).

Eventually, South Africa fell under British rule upon signing the peace treaty of Vereeniging in 1902. Following unification of the Boer and British colonies, several government policies were enacted to entrench white supremacy and racial segregation in South Africa. Racial classification with whites at the top resulted in social separation, political exclusion, economic marginalization, and racial injustices (Marks and Andersson 1987; WHO 1983). In

1923, the African National Congress was formed to peacefully lobby for equal rights for all races. Their efforts were largely unsuccessful, as segregation policies were consolidated under the right-wing National Party when it rose to power in 1948, which marked the official beginning of apartheid. Nelson Mandela, along with many leaders of the ANC, was arrested and imprisoned in 1964. Domestic and international pressure finally resulted in the demise of apartheid in 1990, and the first free elections were held in South Africa in 1994, ushering in a new era with Mandela as president.

Students and staff from the University of Natal, founded in 1910 in Durban, actively protested apartheid policies. In 1950, the first medical school for black students in South Africa was established nearby, later named the Nelson Mandela School of Medicine. The University of Durban-Westville was created in the 1960s with the express intent of providing higher education for students of Indian origin. After the fall of apartheid, these universities merged to form the University of KwaZulu-Natal in 2004, which remains one of the premier academic institutions in South Africa. UKZN sponsors several prominent HIV/AIDS-related research programs that are ongoing today.

3.2 HIV epidemic in Durban and KwaZulu-Natal

Sub-Saharan Africa carries a disproportionate burden of HIV infections when compared to other regions in the world. Based on two national surveys published in 2008 and 2009, South Africa, and specifically the province of KwaZulu-Natal, are at the epicenter of the HIV epidemic with HIV prevalence estimates ranging from 15.8% among the general population over age 2 to 40% among women presenting to antenatal clinics (Health 2009; Shisana et al. 2009) (see Figure 2). With such a considerable prevalence, the odds of having a partner with

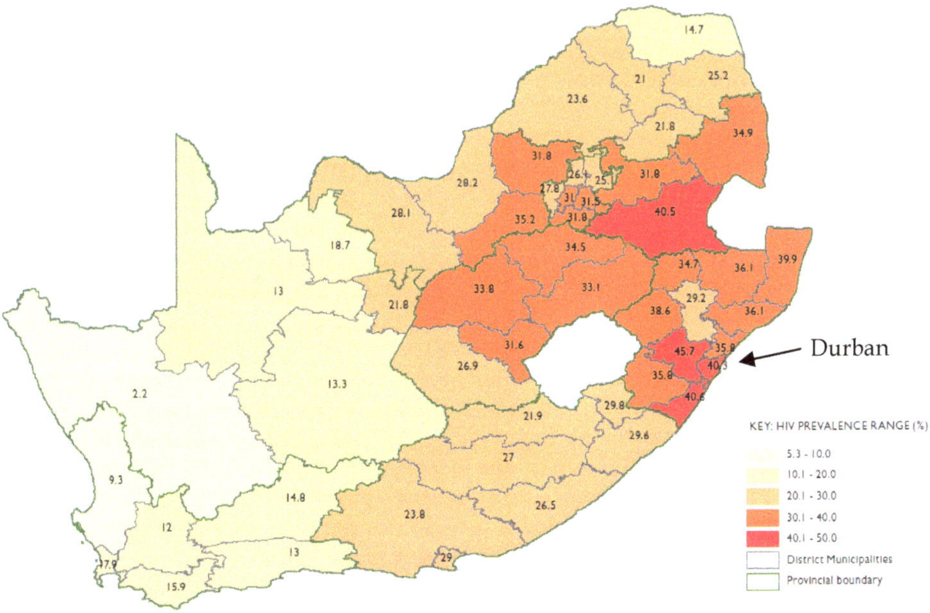

Fig. 2. HIV prevalence by district in South Africa, antenatal clinics, 2008 (Health 2009)

HIV are high, and this has overwhelmed current prevention efforts aimed at discordant couples. In addition to wealth and income disparities, various historical, cultural and political factors have directly and indirectly contributed to these substantial rates.

Until 1988, HIV in South Africa was largely restricted to the homosexual community and hemophiliacs who had received blood transfusions (Abdool Karim et al. 2009; Abdool Karim and Abdool Karim 2005). However, from that point onward, heterosexual transmission became the dominant mode of HIV transmission in South Africa. Using fear, stigma and risk profiling, the apartheid government added to pre-existing prejudices against homosexuals and blacks. After an initially slow introduction of HIV into the heterosexual community, the numbers of individuals with HIV infection grew exponentially from 1990 to 1994. HIV prevalence in pregnant women increased from 0.8% to 7.6% during this period (Ijsselmuiden et al. 1988; Gouws and Abdool Karim 2005). This contributed to a significant rise in the number of perinatal infections. By this time HIV finally became a government priority and condom distribution increased throughout the country.

In the subsequent five years, an even more rapid spread occurred throughout South Africa. In particular, certain areas of rural KZN experienced substantial increases. The main factors identified that fueled the epidemic included migrant laborers, who served as a bridge population between urban and rural community networks (Lurie, Williams, Zuma, Mkaya-Mwamburi, Garnett, Sweat, et al. 2003) and multiple, concurrent partnerships (rural wife and town wife). Also, rape and violence against women increased their susceptibility to HIV (Jochelson, Mothibeli, and Leger 1991; Lurie, Williams, Zuma, Mkaya-Mwamburi, Garnett, Sturm, et al. 2003; Hunter 2005; Wood, Maforah, and Jewkes 1998; Jewkes 2009; Dunkle et al. 2004). During this time, the Treatment Action Campaign was formed to combat the AIDS denialism that had been previously espoused by the government.

In 2003, ART was introduced into the public sector with funding from the US President's Emergency Plan for AIDS Relief (PEPFAR). It took over 5 years after PEPFAR was introduced in South Africa to see decreases in incidence rates, despite one of the largest ART rollouts in the world. Presently, life expectancy in KZN is nearly 50 years for women and 49 years for men (*Statistical Release P0302: Midyear population estimates*). In response to these overwhelming challenges, South Africa's HIV/AIDS and STI National Strategic Plan was launched in 2007 (*The HIV/AIDS Country Scorecard* 2008; HIV & AIDS and STI Strategic Plan for South Africa, 2007-2011 2007). The latest UNAIDS report has shown a sharp decline in the incidence among 18 year olds and women 15-24 years old by 2008 (UNAIDS report on the global AIDS epidemic 2010).

Bringing millions of individuals into care for chronic HIV infection has been a major challenge for South Africa. Despite a developed health care system (8.0% of GDP is spent on health care), the health care system is overwhelmed with the sheer number of individuals infected with HIV. With more than 5.6 million people infected with HIV in South Africa, it is estimated that only 36% of adults and 54% of children eligible for treatment (based upon current WHO criteria that includes CD4 T cells <350 cells/μL) are currently receiving it (Coovadia et al. 2009; UNAIDS report on the global AIDS epidemic 2010). In light of this, it has been no small feat to have over 970,000 individuals on ART.

Poverty in the black population created a general deterioration of health for black South Africans associated with high communicable diseases and violence-related injuries (Packard 1989). Today, over 50% of South Africans live in poverty, more than 40% experience food insecurity, and unemployment remains high (25%) (Rose and Charlton 2002; Ojikutu, Jack, and Ramjee 2007; *Statistical Release P0302: Midyear population estimates*). Government policies have preferentially benefitted the rich, and this has further increased the overall income gap between the wealthy and the poor (Growth, employment and redistribution: a macro-economic framework 1996). However, even when treatment is provided at minimal or no cost, the substantial cost and effort required to travel long distances (and take time away from childcare and subsistence living) becomes a tremendous barrier to regular clinic and pharmacy attendance.

The seeds of the present weakened health care system were sown during the early days of colonization, and through the apartheid era and beyond, government policies further fragmented the health care system. (Coovadia et al. 2009). Traditional healers were marginalized, and health care training and delivery was racially segregated; these factors resulted in disparities in funding, and the doctor-patient ratio differed along racial lines (fewer black providers for more black patients). Similar human resource challenges exist for nursing, and this has been compounded by high rates of HIV infection among health care workers (Statistics 2007 2007; Shisana et al. 2004). The state overtook missionary hospitals that were crucial in the delivery of health care in rural areas and homelands. Also, the government contributes nearly 56% of the national health expenditure to public sector health care services, which treats 80-85% of the population. Conversely, the remaining 15-20% of the population in private health care receive 44% of the national health care expenditure (McIntyre and Dorrington 1990; Goudge 1999). As the government encouraged providers to move to the private sector and removed funding to the public sector, this increased out-of-pocket expenses for poor patients, a significant barrier to care. There are also discrepancies in quality between the public and private systems (Dennison et al. 2007; Schneider et al. 2005; Palmer 1999). Altogether, these factors result in poor integration of services (especially tuberculosis diagnosis and treatment, mental health, and substance abuse counseling), overcrowding, long waiting lists, provider fatigue, and patient dissatisfaction.

4. Comparing Atlanta and Durban

Several aspects about the HIV epidemic in both of these cities make them uniquely comparable and allow the illustration of various important facets of engagement in care. Atlanta and Durban are both mid-sized cities in wealthy countries, yet both are experiencing an HIV epidemic out of proportion to the rest of their respective regions (Table 1). There are significant disparities of income and education in both cities, which provide some explanation for the high prevalence of HIV. A history of racism, substantial migrant and transient communities, cultural denialism of sexual practices, and a thriving commercial sex trade may also contribute to the transmission of HIV in both cities.

	Atlanta MSA	Durban & nearby townships
Population	5.4 million	10.6 million
% of population Black	50%	68%
HIV prevalence	>1%	15.8% to 38.7% (KZN)
Main risk factors for HIV transmission	MSM Heterosexual, IDU	Heterosexual

Table 1. Comparison of population and HIV prevalence of Atlanta and Durban as of 2008 (CDC 2009; Mangla and Gant 2008; Health 2009; Shisana et al. 2009)

Both cities are racially and culturally diverse, which may impede efforts to treat and prevent HIV transmission, and both have gone through changes in the laws and sociopolitical environment for black individuals through the past fifty years. Martin Luther King, Jr., recognized the connection between the struggles of African-Americans and black South Africans living under apartheid rule when he said,

"In this period when the American Negro is giving moral leadership and inspiration to his own nation, he must find the resources to aid his suffering brothers in his ancestral homeland. Nor is this aid a one-way street. The civil rights movement in the United States has derived immense inspiration from the successful struggles of those Africans who have attained freedom in their own nations." (King 1965)

There are also some notable differences between the Atlanta and Durban. About two-thirds of the individuals living with HIV in Atlanta are African-American, but black South Africans comprise an overwhelming majority of individuals with HIV in Durban. HIV transmission in Atlanta occurs primarily through men having sex with men (51%), followed by heterosexual contact (22%), injection drug use, and other means. Transmission in Durban is primarily through heterosexual contact. Also in Atlanta, crack cocaine use contributes indirectly to the spread of HIV (Metsch et al. 2008), whereas in Durban, drug abuse is not a prominent risk factor. In the following three sections, we describe how various institutions, clinics and health care systems have identified ways to overcome barriers to HIV health care and methods to improve adherence to HIV treatment.

5. Engaging in care: access, entry, and retention in clinical care

Based on the social ecological framework, we have identified the three major areas impacting engagement in care are individual, interpersonal, and structural factors (Stokols 1996). Some individual factors that may limit engagement in care include personal health beliefs, substance abuse, homelessness, food insecurity, and competing life priorities. Interpersonal factors that may limit engagement in care include communication with physicians, experiences with health care staff, or the influences of social networks on health behaviors. Structural factors include institutional or systemic factors, economic, cultural and political factors. The lack of health insurance, changes in insurance status based on employment or fluctuations in income, complexity of the health system, and reduction in funding for safety net resources may all limit access, entry and retention into care.

At the political level, local and federal policy has played a pivotal role in the accessibility of HIV treatment. Even despite well-intended efforts, government policies can be complicated or ineffective at delivering or augmenting health care or fail to provide the necessary safeguards for individuals with private insurance. Although it took almost 10 years to enact, the Ryan White CARE Act finally passed in 1990 to provide a safety net of HIV/AIDS clinical care in the US (HRSA). In South Africa, HIV denialism at the highest levels of government, worked against efforts to provide care and reduce transmission, wasting valuable time which undoubtedly led to many unnecessary infections and deaths from HIV/AIDS (Chigwedere and Essex 2010).

5.1 Atlanta

In Atlanta, a patchwork of private providers, hospital clinics, and safety net providers such as Grady Memorial Hospital, the Atlanta Veterans Affairs Medical Center, and county health departments provide the clinical care for persons infected with HIV. An individual's access to medical care and antiretroviral therapy depends on the type of insurance they have, as well as their ability to navigate the system designated for them. Patients who are undocumented (without legal status in the US) rely on the safety nets that have been developed, although their obstacles are even greater than those with legal status. Atlanta is one of the cities in the US eligible for Ryan White part A funds that are directed to the most severely affected EMAs. To qualify for part A funding an EMA must have reported at least 2,000 AIDS cases in the most recent 5 years and have a population of at least 50,000. These Federal funds are then distributed to various sites in the Atlanta EMA by the Ryan White executive committee, which is made up of providers, legislators, patient representatives, and other community stakeholders. Clinical sites must apply each year to the Ryan White funding committee in order to renew their funding. The state-run AIDS Drugs Assistance Programs (ADAP) help to cover the cost of antiretroviral therapy as well as other commonly prescribed medications for HIV patients, but as of fall 2010, funding for the Georgia ADAP fell short of need and a waiting list was created (*HIV Care Program: AIDS Drug Assistance Program*). Individual pharmaceutical companies have now extended assistance for antiretroviral medications for eligible patients on the waiting list, but third-party payer assistance for medications remains one of the most significant hurdles for uninsured patients in care.

The Infectious Diseases Program (IDP) at Grady Memorial Hospital treats 5,000 of the most advanced cases of HIV/AIDS in the Atlanta EMA annually, and it is one of the largest outpatient facilities for HIV-positive individuals in the US. For over twenty years, the IDP has provided integrated and comprehensive HIV health care with over 12 specialty and subspecialty services available on-site including hematology/oncology, neurology, hepatology, dental, ophthalmology, dermatology and metabolic disorders. All HIV-positive patients admitted to Grady Memorial Hospital are tracked by the Social Services department to ensure referral to the appropriate outpatient provider upon discharge and to provide support during hospitalization. Other local hospitals and providers can refer patients to IDP as well.

IDP has made distinct efforts to retain patients in care. Certain populations, such as those who are substance abusers, homeless, and/or have a psychiatric illness were found to be at high risk for virologic failure and subsequent morbidity and mortality from HIV/AIDS. These patients have been targeted for participation in the Transition Center, an open-access part of IDP in which patients can arrive as a walk-in to see a medical or psychiatric provider, attend substance abuse group therapy visits, and see a nutritionist (Cohen et al. 2011). Patients who miss appointments at IDP are contacted by "Client Trackers" who reschedule appointments. Finally, a number of support groups and case management programs run by community-based organizations (*AID Atlanta*) are available for patients to discuss the issues that impact their lives and help patients participate in HIV primary care. Peer navigators, mental health counselors, nurses, and pharmacists all serve as part of the treatment team to guide patients through the health system and the process of self-care needed for HIV management.

5.2 South Africa

Despite the substantial challenges facing patients and health care providers detailed above, there have been tremendous accomplishments in ART delivery and health outcomes. Many programs throughout the country have shown impressive rates of virologic suppression at six months (90-95%) and very low rates of loss to follow up (Boulle et al. 2008; Marconi et al. 2008). These outcomes have remained outstanding even after several years of treatment (Lawn et al. 2008; Rosen, Fox, and Gill 2007). For the small percentage of patients requiring second line therapy, a substantial percentage of patients were able to achieve virologic suppression thereafter (Fox et al. 2010; Murphy et al. 2010). Although encouraging, most of these reports have been from urban clinics with adequate resources to individually and programmatically monitor and manage the large volume of patients initiated on ART. Unfortunately, early data from rural sites with fewer resources have shown more discouraging outcomes (Mutevedzi et al. 2010). Suboptimal adherence to ART has been associated with virologic failure (Nachega et al. 2006; Bisson et al. 2008), drug resistance (Braithwaite et al. 2006), and death (Wood et al. 2002).

Although programmatic monitoring has been required to maintain funding support, it has simultaneously served as a mechanism to assist clinics in assessing, assuring and improving the care delivery processes and quality of the care provided. Some clinical sites have also been fitted with electronic medical records and other electronic systems to improve the workflow and immediate access to necessary data. Another effective systematic change has been the extensive use of counselors, peer navigators, HIV educators and nurses to deliver care for patients who are doing well on treatment, particularly in areas where physician resources are limited (Sanne et al. 2010; Abdool Karim et al. 2009). This approach, known as task shifting, along with down-referral (the decentralization of care to smaller clinics without physicians) has been one way to address the limited human resources relative to the demand (Long et al. 2011; Matovu et al. 2011; Sanne et al. 2010). This approach is consistent with the development of more community-based health centers to improve access, especially in rural areas. In addition to treatment monitoring of patients on a stable regimen, the role for nurse initiation and complete follow up management of patients on ART (NIM-ART) is being assessed in a randomized trial and is being discussed at a national level in order to expand treatment access (Colvin et al. 2010; Uebel et al. 2011; Fairall et al. 2011).

Another intervention being used to improve access and retention in care has been the fast-tracking of patients in desperate need of starting ART (Geng et al. 2011). Similarly, ART initiation in the hospital after initial HIV diagnosis and/or a new opportunistic infection helps to reduce the barriers experienced when patients are discharged from the hospital. This is especially effective when combined with palliative care programs designed to address the multiple symptomatic complaints as well as psychosocial and spiritual needs of the patient. In a busy clinical program, these issues often get overlooked by providers and nurses which can erode trust in the health care team (Sunpath et al. 2011). In East Africa, programs with dedicated staff who use aggressive outreach (by using all available means of transportation) to search for patients within 30 days of a missed visit ultimately have lower lost-to-follow-up rates (Braitstein et al. 2011).

Since 75% of HIV-infected individuals in South Africa use remedies dispensed by traditional healers, it has become increasingly apparent that patients would ultimately benefit from bridging the gap between these disciplines (Shuster et al. 2009). Practitioners of western medicine are now working with traditional healers to assist in HIV education, counseling and testing in the community (Peltzer, Mngqundaniso, and Petros 2006; *Traditional healers in South Africa trained to encourage people to get tested for HIV* 2006). Consequently, this approach has been supported by the South African Department of Public Health (Ojikutu, Jack, and Ramjee 2007).

5.3 Examples of universal health care systems

Various health care systems and clinical settings have created structures to improve the ability of individuals to remain engaged in care. Some health care systems, such as those found in the US Department of Defense (DoD), US Department of Veterans Affairs (VA) and various European countries, have reduced or eliminated the out-of-pocket expenses for patients or have provided financial assistance through the involvement of integrated community-based organizations. In the absence of universal health care, some of the interventions include the use of patient navigators, such as those implemented in clinics across Haiti, comprehensive integrated care centers (the medical home), patient- and family-focused care, optimal use of electronic medical records for tracking and process optimization, community-based specialty care, and interventions specifically targeting drug users or other vulnerable subpopulations.

5.3.1 Vancouver

In contrast to the US, Canada provides a universal health care system for all its residents that covers treatment of HIV. For example, in the province of British Columbia, health care and antiretroviral medications are provided free of charge. Almost as important as eliminating out-of-pocket expenses, this system has virtually eliminated the administrative barriers that accompany similar systems elsewhere when an individual moves in and out of various insurance programs. HIV-positive patients must register with the Drug Treatment Program (DTP) that is coordinated by the British Columbia Center for Excellence in HIV/AIDS. Despite the availability of free health care, investigators in Vancouver found that a significant number of HIV-positive individuals still do not use antiretroviral therapy, and that 40% of people who died from HIV-related causes never initiated ART (Joy et al. 2008). They also found that 16% of individuals waited until their CD4 cell count fell below 50 cells/µl to initiate ART (Joy et al. 2008). The findings in British Columbia demonstrate how access to care alone may not result in optimal health outcomes across all HIV-infected populations, and that multiple factors must be considered when designing interventions to improve health outcomes (Lima et al. 2010; *British Columbia Center for Excellence in HIV/AIDS*).

5.3.2 Military and VA

Most health care in the US is delivered by clinics and hospitals that are privately owned and operated (community-based, academic, corporate-owned) and a smaller percentage are government-based. Since the US is a mixed market system, the payer source is divided between self-pay (12.8%) and third party insurance (87.2%). Third party insurance includes public insurance (46.4% of the total as Medicare, Medicaid and government employee insurance) and private insurance (40.7% of the total) (CMS 2011). Some of the government employee programs such as those associated with the DoD and the VA provide universal access to care for their participants. When care is received at government facilities or other participating facilities, the individual has no (or minimal) out of pocket expenses and does not pay premiums or deductibles. Studies have shown that individuals with HIV in these programs have outcomes equivalent to those reported in clinical trials with high levels of adherence and virologic suppression, as well as low rates of hospitalization and mortality, even among individuals with other significant barriers to care (homelessness, poverty, drug use) (Marconi et al. 2010; Guest et al. 2011). Eliminating out-of-pocket expenses and streamlining health care may result in improved outcomes for HIV patients, even for traditionally marginalized populations.

5.4 Overcoming the barrier of substance abuse

HIV and substance abuse have coexisted since the beginning of the epidemic. Not only does injection drug use provide a direct pathway for HIV transmission via the use of shared blood products, but certain substances, particularly stimulants, have been associated with a high frequency of unprotected sex, providing another pathway for HIV transmission.

Various techniques have been attempted to improve rates of linkage to care among substance abusers, such as coordinated substance abuse, mental health, and medical treatment (Korthuis et al. 2011; Weiss et al. 2011; Cunningham et al. 2011). Targeted outreach programs designed to bring active drug users to engage in medical care have been implemented in many cities in the US and Canada, such as Boston, New Haven, New York, and Vancouver. These outreach programs often partner with community-based harm reduction organizations to provide the needed services in spaces that may be more comfortable for drug users (Cunningham et al. 2007; Bardsley, Turvey, and Blatherwick 1990).

For example, in New York City a partnership between Montefiore Medical Center (academic medical institution) and CitiWide Harm Reduction (community-based organization) was designed to bring HIV-positive drug users into medical care. Medical providers go to single-room occupancy hotels accompanied by the outreach teams from CitiWide to meet potential patients, offer medical services, and educate patients. Immediate needs such as prescriptions for acute illnesses may be written for patients during the outreach, and those who are interested may be referred for primary care services on-site at either CitiWide's walk-in clinic or Montefiore's primary care clinic (Cunningham et al. 2007). Investigators found that patients were more likely to keep same-day or walk-in appointments at CitiWide's walk-in clinic compared with future appointments at Montefiore (Cunningham et al. 2007). These findings emphasize the need to provide care in various ways that facilitate access to care for substance users.

In Massachusetts, a mobile van from the Massachusetts Department of Public Health targets men who have sex with men, in order to diagnose HIV earlier and prevent and treat sexually transmitted infections. Researchers found that men using the mobile van's services reported a variety of substances used, including substance use during sex, and that polysubstance users had higher numbers of male sexual partners, anonymous male sexual partners, and male sexual partners met over the internet in the previous year, when compared with non-polysubstance users (Mimiaga et al. 2008). These findings indicate that mobile van health services are a useful way to target this high-risk group.

5.5 Test, Link to Care, Plus Treat (TLC-Plus)

In order to address many of the challenges in the test-to-treat continuum for HIV infected individuals, the NIH-funded HIV Prevention Trials Network (HPTN) has started a study called TLC-Plus (Test, Link to Care, Plus Treat) in Washington, DC, and Bronx, NY, to evaluate the feasibility of a multifaceted approach to HIV prevention. The study includes a package of interventions that include expanded HIV testing, linkage to care, initiation of ART for those clinically eligible, promotion of high adherence to maintain virologic suppression, and prevention for positives interventions. The study will also assess the patient and provider attitudes toward the initiation of ART in early HIV disease. Outcomes in the intervention communities (Washington, DC, and the Bronx, NY) will be compared to those in the non-intervention communities (Chicago, Illinois, Houston, Texas, Miami, Florida and Philadelphia). This study began enrollment in 2011 and results are expected in approximately 3 years.

5.6 Community-based specialty care

Regular access to a medical provider specialized to treat HIV may be difficult for some HIV-positive patients, and the US Institute of Medicine has recently identified critical shortages in the number of providers specialized to care for HIV-positive individuals (IOM 2011). In addition, some patients may feel that attending an infectious diseases specialty clinic carries a stigma, and they may avoid care for this reason. One way that health systems have circumvented this barrier is to place HIV specialists in community health care settings. For example, Montefiore Medical Center, Bronx, NY, has a hospital-based infectious diseases clinic, as well as several community-based primary care clinics that manage HIV-positive patients by using partnerships between primary care providers and HIV specialists. Investigators found, in a retrospective review comparing those who initiated care in the hospital-based setting versus the community-based setting, that patients initiated ART at similar rates and achieved similar levels of virologic suppression (Chu et al. 2010). The findings here suggest this may be a viable way to provide appropriate HIV specialty care for patients who may find difficulty accessing more centralized care settings, and this may alleviate some of the provider shortages regarding HIV specialists in the US.

6. Medication adherence

After overcoming the hurdles associated with navigating the health care system and understanding the complexities of their disease, individuals with HIV must maintain perfect adherence to difficult regimens requiring multiple doses per day or suffer the consequences of HIV drug resistance and disease progression. Overcoming many psychosocial and physical discomforts related to the diagnosis and disease are paramount to ensuring a steady pace in what would be considered a marathon of necessary therapy. The most common factors associated with poor treatment adherence include untreated depression, active substance abuse, poor insight into disease and treatment, youth, higher pill burden, more frequent dosing and forgetfulness (Nachega et al. 2011). In Sub-Saharan Africa, the cost of ART, lack transportation to the health care facility for refills, and pharmacy stock-outs are additional barriers; stigma and food insecurity were the most prevalent risk factors for poor adherence (Crane et al. 2006; Nachega et al. 2004; Weiser et al. 2003; Weiser et al. 2010).

Various approaches have been undertaken to include incorporation of religious and spiritual counseling, active substance and mental health programs as well as involvement with treatment partners and support groups. Finally, ongoing education and novel techniques to allow the incorporation of pill-taking into activities of daily living have become crucial components for successful HIV treatment.

6.1 United States

In the US, efforts to improve adherence to antiretroviral drug regimens have focused both on individual and structural barriers to optimal adherence. Throughout the past 30 years, as newer HIV drugs are developed and become available on the market, the number of pills needed for a successful regimen has decreased. Now, many patients starting their first regimen can take a single pill (co-formulated tenofovir/emtricitabine/efavirenz, known as Atripla) once a day to achieve virologic suppression. In a meta-analysis of 11 randomized controlled trials, adherence to once-daily regimens was better than to twice-daily regimens (Parienti et al. 2009). The US DHHS Adult and Adolescent Treatment Guidelines have been modified to reflect the impact of barriers to adherence on treatment response, so that regimens with fewer pills are recommended over other regimens (DHHS 2011).

Many HIV clinics have trained staff to counsel patients on medication adherence, which includes reviewing all of the medications taken prior to initiating or changing a regimen, discussing the main side effects, identifying the best ways to take the prescribed medications, and helping patients think about ways to incorporate pill-taking into their lives with contextual and designed reminders. Reminders such as alarms or pill boxes may be coupled with adherence counseling as they have been shown to enhance adherence (Simoni et al. 2006; de Bruin et al. 2010).

For those who are not able to achieve optimal adherence despite individual counseling, some health care systems have developed directly observed therapy (DOT) programs, which are modeled on the adherence programs initially developed for tuberculosis therapy. The idea behind using DOT for HIV therapy is to reduce the risk of viral drug resistance and to achieve virologic suppression, which will provide health benefits to the patient as well as reduce the risk of HIV transmission. There are many varieties of DOT programs in practice, depending on the needs of the patient population and the services available from the health care system. One of the main differences between TB therapy and HIV therapy is that for HIV, the duration of therapy is life-long, and the number of pills or frequency of doses may not decrease over time. However, the overall benefit of DOT on virologic suppression is controversial with studies finding both a lack of benefit and an overall benefit to DOT, with respect to adherence, immunologic, and virologic outcomes (Hart et al. 2010; Myers and Tsiouris 2009; Ford et al. 2009).

One example of a patient-centered DOT program can be found in New York City. Due to the barriers to adherence faced by opioid-dependent HIV-positive patients, a DOT program for HIV therapy was developed to deliver HIV medications at methadone clinics. US federal policies require patients to obtain their methadone doses from one clinic, and at the discretion of the clinic, patients may be required to attend daily or weekly observed dosing appointments. Since the patients may visit the methadone clinic frequently (every day, or at least five to six days per week), HIV medications were coupled with the observed daily methadone dose. Investigators found that patients in the DOT program achieved higher levels of adherence and virologic suppression when assessed after 24 weeks (Berg et al. 2011).

Contingency management, which consists of financial incentives for medication adherence, has also been shown to be efficacious in enhancing participation in substance abuse treatment and for reducing drug use. The use of contingency management for HIV has been shown to be effective (Petry et al. 2010), but the beneficial effect appears to wane after incentives are removed (Rosen et al. 2007). Future studies that incorporate contingency management, patient navigators, and/or peer counseling will need to be tested before contingency management can be considered as a "best practice" for the management of HIV.

6.2 Sub-Saharan Africa

The World Health Organization established several Early Warning Indicators in order to identify how well sites are managing ART usage and adherence. These have directly resulted in optimization of the quality of care and have assisted in the identification of vulnerable clinics (Jordan et al. 2011; Hong et al. 2010). A significant effort has been applied to ensuring high rates of adherence in various clinics throughout Africa and in particular South Africa (Mills et al. 2006). Individual adherence sessions with peer counselors and group education programs provide detailed information on HIV infection, antiretroviral medications, drug interactions, stigma, and adherence techniques (Lawn et al. 2007; Matovu et al. 2011). Many of these programs and support groups work to increase social capital and empower individuals to make health a priority (Achieng et al. 2011). Individuals who do not disclose their HIV status to intimate partners or household members may feel stigmatized and hide their pills for fear of being discovered, and disclosure of HIV status has been proven to improve adherence (Nachega et al. 2004). In Kenya, mobile phone text messages improved ART adherence over standard care (Lester et al. 2010; Pop-Eleches et al. 2011). Various methods of adherence monitoring have been evaluated to determine efficacy (Nachega et al. 2011). Pill counts (Achieng et al. 2011) and pharmacy refill monitoring (Murphy et al. 2011) have been shown to be reliable and inexpensive but not consistent across all settings. Directly observed ART has also been examined with mixed results but overall is costly and labor intensive (Nachega et al. 2010; Hart et al. 2010), as is therapeutic drug monitoring via plasma or hair sampling (van Zyl et al. 2011).

6.3 Haiti

In rural Haiti, a non-governmental organization, Partners in Health, has been working since 1987 to support HIV/AIDS treatment. Among the many barriers to optimal care in Haiti, i.e. poverty, food insecurity, political disruptions, a program was developed to help HIV patients take their medications. *Accompagnateurs*, or community health workers, were people chosen from the local community and trained in medication and symptom management for HIV patients. Since starting this program, patients have experienced an increase in CD4 count and reduction in viral loads, and therefore the accompagnateurs have been identified as a critical component of the clinical care provided for these patients (Koenig, Leandre, and Farmer 2004; Behforouz, Farmer, and Mukherjee 2004).

7. Improving social capital

One important factor to HIV-positive patients achieving optimal health is the ability to leverage social capital. Social capital can be defined as the value that comes from engagement in a social network. Social capital can help HIV patients achieve good health by providing psychological and physical support (e.g. food, shelter, transportation, money for medications). Stigma can inhibit the ability to leverage social capital because it interferes in the individual's willingness to seek help from others in their social network (Bangsberg and Deeks 2010). In a qualitative study conducted in Kenya, Uganda, and Nigeria, researchers found that higher levels of social capital helped HIV-positive patients to prioritize ART adherence and achieve improved health (Ware et al. 2009).

A substantial impact has occurred via the implementation of outreach programs designed to improve the social capital of various disenfranchised populations where stigma, poor health literacy and lack of education stymie those already challenged by competing priorities. Different forms of outreach have been developed, specific to the needs of the marginalized population. These programs have attempted to improve engagement in care and to support those who are living with HIV. For example, programs in Boston (PACT - Prevention, Access to Care and Treatment), San Francisco (PHAST - Positive Health Access to Services and Treatment), and New York City (St. Luke's-Roosevelt Hospital Center's Center for Comprehensive Care) have designed successful outreach programs targeting the patients with the worst levels of engagement in care (Rosenberg 2011). The Community Health Care Van in New Haven provides prevention and treatment services for HIV, hepatitis, substance abuse, and mental illness from a medical van (HRSA). By focusing on the needs of the whole patient, including shelter, food, mental health, and medical comorbidities, and helping them to capitalize on available services and social capital, these programs have helped some of the most vulnerable patients successfully treat their HIV infection.

8. Conclusion

If every HIV-infected individual could know their diagnosis, enter the health care system, start antiretroviral therapy when appropriate and incorporate all the evidence-based preventive health measures into his or her life, we could potentially see a world free of HIV within generations. This is the premise behind the "Test and Treat" strategy (Granich et al. 2009). While this may seem to be a lofty goal, the examples presented here from Atlanta and Durban, as well as those from many other places around the world, suggest that even if the economic resources were made available to implement the "Test and Treat" strategy, there are individual, interpersonal, and structural-level barriers that could limit the impact of such approach (Gardner et al. 2011).

In order to combat the disparities in HIV infection rates and HIV-related morbidity and mortality, creative solutions are necessary. This chapter describes the comparison between the response to the HIV epidemic between Atlanta and Durban, highlighting important similarities and differences between the two cities. Both Atlanta and Durban are located in wealthy countries, yet both have significant racial/ethnic and socioeconomic factors that have led to continued HIV transmission and disparities in HIV outcomes. In each city, individual programs have designed solutions to improve diagnosis and engagement in care. In addition, several other programs around the world have developed their own responses to the HIV epidemic, to deliver care to those who need it within their local contexts.

Focusing on marginalized subpopulations, while difficult, is important both for reducing the disparities in HIV infection and outcomes and also for reducing community-level viral load and subsequent transmission of the virus. These subpopulations of patients may require more intensive resources or specific interventions that successfully engage them in care. For example, several different types of programs in the US, such as targeted outreach in mobile vans, DOT, and variations on the specialty clinic model, have successfully engaged marginalized patients in care. In South Africa, systemic solutions (such as actively seeking out patients who miss appointments and expanding the roles of allied health professionals) and cultural solutions (such as incorporating traditional healers into medical care) are being used to improve engagement in care and ART adherence.

As HIV continues to spread, and as patients live longer, health systems must develop strategies for HIV prevention and continued engagement in care; this will undoubtedly require flexibility and new ideas to be tested and implemented. HIV has been touted as now being a chronic disease, but we must remember that it is an infectious chronic disease. If those infected with HIV have detectable virus circulating in the bloodstream and mucosal surfaces, transmission will continue to occur. Thus, until there is a cure, retaining patients in HIV care over a lifetime is a major challenge for any health care system, particularly for regions that lack universal access to care. Health systems' solutions will also need to address the individual, interpersonal, and underlying structural factors that lead to HIV transmission and the disparities in access to health care. As low- and middle-income countries scale up HIV treatment services, these health systems can serve as models for management of non-communicable diseases as well (Rabkin and El-Sadr 2011). Multiple layers of co-occurring interventions that target individual-level, interpersonal-level, and structural-level factors would address the many aspects of optimal HIV prevention and therapy.

9. References

Abdool Karim, S. S., and Q. Abdool Karim. 2005. *HIV/AIDS in South Africa*. Cape Town: Cambridge University Press.

Abdool Karim, S. S., G. J. Churchyard, Q. Abdool Karim, and S. D. Lawn. 2009. HIV infection and tuberculosis in South Africa: an urgent need to escalate the public health response. *Lancet* 374 (9693):921-33.

Achieng, L., H. Musangi, S. Ong'uti, E. Ombegoh, L. Bryant, J. Mwiindi, N. Smith, and P. Keiser. 2011. Evaluation of methods to promote adherence at an HIV treatment center in central Kenya. Paper read at 18th Conference of Retroviruses and Opportunistic Infections, at Boston, MA.

AID Atlanta. 2011. 2011]. Available from http://www.aidatlanta.org/.

Bangsberg, D. R., and S. G. Deeks. 2010. Spending more to save more: interventions to promote adherence. *Ann Intern Med* 152 (1):54-6; W-13.

Bardsley, J., J. Turvey, and J. Blatherwick. 1990. Vancouver's needle exchange program. *Can J Public Health* 81 (1):39-45.

Behforouz, H. L., P. E. Farmer, and J. S. Mukherjee. 2004. From directly observed therapy to accompagnateurs: enhancing AIDS treatment outcomes in Haiti and in Boston. *Clin Infect Dis* 38 Suppl 5:S429-36.

Berg, K. M., A. Litwin, X. Li, M. Heo, and J. H. Arnsten. 2011. Directly observed antiretroviral therapy improves adherence and viral load in drug users attending methadone maintenance clinics: a randomized controlled trial. *Drug Alcohol Depend* 113 (2-3):192-9.

Bisson, G. P., R. Gross, S. Bellamy, J. Chittams, M. Hislop, L. Regensberg, I. Frank, G. Maartens, and J. B. Nachega. 2008. Pharmacy refill adherence compared with CD4 count changes for monitoring HIV-infected adults on antiretroviral therapy. *PLoS Med* 5 (5):e109.

Boulle, A., P. Bock, M. Osler, K. Cohen, L. Channing, K. Hilderbrand, E. Mothibi, V. Zweigenthal, N. Slingers, K. Cloete, and F. Abdullah. 2008. Antiretroviral therapy and early mortality in South Africa. *Bull World Health Organ* 86 (9):678-87.

Braithwaite, R. S., S. Shechter, M. S. Roberts, A. Schaefer, D. R. Bangsberg, P. R. Harrigan, and A. C. Justice. 2006. Explaining variability in the relationship between antiretroviral adherence and HIV mutation accumulation. *J Antimicrob Chemother* 58 (5):1036-43.

Braitstein, P., J. Daggy, P. Easterbrook, C. Cohen, S. Braithwaite, E. Geng, A. Kambugu, M. Bwana, K. Wools-Kaloustian, and C. Yiannoutsos. 2011. Retaining adults in HIV care: impact of key program characteristics on patient loss to follow-up among adult patients receiving cART in the IeDEA East Africa Consortium. Paper read at 18th Conference of Retroviruses and Opportunistic Infections, at Boston, MA.

British Columbia Center for Excellence in HIV/AIDS. 2011. [cited March 18 2011]. Available from http://www.cfenet.ubc.ca/.

Bulpin, T.V. 1977. Chapter XII: twilight of the republic. In *Natal and the Zulu country*. Cape Town: T.V. Bulpin Publications.

CDC. 2009. HIV surveillance report: diagnoses of HIV infection and AIDS in the United States and dependent areas, 2009.

Chigwedere, P., and M. Essex. 2010. AIDS denialism and public health practice. *AIDS Behav* 14 (2):237-47.

Chu, C., G. Umanski, A. Blank, R. Grossberg, and P. A. Selwyn. 2010. HIV-infected patients and treatment outcomes: an equivalence study of community-located, primary care-based HIV treatment vs. hospital-based specialty care in the Bronx, New York. *AIDS Care* 22 (12):1522-9.

CMS. 2011. CMS Annual Statistics.

Cohen, J., N. Vogenthaler, C. Del Rio, and W Armstrong. 2011. Evaluation of an integrated care program for patients with triple diagnoses: HIV/AIDS, serious mental illness, and substance abuse disorders. Paper read at 18th Conference on Retroviruses and Opportunistic Infections, at Boston, MA.

Colvin, C. J., L. Fairall, S. Lewin, D. Georgeu, M. Zwarenstein, M. O. Bachmann, K. E. Uebel, and E. D. Bateman. 2010. Expanding access to ART in South Africa: the role of nurse-initiated treatment. *S Afr Med J* 100 (4):210-2.

Coovadia, H., R. Jewkes, P. Barron, D. Sanders, and D. McIntyre. 2009. Health in South Africa 1 The health and health system of South Africa: historical roots of current public health challenges. *Lancet* 374 (9692):817-834.

Crane, J. T., A. Kawuma, J. H. Oyugi, J. T. Byakika, A. Moss, P. Bourgois, and D. R. Bangsberg. 2006. The price of adherence: qualitative findings from HIV positive individuals purchasing fixed-dose combination generic HIV antiretroviral therapy in Kampala, Uganda. *AIDS Behav* 10 (4):437-42.

Cunningham, C. O., J. P. Sanchez, D. I. Heller, and N. L. Sohler. 2007. Assessment of a medical outreach program to improve access to HIV care among marginalized individuals. *American Journal of Public Health* 97 (10):1758-61.

Cunningham, C. O., N. L. Sohler, N. A. Cooperman, K. M. Berg, A. H. Litwin, and J. H. Arnsten. 2011. Strategies to Improve Access to and Utilization of Health Care Services and Adherence to Antiretroviral Therapy Among HIV-Infected Drug Users. *Subst Use Misuse* 46 (2-3):218-32.

Das, M., P. L. Chu, G. M. Santos, S. Scheer, E. Vittinghoff, W. McFarland, and G. N. Colfax. 2010. Decreases in community viral load are accompanied by reductions in new HIV infections in San Francisco. *PLoS One* 5 (6):e11068.

de Bruin, M., W. Viechtbauer, H. P. Schaalma, G. Kok, C. Abraham, and H. J. Hospers. 2010. Standard care impact on effects of highly active antiretroviral therapy adherence interventions: A meta-analysis of randomized controlled trials. *Arch Intern Med* 170 (3):240-50.

Dennison, C. R., N. Peer, C. J. Lombard, L. Kepe, N. S. Levitt, K. Steyn, and M. N. Hill. 2007. Cardiovascular risk and comorbid conditions among Black South Africans with hypertension in public and private primary care settings: The HiHi study. *Ethnicity & Disease* 17 (3):477-483.

DHHS. 2011. *Guidelines for the use of antiretroviral agents in HIV-1-infected adults and adolescents*. Department of Health and Human Services, January 10, 2011 2011 [cited March 5 2011]. Available from http://www.aidsinfo.nih.gov/ContentFiles/AdultandAdolescentGL.pdf.

Dunkle, K. L., R. K. Jewkes, H. C. Brown, G. E. Gray, J. A. McIntryre, and S. D. Harlow. 2004. Gender-based violence, relationship power, and risk of HIV infection in women attending antenatal clinics in South Africa. *Lancet* 363 (9419):1415-21.

eHARS Reporting System. 2010. edited by D. o. P. H. Georgia Department of Community Health, HIV Epidemiology Unit. Atlanta.

Fairall, L. R., M. Bachmann, C. Lombard, V. Timmerman, K. Uebel, M. Zwarenstein, A. Boulle, D. Georgeu, C. J. Colvin, S. Lewin, G. M. Faris, R. Cornick, M. Tshabalala, E. Kotze, C. van Vuuren, D. Steyn, and E. D. Bateman. 2011. The effect of task-shifting antiretroviral care in South Africa: a pragmatic cluster randomised trial (STRETCH - streamlining tasks and roles to expand treatment and care for HIV). Paper read at 6th IAS Conference on HIV Pathogenesis, Treatment, and Prevention, at Rome, Italy.

Ford, N., J. B. Nachega, M. E. Engel, and E. J. Mills. 2009. Directly observed antiretroviral therapy: a systematic review and meta-analysis of randomised clinical trials. *Lancet* 374 (9707):2064-71.

Fox, M. P., P. Ive, L. Long, M. Maskew, and I. Sanne. 2010. High rates of survival, immune reconstitution, and virologic suppression on second-line antiretroviral therapy in South Africa. *J Acquir Immune Defic Syndr* 53 (4):500-6.

Gardner, E. M., M. P. McLees, J. F. Steiner, C. Del Rio, and W. J. Burman. 2011. The spectrum of engagement in HIV care and its relevance to test-and-treat strategies for prevention of HIV infection. *Clin Infect Dis* 52 (6):793-800.

Geng, E., W. Muyindike, D. Glidden, M. Bwana, C. Yiannoutsos, P. Braitstein, N. Musinguzi, D. Bangsberg, and J. Martin. 2011. Failure to initiate ART, loss to follow-up and mortality among HIV-infected patients during the pre-ART period in Uganda: understanding engagement in care in resource-limited settings. Paper read at 18th Conference of Retroviruses and Opportunistic Infections, at Boston, MA.

Goudge, J. 1999. The public-private mix. In *South African Health Review 1999*. Durban: Health Systems Trust.

Gouws, E., and Q. Abdool Karim. 2005. Chapter 3: HIV infection in South Africa: the evolving epidemic. In *HIV/AIDS in South Africa*, edited by S. S. Abdool Karim and Q. Abdool Karim. Cape Town: Cambridge University Press.

Granich, R. M., C. F. Gilks, C. Dye, K. M. De Cock, and B. G. Williams. 2009. Universal voluntary HIV testing with immediate antiretroviral therapy as a strategy for elimination of HIV transmission: a mathematical model. *Lancet* 373 (9657):48-57.

Growth, employment and redistribution: a macro-economic framework. 1996. Pretoria.

Guest, J.L., V.C. Marconi, B.K. Agan, G.A. Gandits, A.C. Weintrob, B.G. Hill, J.F. Okulicz, Crum-Cianflone N, and D. Rimland. 2011. Improved mortality after HAART initiation in two cohorts with free access to medical care: experience from the Department of Defense and the Department of Veterans Affairs. Paper read at 15th International Workshop on HIV Observational Databases, at Prague, Czech Republic.

Hart, J. E., C. Y. Jeon, L. C. Ivers, H. L. Behforouz, A. Caldas, P. C. Drobac, and S. S. Shin. 2010. Effect of directly observed therapy for highly active antiretroviral therapy on virologic, immunologic, and adherence outcomes: a meta-analysis and systematic review. *J Acquir Immune Defic Syndr* 54 (2):167-79.

Health, Department of. 2009. 2008 National antenatal sentinel HIV & syphilis prevalence survey. edited by D. o. Health. Pretoria.

HIV & AIDS and STI Strategic Plan for South Africa, 2007-2011. 2007. edited by D. o. Health. Pretoria.

HIV Care Program: AIDS Drug Assistance Program. 2011. [cited March 18 2011]. Available from http://health.state.ga.us/programs/stdhiv/adap.asp.

The HIV/AIDS Country Scorecard. 2011. 2008 [cited March 2011]. Available from http://aidsaccountability.org/.

Hixson, B. A., S. B. Omer, C. del Rio, and P. M. Frew. 2011. Spatial clustering of HIV prevalence in Atlanta, Georgia and population characteristics associated with case concentrations. *J Urban Health* 88 (1):129-41.

Hong, S. Y., A. Jonas, E. Dumeni, A. Badi, D. Pereko, A. Blom, V. S. Muthiani, A. N. Shiningavamwe, J. Mukamba, G. Andemichael, R. Barbara, D. E. Bennett, and M. R. Jordan. 2010. Population-based monitoring of HIV drug resistance in Namibia with early warning indicators. *J Acquir Immune Defic Syndr* 55 (4):27-31.

HRSA. 2011. *The HIV/AIDS program home: caring for the underserved*. U.S. Department of Health and Human Services, Health Resources and Services Administration [cited January 27 2011]. Available from http://hab.hrsa.gov.

2011. *Outreach: engaging people in HIV care* 2011]. Available from http://hab.hrsa.gov/tools/HIVoutreach/.

Hunter, M. 2005. Cultural politics and masculinities: Multiple-partners in historical perspective in KwaZulu-Natal. *Cult Health Sex* 7 (4):389-403.

Ijsselmuiden, C. B., M. H. Steinberg, G. N. Padayachee, B. D. Schoub, S. A. Strauss, E. Buch, J. C. Davies, C. de Beer, J. S. Gear, and H. S. Hurwitz. 1988. AIDS and South Africa--towards a comprehensive strategy. Part I. The world-wide experience. *S Afr Med J* 73 (8):455-60.

IOM. 2011. HIV screening and access to care: health care system capacity for increased HIV testing and provision of care. Washington, DC: Institute of Medicine.

Jewkes, R. 2009. Women and HIV. In *HIV/AIDS in South Africa 25 years on: a psycho-social perspective*, edited by P. Rohleder, L. Swartz, S. Kalichman and L. Simbayi. New York: Springer.

Jochelson, K., M. Mothibeli, and J. P. Leger. 1991. Human immunodeficiency virus and migrant labor in South Africa. *Int J Health Serv* 21 (1):157-73.

Jordan, M., K. Kelley, A. Saadani Hassani, Y. Obeng-Aduasare, and S. Bertagnolio. 2011. Monitoring ART: clinic and program performance using WHO HIV drug resistance early warning indicators in 21 countries. Paper read at 18th Conference of Retroviruses and Opportunistic Infections, at Boston, MA.

Joy, R., E. F. Druyts, E. K. Brandson, V. D. Lima, C. A. Rustad, W. Zhang, E. Wood, J. S. Montaner, and R. S. Hogg. 2008. Impact of neighborhood-level socioeconomic status on HIV disease progression in a universal health care setting. *J Acquir Immune Defic Syndr* 47 (4):500-5.

Kalichman, S. C., C. Cherry, C. Amaral, D. White, M. O. Kalichman, H. Pope, C. Swetsze, M. Jones, and R. Macy. 2010. Health and treatment implications of food insufficiency among people living with HIV/AIDS, Atlanta, Georgia. *J Urban Health* 87 (4):631-41.

King, M.L. 2011. *Martin Luther King: speech about South Africa* 1965 [cited April 4 2011]. Available from http://www.racismreview.com/blog/2011/01/17/mlk-speech-about-south-africa/.

Koenig, S. P., F. Leandre, and P. E. Farmer. 2004. Scaling-up HIV treatment programmes in resource-limited settings: the rural Haiti experience. *AIDS* 18 Suppl 3:S21-5.

Korthuis, P. T., M. J. Tozzi, V. Nandi, D. A. Fiellin, L. Weiss, J. E. Egan, M. Botsko, A. Acosta, M. N. Gourevitch, D. Hersh, J. Hsu, J. Boverman, and F. L. Altice. 2011. Improved quality of life for opioid-dependent patients receiving buprenorphine treatment in HIV clinics. *J Acquir Immune Defic Syndr* 56 Suppl 1:S39-45.

Lawn, S. D., A. D. Harries, X. Anglaret, L. Myer, and R. Wood. 2008. Early mortality among adults accessing antiretroviral treatment programmes in sub-Saharan Africa. *AIDS* 22 (15):1897-908.

Lawn, S. D., R. Kaplan, R. Wood, and L. G. Bekker. 2007. Promoting retention in care: an effective model in an antiretroviral treatment service in South Africa. *Clin Infect Dis* 45 (6):803.

Lester, R. T., P. Ritvo, E. J. Mills, A. Kariri, S. Karanja, M. H. Chung, W. Jack, J. Habyarimana, M. Sadatsafavi, M. Najafzadeh, C. A. Marra, B. Estambale, E. Ngugi, T. B. Ball, L. Thabane, L. J. Gelmon, J. Kimani, M. Ackers, and F. A. Plummer. 2010. Effects of a mobile phone short message service on antiretroviral treatment adherence in Kenya (WelTel Kenya1): a randomised trial. *Lancet* 376 (9755):1838-45.

Lima, V. D., K. J. Lepik, W. Zhang, K. A. Muldoon, R. S. Hogg, and J. S. Montaner. 2010. Regional and temporal changes in HIV-related mortality in British Columbia, 1987-2006. *Can J Public Health* 101 (5):415-9.

Long, L., A. Brennan, M. P. Fox, B. Ndibongo, I. Jaffray, M. Maskew, P. MacPhail, I. Sanne, and S. Rosen. 2011. Shifting management of stable ART patients from doctors to nurses in South Africa: excellent outcomes and lower costs. Paper read at 18th Conference of Retroviruses and Opportunistic Infections, at Boston, MA.

Longerbeam, A. 2010. Putting faces to the statistics: child sex trafficking in Atlanta. *Change*, http://news.change.org.

Lurie, M. N., B. G. Williams, K. Zuma, D. Mkaya-Mwamburi, G. P. Garnett, M. D. Sweat, J. Gittelsohn, and S. S. Karim. 2003. Who infects whom? HIV-1 concordance and discordance among migrant and non-migrant couples in South Africa. *AIDS* 17 (15):2245-52.

Lurie, M. N., B. G. Williams, K. Zuma, D. Mkaya-Mwamburi, G. Garnett, A. W. Sturm, M. D. Sweat, J. Gittelsohn, and S. S. Abdool Karim. 2003. The impact of migration on HIV-1 transmission in South Africa: a study of migrant and nonmigrant men and their partners. *Sex Transm Dis* 30 (2):149-56.

Mangla, A., and Z. Gant. 2008. Georgia HIV/AIDS surveillance summary. edited by G. D. o. P. Health and G. D. o. C. Health.

Marconi, V. C., G. A. Grandits, A. C. Weintrob, H. Chun, M. L. Landrum, A. Ganesan, J. F. Okulicz, N. Crum-Cianflone, R. J. O'Connell, A. Lifson, G. W. Wortmann, and B. K. Agan. 2010. Outcomes of highly active antiretroviral therapy in the context of universal access to healthcare: the U.S. Military HIV Natural History Study. *AIDS Res Ther* 7 (1):14.

Marconi, V. C., H. Sunpath, Z. Lu, M. Gordon, K. Koranteng-Apeagyei, J. Hampton, S. Carpenter, J. Giddy, D. Ross, H. Holst, E. Losina, B. D. Walker, and D. R. Kuritzkes. 2008. Prevalence of HIV-1 drug resistance after failure of a first highly active antiretroviral therapy regimen in KwaZulu Natal, South Africa. *Clin Infect Dis* 46 (10):1589-97.

Marks, S., and N. Andersson. 1987. Issues in the political economy of health in Southern Africa. *J South Afr Stud* 13 (2):177-86.

Matovu, F., D. Wabwire, J. Nakibuuka, M. Mubiru, D. Bagendra, P. Musoke, and M.G. Fowler. 2011. Efficacy of using peer counselors and nurses to support adherence to HAART among HIV-1-infected patients at the Prevention of MTCT Program, Mulago Hospital, Kampala, Uganda: a randomized non-inferiority interventional trial. Paper read at 18th Conference of Retroviruses and Opportunistic Infections, at Boston, MA.

McIntyre, D. E., and R. E. Dorrington. 1990. Trends in the distribution of South-African health-care expenditure. *South African Medical Journal* 78 (3):125-129.

Metsch, L. R., M. Pereyra, S. Messinger, C. del Rio, S. A. Strathdee, P. Anderson-Mahoney, E. Rudy, G. Marks, L. Gardner, and Artas Study Grp. 2008. HIV transmission risk behaviors among HIV-infected persons who are successfully linked to care. *Clinical Infectious Diseases* 47 (4):577-584.

Mills, E. J., J. B. Nachega, I. Buchan, J. Orbinski, A. Attaran, S. Singh, B. Rachlis, P. Wu, C. Cooper, L. Thabane, K. Wilson, G. H. Guyatt, and D. R. Bangsberg. 2006. Adherence to antiretroviral therapy in sub-Saharan Africa and North America: a meta-analysis. *JAMA* 296 (6):679-90.

Mimiaga, M. J., S. L. Reisner, R. Vanderwarker, M. J. Gaucher, C. A. O'Connor, M. S. Medeiros, and S. A. Safren. 2008. Polysubstance use and HIV/STD risk behavior among Massachusetts men who have sex with men accessing Department of Public

Health mobile van services: implications for intervention development. *AIDS Patient Care STDS* 22 (9):745-51.

Murphy, R. A., H. Sunpath, Z. Lu, N. Chelin, E. Losina, M. Gordon, D. Ross, A. D. Ewusi, L. T. Matthews, D. R. Kuritzkes, and V. C. Marconi. 2010. Outcomes after virologic failure of first-line ART in South Africa. *AIDS* 24 (7):1007-12.

Murphy, R., H. Sunpath, C. Castilla, S. Ebrahim, R. Court, H. Nguyen, D. R. Kuritzkes, V. C. Marconi, and J. B. Nachega. 2011. Adherence to second-line ART and long-term virologic outcomes in South Africa. Paper read at 18th Conference of Retroviruses and Opportunistic Infections, at Boston, MA.

Mutevedzi, P. C., R. J. Lessells, T. Heller, T. Barnighausen, G. S. Cooke, and M. L. Newell. 2010. Scale-up of a decentralized HIV treatment programme in rural KwaZulu-Natal, South Africa: does rapid expansion affect patient outcomes? *Bull World Health Organ* 88 (8):593-600.

Myers, J. E., and S. J. Tsiouris. 2009. Is there a place for directly observed therapy in HAART? *Lancet* 374 (9707):2030-2.

Nachega, J. B., R. E. Chaisson, R. Goliath, A. Efron, M. A. Chaudhary, M. Ram, C. Morroni, H. Schoeman, A. R. Knowlton, and G. Maartens. 2010. Randomized controlled trial of trained patient-nominated treatment supporters providing partial directly observed antiretroviral therapy. *AIDS* 24 (9):1273-80.

Nachega, J. B., M. Hislop, D. W. Dowdy, M. Lo, S. B. Omer, L. Regensberg, R. E. Chaisson, and G. Maartens. 2006. Adherence to highly active antiretroviral therapy assessed by pharmacy claims predicts survival in HIV-infected South African adults. *J Acquir Immune Defic Syndr* 43 (1):78-84.

Nachega, J. B., V. C. Marconi, G. U. van Zyl, E. M. Gardner, W. Preiser, S. Y. Hong, E. J. Mills, and R. Gross. 2011. HIV Treatment Adherence, Drug Resistance, Virologic Failure: Evolving Concepts. *Infect Disord Drug Targets.*

Nachega, J. B., D. M. Stein, D. A. Lehman, D. Hlatshwayo, R. Mothopeng, R. E. Chaisson, and A. S. Karstaedt. 2004. Adherence to antiretroviral therapy in HIV-infected adults in Soweto, South Africa. *AIDS Res Hum Retroviruses* 20 (10):1053-6.

The New Georgia Encyclopedia. 2011. [cited April 1 2011]. Available from http://www.georgiaencyclopedia.org/.

Ojikutu, B., C. Jack, and G. Ramjee. 2007. Provision of antiretroviral therapy in South Africa: unique challenges and remaining obstacles. *J Infect Dis* 196 Suppl 3:S523-7.

Packard, R. 1989. *Preindustrial South Africa: a virgin soil for tuberculosis? White plague, black labour tuberculosis and political economy of health and disease in South Africa.* Pietermaritzburg: University of Natal Press.

Palmer, N. 1999. Patient choice of a primary health care provider. In *South African health review*. Durban: Health Systems Trust.

Parienti, J. J., D. R. Bangsberg, R. Verdon, and E. M. Gardner. 2009. Better adherence with once-daily antiretroviral regimens: a meta-analysis. *Clin Infect Dis* 48 (4):484-8.

Peltzer, K., N. Mngqundaniso, and G. Petros. 2006. HIV/AIDS/STI/TB knowledge, beliefs and practices of traditional healers in KwaZulu-Natal, South Africa. *AIDS Care* 18 (6):608-13.

Petry, N. M., J. Weinstock, S. M. Alessi, M. W. Lewis, and K. Dieckhaus. 2010. Group-based randomized trial of contingencies for health and abstinence in HIV patients. *J Consult Clin Psychol* 78 (1):89-97.

Pop-Eleches, C., H. Thirumurthy, J. P. Habyarimana, J. G. Zivin, M. P. Goldstein, D. de Walque, L. Mackeen, J. Haberer, S. Kimaiyo, J. Sidle, D. Ngare, and D. R. Bangsberg. 2011. Mobile phone technologies improve adherence to antiretroviral treatment in a resource-limited setting: a randomized controlled trial of text message reminders. *AIDS* 25 (6):825-834.

Rabkin, M., and W. M. El-Sadr. 2011. Why reinvent the wheel? Leveraging the lessons of HIV scale-up to confront non-communicable diseases. *Glob Public Health* 6 (3):247-56.

Rose, D., and K. E. Charlton. 2002. Quantitative indicators from a food expenditure survey can be used to target the food insecure in South Africa. *J Nutr* 132 (11):3235-42.

Rosen, M. I., K. Dieckhaus, T. J. McMahon, B. Valdes, N. M. Petry, J. Cramer, and B. Rounsaville. 2007. Improved adherence with contingency management. *AIDS Patient Care STDS* 21 (1):30-40.

Rosen, S., M. P. Fox, and C. J. Gill. 2007. Patient retention in antiretroviral therapy programs in sub-Saharan Africa: a systematic review. *PLoS Med* 4 (10):e298.

Rosenberg, T. 2011. A housecall to help with doctor's orders. *New York Times*, February 28.

Russell, G. 1899. *The history of old Durban and reminiscences of an emigrant of 1850.*

Sanne, I., C. Orrell, M. P. Fox, F. Conradie, P. Ive, J. Zeinecker, M. Cornell, C. Heiberg, C. Ingram, R. Panchia, M. Rassool, R. Gonin, W. Stevens, H. Truter, M. Dehlinger, C. van der Horst, J. McIntyre, and R. Wood. 2010. Nurse versus doctor management of HIV-infected patients receiving antiretroviral therapy (CIPRA-SA): a randomised non-inferiority trial. *Lancet* 376 (9734):33-40.

Schneider, H., N. Chabikuli, D. Blaauw, I. Funani, and R. Brugha. 2005. Sexually transmitted infections -- factors associated with quality of care among private general practitioners. *S Afr Med J* 95 (10):782-5.

Shillington, K. 2005. Central and Southern Africa: Cetshwayo (c. 1826-1884). In *Encyclopedia of African history*, edited by K. Shillington. New York: Fitzroy Dearborn Taylor & Francis Group.

Shisana, O., E. J. Hall, R. Maluleke, J. Chauveau, and C. Schwabe. 2004. HIV/AIDS prevalence among South African health workers. *S Afr Med J* 94 (10):846-50.

Shisana, O., T. Rehle, L.C. Simbayi, K. Zuma, S. Jooste, V. Pillay-van-Wyk, N. Mbelle, J. Van Zyl, W. Parker, N.P. Zungu, S. Pezi, and SABSSM III Implementation Team. 2009. South African national HIV prevalence, incidence, behavior, and communication survey, 2008: a turning tide among teenagers? Cape Town: HSRC Press.

Shuster, J. M., C. E. Sterk, P. M. Frew, and C. del Rio. 2009. The cultural and community-level acceptance of antiretroviral therapy (ART) among traditional healers in Eastern Cape, South Africa. *J Community Health* 34 (1):16-22.

Simoni, J. M., C. R. Pearson, D. W. Pantalone, G. Marks, and N. Crepaz. 2006. Efficacy of interventions in improving highly active antiretroviral therapy adherence and HIV-1 RNA viral load. A meta-analytic review of randomized controlled trials. *J Acquir Immune Defic Syndr* 43 Suppl 1:S23-35.

Statistical Release P0302: Midyear population estimates. 2011. [cited March 2011]. Available from http://www.statssa.gov.za/.

Statistics 2007. 2007. Pretoria.

Stokols, D. 1996. Translating social ecological theory into guidelines for community health promotion. *Am J Health Promot* 10 (4):282-98.

Sunpath, H., C. Edwin, N. Chelin, S. Nadeasn, K. Gate, R. Maharaj, R. Court, Y. Moosa, and R. Murphy. 2011. Operationalizing early inpatient ART during hospitalization with acute opportunistic infection in South Africa. Paper read at 18th Conference of Retroviruses and Opportunistic Infections, at Boston, MA.

Traditional healers in South Africa trained to encourage people to get tested for HIV. March 2011 2006. Available from http://www.medicalnewstoday.com/articles/39305.php.

Uebel, K. E., L. R. Fairall, D. H. van Rensburg, W. F. Mollentze, M. O. Bachmann, S. Lewin, M. Zwarenstein, C. J. Colvin, D. Georgeu, P. Mayers, G. M. Faris, C. Lombard, and E. D. Bateman. 2011. Task shifting and integration of HIV care into primary care in South Africa: The development and content of the streamlining tasks and roles to expand treatment and care for HIV (STRETCH) intervention. *Implement Sci* 6 (1):86.

UNAIDS report on the global AIDS epidemic. 2010. Joint United Nations Programme on HIV/AIDS.

United States Census. 2011. U.S. Census Bureau [cited January 27 2011]. Available from http://www.factfinder.census.gov.

van Zyl, G. U., T. E. van Mens, H. McIlleron, M. Zeier, J. B. Nachega, E. Decloedt, C. Malavazzi, P. Smith, Y. Huang, L. van der Merwe, M. Gandhi, and G. Maartens. 2011. Low lopinavir plasma or hair concentrations explain second line protease inhibitor failures in a resource-limited setting. *J Acquir Immune Defic Syndr.*

Ware, N. C., J. Idoko, S. Kaaya, I. A. Biraro, M. A. Wyatt, O. Agbaji, G. Chalamilla, and D. R. Bangsberg. 2009. Explaining adherence success in sub-Saharan Africa: an ethnographic study. *PLoS Med* 6 (1):e11.

Weiser, S. D., D. M. Tuller, E. A. Frongillo, J. Senkungu, N. Mukiibi, and D. R. Bangsberg. 2010. Food insecurity as a barrier to sustained antiretroviral therapy adherence in Uganda. *PLoS One* 5 (4):e10340.

Weiser, S., W. Wolfe, D. Bangsberg, I. Thior, P. Gilbert, J. Makhema, P. Kebaabetswe, D. Dickenson, K. Mompati, M. Essex, and R. Marlink. 2003. Barriers to antiretroviral adherence for patients living with HIV infection and AIDS in Botswana. *J Acquir Immune Defic Syndr* 34 (3):281-8.

Weiss, L., J. Netherland, J. E. Egan, T. P. Flanigan, D. A. Fiellin, R. Finkelstein, and F. L. Altice. 2011. Integration of buprenorphine/naloxone treatment into HIV clinical care: lessons from the BHIVES collaborative. *J Acquir Immune Defic Syndr* 56 Suppl 1:S68-75.

WHO. 1983. Apartheid and health. Geneva: World Health Organization.

2010. *Towards universal access: scaling up priority HIV/AIDS interventions in the health sector* 2010 [cited November 30 2010]. Available from http://www.who.int/topics/hiv_aids/en/.

Wood, E., J. S. Montaner, K. Chan, M. W. Tyndall, M. T. Schechter, D. Bangsberg, M. V. O'Shaughnessy, and R. S. Hogg. 2002. Socioeconomic status, access to triple therapy, and survival from HIV-disease since 1996. *AIDS* 16 (15):2065-72.

Wood, K., F. Maforah, and R. Jewkes. 1998. "He forced me to love him": putting violence on adolescent sexual health agendas. *Soc Sci Med* 47 (2):233-42.

Yee, Daniel. 2007. FAA: Atlanta airport is nation's busiest. *USA Today*.

3

Is It Possible to Implement AIDS' Prevention in Primary School?

Dominique Berger
PAEDI, EA 4281, Claude Bernard University - Lyon 1 - IUFM
France

1. Introduction

In France, health education is included in the primary school science curriculum. A part of this curriculum is called "human body and health education" (MEN, 2002). A quantitative study of teachers' practices showed that teachers focus mainly on nutrition, hygiene, and dental health (Jourdan, & al., 2002). In the curriculum, the topic "Reproduction of living beings and sexuality education" concerns children aged 9-11 (Key Stage 2). Teachers often acknowledge that teaching about sexuality education and prevention of sexually transmitted diseases is difficult, because they do not feel comfortable with the subject matter. In a previous study (Jourdan et al., 2002), it had been shown that sexuality and AIDS were tackled by only 8 teachers out of 286 that were involved in the study. However, the curriculum guidelines of the French ministry of education (MEN, 2003) and the World Health Organisation (WHO) texts insist on the necessity for implementing early sexuality education and HIV/AIDS prevention programs, particularly in primary schools (WHO, 1999, 2004a). In this context, developing exchanges of experiences and partnership between teachers and health educators (school health services and health education NGOs) seems to be quite relevant.

The nature of health education in schools also implies taking ethical considerations into account. The aim is not to promote a new secular morality defining "good" (healthy) and "bad" (risky) behaviours, but to prepare the children for responsible citizenship. Hence teachers in health education should not attempt to impose norms of acceptable behaviours, but should taking into account children's peculiarities, expectations, needs, and also their representations. Children's representations are thought to provide coherent models to represent learner reasoning when faced with a problematic situation (Jodelet, 1991; Farr, 1997). The construction of these representations is rather complex as this phenomenon depends on the values and beliefs shared by a social group, and which give rise within a social groupto a common outlook manifested during social interactions. As these representations are linked to an individual's emotional responses as well as the cultural and social group(s) the individual belongs to, they constitute a decisive element in his/her relationships with the world, and are resistant to change. Representations therefore seem very essential (Fischer, 2001), are closely linked to behaviour (Abric, 1997), and cannot be changes as readily as knowledge.

Any programme attempting to change representations should not only take into consideration the relevant knowledge, but also the social and cultural aspects of the children's daily environment. (Doise & Mugny, 1997). The interest of taking into account pupils' representations in an HIV/AIDS education programme for children under twelve has been already justified (Fassler, Mc Queen, Ducan & Copeland (1989; Ferron, Feard, Bon, Spyckerelle, & Deschamps,1989; Thomas, 1991; Sly. Eberstein, Quadano, & Kistner, 1992; Schaalma, Kok, & Peters, 1993; Shonfeld et al., 1993; Kelly, 1995; WHO, 1999, 2004a, 2004b). This chapter presents a collaborative research project attempting to identify and study the initial representations of 9 and 10 year-old pupils relating to aids and to examine the impact of an early educational programme on regular teacher's activities and interventions of health educators.

Some of the initial results of the study have been already reported in a French journal for teachers (Berger, Collet, Laquet-Riffaud, & Jourdan, 2003).

2. Methodology

Most evaluations of health education programs are usually quasi-experimental designs, but to study health education other designs seem more appropriate (Victoria, Habicht, & Bryce 2004). In our context, using a controlled randomized study design as a method for assessing the effects of the implementation of a programme would be excessively difficult. The impact of the intervention on the children's social environment means that attempting to use a control group would be delusive, and that attaining true randomisation would be virtually impossible (Tones & Tilford, 2001). This situation results from the complex nature of causal chains in public health interventions.

In spite of their limits, several authors have concluded in favour of collaborative research designs aiming at determining exactly what content and what tools would be most suitable for health education (Darroch, & Silverman, 1989; Heymans, 1993). Associating all agents in the design and implementing the programme based on collaborative research design makes it possible to make the interactions between researcher and agents more visible and transparent (Martinand, 2003; Merini, 2005). These would be otherwise masked and confounding factors.

The data for the present study concern the two sides of the collaborative research. On one hand, an account of the general course of the study is provided and, on the other hand, the results from two questionnaires (pre- and post-questionnaire) that were used to collect information on pupils' representations are compared and analyzed.

2.1 Programme

The model on which this study is based relates to the "allosteric learning model" described by Giordan (1995). This socio-constructivist model assumes that learners build knowledge from their own lives, and learn through their mental representations that depend on their social and biological experiences, and their dispositions.

Learning is a highly active mental process that operates in an integrative mode through the conflict between what a learner has in his/her mind and what (s)he can identify and understand from his/her environment. When a learner develops a new model, all his/her mental models must be reorganized based on an interaction between the pre-existing representations and new information from environmental sources (Giordan, 2000). Health education requires the teacher to take the pupils' representations into account and to help them construct new and more relevant ones. Moreover, each child's environment must be taken into account in the programme as children's representations are not only based on what they learned at school, but also on all the other aspects of their lives (Downie, Tannahill, & Tannahill, 1996).

The research programme was developed by the Auvergne I.U.F.M. (Teachers' Training Institute), the I.N.R.P. (National Institute for Pedagogical Research) and the School of Medicine at the University of St Etienne, in partnership with the local School Health Services. The research design was regularly approved and evaluated
by a pilot committee, which defined its ethical framework on the basis of the texts published by the French Society of Public Health. This pilot committee included representatives of parents' associations, Regional Health Authorities (DDASS), the School of Medicine, the Training Institute, primary teachers, the heads of the schools concerned, and the technical advisers of school health services. The implementation of the project in each school involved its approval by the school council, a meeting with the parents, the training of those involved, and the action in the classroom.

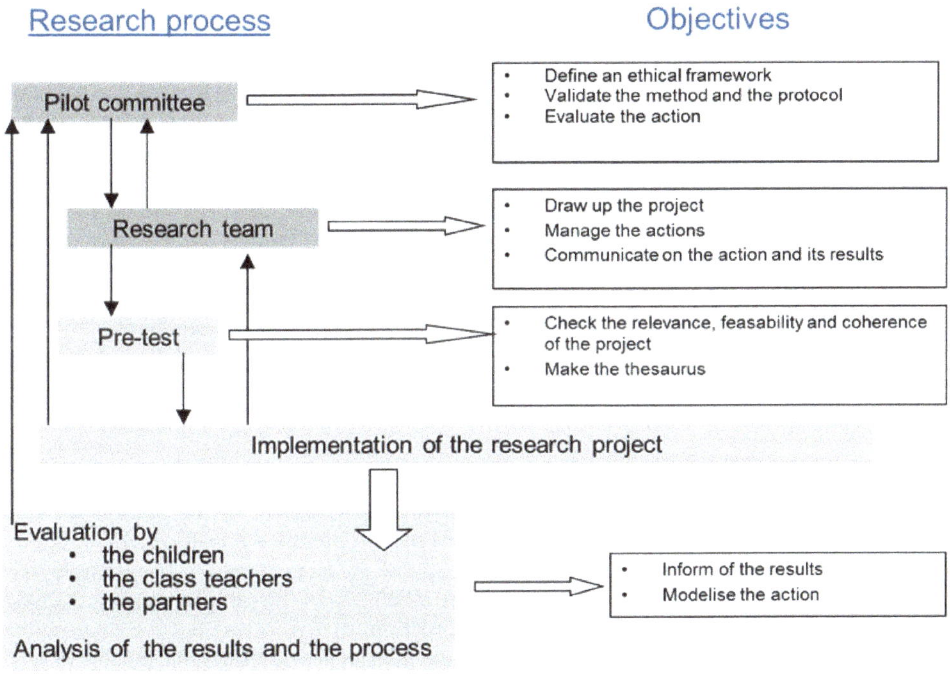

Fig. 1. Research's design

Figure 1 presents the collaborative research design founded on six principles:

1. Insure complementarily between regular teacher's activities and interventions of health educators.
2. Thoroughly preparing the context of the project by involving the families, teachers, and school health services in the comprehensive approach. These partners actively participated in the design of the study (questionnaire, interventions in the classrooms, relationship with the population).
3. Inclusion of all the classes at each school level investigated.

4. Working with groups of children of adapted size (no more than 15).
5. Separating children into groups according to gender (separating girls from boys).
6. Using a participatory activity design with games and tools that favour high rates of participation.

The programme was developed on the basis of previous studies, (see Kirby, 2002 and UNAIDS, 1997). It was first piloted in a school during the school year preceding the study. The team that worked at each site was composed of six people (three per single-sex half group). Two persons from the research team, two representatives of school health services (a nurse and a doctor), and two observers who were to evaluate the teaching project and the way it was implemented.

Evaluation of the process was carried out using the following indicators:

- For the pilot committee, the number of meetings that were held was compared with the scheduling and the number of participants in each category (parents, teachers, doctors, and nurses). There were three interviews with all the members of the pilot committee, one before the project, one between the two sessions, and one after the results of the project had been made available.
- For the school health services, an individual and anonymous questionnaire was used. It dealt with the form of the action, its pedagogical value, and the analysis of the elements benefiting health education in schools. Fourteen school nurses and 14 school doctors were interviewed.
- For the school staff, the same type of individual and anonymous questionnaire was used. All the teachers and heads of schools involved in the programme (28) were interviewed.
- The participation of the parents was measured for every meeting, and analysed in relation to the age group of the pupils and to the socio-economic status of the schools. Twenty interviews were carried out with parents from 4 categories of schools.
- Each session was evaluated by an outside observer, using a grid including items relating to the way the session went, the interactions between adults and children, the involvement of the children, and the amount of time they spoke.

2.2 Population

The study was performed in the south east of France (the regions of the Loire and Haute Loire) in 1998-2000. It concerned pupils in "Cours moyen première année" (CM1) et "Cours moyen deuxième année" (CM2), which correspond to Key Stage 2. The sample was composed of 10 schools and 18 classes. Due to the small size of the sample, its characteristics do not correspond to those of the reference population, that is, it was not a representative sample. Nevertheless, schools corresponding to the main types of school in the country were selected (small size / large size; rural / urban; privileged / under-privileged). The research team asked teachers if they were willing to cooperate in the study. All the teachers that were questioned volunteered to have their class take part in the project. The overall results of the investigation concern 353 children. Among the participating children, 54% were girls and 46% were boys, while 31% and 69% of them came from CM1 and CM2, respectively. The total sample can be divided into 4 sub-groups depending on the social environment of the school. This classification was established using the criteria of the National Institute of Statistics and Economic Studies (INSEE 2003), that is to say, on the basis of the head of the family's profession. Population A (14%) was severely under-privileged (coming from schools classified as "educational priority zones"). Population B (31%) was relatively under-

privileged. Population C (30%) was quite privileged, and D (25%) was highly privileged. This classification brought out variations in the number of children per family. For Population A, there was an average of more than 4 children, for B and C, there was an average of 1.7, and for D, an average 1.5 of children per family. The children from Population A were the only ones to have parents with a significant age difference. The father was on average 10 years older than the mother, whereas, in the other sub-categories, the father was on average no more than 3.5 years older than the mother. However, the average age of the mothers in the four sub-populations was the same (35 years).
The children classified in A were generally older than those in the other sub-populations and faced more difficulties at school. Sixty percent of them repeated a year at least once (16% for the other groups).

2.3 Questionnaire

Due to the age of the pupils, it was not possible to use either the same questionnaire for adolescents and adults, or a multiple choice questionnaire to determine, as it was done with adolescents, the way the children represented modes of infection. Indeed, unfamiliar words, coming from adult or adolescent vocabulary about sexuality, inhibited communication with young children (WHO, 1999). However, we designed a new questionnaire based on pre-existing ones, but in which the vocabulary had been modified based on the results obtained in the pilot study. Thus, in spite of the fact that it made the questions harder to analyse, we used many open questions, sometimes along with closed questions. Using only closed questions would not have enabled us to grasp the complexity of the representations of AIDS in young children.
The validation of the questionnaire (understanding of the questions, coherence between writing questionnaire, and interview) was carried out at the end of the pilot study with a sample of children, who first filled in the questionnaire and then were interviewed. The questionnaire had 22 questions covering 7 aspects:

- Initial representations of the HIV pandemic.
- An assessment of communication about AIDS.
- Knowledge about AIDS
- Modes of infection and protection.
- Determining how close the subject feels the epidemic to be.
- An evaluation of the representations of the possibilities of living with an affected person.
- An evaluation of social and individual representations of solidarity towards affected people. The same questionnaire was applied for both the pre-test and the main test following intervention (series 1 and 2).

For the analysis of our pilot investigation, we started by devising a thesaurus. Each answer was put in a lexical category and coded. This made it possible to take subtle differences into account. The total number of words was 255, and the number of items we added to the first version of the thesaurus after our first processing was low (< 10%). These precautions were taken in order to standardize the data acquired from the questionnaires and reduce any distortion in interpretation.

2.4 Teaching approach

We initially attempted to measure the impact of early preventive action on children's representations. The protocol was composed of two interventions in the course of the school year, one at the beginning and one at the end, at least six months later. Between the two interventions, the regular teachers worked on health education with the pupils ("normal" biology course including sexuality education). The two sessions were designed with the same pedagogical structure, which had two requirements, that is, to collect useful evidence from the questionnaires, and to put the children in a position where they were actors in their own learning process. The two sessions were structured as follows: A short presentation of the team and the framework, a question-writing time, a presentation about HIV/AIDS, work in small single-sex groups on the answers to the questions asked without the teachers, a game (a card-game for the first, and role-playing for the second), and, finally, the collective writing of a text for the teacher and the families.

2.5 Presenting the questionnaire

The questionnaire was intended to characterize children's initial representations and it was anonymous. After the pre-test, it appeared to be necessary, in order to attain this goal, to break away from the school environment and the behaviour it induces, especially in relation to writing. So, in the instructions for the procedure, we stressed that neither spelling nor the quality of the writing were important. What we were interested in was what the children thought, and in having them express their ideas in their own words. The intent was not to make things hard for the children by asking them to write, but simply to obtain their answers so we could analyse them and associate them with representations. We also explained that we would not give any further explanations about the meaning of the questions, as, we were afraid that in doing so, we could influence the answers. In order for all the children to be able to fill in the questionnaire as best as they could, we chose a collective approach. Each question was read out aloud and timed. Thus, we were able to include all the questionnaires in the analysis process, even those from children with serious literacy problems.

2.6 Information provided

This presentation was intended to provide precise and complex scientific information, and to give unity to sketchy and fragmentary representations, re-situating them in a context, and bringing out the link between the illness, the people, forms of behaviour, and oneself.

2.7 The children's questions

After children had filled in the questionnaire, they were invited to ask any questions they wanted to freely and anonymously, so that the educators could answer them in the second part of the session. Another form had been prepared for this and annexed to the questionnaire. Our aim here was to make the children put their questions in written form before the informational presentation, as well as to give us a representative body of questions, and to define these precisely before providing answers.

While the children were at break, their questions were written out again, with no modification whatsoever. After break, the children were put in single-sex groups in separate rooms without their regular teachers so as to make it easier for the children to express themselves more freely on private issues pertaining to genitalia and sexuality. The presence of fellow pupils of the opposite sex and of the regular teacher that pupils will continue to study with could discourage the children from discussing these issues openly. The health educator then read out a question and asked the group to respond, only taking part to give clarification, to substantiate an answer, to get the children talking again, or to regulate the

exchanges and make sure that everyone participated. This process was repeated for each question that had been asked by the children prior to the break.
Our ethical approach was to use only the vocabulary from the presentation or that was used by the children, excluding any words or expressions coming from adolescent or adult vocabulary, particularly in the field related to the management of sexuality. This was essential as we found that use of unfamiliar sexuality related terms coming from adult or adolescent vocabulary inhibited communication and thwarted our objectives. However, by using in our answers exactly the same expressions and words that the children used to formulate their questions, which were sometimes very direct questions about sexual practices, we could show the children that any subject can be tackled with them. The educator's role was mainly to get the discussion going, to modify, or to substantiate the representations by clarifying points, and, if necessary, to offer extra help in completing fragmentary or sketchy knowledge.

2.8 Teaching tools

The card game in the first session: The card game was devised for this experiment and for this particular group. It was based on an approach developed for adolescents (Ricard, 2000) and on the results of the pilot study. It included situations in daily life concerning both close relationships with affected people and more distant situations, so as to enable the children to express their certainties and doubts, and the rumours they had heard. The rules were simple. Each child was given some cards. He read out what was written on the card, showed it to the group, and put it down on one of three cards which indicated no risk, I do not know, or high risk. The child explained his choice and then asked the group to say what they thought. This approach enabled us to involve all the children, even the shyest, and gave them an opportunity to express themselves.
Role playing game in the second session: The aim of this activity was to get the pupils to talk about HIV/AIDS while adopting a point of view different from their own. They had to take the role of parents, teachers, and children in concrete situations. This game is intended to put the children in a situation where they could express and become aware of their own representations of the pandemic, the risk of infection, and the ways of protecting themselves. This projected identification had a powerful emotional component.
Final written work: The children dictated to the educator an account of what they had done, or of the ideas and things which they felt to be important, and which they, therefore, wanted to share with their families and class teacher. The advantage this strategy had over an individual account was that it did not put the children in a difficult school situation by asking them to write. It also made it possible to summarize what was essential.

3. Results

3.1 Statistical analysis

The questionnaires were processed by the statistics department at the St Etienne School of Medicine, according to the thesaurus drawn up during the pre-test, using Epi info 5.01 and SPSS. The level of estimated statistical significance applied for the tests was $p. < 0.05$. When the size of samples was small, the adjusted Khi2 (Yates method) was used and, if the size of one of the samples was beneath 5, we kept the results given by Fisher's test. The analysis was only univariate. The questions asked by the children were analysed using the method of

the "analysis of content" (Bardin, 1993). We therefore put the answers together according to their semantic structure, and observed combined frequency indicators (co-occurrence analysis), which enabled us to establish links between the data (Microsoft Access).
The data described here focus on a comparative study of the results of the two questionnaires. However, the programme was also assessed by the pilot committee, the school medical staff, the teachers and the parents.

3.2 Evaluation of the process

The pilot committee: The committee supervised the research activities all the way throughout the entire project. They met before the sessions to validate the protocol and also defined an ethical framework based on respecting people, and respecting the convictions of the children and their families. After the first session, the results of the first set of data were presented, as well as a report written by observers from outside the team about the way the ethical framework had been respected, and how the sessions had gone and been managed. Once the whole protocol had been applied, the different results and analyses were presented and discussed. All members of the committee attended regularly, including parents' associations. In the interviews at the end of the project, the committee members declared that their opinions had been taken into account.
Medical staff: The evaluation of the schools' medical staff (school doctors and nurses) was carried out through an anonymous individual questionnaire. The entire data set obtained by this questionnaire cannot be analysed here. The results show that the medical staff found the organization relevant. After the experiment, they admitted that they felt more comfortable about tackling the issues of AIDS and sexuality in a comprehensive approach to health education for young pupils. They expressed their need for training, to update their knowledge about HIV, to learn how to teach health education, and to develop their theoretical and pedagogical background. Teachers: For the teachers, an anonymous individual questionnaire was also used. Teachers said they were in favour of this kind of intervention in schools, insisting on how advantageous it was to build up partnerships with competent professionals who have been trained for such actions with children, not with a view of making up for insufficiencies or to replace the class teacher, but to working with the teacher on a common project that is part of their syllabus. Before the intervention, most teachers found it hard or even impossible to talk about such matters with their pupils, although they were well aware of the need for it. The reasons they put forward for this were: (a) They did not have enough knowledge about the disease, the way it is caught, and what protection can be used. (They considered that the only information they had was from the media, and deemed this to be inadequate for giving precise information to children). (b) They were afraid of how the parents might react as they considered this topic to a delicate or sensitive subject. (c) They found it hard to tackle questions about sexuality with children. (d) They were worried that they might be asked questions that they could not answer. Moreover, they all stated that they had changed the way they considered having HIV positive children in their school, and felt better prepared to tackle the issue with parents and colleagues.
The parents: Parental attendance at meetings organized in each school before the interventions varied enormously in relation to the social category involved. Families from the most under-privileged social categories attended less than the others. The aims of the meetings were to present the collaborative research project, answer any questions, and give an account of the results. Right from the start, we noted that it was not really possible to get

parents from the most underprivileged schools involved, and the number of parents present was always very low. However, there was a high attendance rate for parents from more privileged schools. As a result of these meetings, it was obvious that very few parents were against early AIDS prevention, and there was not any obvious and definite opposition. The observations made by parents mainly concerned their desire that family religious and philosophical beliefs be respected.

3.3 Analysis of the questions asked by the children

We were able to study 350 forms. The variables which we used were gender (190 girls and 160 boys), the class at school (114 CM1 and 236 CM2), and the social class (highly privileged 88, quite privileged 103, quite underprivileged 109, and seriously underprivileged 50). Only the first ten questions asked by each child were taken into account and analysed. During the first session, the children asked a total of 1267 questions, and during the secon 759. Thus, there was a drop of 40% ($p.<10$- 3). The average number of questions asked in the first series was 3.62 per child, and for the second 2.16. In the first session, 95.7% of the children asked at least one question, and 73.7% in the second. The number of questions asked per pupil goes down significantly faster in the second series than in the first ($p.<10$-3). Between the two sessions, there was a significant increase ($p <10$- 3) of the number of children not asking any questions, rising from 19 in the first series to 96 in the second.
The analysis of the questions showed that the changes varied according to the item concerned. There was little or no change for the questions about the disease, "love and sexuality," anxiety, the fight against AIDS, and living with the virus. There was a significant decrease in the number of questions concerning the modes of infection ($p.<10$-3) and protection behaviours ($p.=0.025$). The questions on protection, anxiety, attempts to understand, and even the questions on modes of infection, go down much more for the boys than for the girls. The children coming from severely underprivileged families still asked a lot of questions ($p.=0.03$), as did those from a highly privileged background ($p =0.04$).

3.4 Analysis of the questionnaires

The pupils were required to complete the questionnaire before session 1 and before session 2. The results are shown in Table 1. For the closed questions, the results are expressed as percentages of the total number of questionnaires taken into account in the analysis. For open-ended questions, the responses have been grouped into different items and are expressed as percentages of the total number of questionnaires including an answer to the concerned question (data are given in Table 1 only if the items are cited in more than 5 % of the cases in session 1 or 2). For multiple choice questions, the total percentage could exceed 100, because children were allowed to give more than one answer. When a significant impact of gender, age, or social status on the responses was observed, it is indicated. When a significant difference was observed between second and first session, the data are in bold print.
The analysis of the first questionnaire gives an overview of the initial representations of the pupils. The results are shown in Table 1.The comparison between pre- and post-questionnaires guided us to identify where a modification of representations was observed. The analysis was performed taking into account five points: (a) knowledge about AIDS, (b) communication about AIDS, (c) knowledge about the disease, (d) knowledge about modes of infection and protection, and (e) relationships with affected people (the analysis of the other parts of the questionnaire are not shown in this article).

3.5 Knowledge about AIDS

The analysis of the first questionnaire (pre-test) indicated that more than 92% of the children had information about AIDS, while, six months later, this percentage increased to 98% for the second questionnaire. The main source of information was television (88%) followed by the family (25%). However, these results (Question 2) were inconsistent with the results from another question (Question 4), where more than 65% of the children stated that they had talked about AIDS with their families. The only source of information which changed significantly between the two questionnaires was the school (*p.*<10-3). Children mainly associated AIDS with words suggesting, Illness, Death, and Sexuality. They also mentioned, to a lesser extent, condoms, blood as a vector for infection, taking drugs, and finally prevention, and solidarity. The intervention did not trigger any substantial change in initial associations with Illness/Death/Sex, but it nevertheless allowed most children, who had not ever discussed the subject, to be involved in discussions about AIDS. Three-quarters of those who did not mention anything initially, did contribute after the intervention. Thus, the highly privileged group D referred initially to sex and sexuality more than the severely underprivileged group (*p.*<10-3). But, this difference was much smaller at the end of the session (*p.*=0.05).

3.6 Communication about AIDS

Figure 2 shows the differential influence of socioeconomic status on the impact of communication about AIDS with adults (Have you ever talked about AIDS with adults?) and in the family (Have you talked about AIDS in your family?). While an increase incommunication with adults was observed for all 4 groups, it was limited to the

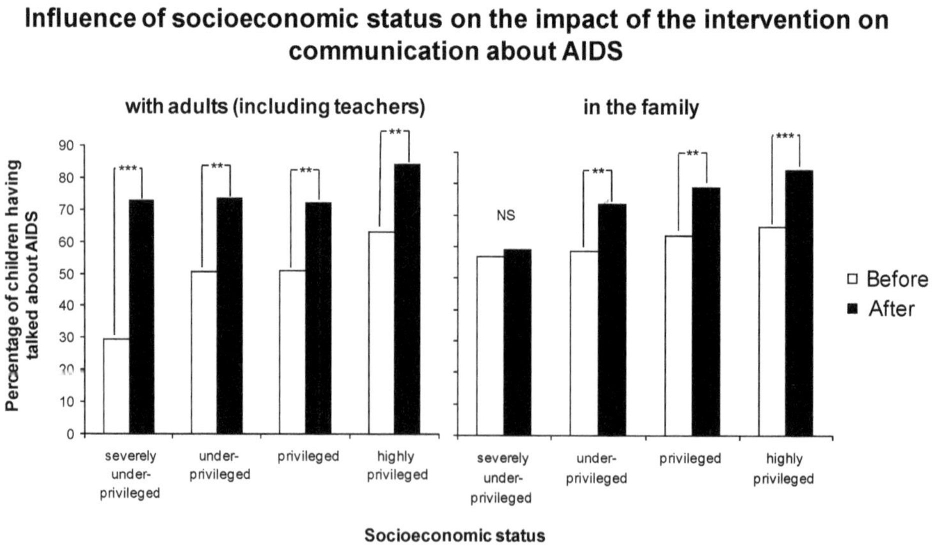

(* *p.* < 0.05 ** *p.*< 0.01, *** *p.* < 0.001).

Fig. 2. Influence of Socioeconomic Status on the Impact of the Intervention on Communication about AIDS.

underprivileged, privileged and highly privileged groups for communication inside the family. Results are expressed as percentages of the total number of questionnaires including an answer to the question.

Pupils also exchanged on the topic of AIDS with adults, with friends and at school. Fifty-one percent of the children had talked about AIDS with adults before the intervention. At the end, 76 % of them have talked about the subject with adults, either before the first session or between the two sessions. The intervention did not bring on a significant increase in discussion of AIDS within the family in the severely underprivileged group (p.=0.3 49%), unlike in the other groups, where there was a significant increase of 74%, 79% and 85%, for groups B, C and D with p=0.01, p.=0.01, and p=.001, respectively, indicating that communication between the pupils was also enhanced. (clarify the meaning)

3.7 Knowledge about the disease

Before the intervention, more than half of the children associated AIDS with a fatal illness. On a scale ranging from 0 to 10, the children rated the dangerousness of AIDS at more than 8. Population A alone stands out by assessing its gravity at less than 8 (p.=0.007). The illness which is symbolically associated with AIDS is cancer.

Infectious illnesses are not often quoted, and only 5% of the children mention Hepatitis B. After the intervention, we found that references to infectious diseases dropped considerably, and associations with childhood illnesses disappeared. Two-thirds of the children stated that they knew what a virus is, and were able to give a relevant explanation, with a definition based on one of three 'concepts,': a microbe, an illness, or a vector of an illness. However, only one-third knew what HIV positive means.

3.8 Modes of infection and protection

Before the intervention, 88% of the children associated AIDS with a transmissible disease and 97% after the intervention. The change was slight but significant. In the pre-test, 74% of the children correctly answered the question "What gives you AIDS ?" and in the post-test 89%. For the children, AIDS is transmitted by vectors: secretions (sperm), sex, drugs, and the HIV virus; and by behaviour: sexuality, drug addiction, and medical practices related to the handling of blood, such as, transfusion and giving blood. Drug addiction was scarcely mentioned, and references to syringes or exchanging syringes were very uncommon. Similarly, references to materno-foetal transmission, and to incorrect vectors, such as, saliva, mosquitoes, daily actions, morality, or God, were almost non-existent. The lexical field used was fairly limited, but it was wider in the second session. The question was put in such a way as to give the children the possibility of replying by designating supposedly high-risk groups (homosexuals, prostitutes, drug-addicts, dirty people, and others).

The pupils did not consider that people identified as 'deviant' were responsible for beginning the infection. As far as modes of infection are concerned, after the intervention there was a modification concerning the answers about vectors of infection, and those about behaviour. Representations definitely became clearer. Before the sessions, more than half the children explained that contamination came from vectors: sex (1/2) and drugs (3/4), but after the session, they referred to "dangerous" behaviour (90% sexuality and 50% also mentioned drug addiction).

Preventive action modified representations concerning modes of infection (p.=0.001). However, this reversal was less obvious for the very underprivileged social categories (p.=0.03).

In order to know whether an individual may have been infected, more than half the children suggested active solutions, such as, having a test, or going to see a doctor. Fifteen percent suggested passive solutions, waiting for the symptoms to appear, or waiting till you feel ill. The girls suggested fewer active solutions than the boys ($p.$=0.013), and the severely underprivileged children fewer than the highly privileged ($p.$=0.049). After the intervention, reference to detection increased considerably (p =0.002), and there was less mention of adopting a passive stance or waiting for symptoms to appear (p =0.016).
Prior to the intervention, 68 % of the children suggested the condom as a way to be protected, and this percentage increased to 91% afterwards. The intervention mainly gave rise to a considerable increase in references to condoms, protection, and avoidance. There were no statistically significant difference related to age, sex, or social status in this increase.

3.9 Relationship with affected people

One out of two children had heard of someone who had or had had AIDS, both before and after the intervention. Only one in ten had heard of it through a channel other than television. Before the intervention, 64% of the children thought it was dangerous to live with an HIV positive person. Twenty-nine percent continued to think so, even after the intervention, but there was a significant change in the way infected people are seen and in the perception of the absence of risk of infection in everyday life.

4. Discussion

The aim of our study was to identify the initial representations of pupils on AIDS/HIV and to analyse the impact of an educational programme based on regular teacher's activities and interventions of health educators on these representations, on communication about AIDS/HIV, and on the way in which infected people are seen. The main novel features of our study were its target (young pupils aged 9 and 10), the close partnership between teachers and health educators, the involvement of parents, and the fact that it was based on a learner-centred model (the allosteric model as described by Giordan, 1995). First, we are going to discuss the relevance of such a research design and, secondly, we will analyse the pupils' initial representations on AIDS/HIV and the impact of the program. Finally, the issue of communication about AIDS in the family and with peers will be addressed.
The main characteristic of collaborative research is the close involvement of the target population in the development and management of the program, or, in other words, the proximity between researchers and actors (Martinand, 2003; Merini, 2005). It also aims at an improvement of practices here and now. Our study shows the interest of such a design in AIDS/HIV prevention. Indeed, the actors (teachers, parents, doctors, nurses etc.) were highly involved in the programme throughout the two years it took place. The intervention was conducted in a coherent manner in relateion to the educational environment of the pupils. In addition, the design lead us to take into account the ethical issues linked to preventive intervention (respect for people, cultures, family upbringing etc.) Nevertheless, we must also underline the limits of such a design. It was time consuming and the involvement of the severely under-privileged group was lower than that of the other groups.
As described in previous studies (e.g., Anochie & Ikpeme, 2003), the analysis of the initial questionnaires indicated that 9- and 10-year-old children did have representations of the HIV pandemic, the people affected, and the modes of infection and protection, but they had incomplete information on the subject. More than half of the pupils associated AIDS with a

fatal illness as serious as, or more serious than cancer, transmitted by 'sex,' and 'caught' especially by adolescents and adults. They thought the illness could be avoided by putting on a condom (68 %), and detected by 'tests' or going to 'see a doctor' (80%). The content of their scientific statements was still at times completely or partially incomprehensible, as they could not fit them into a more general conceptual framework of knowledge, which would allow overall understanding (Kirb, Short, Collins, Rugg, Kolbe, Howard, 1994; Kirby, 1995; UNAIDS 1997). It can be noted that the highly privileged group D refered to sex and sexuality more than the severely underprivileged group A. It was also evident that the severely underprivileged children generally used a much more limited lexical field than the others. This observation was evident in the questionnaire as well as in the analysis of the transcripts of work in sub-groups. This lexical limitation seemed to have interfered with establishing complex representations, and these pupils were not able to avoid reductive over-simplification.

At the end of the session, more children answered most of the open questions, and did so using more words. The lexical field concerning biomedical knowledge was of higher qualityRegarding modes of infection, we found the focus on vectors of infection decreased whereas attention tobehaviour increased. Before the sessions, more than half the children explained that contamination came from vectors, such as sex or drugs, but, after the session, they mainly referred to dangerous behaviour (sexuality, drug-addiction). Regarding protection, the study showed the interventions had had considerable impact. At the end of the sessions, only 8 children answered that you cannot avoid catching AIDS. There was a 150 % increase in the number of children stating that "the condom protects you from HIV infection" and three times more children spoke about protective behaviour.

These data have to be interpreted with precaution, because it is well known that there is no direct link between knowledge and behaviours (e.g., UNAIDS, 1997). In addition to the influence of socioeconomic status on children's representations, we observed an influence of age and gender. The representations of the 10- year-olds were more relevant than those of the 9- year-olds, who are still quite childish,. Researchers working on representations in children of different ages have made similar observations (BMA, 1997; UNAIDS 1997; Brown 1990). However, most authors found little difference between girls and boys (du Guerny &Sjoberg, 1993; Guthrie, Wallace, Doerr, Janz, Schottenfeld, Selig, 1996; Prah Rugger, 2004; UNAIDS, 2004).

The study also investigated communication about AIDS. People with whom pupils speak about AIDS were mainly their families and peers. Nevertheless, in the second questionnaire, only 1 % to 4 % of them stated that they had never heard their friends talking about AIDS. In a study performed with primary school children (11-yearsold), Anochie and Ikpeme (2003) found that friends were not an important source of information for pupils (4 %). It is not easy to interpret this statement, as, in question 3, 44% of the same children stated that they have talked about AIDS with other children. Perhaps this contrast indicates that other pupils are not considered to be a worthy source of information, bu comparison to other sources, which they see as more knowledgeable. It is highly likely that the children hear more about AIDS through the media than from their friends, which caused them to underestimate the importance of the information they got from their peers. Moreover, the children appear to have discounted this information as not being serious and, therefore, not worth mentioning, in comparison with information given by experts on the TV, 'which tells the truth.' This interpretation also proved to be valid with the analysis of the work done in the sub-groups of the study.

About 62% of the children have talked about AIDS in their families before the intervention, whatever their age, sex, or social origin. In the second series, 76 % of them have talked about the subject with their families, either before the first session or between the two. But our intervention did not bring any significant increase in communication within the family in the severely underprivileged group. These data show how hard it is to get a family to talk about AIDS, particularly for the severely underprivileged, and raises the question of family communication in the field of health education. It is likely that the intervention triggered discussion in families where there was a readiness for this. Our analysis shows that more than 90% of the families of the underprivileged group were of foreign origin (North African and Turkish). Talking about sexuality, especially with boys, in a cultural framework that was profoundly steeped in tradition, meant adopting a new Western-style cultural position. Thus it was difficult to talk about such a private subject in the family. Their priority was apparently to not deny their origins, and to preserve their identity, so as not to be swallowed up by integration, which was experienced as culturally destructive. As a result, no standard model of intervention could be put forward because the cultural dimension was a significant variable in actions and their impact (Rosenthal, 1990; Tones & Tilford, 2001; WHO 1997, 2004a, 2004b). The whole community must really be involved when the intervention occurs in a multicultural environment.

The analysis of the interviews indicated that communication about AIDS in families and between friends was related to an external stimulus, generally the media (but sometimes school). Television news and special programmes made families react. Families who tackled the issue without any direct link with the media were only few and far between. When they did, it was more frequently to warn children about the risks of sex and drugs than to incorporate this into a more general discussion about exclusion, life, its risks and the management of these risk, or about sexuality and pleasure.

The cross analysis of the questions showed that when the question of the integrating an HIV positive person in different situations was raised, the attitude of children from families where AIDS was discussed was no different from that of children from backgrounds where it was not. So, it would seem that the family message did not focus on the integration of infected persons. Nor was it a message of exclusion. It was likely that the parents' message did not concern infected people. The reality of the infected person remained largely virtual. Information mainly came from the mass media and television, and contact with sufferers in their daily lives was rare.

5. Conclusion

This study shows an evolution in the representations of pupils about HIV/AIDS. The intervention led them to build new representations that take more objective facts into account. These results are interesting but have to be discussed, as it is well known that there is no one to one link between knowledge and behaviour. The mere provision of knowledge is not enough if the aim is a relevant scientific education, but the educational process here includes helping children "to clarify their values in relation with themselves, health, health-influencing behaviours" (Downie et al., 1996). In addition, such an intervention makes it possible to talk much more about a much broader spectrum of themes related to health. In working on HIV/AIDS prevention and sexuality education, numerous other aspects of science education are tackled, and mainly the status of science in relation to everyday life (nature of science and scientific knowledge, application of science concepts, values that underlie science etc.) By providing an HIV/AIDS education programme, it is only possible to promote a comprehensive health approach (St Leger & Nutbeam, 1999), if the whole educational environment is involved, if the intervention is really learner-centred, if the programme is sufficiently open and does not aim at enforcing some form of behaviour, and if the ethical framework is clearly defined. Such an approach, to be effective, must take into account the complexity of health, and the factors which influence it, but also actual science education theory and practice. This last point is decisive as one of the most important difficulties in implementing relevant programs is, in addition to taking into account cultural and social diversity, the involvement of teachers and school staff (Ayo-Yusuf, 2001; Han & Weiss, 2005).

6. Annex

	SESSION 1		SESSION 2	
	Responses	Impact of gender, age or social status	Responses	Impact of gender, age or social status
General representation of HIV/AIDS				
Have you already heard of AIDS ?	Yes : 92 % No : 8 %	No gender, age or social influence	Yes : 98 % No : 2 %	No gender, age or social influence
If yes, where ?	Media (TV radio) 88 % Family 25 % Doctor 7 % School 7 % Friends 1 %	The number of non responders is higher in the group of young pupils: CM1 / CM2 (19 vs 5 %) * The parents are less often cited by pupils in group A than pupils in groups C* and D * No gender influence	Media (TV radio) 90 % **School 38 %** + Family 33 % Doctor 2 % **Friends 4 % +** (the increase is only significant in the older group CM2)	The number of non responders is higher in the group of young pupils : CM1 (7 vs 2 %) * The parents are less often cited by pupils in group A (8 %) than pupils in groups C (16 %)* and D (14 %) * No gender, age or social influence
What does AIDS make you think of ? Write three words	Disease ou illness ? : 42 % Death : 34 % Sexuality 9 % Protection behaviour 4 %	Concerning the item « sexuality », boys outnumbered girls (12 vs 7 %)* Pupils in group D give more words about sex than C, B and A * No age influence	Disease ou illness ? : 46 % **Death : 26 %** + Sexuality : 11 % Protection behaviour 7 %	Pupils in group D give more words about sex than C, B and A * No age or gender influence
Communication about AIDS				
Have you ever talked about AIDS with adults ?	Yes : 51 % No : 49 %	Pupils in group A (29 %) had spoken less about AIDS with adults than groups B50% C51 % and D* 63 % No gender or age influence	**Yes : 76 % No : 24 %** +	The impact of the interventions is not significant for the group A 49% but it is for the other's B 74 %*,C79%* and D 85%*. No gender or age influence
with other children ?	Yes 44 % No : 56 %	No gender, age or social influence	**Yes : 75 % No : 25 %** ++	No gender, age or social influence
if yes, with whom ?	Parents 65 % Brothers and sisters 14% Uncles, aunts,	Pupils in group A had spoken less about AIDS with theirs parents than group D *	Parents 65 % Brothers and sisters 17% **Uncles, aunts, cousins 15 %** +	Pupils in group A had spoken less about AIDS with their parents, uncles, aunts and cousins than

	cousins 10 % Friends 45 %	No gender or age influence	**Friends 65 %** +	groups B, C and D * The increase in family communication is better in the higher social group. There is no change in group A*. No gender or age influence
Have you talked about AIDS in your family ?	Yes 62 % No 38 %	No gender, age or social influence	**Yes 76 % No 24 %** +	There is an influence of social status on the impact of the training session : the increase in communication is limited to groups C, D and E* No gender or age influence
Knowledge about HIV/AIDS				
Do you known what "Virus" means?	Yes 65% No 35%	No social, age or gender incidence	Yes 67% No 33%	No gender, age or social influence
Can you explain what Virus means ?	Disease 54% Microbe 31 % Vector 14%	Large number of non-responders (32% of children asking yes to the previous question) There is a gender difference, girls link "virus" with illness and boys with microbe.* No social or age incidence	Disease 44% Microbe 36 % Vector 20 %	Large number of non-responders (47% of children asking yes to the previous question) No gender, age or social influence
Do you known what "HIV positive" means ?	Yes 35 % No 65 %	Girls says yes more often then boys (41% vs 28%)* No social or age incidence	**Yes 65 % No 35 %** +	No gender, age or social influence
Can you explain what means HIV positive means ?	Someone who is sick (AIDS) 52% Someone who has the HIV virus but is not sick 33 %, Someone with serious disease having no link with Aids 13%	Large number of non-responders (63% of children asking yes to the previous question) Pupils in group A had spoken more about serious diseases without link with AIDS (A 33%, B 3%, C19%, D 9%)*	Someone who is sick (AIDS) 49% **Someone who has the HIV virus but is not sick 51 %** + **Someone with serious disease having no link with Aids 0%**	Large number of non-responders (40% of children asking yes to the previous question) There are more responses concerning the virus in the older group (CM2) 36% than in the younger one (CM1) 15% * No social or gender difference
How can we know if we are HIV positive ?	Active solutions 80% Passive solutions 20% 7 children said there is no way to know if you are HIV positive	Difference with group A (72%) who suggest fewer active solutions than B 81%, C 78%, D 87%* No gender or age influence	**Active solutions 93% Passive solutions 7%** + **no children said there is no way to know if you are HIV positive**	Girls suggested fewer active solutions than boys * Group A suggest fewer active solutions than the others group*
Assessment of modes of infection and protection				
Is AIDS a transmissive illness?	88% of the pupils consider AIDS as a transmissive disease	No gender, age or social influence	**97 % of the pupils consider AIDS as a transmissive disease** +	No gender, age or social influence
If yes ? What gives you AIDS?	Number of words per pupil = 1.28 Things (sperm, secretions, drugs) 58 %	Pupils in group D give more words about sex 66% , than C 55%, B 55% and A 28%* There are more responses	**Number of words per pupil = 1.72** + **Things (sperm, secretions, drugs) 36 %** +	No gender, age or social influence

	Behaviour (sexual intercourse, using drugs...) 28% Condition (illness, poverty...) 6% God, evil, sin, fate 5%	with older pupils (CM2) 90% than younger (CM1) 76% No gender difference	**Behaviour (sexual intercourse, using drugs...) 59%** $^{+}$ Condition (illness, poverty...) 3% **God, evil, sin, fate 0%**	
Is AIDS an illness we can avoid?	Yes : 90% No: 10%	No gender, age or social influence	**Yes : 98% No: 2%** $^{+}$	No gender, age or social influence
How can you protect yourself? 3 words	Number of words used : 1.05 Using condom : 68% Avoidance behaviour : 11 % Protection behaviour : 5 %	No gender, age or social influence	**Number of words used : 1.37** $^{+}$ **Using condom : 91 %** $^{+}$ Avoidance behaviour : 6 % Protection behaviour : 3 %	No gender, age or social influence.
At what age can you get Aids ?	Teenagers : 45 % Throughout life : 24% Childhood : 15 % Adult : 9 % (Never : 1%)	No gender, age or social influence	**Teenagers : 32 %** $^{+}$ **Throughout life : 40%** $^{+}$ Childhood : 16 % **Adult : 2%** $^{+}$ (Never : 0%)	No gender, age or social influence
Life with affected people				
Have you heard of anyone with AIDS?	Yes 47% No : 56 %	No gender, age or social influence	Yes 46% No 54%	No gender, age or social influence
If yes, where?	Media 81% Family: 11%	No social, age or gender incidence	Media : 87% Family : 6%	No gender, age or social influence
Can you live with someone with AIDS without any risk for yourself?	Yes 36% No 64 %	No gender, age or social influence	**Yes 71% No 29%** $^{+}$	No gender, age or social influence
Is there a risk for me if a classmate is HIV positive?	No : 59% Yes 41%	No gender, age or social influence	**No 86% Yes 14%** $^{+}$	No gender, age or social influence

Table 1. Analysis of the responses to the questionnaire. The pupils had to fill it in before session 1 and before session 2. The results are shown as follows. Closed questions: results are expressed as percentages of the total number of questionnaires taken into account in the analysis. Open questions: the responses are put together in different items; results are expressed as percentages of the total number of questionnaires including a response to the concerned question (data are given in the table only if the items are cited in more than 5 % of the cases in session 1 or 2). For multiple choice questions, the total percentage could exceed 100 because children were allowed to give more than one answer. When a significant impact of gender, age or social status on the responses is observed, it is indicated in the table. When a significant difference was observed between second and first session, the data are in bold print. CM1: young group (age 9), CM2 old group (age 10), A : severely under-privileged B : relatively under-privileged C : quite privileged, and D : highly privileged. Statistical significance : Impact of sex, age or social status on responses in session 1 or session 2 : * $p < 0.05$. difference between session 2 and session 1 : $^{+}$ $p < 0.05$.

7. Acknowledgments

Author thank Rémi Collet, Didier Jourdan and Crane Rogers for there contribution to the research.

8. References

Abric, J-C. (1997). *Pratiques sociales et représentations* (2nd edition). PUF. Paris.

Anochie, I., & Ikpeme, E. (2003). AIDS awareness and knowledge among primary school children in Port Harcourt metropolis. *Niger Journal of Medicine, 2003 (1),* 27-31.

Ayo-Yusuf, I., Naidoo, S., Chikte, U. M. (2001). The role of primary school teachers in HIV prevention in South Africa. *SAD, (12),* 596-598.

Bardin L. (1993). *L'analyse de contenus*, PUF, Paris.

Berger D., Collet R., Laquet-Riffaud A., & JOURDAN D. (2003). Quelles représentations les enfants ont-ils du SIDA ? Contribution d'une recherche-action en éducation pour la santé auprès de classes de CM1 et CM2. *En question. 48*. 1- 29.

BMA Foundation for AIDS. (1997) *Using effectiveness research to guide the development of school sex education.* London: British Medical Association.

Brown M. D., Nassau J. H., & Barone V. J. (1990). Differences in A.I.D.S. knowledge and attitudes by grade level. *Journal of School Health. (60)6,* 270-275.

Darroch J., & Silverman J. (1989). What public school teachers teach about preventing pregnancy, A.I.D.S. and S.T.D. *Family Planning Perspective, (21)2,* 65- 73.

Des Jarlais D., Lyles C., Crepas N., & TREND group (2004). Improving the reporting quality of nonrandomized evaluations of behavioural and public health interventions: The TREND statement. *American Journal of Public Health, 94(3),* 361-366

Doise W., & Mugny J.P. (1984). *Le développement social de l'intelligence.* Oxford: Pergamon Press.

Downie R. S., Tannahill C., & Tannahill A. (2004). *Health promotion: Models and values* (2nd edition). Oxford: Oxford Press.

Du Guerny J, & Sjöberg E. (1993) Inter-relationship between gender relations and the HIV/AIDS epidemic: Some possible considerations for policies and programmes. *AIDS, 7,* 1027-34. 238 *Representatives of HIV/AIDS in Children*

Farr R. (1997). Les représentations sociales. In *Psychologie sociale.* S. Moscovici. (dir.) PUF Editor Paris.

Fassler D., MC Queen K., Ducan P., & Copeland L. (1990). Children's perceptions of A.I.DS. *J. Am. Acad. Child adolesc. Psychiatry.* (29)3, 459-462.

Ferron C., Feard S., Bon N., Spyckerelle Y., & Deschamps J-P. (1989). L'enfant et le SIDA, connaissance et représentation, *revue française de pédiatrie* (XXV), 195-209.

Fischer G.N. (2001). *Les concepts fondamentaux de la psychologie sociale.* Paris: Dunod Editor.

Giordan A. (1995). New models for the learning process: Beyond constructivism. *Prospects* (XXV) 1.

Giordan A. (2000) Health Education, Recent and Future Trends. *Mem Inst Oswaldo Cruz.* (95), suppl. I: 53-58.

Guthrie BJ, Wallace J, Doerr K, Janz N, Schottenfeld D, & Selig S. (1996). Girl Talk: Development of an intervention for prevention of HIV/AIDS and other sexually transmitted diseases in adolescent females. *Public Health Nursing* (13), 318-30.

Han SS, & Weiss B. (2005) Sustainability of teacher implementation of schoolbased mental health programs. *J Abnorm Child Psychol.* (33)6. 665-79.

Heymans A. (1993). Prévention, sexualité, SIDA qu'en est-il pour les enfants ? in *Les jeunes face au SIDA de la recherche à l'action* A.N.R.S. Editor. Paris. 94-100.

INSEE (2004). Nomenclatures et codes. Les nomenclatures des professions et catégories socioprofessionnelles; Liste des catégories socioprofessionnelles agrégées 2003. *La documentation Française.* Paris.

Jodelet D. (1991). *Les représentations sociales.* Paris: PUF Editor.

Jourdan, D., Piec, I., Aublet-Cuvelier, B., Berger, D., Lejeune, M. L., Laquetriffaud, A., Geneix, C. & Glanddier, P. Y. (2002). Education à la santé à l'école: pratiques et représentations des enseignants du primaire. *Santé Publique,* 14, 403-423

Kelly J. (1995). Advances in HIV/AIDS education and prevention. *Family Relations. 44,* 345-52.

Kirby D, Short L, Collins J, Rugg D, Kolbe L, & Howard M, (1994). School-based programs to reduce sexual risk behaviors: A review of effectiveness. *Public Health Reports, 109,* 339-60.

Kirby D. (1995) *A review of educational programs designed to reduce sexual risk-taking behaviors among school-aged youth in the United States.* ETR Associates. Santa Cruz.

Kirby, D. (2002). Effective approaches to reducing adolescent unprotected sex, pregnancy, and childbearing. *J. Sex. Res, 39(1),* 51-7.

Martinand J.L., (2003). Les savoirs entre pratique, formation et recherche. *Recherche et Formation* (40).

Merini C. (2005). Travail conjoint et professionnalité enseignante *Rapport d'étude IA 92-UIMM Mai 2005* ADASE, Paris.

MEN (Ministère de l'éducation nationale) (2002) BO hors série nÆ1 du 14 février 2002

MEN (Ministère de l'éducation nationale) (2003) L'éducation à la sexualité dans les écoles, les collèges et les lycées BO n°27 du 17 février 2003

Prah Ruger J. (2004) Combating HIV/AIDS in developing countries BMJ (121)329;121-122.

Ricard E. (2000) Sida que savons-nous? 33 cartes pour en parler. *Transcriptase Sud.* (3)19-20.

Rosenthal D, Moore S, & Brumen I. (1990) Ethnic group differences in adolescents. *Australian Journal of Social Issues,25,* 220-39.

Schaalma H, Kok G., & Peters L. (1993). Determinants of consistent condom use by adolescents: The impact of experience of sexual intercourse. *Health Education Research, 8,* 255-69.

Schonfeld D. J., Johnson S. R., Perrin E. C., O'hare L. L. & Cicchetti D. V. (1993). Understanding of A.I.D.S. by elementary school children - A developmental survey, *Pediatrics.* (92)3, 389-395.

Sly D. F., Eberstein I. W., Quadano D., & Kistner J. A. (1992). Young children's awareness, knowledge & beliefs about A.I.D.S.: observations from a pretest, *A.I.D.S. education & prevention. 4(3),* 227-239.

ST Leger, L. AND Nutbeam, D. (1999) Evidence of Effective Health Promotion in Schools. In Boddy, D. (ed). *The Evidence of Health Promotion Effectiveness: Shaping Public Health in a New Europe.* European Union, Brussels.

THOMAS P. (1991). "Chat-SIDA", une recherche-action en éducation pour la santé avec des enfants de CM2 d'Argenteuil. *Thesis for the C.E.S. de psychiatrie. U.E.R. de médecine Broussais/Hôtel-Dieu.* Université Paris VI.

Tones K. & Tilford S. (2001). *Health Promotion effectiveness, efficiency and equity* (third edition). Cheltanham: Nelson Thornes Editor.

UNAIDS (1997). Influence de l'éducation en matière de VIH et de santé sexuelle sur le comportement sexuel des jeunes: un bilan actualisé. Geneva.

UNAIDS (2004). AIDS and girls education. Geneva VICTORIA C. G., HABICHT J. P., & BRYCE J. (2004). Evidence-based public health moving beyond randomized trials. *Am. J. Public Health.* (94) 400-405.

WHO. (1999), Preventing HIV/AIDS/STI and related discrimination an important responsability of health promoting schools. *WHO information series on school health.* WHO Editor Geneva.

WHO. (2004a). Guide to Monitoring and Evaluating National HIV/AIDS Prevention Programmes for Young People - Addendum to the UNAIDS *"National AIDS Programmes: A Guide to Monitoring and Evaluation"*. Geneva.

WHO. (2004b). Participatory Learning Activities from the EI/WHO Training and Resources Manual on School Health and HIV and AIDS Prevention. Geneva.

WHO. (1997). *Promoting health trough school.* Geneva

4

The Role of the Private Sector in HIV and AIDS Interventions in Developing Countries: The Case of Lesotho

Zitha Mokomane and Mokhantšo Makoae
Human Sciences Research Council of South Africa
South Africa

1. Introduction

The HIV and AIDS pandemic enters its fourth decade of expansion having undermined every aspect of society. This is particularly the case in sub-Saharan Africa, which remains the most heavily affected region, accounting for 72% of all new infections in 2008, and for 68% of the global number of people living with HIV in 2009 (United Nations, 2010; UNAIDS, 2010). UNAIDS further reports that during 2009 alone an estimated 1.3 million adults and children died as a result of AIDS in sub-Saharan Africa and that more than 15 million have died in the region since the beginning of the epidemic in the early 1980s (UNAIDS, 2008; 2010).

The impact of the epidemic in sub-Saharan Africa is widely felt in, among others, the health, education, agriculture, mining, transport and other production sectors. Furthermore, to the extent that the vast majority of people living with HIV and AIDS are between the ages of 15 and 49 years—in the prime of their working lives (International Labour Organisation, 2006), the epidemic weakens economic activity through decreased productivity due to absenteeism resulting from sickness, caring for family and dependents; and organizing and attending funerals; low morale at work due to losing family, friends and colleagues; increased costs due to rising health insurance, sick leave, funeral costs, recruiting and training skilled workers; and reduced labour supply due to increased mortality (Phororo, 2003; Sidhu, 2008). Government income also declines as tax revenues fall and governments are pressured to increase their spending to deal with the expanding epidemic (Avert, 2011).

It is largely against this background that the 2001 United Nations Declaration of Commitment on identified the private sector as an essential part of the national and global responses to [HIV and AIDS]. In line with this Declaration, and as the epidemic continues to affect the working population, the private sector in Africa has over the past years scaled up its response by complementing the work of the traditional public sector and civil society actors (Sidhu, 2008). Progressive companies throughout the region are putting in place a wide range of HIV and AIDS prevention, care, and treatment programmes. These include education and awareness campaigns; training of peer educators; distribution of condoms; promotion of HIV testing; and treatment of, and protection against, other sexually transmitted infections (Rosen et al, 2007). The prevention programmes are typically designed to reduce the incidence of the epidemic in the workplace. Care and treatment programmes, on the other hand, are often meant to support employees who are infected with HIV and who have AIDS, with the objective of keeping these employees in the workforce, and delaying or avoiding the costs of AIDS (Rosen & Simon, 2003; Rosen et al, 2004; George et al, 2009)

An example of the African private sector engagement in national HIV and AIDS response is that of the Private Sector Coalition Against AIDS in Lesotho (PSCAAL) initiative that operated between 2002 and 2006 in the Southern African Kingdom. The main goal of the initiative—which was managed by CARE South Africa-Lesotho (hereafter to be referred to as 'CARE')—was to facilitate a partnership among private sector companies in the fight against HIV and AIDS in an environment characterized by a large female workforce and rural-urban migration. Largely based on evidence showing that HIV and AIDS was a serious threat to production in the textile industry (Ruscombe-King, 2008; UNAIDS, 2008), various companies in the textile sector formed part of the sites where PSCAAL activities were undertaken.

The activities included providing peer education for the workforce to raise awareness about, and increase demand for, HIV prevention services. Peer education is commonly used for promoting sexual and reproductive health, especially with regards to HIV prevention among youth by enhancing social learning and providing psychosocial support (Population Council, n.d; Swartz et al, 2010). A group of individuals recruited from among the target population is used as peer educators or agents of change in order to change social norms among peer targets (Chandan et al, 2008:12). The PSCAAL programme implementation involved: (1) training workers to conduct peer education and provide peer counselling to their colleagues in order to influence behaviour change; (2) facilitating the provision of care and support through formation of support groups to encourage workers to talk about HIV and AIDS; (3) using mobile services to encourage workers to utilise voluntary counselling and testing (VCT) services at the workplace; and (4) providing training in workplace HIV and AIDS policies to assist companies to institutionalise their response to the epidemic. Overall, PSCAAL's approach was based on the assumption that exposure of workers to the programme activities would lead to "a shift from risk behaviours contributing to HIV and AIDS towards risk-avoiding strategies in the workforce" (Hanisch, 2006).

This chapter assesses the extent to which PSCAAL's activities enhanced HIV and AIDS knowledge and behaviour changes among the female textile workers. The differences between workers who participated in the peer education programme (PEP) and those who did not participate are examined in terms of: (1) knowledge of HIV and AIDS; (2) preventive behaviour measured as uptake of HIV testing and consistent condom use; (3) attitudes towards HIV; and (4) level of self-efficacy in relation to HIV prevention. The opportunities which PSCAAL could have lost through their programming are also explored and recommendations for more effective private sector engagement in sub-Saharan Africa are given. Unlike previous studies that generally used secondary data to explore these issues, this current study obtained empirical data from workers themselves, and obtained their perspectives on the factors that increase their vulnerability to HIV and the suitability of available support and services.

2. Background

Lesotho is one of the five countries with the highest HIV prevalence in the world with about 23.6% of adults infected in 2008 (National AIDS Commission, 2008). Consistent with the global pattern, women are disproportionately affected by HIV and AIDS, accounting for 57% of the total HIV-positive cases in Lesotho in 2007 (Khobotlo et al., 2009; UNAIDS, 2009), and most infections occur among young women aged 15-24 years. According to (Khobotlo et al, 2009), in 2007 young women had an HIV prevalence of 14.3% compared to 5.6% among men of the same age. Several factors underlie this pattern. These include the migration of young women from rural to urban to seek employment, particularly in the apparel industry. This was a major livelihood strategy following mass retrenchment of male workers from South African mining industry in the 1990s. While the women's migration certainly contributed to family welfare through food security, it also increased the women's vulnerability to HIV infections, as has been established in the literature. That is, although the causation patterns behind the population mobility/HIV connection are complex, it is shown that migration can create situations that increase people's vulnerability and risks (Brummer, 2002; Santis et al, 2007). The most commonly cited post-migration characteristic is separation from a regular partner and family. This view posits that a new social environment can result in a lack of social support which, in turn, can be linked to risk-taking behaviour (Campbell, 2001). Another view is that by leaving their homes, migrants also leave their familiar environment with traditional norms and values and the anonymity of being a foreigner can increase risky sexual activities (Decosas et al, 1995; Girdker-Brown, 1998).

Lesotho also has a long history of gender inequalities couched in the laws, traditions and social norms that shape relationships between males and females in different contexts. Despite increased female educational attainment, recent legislative reviews, and the country's ratification of international and regional commitments such as the 1995 Convention on the Elimination of All Forms of Discrimination against Women (CEDAW) and the Southern Africa Development Community (SADC) Addendum on the Prevention and Eradication of Violence against Women and Children, the low status of women in society has remained almost unchanged (Makoa 1997), and gender inequalities continue to affect majority of women and to influence relationships between men and women. For example, although the Government of Lesotho enacted the Legal Capacity of Married Persons Act 9 of 2006 which provides women equality in marriage, inheritance and other spheres (Dube, 2008), the previous common-law principle of marital power which reduced women to minors and gave husbands control over women is still entrenched in various patriarchal institutions in the society. Overall, therefore, gender-related socio-cultural and economic inequalities as well as financial insecurity affect women negatively and may increase their vulnerability to HIV transmission (Ministry of Health and Social Welfare, 2004).

There is also wide empirical evidence showing that the socioeconomic determinants of HIV infection include the level of education and responsiveness to information intended to prevent the spread of HIV. De Walque (2007), for example, identifies several studies conducted in Africa showing a negative relationship between HIV prevalence and educational status. Low educational attainment can therefore be seen as one of the characteristics of the textile work force in Lesotho. It is estimated that more than one third of the 45 000 mainly Basotho women workers in the textile industry (44.0% of females) and about 35.6% employees are infected with HIV and that more than 2 000 workers in the industry are killed by AIDS annually (ALAFA, 2006; UNAIDS, 2008). To this end, the PSCAAL intervention was crucial because unlike most peer education interventions that target adolescents and youth, the target population was young female adults, most of them

in stable sexual relationships, who worked in the textile industry. The goal was to help participants develop the knowledge, attitudes, beliefs and life-skills required to engage in healthy behaviours that provide a buffer from HIV risk factors.
As part of the national response to the AIDS epidemic, the Government of Lesotho has adopted a multi-sectoral approach to address HIV and AIDS in the thematic areas of prevention; treatment, care and support; impact mitigation; and management and coordination. However, lack of a coordinated and adequately resourced response strategy for almost two decades of the epidemic led to the epidemic spreading and deepening poverty. PSCAAL was therefore implemented by CARE South Africa-Lesotho to enhance the response of the private sector to HIV and AIDS as part of CARE's strategy to address the epidemic as a developmental problem (Colvin, Lemmon & Naidoo, 2006).

3. Methodology

3.1 Study design

The data used are drawn from the results of a cross-sectional knowledge, attitudes, beliefs and practices study conducted between April and June 2008 among female workers in two textile factories that had participated in the PSCAAL programme in the Lesotho capital, Maseru. The study was done as part of the CARE's *'Gender, Sex and Power'* project - a research project undertaken to understand how strategies to reduce risk and promote empowerment of women were creating durable changes in their health behaviour (CARE International, 2007).

3.2 Data collection

Data was collected using a combination of quantitative and qualitative methods, namely:

i. *Interviews.* These entailed the administering of questionnaires designed to collect information on the female workers' demographic and socio-economic characteristics, as well as their awareness of HIV and AIDS; uptake of HIV testing; decision-making in sexual relationships; gender equality beliefs; and sense of self-efficacy. Interviews were conducted in the vernacular (Sesotho), and respondents were selected using purposive sampling, based in the consent and availability of the workers during their lunch break and after work in the evenings. This sampling procedure yielded a total of 186 respondents.

ii. *Focus group discussions.* A total of four focus group discussions (FGDs), two in each factory, were conducted. In each factory, one group consisted of with women who participated in the peer education programme (including peer educators) and those who did not. Each group had seven participants who were recruited with the assistance of the peer educators. The purpose of the FGDS was to enable women discuss what they considered as important practices and the factors that produce the reported behaviours following a guided conversation.

iii. *Key informant interviews.* These entailed semi-structured interviews with service providers who worked with CARE during the time of PSCAAL, human resource managers of the studied factories, personnel officers who were also HIV and AIDS focal persons at the workplace, and a health care provider in an onsite clinic at one of the factories where PSCAAL had peer education activities. These interviews were aimed at obtaining an outsider's perspective on HIV risk in these settings.

Method triangulation was pursued by following up in focus groups and key informant interviews issues which workers raised in one-to-one interviews. For example, questions about HIV risk and access to treatment for people living with HIV and a range of factors which could influence access were pursued with different sources. This approach helped to validate the data across different sources and contexts of interviewing.

3.3 Data analysis

The data analysis was guided by the main goal of the study: to understand if there were differences between women who participated in PSCAAL's peer education programme (PEP) at the workplace and those who did not participate in the PEP, with particular respect to the kind of critical decisions related to the prevention of HIV infection that the different categories of women make in their sexual relationships.

Quantitative analysis using SPSS provided characterization of the studied population in terms of the following domains: socio economic and household characteristics, work and finances; HIV and AIDS awareness; HIV testing; access to care; stigma and discrimination; decision making in sexual relationships; gender equality beliefs and norms; gender violence; self efficacy and sense of community. Univariate analyses were used to show patterns in the data, while bivariate analyses were carried out to determine associations between the independent variable (participation in the PEP) and selected dependent variables within the specified domains. Qualitative data from the FGDs and the key-informant interviews was analysed thematically. The qualitative and quantitative results were synthesized to illustrate core issues to the participants' vulnerability to HIV infection.

4. Findings

4.1 Study population

Table 1 shows descriptive statistics for the study population. The key findings are that the majority (126 of the 186 women who were interviewed) had participated in the PEP, and were young, with over 70% aged below 35 years. Over half (51.6%) of the PEP participants were married, compared with 36.7% of non-participants. There was no difference between PEP participants and non-participants in terms of educational attainment: majority (61.9% and 61.7% respectively), had secondary school education and above, while about 38% of each sub-group had primary education or less. More than 70% of women in the two groups earned an average of M800 (approximately US$80) per month.

4.2 Knowledge about HIV and AIDS and HIV prevention services

Sound knowledge about HIV has been widely documented as an essential pre-requisite albeit, often insufficient, condition for adoption of behaviours that reduce the risk of HIV transmission (UNAIDS 2009). It was therefore expected that the impact of the PEP's component of raising HIV and AIDS awareness among the female textile workers would be reflected in a high number of PEP participations who had knowledge about the epidemic and showed the ability to apply the information obtained in ways which prevented HIV infection.

The study results showed that, overall, knowledge about HIV and AIDS was high among all workers, with 99.2% of PEP participants stating that they had ever heard of HIV or AIDS. The corresponding figure for non-participants was 96.6 %. Although the results were not

Characteristic	Participants	Non-Participants
Age Group (years)		
18-25	15.1	20.0
26-29	31.0	28.3
30-34	25.4	23.3
35-39	20.6	15.0
40+	7.9	13.3
Highest Education	0.8	1.7
Never attended school	37.3	36.7
Primary school	35.7	46.7
Secondary school	23.8	13.3
High school	2.4	1.7
Post-high school	20.6	35.0
Marital Status	51.6	36.7
Never married	15.1	15.0
Married	12.7	13.3
Divorced/Separated/Deserted	52.8	48.3
Widowed	1.6	1.7
Position in Factory	39.0	43.3
Skilled Worker	6.5	6.7
Administrator/receptionist	82.4	73.3
/personnel	16.8	26.7
Unskilled worker	0.8	0.0
Supervisor		
Monthly Wage		
Less than M800		
M800-M1200		
More than M1200		
Total (%)	**100**	**100**
(N)	**126**	**60**

Table 1. Percentage distribution of sample by selected background characteristics

statistically significant, discussions with PEP participants suggested that they tended to have more accurate information and had developed a particular consciousness about HIV and AIDS which helped them behave differently by avoiding risk behaviours and being proactive in obtaining care services and support. For example, one of the interviewed peer educators identified the differences between PEP and non-PEP participants as the varying breadth and depth of information which, for the former, included other health issues not just HIV and AIDS, risk factors such as intimate partner violence and women abuse; as well as the ability to apply the acquired knowledge about HIV transmission and prevention in their intimate relationships.

"It has helped me a lot because I have acquired a lot of privileged information. For example, I know that condoms are not only used as a protection against HIV/AIDS and as a means of birth control, but can also be used to prevent transmission of STIs…Some [non-peer education participants] might have knowledge, but most might not… For example, if I am married to an abusive husband who does not treat me well, I know where I can go to get help" (Peer Educator, PEP participants' focus group).

Although women in focus groups for non-PEP also displayed similar knowledge about prevention of HIV infection, their discussions also indicated a strong inclination to take their social and cultural roles into consideration when they make decisions in sexual relationships.

An empowered woman is a woman who looks after the needs of her children, for example, who sees that her children are properly fed and well clothed, especially during cold winter. A woman who looks after the affairs of her family; who takes good care of her husband and children ... who does not wash her linen in public, who respects her husband and humbles herself and discusses things with husband... (Non-PEP focus group)

Analysis of the quantitative data also suggested that women who had participated in the PEP were significantly more likely to know where to obtain most of the essential HIV and AIDS services such as condoms and VCT services (Table 2)

HIV/AIDS service	Participants	Non-Participants
1. Information on HIV and AIDS**	81.0	61.7
2. Condoms**	93.7	85.0
3. VCT services*	92.9	68.3
4. Health monitoring services for HIV and AIDS[NS]	79.4	65.0
5. Medical treatment for opportunistic infections[NS]	81.0	71.7
6. ARVs**	91.3	71.2
Total (N)	**126**	**60**

Note: *:p<0.000 ** p<0.05 NS: Not statistically significant

Table 2. Proportion of sample who know where to obtain essential HIV/AIDS information and services, by PEP participation

Furthermore, PEP participants were also more likely than non-participants (97.6% and 91.7% respectively) to be of the correct view that knowing one's HIV status was imperative. While this result was not statistically significant, the advanced reasons were significant, with those who had participated in the PEP more likely to state the more important advantages of HIV testing: to protect oneself and to prevent infecting others (UNAIDS, 2009). Table 3 shows these results.

Reason	Participants	Non-Participants
So that I can take care of myself	55.2	40.0
To avoid being infected	8.0	10.0
To avoid infecting sexual partners	7.2	3.3
So that I can live longer	8.8	6.7
Avoid mother-to-child transmission	3.2	3.3
Other	17.6	36.7
Total (%)	**100**	**100**
(N)	**125**	**60**

Note: p<0.05

Table 3. Percentage distribution of sample by perceived importance of HIV testing, and PEP participation

4.3 HIV testing

Consistent with their relatively greater recognition of the importance of testing, PEP participants were significantly more likely to have had tested for HIV and also to have used an STI treatment centre in the six months preceding the survey (Table 4).

HIV/AIDS service	Participants	Non-Participants	Total
Tested for HIV**	90.7	9.3	**43**
Used STI services**	100.0	0.0	**13**
Used TB servces[NS]	88.9	11.1	**9**

Note: ** $p<0.05$ NS: Not statistically significant

Table 4. Proportion of sample who know at least one source of HIV/STI service and who utilized an HIV/STI service in the last six months by PEP participation

The above results were further affirmed in the key informant interviews and FGDs. For example:

"There is increase in the uptake of HIV testing among the workforce; workers are interested in knowing their HIV status following their exposure to peer education. More people come early even before they fall ill. Also because things have changed in HIV care – rapid testing ensures they know their status immediately. They make follow-ups after testing HIV positive and they willingly seek CD4 count assessment" (VCT service provider, key informant interview)

We have lists of many people who wish to test because after talking to them, they now have understanding about the infection…It is easy for us even to tell our partners that we went for HIV test because we talk about it in our families (Participant, PEP participants' focus group)

4.4 Attitudes towards HIV

In general there seemed to be a positive attitude towards HIV and AIDS among the workers interviewed (both PEP participants and non-participants). For example, over 70% agreed with the statement that HIV was a terminal illness (Table 5) as opposed, presumably, to being a 'death sentence'. Other indicators of positive attitudes include high proportion who stated their ability to talk to various people about HIV and AIDS, their willingness to inform family members in case of a positive test, as well as the relatively high proportions that disagreed, or strongly disagreed, with negative statements such as "HIV/AIDS is punishment for bad behaviour" and "people with HIV or AIDS should feel ashamed of themselves", among others. It is noteworthy, however, that women who participated in the PEP were generally less likely to agree with negative statements, even though the results were not statistically significant.

4.5 Condom use

Condom use is an important measure of protection against HIV. Its maximum protective effect is, however, achieved when the use is consistent rather than occasional (UNAIDS, 2009). The study results show that women who participated in the PEP were significantly more likely than those who did not participate to be the final decision-makers regarding condom use in their sexual relations. They were also more likely to be confident in obtaining condoms without feeling embarrassed; to refuse to have sex with their partners without a condom; and to suggest an HIV test to their partners and others (Table 6).

Indicators of attitudes to HIV and AIDS	Participants	Non-Participants
Strongly agreed/agreed		
HIV infection is a terminal illness[NS]	77.8	78.3
I would tell a fellow support group member if I tested HIV positive[NS]	71.0	74.6
I would tell a member of my family if I tested HIV positive	91.3	95.0
I can talk freely to others about HIV and AIDS	92.7	84.7
I can encourage my family member or close friend to test for HIV	93.6	93.3
Strongly disagreed/disagreed		
HIV/AIDS is punishment for bad behaviour[NS]	82.5	78.0
I would be ashamed if a family member/close friend had HIV/AIDS[NS]	86.5	86.7
People with HIV or AIDS should feel ashamed of themselves**	89.7	88.3
I would not tell anyone if I tested HIV positive[NS]	69.0	55.9
I would be worried to take ARVs in the presence of other people who don't know about my HIV status[NS]	71.8	60.0
Total (%)	**100**	**100**
N	**126**	**60**

Note: ** $p<0.05$ NS: Not statistically significant

Table 5. Percentage of sample who agreed and disagreed with various indicators of attitudes to HIV and AIDS, and PEP participation

Although the PEP participants were undoubtedly more aware that practising safer sex by using condoms consistently prevented HIV transmission, evidence from the key informant interviews and focus groups, however, shows that many of these women, just like their counterparts who did not participate in the PEP, are often placed at a higher risk of HIV infection through inconsistent use of condoms. For example, a nurse clinician mentioned that there were many workers who sought treatment for sexually transmitted infections (STI) because they did not use condoms consistently and re-infections were common. Overall condoms were perceived as an important factor which could influence women's access to material support or stability in their marriage and other sexual relationships. It was also alleged that there was a tendency among some men to use material support as bait to access unprotected sex.

In the focus group discussions, the women workers were generally depicted as constantly in search of men who were prepared to assist them financially. These men—many of whom belonged to similarly vulnerable communities such as the taxi industry, uniformed services and migrant mine workers—were powerful in relationships; they cohabited with their lovers and dictated the use of a condom - usually insisting on non-use if they supported women materially. The following statements illustrate:

Women mainly see policemen, soldiers and taxi drives with the expectation that police and army men earn a lot of money.... Taxi drivers are simply favoured because they provide lift to and from work.

Indicator of decision-making in sexual relationships	Condom use in last six months							
	Participant				Non-Participant			
	All or most of the time	Some-times	Rarely or Never	*N*	All or most of the time	Some-times	Rarely or Never	*n*
Final decision-maker on condom use**								
Participant	67.6	13.5	18.9	37	42.9	50.0	7.1	14
Partner	16.7	25.0	58.3	12	40.0	20.0	40.0	5
It's a joint decision	53.8	23.1	23.1	26	33.3	46.7	20.0	15
Can refuse sex if not feeling wellNS								
Always	56.6	18.9	24.5	53	40.9	45.5	13.6	22
Sometimes	30.8	30.8	38.5	13	22.2	44.4	33.3	9
Never	58.3	0.0	41.7	12	40.0	40.0	20.0	5
Likely reaction if partner refuses condom*								
Refuse to have sex with him	66.1	16.1	17.9	56	41.7	50.0	8.3	24
Persuade him to use a condom	50.0	25.0	25.0	4	28.6	28.6	42.9	7
Surrender and agree to have sex without condom	10.5	21.1	68.4	19	20.0	40.0	40.0	5
Can convince partners to use condoms*								
Always	60.9	20.3	18.8	64	52.9	32.4	14.7	34
Sometimes	18.2	45.5	36.4	11	12.5	62.5	25.0	8
Never	16.7	16.7	66.7	18	0.0	33.3	67.7	3

Note: * p<0.000 ** p<0.050 NS: Not statistically significant n: total

Table 6. Proportion of sample by selected indicators of sexual decision-making and negotiation, by condom use in last six months

The problem is that if these men refuse to use condoms, the women cannot refuse them sex because they have received material support from them…but the women here are also promiscuous (Focus group, peer education participants).

"We don't use condoms; that is why there are a lot of unwanted pregnancies, STIs and HIV/AIDS. More often, when a man dies of AIDS, the wife also follows and the girlfriends too" (FG2 -non peer education).

The poor economic situation of the textile female workers as shown by low monthly wages (Table 1) and myriad responsibilities they had within the household (see Table 7) provide part of the answer to why their knowledge about HIV transmission did not produce the intended behavioural changes. A compelling body of evidence has shown that women living in poverty, or facing the threat of poverty, may be particularly vulnerable to sexual exploitation through the need to trade or sell sex, or to engage in multiple concurrent relationships, in order to survive (Epstein, 2007). Indeed some women entered into relationships with the expectation that men would augment their budgets:

"We earn very little money here, this is what makes us easy prey and exposed to HIV infection. For example, if a man tells you he will drive on Mpilo Boulevard (an expression used to describe unprotected sex), just because you are at the mercy of this person, you agree to have unsafe sex in expectation that he will not withhold his money or other favours" (FG1- non peer education participants)

"There's even a common saying that if a man visits his girlfriend, especially those who work in the factories, he should use a braai pack (frozen chicken portions) to knock on the girlfriend's door. This compromised many women's life because they could not refuse to have unprotected sex for fear that the boyfriend would leave. But our education and encouragement have changed a lot of women's attitudes and views" (Peer educator)

Characteristic	%
Number of children	
0	18.4
1	35.1
2	27.0
3+	19.5
Number of dependents	2.2
0	8.6
1	12.4
2	20.0
3	20.5
4	13.5
5	22.7
6+	19.9
Type of accommodation	66.6
Own house	9.7
Rented house/backyard	0.5
Parent's house	1.6
Cohabiting	1.6
Relative's house	96.7
Other	75.5
Main responsibility in household	59.8
Food	35.9
Clothing	41.3
Rent	58.2
Health care	39.1
Transport	
School fees	
Insurance/Funeral policy	
Total (%)	**100**
(N)	**186**

Table 7. Percentage distribution of sample by selected socioeconomic indicators

5. Conclusion

The PSCAAL programme was intended to influence behaviour change among women who worked in the textile industry through an HIV and AIDS peer education and support programme which provided information and voluntary counselling and testing services. The overall pattern that emerged from this study indicates that most women who participated in the programme had relatively higher knowledge about HIV and AIDS, and seemed to be more aware of the sources of essential HIV and AIDS prevention and treatment services, as well as the importance of preventive behaviours such as HIV testing and consistent condom use. Despite these achievements, the skills the women learned in the peer education programmes do not seem to have trickled down to the traditionally entrenched gender beliefs, or to have enhanced the programme participants' self efficacy in their sexual relationships. For example, majority of women who participated in peer education programmes were, just like their counterparts who did not participate in the programme, not the main decision-makers regarding condom use; their partners were. By the same token, more than a third of all women (both participants and non-participants) stated that they would surrender if their partners refused to use a condom, and their main reason was that they feared that their partners would use violence. Qualitative evidence shows that this can be largely attributed to skewed gender relations and women's lower economic status, as well as individualized approaches that target women and disregard the socioeconomic context of heterosexual relationships through which HIV infection mostly occur. These barriers have been noted in other sub-Saharan countries that have similarly high HIV prevalence like Lesotho, and have also been noted in the Millennium Project task Force report which stated, in part, that "Prevention and care programs will fail if they ignore the underlying determinants of the epidemic: poverty; gender inequality; and social dislocation" (Nelson, 2005:20).

Against this background, it is imperative for HIV and AIDS interventions in African countries to be framed with an in-depth understanding of the multifaceted nature of the contextual factors that increase HIV vulnerability, and build women's and families' resilience to the socioeconomic factors which influenced their vulnerability to HIV transmission and the impact of AIDS. Private companies and business have a unique role to play in this regard since they interact with people living and affected by HIV and AIDS directly through employment relations, and indirectly through customers, employees' families, and community members (Nankobogo, 2007). It should be recognised, however, that the core business of many private sector organisations is not HIV and AIDS, and their range of activity often extends beyond the scope of national HIV and AIDS strategic framework. As Nelson (2005:11) cautions, "The core business of business is, and must remain, the profitable production of goods and services … (and) it is important not to create unrealistic expectations of what activities business can undertake in the fight against HIV/AIDS".

Nonetheless, the private sector can still make meaningful contributions that can help in achieving greater scale in national and community-level efforts against HIV infection and AIDS (Nelson, 2005). Drawing on the International Business leaders Forum Spheres of influence model and the Global Business Coalition's business action model, Nelson summarised the various ways in which the private sector can be involved into six 'building blocks of corporate engagement": (1) demonstrate good workplace programmes to other companies; (2) Extend internal programmes along corporate value chains; (3) share core competencies and assets with other sectors; (4) make strategic philanthropic donations; (5) help build effective institutions; and (6) engage in public policy dialogue. Given the findings of this study on which this chapter is based, three of these building blocks are, perhaps, the most relevant for sub-Saharan African:

1. *Demonstrate good workplace programmes to other companies.* Workplace programmes in developing countries focus primarily in promoting behaviour change (Sai, 1995) through for example, creating awareness, and encouraging the workforce to undertake HIV testing and seek treatment. While these programmes are critical, they may have limited benefits in sub-Saharan Africa given the evidence that structural socio-economic and cultural factors are the key pathways of HIV transmission in the region. Therefore in addition to enhancing workers' health literacy and ability to obtain, process and understand basic health information and services needed to make appropriate health decisions (Sanders, 2007) in the context of HIV and AIDS, management in industries that employ women need to consider the broader socio-cultural factors that influence women's vulnerability. For example, to the extent that gender relations are to a large extent influenced by women's low economic status, female workers should be empowered economically by paying wages that take into account the cost of living in a country. Employers could also consider developing investment funds with the employees. There is also need to strengthen monitoring and evaluation of workplace programmes (Weston, et al, 2007) and to share the evidence of effectiveness with other companies particularly small and medium enterprises and those that are just straying out (Nelson, 2005).
2. *Share core competencies and assets.* Unique skills and capacities such as logistics and distribution resource management, communication and marketing that can be used effectively and creatively to respond to HIV and AIDS in behaviour change campaigns, procurement and distribution of commodities and information materials, and improved management of programmes. The private sector can share these competencies through effective partnerships with civil society, community organisations and the public sector. Not only will such partnerships contribute to the private sector's economic case for tackling HIV and AIDS, but they also have a business case. Studies indicate that employees strongly appreciate when their company and senior management are involved in social causes, and indeed, many companies working in high HIV prevalence countries have improvements in productivity, morale and staff turnover when they take an active, visible role in the AIDS response (UNAIDS, 2011).
3. *Help build effective institutions*, particularly Business Coalitions against HIV and AIDS. These Coalitions can be described as organisations of business that work together to address the issue of HIV and AIDS, and may include sectoral associations, chambers of commerce, labour unions, employer federations and other groups of companies that have committed themselves to addressing the issue of HIV and AIDS (Sidhu, 2008). National Business collation remove the need for private sector companies to act in isolation by providing a forum for cooperation and partnership, serving as a interlocutors between the private and public sector responses to HIV and AIDS (Nankobogo, 2007; Sidhu, 2008). Although Business Coalitions are a relatively new concept around the world, and still need more support to strengthen their organizations and fulfill their visions, their positive impact is already being felt in some countries (Sidhu, 2008). Therefore, given that as of January 2008, there were 25 national Business Coalitions in Africa and four were scheduled for launch in 2008/2009 (see Sidhu, 2008),

there should be increased advocacy for African business involvement in HIV and AIDS prevention through participation in local business coalitions. Through these coalitions private sector companies can for example, be linked with AIDS service organisations that are more experienced and better equipped to provide a range of HIV and AIDS related services such as information and prevention campaigns, and mitigation and care measures -such as medical and home-based care and financial advice—for those infected and affected by the epidemic (GTZ, 2005).

6. Acknowledgments

The research project on which this chapter is based was funded by the Ford Foundation and commissioned by CARE South Africa-Lesotho to the Human Sciences Research Council of South Africa, The authors wish to thank Ms Palesa Ndabe for supervising the collection and data capturing in Lesotho.

7. References

ALAFA. (2006). *Bono Attends Launch of ComMark's ALAFA (Apparel Lesotho Alliance to Fight AIDS) Project in Lesotho.* Press Release, 16 May 2006. Retrieved from www.alafa.info.

Avert (2011). *The Impact of HIV & AIDS in Africa.* Retrieved from www.avert.org/aids-impact-africa.htm.

Brummer, D. (2002). *Labour migration and HIV/AIDS in Southern Africa.* International Organization for Migration Regional Office for Southern Africa: Pretoria.

Campbell, C. (2001). Going underground and going after women: masculinity and HIV transmission amongst black workers on the gold mines, In: R. Morrell (Ed.), *Changing Men in Southern Africa,* University of Natal Press and Zed Books, Pietermaritzburg and London:

CARE International (2007). Gender, Sex and the Power to Survive: Impact and Implications of Empowering Women at Risk of HIV and AIDS. *Proceedings of CARE's Gender, Sex and Power' Project Meeting,* New Delhi, India, October 2007.

Chandan, U., Cambanis, E., Bhana, A., Boyce, G., Makoae, M., Mukoma, W. & Phakati, S. (2008). *Evaluation of My Future Is My Choice (Mfmc) Peer Education Life Skills Programme in Namibia: Identifying Strengths, Weaknesses, and Areas of Improvement*: UNICEF, Namibia.

Colvin, M., Lemmon, G. & Naidoo, J. (2006). *Private Sector Response to HIV and AIDS in Lesotho.* ComMark Trust, HLSP, Edinburgh.

De Walque, D. (2007). How does the impact of an HIV/AIDS information campaign vary with educational attainment? Evidence from rural Uganda. *Journal of Development Economics*, Vol. 84, pp. 686–714.

Decosas, J.F., Kane, J.K., Anarfi, K.D., Sodji, K.D. and Wagner, H.U. (1995). Migration and AIDS, *The Lancet*, Vol. 346, No. 8978, pp. 826-828

Dube, B.A. (2008). *The Law and Legal Research in Lesotho.* Retrieved from www.nyulawglobal.org/globalex/lesotho.htm

Epstein, H. (2007). *The Invisible Cure. Africa, The West, and the Fight Against AIDS*, Farrar, Strauss & Giroux, New York.

George, G.; Gow, J., & Whiteside, A. (2009). HIV/AIDS in Private Sector Companies: Cost Impacts and Responses in Southern Africa. *HIV Therapy*, Vol. 3, No. 3, pp. 293-300.

Girdler-Brown, B. (1998). Migration and HIV/AIDS: Eastern and Southern Africa, *International Migration*, Vol. 36, No. 4., pp. 513-515.

GTZ (2005). *HIV/AIDS and Private Sector Promotion: fact Sheet.* Retrieved from www. gtz.de.

Hanisch, D. (2006). *Impact Assessment – Report on Focus Group Discussions with Peer Educators.* PSCAAL Project Workplace Outreach Component. CARE Lesotho, Maseru.

International Labour Organisation. (2006). *Press Release ILO/06/56.* International Labour Organisation, Geneva.

Khobotlo M., Tshehlo,R., Nkonyana, J., Ramoseme, M., Khobotle, M., Chitoshia, A., Hildebrand, M., & Fraser, N. (2009). Lesotho: *HIV Prevention response and Modes of Transmission Analysis.* Lesotho National AIDS Commission, Maseru, Lesotho.

Makoa, F.K. (1997). Gender and Politics: A Note on Gender Inequality in Lesotho, *Journal of Social Development in Africa,* Vol. 12, No. 1, pp. 5-14.

Ministry of Health and Social Welfare. (2004). *Lesotho Demographic & Health Survey.* Ministry of Health and Social Welfare, Maseru.

Nankobogo, F. (2007). The Role of Private Sector in the Fight Against HIV/AIDS in sub-Saharan Africa. Thematic Stakeholder Consultations, Bamako, Mali, 10-12 December 2007.

National AIDS Commission (2008). *Lesotho UNGASS Country Report, January 2006-December 2007.* Maseru, National AIDS Commission. Retrieved from www.nas.org.ls.

Nelson, J. (2005). Building Public Sector Capacity to Adress HIV/AIDs: the Role of the Private Sector. Corporate Social Responsibility Initiative Working Paper No. 8. Cambridge, MA: John F. Kennedy School of Government, Harvard University.

Phororo, H. (2003). *HIV/AIDS and the Private Sector in Namibia: Getting the Small Businesses on Board.* Hanns Seidel Foundation Namibia, Occasional Paper No. 3/2003

Population Council (n.d) Peer Education and HIV/AIDS. Past experiences, future directions. Horizons. Retrieved from www.popcouncil.org.

Rosen, S. & Simon, J.L. (2003). Shifting the Burden: The Private Sector's Response to the AIDS Epidemic in Africa. *Bulletin of the World Health Organisation,* Vol. 8, No. 10, pp.131-139.

Rosen, S.; Feeley, F.; Connelly, P.; & Simon, J. (2007). The Private Sector and HIV/AIDS in Africa: Taking Stock of 6 Years of Applied Research. *AIDS,* Vol. 21, suppl 3, pp. S41-S51.

Rosen, S.; Vincent, J.R.; Macleod, W.; Fox, M.; Thea, D.M. and Simon, J.L. (2004). *AIDS,* Vol. 18, No. 2, pp. 317-324.

Ruscombe-King, R (2008). *HIV and AIDS in Lesotho, 2008,* Retrieved www.avert.org/aids-lesotho.htm.

Sai, K. (1995). AIDS and the private sector: the burden and the responsibility. *AIDScaptions,* Vol. 2, No. 1, pp. 4-8.

Sanders, L. M., Thompson, V.T., & Wilkinson, J. D. (2007) Caregiver Health Literacy and the Use of Child Health Services. *Pediatrics* Vol. 119; pp. e86-e92.

Santis, W., Rosenblum, L., Vince, W.C. et al. 2007. *Involving young people in efforts to combat HIV and AIDS in Africa: the importance of income-generating strategies* Newton, MA: Education Development Center (EDC).

Sidhu, I.K. (2008). *Business Coalitions Tackling AIDS: A Worldwide Review*. Retrieved from http://data.unaids.org.

Swartz, S., Van der Heijden, I., Makoae, M., Richter, L., Rozani, A., Runciman, T. & Ndimande, N. (2009). *With a little help from my friends': exploring the impact of peer-led HIV intervention and psychosocial support groups for orphaned and vulnerable children in South Africa.* (Report produced for the Harvard Centre for the Support of Peer Education, 31 March). Retrieved from www.hsrc.ac.za.

UNAIDS. (2008). *2008 Report on the Global AIDS Epidemic*. Retrieved from www.unaids.org.

UNAIDS. (2009). *Monitoring the Declaration of Commitment on HIV/AIDS: Guidelines on Construction of Core Indicators, 2010 Reporting*. UNAIDS, Geneva.

UNAIDS. (2010). *UNAIDS Report on the Global Aids Epidemic 2010*. UNAIDS , Geneva

UNAIDS. (2011). *Civil Society and Private Sector Division*. Retrieved from www.unaids.org.

United Nations. (2010). *Millennium Development Goals Report: 2010*. United Nations, New York.

Weston, M.D., Churchyard, G.J., Mametja, D., McIntyre, J.A., & Randera, F. (2007). Business and AIDS: sectoral challenges and opportunities. AIDS, Vol. 21, Suppl 3, pp. S85-S89.

Part 2

Prevention of Mother to Child Transmission of HIV (PMTCT)

5

Antenatal Screening and HIV-Pregnancy: Strategies for Treatment

Ali A. Al-Jabri[1], Abdullah A. Balkhair[2],
Mohammed S. Al-Balosh[3] and Sidgi S. Hasson[3]
[1]*Head of Immunology Division, Department of Microbiology and Immunology, College of Medicine and Health Sciences, Sultan Qaboos University, Muscat,*
[2]*Head of Infectious Diseases Unit, Department of Medicine, Sultan Qaboos University Hospital,Muscat,*
[3]*Department of Microbiology and Immunology, College of Medicine and Health Sciences, Sultan Qaboos University, Muscat,*
Oman

1. Introduction

More than half of all people living with HIV are women and girls (WHO & UNAIDS, 2010). In sub-Saharan Africa, more women than men are living with HIV, and young women aged 15–24 years are as much as eight times more likely than men to be HIV positive (WHO & UNAIDS, 2010). In developed countries, the women who are intravenous drug users, partners of drug users or bisexual men, or involved in sex work are more likely to be positive for HIV (WHO & UNAIDS, 1999). There are higher proportions of young women than young men who acquired HIV infection through sex. Their exposure to the virus at an earlier age, coupled with physiological and sociological factors increases their risk (WHO & UNAIDS, 1999).

Globally, HIV is the leading cause of death in women of reproductive age. Since nearly all HIV infections in children are acquired from their mothers, the global epidemiology of HIV in children reflects that of HIV in women. Nearly all such infections can be prevented by programs providing highly effective antiretroviral therapy (ART) and antiretroviral (ARV) prophylaxis interventions.

There are tremendous efforts to control HIV/AIDS and reduce the mortality and morbidity rates by improving the accessibility to ART to all HIV- infected patients, trying to eradicate the virus from reservoirs of infection and designing an effective vaccine that can elicit protective antibody response as well as cell mediated response against HIV (Al-Jabri & Al-Enzi, 2009). An important step in the fight against HIV/AIDS is to perform antenatal screening and counseling.

2. The importance of antenatal screening and counseling

HIV testing of individuals should be undertaken only when they are informed about the test and should be entirely voluntary. HIV testing and counseling enable women to learn whether they are infected, understand their HIV status and make more informed choices for the future. HIV testing and counseling also provide essential knowledge and support: they enable uninfected women to remain so, enable those infected with HIV to plan for the future and prevent HIV transmission to others. Those who are infected can also benefit from available care, treatment and support services. Knowledge of HIV infection leads to initiate ART for the long-term treatment of women living with HIV and intervenes with the transmission of HIV infections to infants and young children.

HIV testing in pregnancy is important for many reasons, but this must be balanced against the possible risks of stigmatization, discrimination and violence. Voluntary counseling and testing should be encouraged for pregnant women and couples. Post-test counseling is extremely important following a diagnosis of HIV and should include information about pregnancy-related issues and the risk of mother to child transmission (MTCT). Counseling is also important for HIV-negative women as it provides an opportunity for risk-reduction.

HIV-infected women who know their sero-status are able to make informed choices about their reproductive lives and, if pregnant, to access specific interventions, such as ARV drugs and infant-feeding counseling and support, which can significantly reduce the risk of MTCT of HIV. Currently, the majority of people infected with HIV unaware of their status and cannot receive the services they actually need.

A key factor limiting the scale-up of MTCT programs is lack of knowledge of HIV status (Al-Jabri et al. 2010). Increasing the availability and acceptability of HIV testing and counseling services, with no dough, will encourage more women to know their status, providing a gateway to MTCT interventions (Bolu et al. 2007). Key factors contributing to the scale-up of testing and counseling include a policy of provider-initiated testing and counseling with the right to refuse testing; group pretest counseling; rapid HIV testing; innovative staffing strategies; and community and male involvement. Integration of testing and counseling within the community and all maternal and child health settings are critical for scaling-up and for linking women and their families to care and treatment services (Bolu et al. 2007).

3. Strategies for treatment

Three types of interventions should be tackled by any program concerned with prevention of MTCT: primary prevention of HIV in women; prophylaxis with ARV drugs in breastfeeding infants and prophylaxis with ARV drugs for lactating mothers.

Taking ARV treatment can reduce the risk of MTCT. There are two different ways in which drugs can act. First, they may reduce the viral load so the baby is exposed to less of the virus while in the uterine and during childbirth. The aim of HIV treatment is to decrease the viral load <50 copies/ml. Second, the drugs may cross the placenta and enter the baby's body, where they can prevent the virus from ever taking hold.

One of the key attainments in HIV research was the demonstration by the Pediatric AIDS Clinical Trials Group 076 (PACTG 076) that administration of zidovudine to the pregnant woman and her infant could reduce the risk of perinatal transmission (PT) by nearly 70% (Connor et al. 1994). Following the results of PACTG 076, implementation of the zidovudine regimen coupled with increased antenatal HIV testing and counseling rapidly resulted in significant declines in HIV transmission (CDC, 2006). Subsequent clinical trials and observational studies showed that combination ARV prophylaxis (initially dual and then triple combination therapy) given to the mother antenatally was associated with further declines in transmission to less than 2% (Cooper et al. 2002, WHO 2010).

4. Mechanisms of action of ARV prophylaxis in reducing perinatal transmission of HIV

There are a number of mechanisms through which zidovudine or other ARV drugs can reduce PT. One central mechanism is by decreasing maternal viral load in the blood and genital secretions via antenatal drug administration, particularly in women with high viral loads. However, ARV drugs have been shown to reduce the risk of transmission even among women with HIV RNA levels <1,000 copies/ml (Ioannidis et al. 2001). Additionally, the level of HIV RNA at delivery and receipt of antenatal ART are each independently associated with the risk of transmission, suggesting that ARV prophylaxis does not work solely through reduction in viral load (Sperling et al. 1996).

An additional mechanism of protection is pre-exposure infant prophylaxis provided by administration of ARV drugs that cross the placenta from the mother to the infant, resulting in adequate systemic drug levels in the infant. This mechanism of protection is particularly significant during the infant's passage through the birth canal, a time of rigorous exposure to maternal genital tract virus. Post-exposure infant prophylaxis is provided through administration of drug to the infant after birth. This mechanism protects the infant from cell-free or cell-associated virus that might have obtained access to the fetal/infant systemic circulation. This can occur through maternal-fetal transfusion during uterine contractions in labor or through systemic dissemination of virus swallowed by the infant during passage through the birth canal.

It is predictable that efficacy of ARV drugs in reducing PT is multi-factorial, and each of these mechanisms is contributory. The efficacy of ARV regimens administered only during labor and/or to the newborn in reducing PT demonstrates the importance of the pre- and post-exposure components of prophylaxis in reducing PT (Wade et al. 1998).

5. Perinatal transmission of HIV and maternal viral load

In PACTG 076, antenatal maternal HIV RNA copy number was associated with HIV transmission in women receiving placebo. In women receiving zidovudine, the relationship was markedly attenuated and no longer statistically significant (Sperling et al. 1996). An HIV RNA threshold below which there was no risk of transmission was not identified; zidovudine was effective in reducing transmission regardless of maternal HIV RNA copy number (Shapiro et al. 1999). Other data from larger numbers of zidovudine-treated, HIV-infected pregnant women indicate that HIV RNA levels correlate with risk of transmission even in women treated with ARV agents (The European Collaborative Study, 1999).

Although the risk of PT in women with undetectable HIV RNA levels appears to be extremely low, transmission from mother to infant has been reported among women with all levels of maternal HIV RNA. Additionally, although HIV RNA may be an important risk factor for transmission, other factors also appear to play a role (Mock et al. 1999). Although there is a general correlation between viral load in plasma and in the genital tract, discordance has also been reported, particularly between HIV proviral load in blood and genital secretions, especially in the presence of other genital tract infections (Hart et al. 1999).

The use of ARV drugs during pregnancy for prevention of PT should be discussed with and offered to all infected pregnant women regardless of their HIV RNA level. Results of epidemiologic and clinical trials suggest that women receiving potent combinations of ARV drugs that effectively reduce HIV RNA to <1,000 copies/ml or undetectable levels have very low rates of PT (Cooper et al. 2002). However, because transmission can occur even at low or undetectable HIV RNA copy numbers, HIV RNA levels should not be a determining factor when deciding whether to use ARV drugs for prevention of PT. Additionally, the efficacy of ARV drugs is not solely related to lowering viral load (Cooper et al. 2002; Ioannidis et al. 2001). Therefore, ARV prophylaxis should be given even to women who have a very low or undetectable viral load on no therapy.

6. Intrapartum ARV therapy/prophylaxis

6.1 Women who have received antepartum ARV drugs

The PACTG 076 results and subsequent epidemiologic studies have proven the efficacy of the three-part zidovudine chemoprophylaxis regimen alone or in combination with other ARV agents. The PACTG 076 zidovudine regimen includes a continuous intravenous infusion of zidovudine during labor (initial loading dose of 2 mg/kg intravenously over 1 hour, followed by continuous infusion of 1 mg/kg/hour until delivery). Therefore, intravenous zidovudine during the intrapartum period should be discussed with and recommended to all HIV-infected pregnant women. For a scheduled cesarean delivery, intravenous zidovudine should begin 3 hours before surgery, according to standard dosing recommendations. Women receiving fixed-dose combination regimens that include zidovudine (e.g., the zidovudine/lamivudine combination) should have zidovudine administered intravenously during labor while other ARV components are continued orally (e.g., if a woman is receiving zidovudine/lamivudine during pregnancy, zidovudine should be given intravenously and lamivudine should be given orally during labor).

If known or suspected zidovudine resistance or toxicity has precluded antenatal use of zidovudine, intrapartum zidovudine according to the PACTG 076 protocol should still be recommended unless a woman has a documented history of hypersensitivity. This intrapartum use of the drug is recommended due to the unique characteristics of zidovudine and its proven record in reducing PT.

There is a pharmacologic antagonism between zidovudine and stavudine, and therefore these drugs should not be co-administered during labor. Women who are receiving an antepartum stavudine-containing regimen should discontinue stavudine during labor while intravenous zidovudine is being administered, with other components of the regimen continued orally.

6.2 Women who have received antepartum ARV drugs but have suboptimal viral suppression near delivery

Women who have received ART may not achieve complete viral suppression by the time of delivery due to factors such as poor adherence, viral resistance, or late entry into care. Regardless of the reason, all women who have HIV RNA levels >1,000 copies/ml near the time of delivery should be offered a scheduled cesarean delivery at 38 weeks, which may significantly reduce the risk of transmission.

The addition of single-dose nevirapine during labor has not been shown to reduce PT of HIV in this group of women. The PACTG 316 study, conducted in women in the United States, Europe, Brazil, and the Bahamas who were receiving ARV drugs during pregnancy (primarily combination therapy), showed that the addition of single-dose nevirapine did not reduce the risk of MTCT of HIV even in the setting of maternal viremia but was associated with the development of nevirapine resistance in 15% of women with detectable HIV RNA postpartum (Cunningham et al. 2002). However, the number of women with detectable HIV RNA at delivery, and especially with HIV RNA >10,000 copies/ml, was small and may have been insufficient to allow assessment of a possible benefit of single-dose nevirapine in this subgroup. Given the risk of development of resistance and the lack of data to suggest added efficacy, addition of single-dose nevirapine when a woman has received antepartum drugs is generally not recommended.

6.3 Women who have not received antepartum ARV drugs

All HIV-infected women who have not received antepartum ART should have intravenous zidovudine started immediately to prevent PT of HIV. Although intrapartum/neonatal ARTs will not prevent PT that occurs before labor, most transmission occurs near to or during labor and delivery. Pre-exposure prophylaxis for the fetus can be provided by giving the mother a drug that rapidly crosses the placenta to produce systemic ARV drug levels in the fetus during intensive exposure to HIV in maternal genital secretions and blood during birth. In general, zidovudine and other NRTI drugs as well as NNRTI drugs cross the placenta well, although protease inhibitors drugs do not.

Epidemiologic data indicate that intravenous maternal intrapartum zidovudine followed by oral zidovudine for 6 weeks for the infant significantly reduces transmission compared to no treatment (Wade et al. 1998). In a New York State cohort study, transmission rates were 10% with intrapartum and neonatal zidovudine compared with 27% without zidovudine, a 62% reduction in risk (Wade et al. 1998). The PETRA study demonstrated that intrapartum prophylaxis alone, without an infant post-exposure prophylaxis component, is not effective in reducing PT (Petra Study Team, 2002).

Whether the addition of other ARV drugs to the intravenous intrapartum/newborn zidovudine regimen when no maternal antepartum drugs have been received increases efficacy in preventing PT has not been directly studied. Several intrapartum/neonatal prophylaxis regimens have been found to be effective in international studies. These include oral zidovudine/lamivudine during labor followed by one week of oral zidovudine/lamivudine to the infant and single-dose intrapartum/newborn nevirapine (Petra Study Team, 2002). However, none of these regimens has been compared to intravenous zidovudine combined with 6 weeks of infant zidovudine prophylaxis.

Studies need to address whether adding drugs to the intravenous intrapartum/newborn zidovudine regimen will enhance efficacy in reducing PT. In the absence of data, some experts feel additional drugs may be warranted. One option is to add the single-dose intrapartum/newborn nevirapine regimen to the intravenous/6-week infant zidovudine regimen. Although single-dose nevirapine did not provide additional efficacy when added to antepartum combination ARV regimens in PACTG 316, in this situation, no maternal antepartum therapy has been given. Theoretical advantages of combining the zidovudine and nevirapine intrapartum/neonatal regimens include the known short-term safety of each regimen alone, excellent tranplacental passage of both drugs, greater antiviral activity of nevirapine compared to zidovudine, as well as the activity of nevirapine against extracellular and intracellular virus (Musoke et al. 1999) and the known synergy of zidovudine and nevirapine in inhibiting HIV replication *in vitro* (Koup et al. 1993). However, single-dose nevirapine is associated with the development of nevirapine -resistant virus (Jourdain et al. 2004).

Studies have shown that nevirapine resistance after intrapartum administration of single-dose nevirapine can be substantially reduced (but not eliminated) by using a short postpartum course of ARV agents from alternate classes (a "tail"). There is no current consensus about the exact duration or composition of the ARV tail. Several trials in Africa have found 3 to 7 days of maternal/infant postpartum zidovudine/lamivudine to be effective (Chaix et al. 2006; McIntyre et al. 2009). Development of resistance to zidovudine or lamivudine given for a short period in this setting is rare (Mandelbrot et al. 2001).
More recent studies have found that 7 days of tenofovir/emtricitabine (TEmAA ANRS 12109 Study Group, 2009), 7 days of zidovudine/didanosine/lopinavir-ritonavir (Van Dyke et al. 2009), and 30 days of zidovudine/didanosine or zidovudine/didanosine/lopinavir-ritonavir (Lallemant et al. 2010) all appear to be effective at reducing the development of nevirapine resistance.

7. The efficiency of current anti-HIV treatments

The efficacy of ARV drugs in preventing MTCT of HIV varies with the type of regimen used and the duration over which it is given. Combination regimens which include different types of ARV drugs are more efficacious than monotherapies as discussed above. It is well known that monotherapies can lead to ARV resistance in the virus, which may limit future therapeutic options when treatment is needed. According to the 2010 WHO treatment guidelines it is recommended that pregnant women living with HIV and their exposed infants receive combination therapy rather than single-dose nevirapine. ARV prophylaxis is also recommended during breastfeeding in settings where breastfeeding is judged to be the safest infant feeding option. In addition, all women eligible for treatment under WHO guidelines should receive an appropriate combination therapy for their own health (WHO, 2010).

8. Practice and procedures

Three types of interventions should be tackled by any program concerned with prevention of mother-to-child transmission of HIV: primary prevention of HIV-1 in women; prophylaxis with ARV drugs in breastfeeding infants and prophylaxis with ARV drugs for lactating mothers. Administration of zidovudine to the pregnant woman and her infant could reduce the risk of perinatal transmission by nearly 70%. Combination ARV prophylaxis given to the mother antenatally is associated with further declines in transmission to <2%. Combination regimens are more effective than single-drug regimens in reducing perinatal transmission.

9. Chapter key facts

- Zidovudine administration to the pregnant woman and her infant can reduce the risk of perinatal transmission by nearly 70%.
- Combination regimens are more effective than single-drug regimens in reducing perinatal transmission. A longer three-part regimen given antenatally, intrapartum, and postpartum is superior in preventing perinatal transmission than a shorter two-part antepartum/intrapartum or intrapartum/postpartum regimen.
- The standard recommendation for infant prophylaxis in the absence of maternal antenatal and intrapartum therapy is six weeks of infant zidovudine. The addition of

single-dose intrapartum nevirapine is generally not recommended for women who are receiving the standard recommended antenatal antiretroviral prophylaxis regimens.

- Antiretroviral prophylaxis should be given to women who have a very low or undetectable viral load on no therapy.
- Intravenous zidovudine during the intrapartum period should be discussed with and recommended to all HIV-infected pregnant women.

10. Summary points of chapter

- HIV is the leading cause of death in women of reproductive age.
- HIV testing and counseling should be undertaken and should be entirely voluntary.
- Three types of interventions should be tackled by any program concerned with prevention of mother-to-child transmission: primary prevention of HIV in women; prophylaxis with antiretroviral drugs in breastfeeding infants and prophylaxis with antiretroviral drugs for lactating mothers.
- Taking antiretroviral treatment can reduce the risk of mother-to-child transmission.
- Administration of zidovudine to the pregnant woman and her infant could significantly reduce the risk of perinatal transmission.
- Combination antiretroviral prophylaxis (initially dual and then triple combination therapy) given to the mother antenatally can further declines the transmission significantly.
- Regardless of the reason, all women who have HIV RNA levels >1,000 copies/ml near the time of delivery should be offered a scheduled cesarean delivery at 38 weeks, which may significantly reduce the risk of transmission.
- Given the risk of development of resistance, addition of single-dose nevirapine when a woman has received antepartum drugs is generally not recommended.

11. Definitions and explanations of words and terms

Antenatal	Before birth
Antepartum	Before labour or child birth
Antiretroviral	Drugs used for the treatment of antiretroviral infections
Antiretroviral Therapy	Drugs used against retroviruses such as HIV
Intrapartum	During labour and delivery or childbirth
Intravenous	Occurring or introduced to within a vein or veins usually by means of injection
Labour	The process of child birth
Microbicides	An agent destructive to microbes
Monotherapy	Single drug treatment
Mother to child transmission	Is the transfer of an agent (e.g. HIV) from the mother to her unborn or born baby
Perinatal	Occurring during , or pertaining to, the periods before, during, or after the time of birth i.e. before delivery from

	the 28th week of gestation through the first 7 days after delivery
Pharmacologic Antagonism	Opposition in action of drugs
Prophylaxis	Protection treatment against disease
Viral Resistance	The development of mutation within the virus genome that leads to the virus becoming resistance to the drug treatment

12. List of abbreviations

ART	Antiretroviral Therapy
ARV	Antiretroviral
PT	Perinatal Transmission
RNA	Ribonucleic acid
UNAIDS	United Nations AIDS
NRTI	Nucleoside reverse transcriptase inhibitors
NNRTI	Non-nucleoside reverse transcriptase inhibitors

13. References

Al-Jabri, A.A. and F.Q. Alenzi. 2009. Vaccines, virucides and drugs against HIV/AIDS: Hopes and optimisms for the future. The Open AIDS Journal 3: 1-3.

Al-Jabri A.A. Al-Muharrmi Z.K., Balkhair A.A. and Ganguly S. 2010. The importance of antenatal screening of HIV among pregnant women. Saudi Medical Journal 31:64-8.

Bolu, O.O. and V. Allread, T. Creek, E. Stringer, F. Forna, M. Bulterys and N. Shaffer. 2007. Approaches for scaling up human immunodeficiency virus testing and counseling in prevention of mother-to-child human immunodeficiency virus transmission settings in resource-limited countries. Am J Obstet Gynecol. 197:S83-9.

CDC. 2006. Achievements in public health. Reduction in perinatal transmission of HIV infection--United States, 1985-2005. MMWR Morb Mortal Wkly Rep. 55:592-597.

Chaix, M.L. and D.K. Ekouevi, F. Rouet, B. Tonwe-Gold, I. Viho, L. Bequet, G. Peytavin, H. Toure, H. Menan, V. Leroy, F. Dabis, C. Rouzioux; Agence Nationale de Recherches sur le SIDA Ditrame Plus Study Group. 2006. Low risk of nevirapine resistance mutations in the prevention of mother-to-child transmission of HIV-1: Agence Nationale de Recherches sur le SIDA Ditrame Plus, Abidjan, Cote d'Ivoire. J. Infect. Dis. 193:482-487.

Cooper, E.R. and M. Charurat, L. Mofenson, C. Hanson, J. Pitt, C. Diaz, K. Hayani, E. Handelsman, V. Smeruglio, R. Hoff and W. Blattner. 2002. Combination antiretroviral strategies for the treatment of pregnant HIV-1-infected women and prevention of perinatal HIV-1-transmission. JAIDS. 29:484-494.

Connor, E.M. and R.S. Sperling, R. Gelber, P. Kiselev, G. Scott, M.J. O'Sullivan, R. Van Dyke, M. Bey, W. Shearer, R.L. Jacobson, E. Jimenez, E.O'Neill, B. Bazin, J-F. Delfraissy, M. Culnane, R. Coombs, M. Elkins, J. Moye, P. Stratton and J. Balsley. 1994. Reduction of maternal-infant transmission of human immunodeficiency virus type 1 with Zidovudine treatment. N. Engl. J. Med. 331:1173-1180.

Cunningham, C.K. and M.L. Chaix, C. Rekacewicz, P. Britto, C. Rouzioux, R.D. Gelber, A. Dorenbaum, J.F. Delfraissy, B. Bazin, L. Mofenson and J.L. Sullivan. 2002. Development of resistance mutations in women receiving standard antiretroviral therapy who received intrapartum nevirapine to prevent perinatal human immunodeficiency virus type 1 transmission: a substudy of pediatric AIDS clinical trials group protocol 316. J. Infect. Dis. 186:181-188.

Hart, C.E. and J.L. Lennox, M. Pratt-Palmore, T.C. Wright, R.F. Schinazi, T. Evans-Strickfaden, T.J. Bush, C. Schnell, L.J. Conley, K.A. Clancy and T.V. Ellerbrock. 1999. Correlation of human immunodeficiency virus type 1 RNA levels in blood and the female genital tract. J. Infect. Dis. 179:871-882.

Ioannidis, J.P. and E.J. Abrams, A. Ammann, M. Bulterys, J.J. Goedert, L. Gray, B.T. Korber, M.J. Mayaux, L.M. Mofenson, M.L. Newell, D.E. Shapiro, J.P. Teglas and C.M. Wilfert. 2001. Perinatal transmission of human immunodeficiency virus type 1 by pregnant women with RNA virus loads <1000 copies/ml. J. Infect. Dis. 183:539-545.

Jourdain, G. and N. Ngo-Giang-Huong S. Le Coeur, C. Bowonwatanuwong, P. Kantipong, P. Leechanachai, S. Ariyadej, P. Leenasirimakul, S. Hammer, M. Lallemant; Perinatal HIV Prevention Trial Group. 2004. Intrapartum exposure to nevirapine and subsequent maternal responses to nevirapine-based antiretroviral therapy. N. Engl. J. Med. 351:229-240.

Koup, R.A and F. Brewster, P. Grob and J.L. Sullivan. 1993. Nevirapine synergistically inhibits HIV-1 replication in combination with zidovudine, interferon or CD4 immunoadhesin. AIDS. 7:1181-1184.

Lallemant, M. and N. Ngo-Giang-Huong G. Jourdain, P. Traisaithit, T.R. Cressey, I.J. Collins, T. Jarupanich, T. Sukhumanant, J. Achalapong, P. Sabsanong, N. Chotivanich, N. Winiyakul, S. Ariyadej, A. Kanjanasing, J. Ratanakosol, J. Hemvuttiphan, K. Kengsakul, W. Wannapira, V. Sittipiyasakul, W. Pornkitprasarn, P. Liampongsabuddhi, K. McIntosh, R.B. Van Dyke, L.M. Frenkel, S. Koetsawang, S. Le Coeur, S. Kanchana; PHPT-4 Study Team. 2010. Efficacy and safety of 1-month postpartum zidovudine-didanosine to prevent HIV-resistance mutations after intrapartum single-dose nevirapine. Clin. Infect. Dis. 50:898-908.

Mandelbrot, L. and A. Landreau-Mascaro, C. Rekacewicz, A. Berrebi, J.L. Bénifla, M. Burgard, E. Lachassine, B. Barret, M.L. Chaix, A. Bongain, N. Ciraru-Vigneron, C. Crenn-Hébert, J.F. Delfraissy, C. Rouzioux, M.J. Mayaux, S. Blanche; Agence Nationale de Recherches sur le SIDA (ANRS) 075 Study Group. 2001. Lamivudine-zidovudine combination for prevention of maternal-infant transmission of HIV-1. JAMA. 285:2083-2093.

McIntyre, J.A. and M. Hopley, D. Moodley, M. Eklund, G.E. Gray, D.B. Hall, P. Robinson, D. Mayers and N.A. Martinson. 2009. Efficacy of short-course AZT plus 3TC to reduce nevirapine resistance in the prevention of mother-to-child HIV transmission: a randomized clinical trial. PLoS Med. 6:e1000172.

Mock, P.A. and N. Shaffer, C. Bhadrakom, W. Siriwasin, T. Chotpitayasunondh, S. Chearskul, N.L. Young, A. Roongpisuthipong, P. Chinayon, M.L. Kalish, B. Parekh and T.D. Mastro. 1999. Maternal viral load and timing of mother-to-child HIV transmission, Bangkok, Thailand. Bangkok Collaborative Perinatal HIV Transmission Study Group. AIDS. 13:407-414.

Musoke, P. and L. Guay, D. Bagenda, M. Mirochnick, C. Nakabiito, T. Fleming, T. Elliott, S. Horton, K. Dransfield, J.W. Pav, A. Murarka, M. Allen, M.G. Fowler, L. Mofenson, D. Hom, F. Mmiro and J.B. Jackson. 1999. A phase I/II study of the safety and pharmacokinetics of nevirapine in HIV-1-infected pregnant Ugandan women and their neonates (HIVNET 006). AIDS. 13:479-486.

Petra Study Team. 2002. Efficacy of three short-course regimens of zidovudine and lamivudine in preventing early and late transmission of HIV-1 from mother to child in Tanzania, South Africa, and Uganda (Petra study): a randomised, double-blind, placebo-controlled trial. Lancet 359:1178-1186.

Shapiro, D.E. and R.S. Sperling and R.W. Coombs. 1999. Effect of zidovudine on perinatal HIV-1 transmission and maternal viral load. Lancet 354:156; author reply 157-158.

Sperling R.S. and D.E. Shapiro, R.W. Coombs, J.A. Todd, S.A. Herman, G.D. McSherry, M.J. O'Sullivan, R.B. Van Dyke, E. Jimenez, C. Rouzioux, P.M. Flynn and J.L. Sullivan. 1996. Maternal viral load, zidovudine treatment, and the risk of transmission of human immunodeficiency virus type 1 from mother to infant. Pediatric AIDS Clinical Trials Group Protocol 076 Study Group. N Engl J Med. 335:1621-1629.

TEmAA ANRS 12109 Study Group. 2009. Tolerance and viral resistance after single-dose nevirapine with tenofovir and emtricitabine to prevent vertical transmission of HIV-1. AIDS 23:825-833.

The European Collaborative Study. 1999. Maternal viral load and vertical transmission of HIV-1: an important factor but not the only one. AIDS 13:1377-1385.

Van Dyke, R. and G. Jourdain and D. Shapiro. 2009. A Phase II Study of the incidence of nevirapine resistance mutations in HIV-infected Thai women receiving a single intrapartum dose of NVP followed by a postpartum tail of ZDV/ddI or ZDV/ddI/LPV/r: IMPAACT P1032. Paper presented at: 16th Conference on Retroviruses and Opportunistic Infections; February 8-11, 2009; Montreal, Canada. Abstract 95aLB.

Wade, N.A. and G.S. Birkhead, B.L. Warren, T.T. Charbonneau, P.T. French, L. Wang, J.B. Baum, J.M. Tesoriero and R. Savicki. 1998. Abbreviated regimens of zidovudine prophylaxis and perinatal transmission of the human immunodeficiency virus. N. Engl. J. Med. 339:1409-1414.

WHO & UNAIDS. 2010. Global Report, UNAIDS report on the global AIDS epidemic.

WHO & UNAIDS. 1999. HIV in pregnancy. WHO/CHS/RHR/99.15, UNAIDS/99.35E.

WHO. 2010. Antiretroviral drugs for treating pregnant women and preventing HIV infection in infants: towards universal access 2010 http://www.who.int/hiv/pub/mtct/antiretroviral2010/en/index.html

Effectiveness of the Regular Implementation of the Mother to Child Transmission Plus (MTCT-Plus) Program in Burkina Faso, West Africa

Fabio Buelli[1,2,5], Virginio Pietra[2,3], Richard Fabian Schumacher[2,4], Jacques Simpore[3], Salvatore Pignatelli[2,3], Francesco Castelli[1,2] and the ESTHER-Brescia Study Group
[1]*Institute for Infectious and Tropical Diseases, University of Brescia, Brescia,*
[2]*Medicus Mundi Italy, Brescia,*
[3]*St. Camille Medical Center, Ouagadougou,*
[4]*University Children's Hospital, Brescia,*
[5]*Ph.D. in Appropriate Methods and Technologies for International Development Co-operation, University of Brescia (A. Archetti Fund),*
[1,2,4,5]*Italy*
[3]*Burkina Faso*

1. Introduction

Since the 90s, many developing countries have introduced health strategies aimed at reducing Mother-to-Child transmission rate of HIV. These strategies (PMTCT - Prevention of Mother-to-Child Transmission) are based on (i) adequate counselling for HIV voluntary testing during antenatal care visits, (ii) single dose or a short antiretroviral therapy treatment to the mother and the newly-born baby (WHO, 2001; WHO, 2004; WHO, 2006) and (iii) formula feeding or (iv) exclusive breast-feeding with early weaning (WHO, 2003a; WHO, 2006).

During the last years, thanks to the increase of the PMTCT program coverage, the aim of the program was enlarged to address the needs of all the family members of the HIV-positive women detected by the program. The World Health Organization (WHO) then introduced the Mother-to-Child Transmission Plus (MTCT-plus) program aimed at promoting health, eventually including the use of Highly Active Antiretroviral Treatment (HAART) for the infected mothers, their children, even those whose father is different from the current partner, and the partners themselves (WHO, 2003b).

Aims of the program are, therefore, (i) to reduce HIV vertical transmission rates through specific antiretroviral therapies for the HIV-infected pregnant women, (ii) to involve a larger number of children and partners in the early stage of the disease and (iii) to increase the children survival rates by improving the HIV-positive mothers' life expectancy. (Berer, 1999; Brahmbatt et al, 2006). Psychosocial and nutritional supports and family planning are also integral components of MTCT-plus activities. Programs also focus on health education, including best breastfeeding practices to reduce transmission risk and nutrition.

Another important expectation of the program is to raise awareness and acceptability of HIV testing and early antiretroviral therapy, thus curbing the incidence of overt AIDS.
Since 2003, many MTCT-plus programs have been implemented in HIV endemic developing countries, yielding conflicting results in different settings (Tonwe-Gold et al, 2009).
In Burkina Faso, where a stable HIV-prevalence of 1.8% is recorded (UNAIDS, 2006), the PMTCT program started in 2002 and the MTCT-plus program was introduced later on thanks to the World Bank (TAP-Treatment Acceleration Program) and the Global Fund funding, which increased the availability of antiretroviral drugs.
Aim of our work is to describe the achievements and the constraints faced by the real-life implementation of MTCT-plus program at the St. Camille Medical Center in Ouagadougou, Burkina Faso.

2. Methods

Study site: St. Camille Medical Center (SCMC) in Ouagadougou, Burkina Faso, a large mother and child health center, where more than 3000 deliveries take place every year (picture 1). Prevention and care of HIV infection have been carried out since 2002 at the center (WHO 2004). Thanks to a collaborative agreement, physicians from the University of Brescia and from the Spedali Civili General Hospital in Brescia (Italy) have been working in the Center to support local staff and anti-HIV activities.

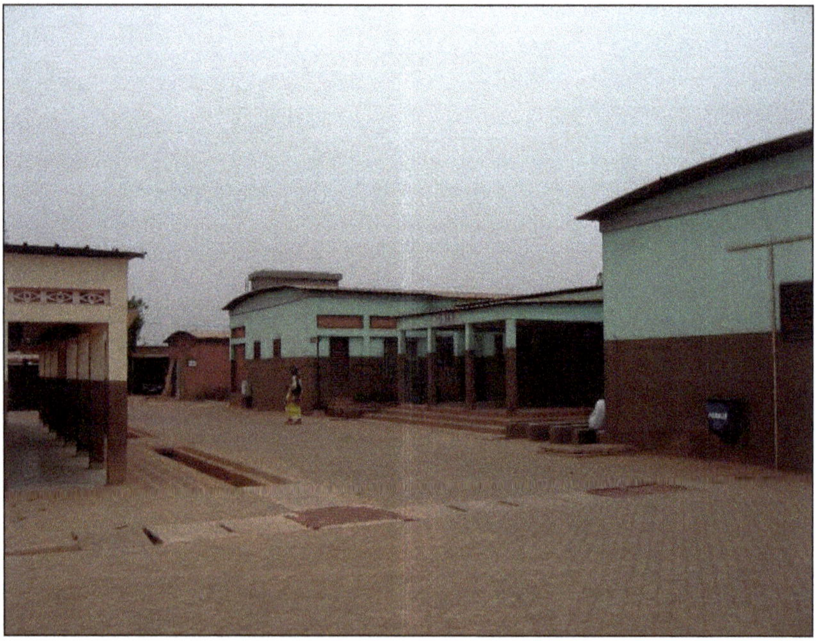

Fig. 1. St. Camille Medical Center

Voluntary Counselling and Testing (VCT): VCT is offered at St. Camille Medical Center to all pregnant women during their prenatal visit (opt-in strategy). Counselling involves an individual pre-test and post-test, conducted during the same morning by specially trained midwives. All women are also asked to invite their partners to undergo the test. Moreover, HIV positive women are invited to test all the children had from previous pregnancies. Should the partner test HIV-infected, possible co-wives are also invited by the partner to undergo the test.

Screening test: after informed consent, serological screening is immediately performed by two sequential rapid tests (Determine® and Genie-II®) (Koblavi-Dème et al, 2001) to avoid loss to follow-up and assure adequate post-test counselling. In case of conflicting results, an additional ELISA test is also performed. Polymerase Chain Reaction (PCR) test, available at the Center, is used to detect infection in young children under 18 months (Simporé et al, 2006).

Patients management and PMTCT protocol: The national guidelines applied by the Center followed the indications provided by WHO during the study period (WHO, 2003c; WHO, 2006) both with regard to PMTCT protocols, and to the indications for therapy and for any immunological assessment.

Nevertheless, until 2006, access to treatment has resulted in waiting lists so that even women in need of therapy have made only prophylaxis in pregnancy, starting HAART after delivery.

From 2006 onwards, all women in need of therapy started HAART during pregnancy. Prophylaxis, including the breast-milk substitutes, were provided for free, while for HAART a contribution of 3 USD per month was asked (table1).

	During pregnancy	**During delivery**	**After delivery**
Protocol	**AZT** (300 mg x 2/day from 28° week of pregnancy)	**NVP** (200 mg single dose) + **AZT/3TC** (300mg/150mg)	**Mother: AZT/3TC** (300/150mg x 2/day for 1 week) **Newborn : NVP** (2mg/kg single dose) + **AZT** (4mg/kg X 2 / day for 1 week)

Table 1. PMTCT protocols (prophylaxis)

3. Results

From 1st May 2002 to 30th September 2008, 20,040 deliveries took place at SCMC and 4,028 (20.1%) VCT were carried out in pregnant women, with a seropositivity rate of 20.5% (826/4028). These 826 HIV+ pregnant women were enrolled in the PMTCT program.

Only 354 HIV+ pregnant women (42.8%) were enrolled in our MTCT-plus programme while the remaining 472 women were included in other centers' programs according to their living area and centers availability.

Catholic religion was declared by 40.4% of the sample (143/354), while the majority of the sample (185/354, 52.3%) declared to be Muslim, as it is the case for the routine attendance of the Mother-and-Child (MCH) clinic in this predominantly Muslim country.

As to the educational level, 102/354 (28.8%) attended the primary school (including Koranic school), while 35.6% attended the secondary school (126/354). Only 10 women (2.8% of the

sample) attended higher level schools. A remarkable part of the sample (32.8%, 116/354) declared to be illiterate.
As many as 129/354 women (36.4%) could only speak the local language (Mòoré), including 15 women who declared Koranic school. The remainig 63.6% (225/354) could also speak French. Most women were married (246/354; 69.5%), while 77/354 (21.8%) declared to be unmarried, but with a steady partner. The remaining 18/354 (5.1%) declared to be divorced and 13/354 (3.7%) declared to be widows, 3 of whom married again. (Table 2).

	Number	%
Religion		
- Catholic	143/354	(40.4%)
- Muslim	185/354	(52.3%)
- Others	26/354	(7,3%)
Language		
- French and local language	225/354	(63.6%)
- Only local language	129/354	(36.4%)
Civil Status		
- Married	246/354	(69.5%)
- Unmarried (steady partner)	77/354	(21.8%)
- Divorced	18/354	(5.1%)
- Widows	13/354	(3,7%)
Educational Level		
- Illiterate	116/354	(32.8%)
- Primary School	102/354	(28.8%)
- Secondary school	126/354	(35.6%)
- Higher school level	10/354	(2.8%)

Table 2. Description of the female population

After counseling, 182/344 living partners (52.9%) accepted to undergo the test and 115/182 (63.2%) tested positive. Among those partners who did not accept HIV testing, 82/162 (50.6%) were not informed by the woman, 29/162 (17.9%) were informed but refused to undergo the test, while for the remaining 51/162 (31.5%) information was not available.
Polygamic families in our sample had very low acceptance rate to the test (just 1/46 of the co-wives was tested, 2.1%, with negative result).
Out of the 115 HIV-infected partners, only 36 (31.3%) accepted to be followed at the St. Camille Medical Center, while the remaining 79 did not show up anymore.
The average age of our HIV+ patient cohort (390 in total, 354 women and 36 partners) was 32.3 years old (SD ± 6.3 years old) with a significant difference ($p < 0,01$) between women (31.5 years old) and their partners (40.8 years old).
At the end of September 2008, we counted 647 living children for the women enrolled in the program, considering all the children had before (348, 53.8%) and those delivered in the current and/or in a later pregnancy (299, 46.2%). As many as 249 dead children were also reported with an overall average of 2.5 children per woman.
The 17.8% (63/354) of our pregnant women was at the first pregnancy at the moment of enrollment.

Furthermore, a significant proportion of pregnant women (48/354) declared not having other living children due to the negative outcome (abortion) of previous pregnancies or to the death of previous children.
HIV testing was carried out in 186/348 (53.4%) children had from previous pregnancies, with a HIV prevalence rate of 10.2% (19/186) and in 231/299 children delivered under the PMTCT program, with a HIV prevalence rate of 4.3% (10/231). In our study, we did not observe any neonatal infection from that sub-set of mother who underwent HAART during pregnancy after 2006 (Simporé et al, 2007).
Out of the 29 HIV infected children, 20 are currently followed at the St. Camille Medical Center, 4 are followed by other centers and 5 are lost to follow-up.
At the time of enrolment most adult people in our sample (354 women and 36 men) were in the early stages of infection: 315/354 (88.9%) women and 25/36 (69.4%) partners were in stages WHO-1 or WHO-2, while only 39/354 (11%) women and 11/36 (30.5%) partners were in stage WHO-3 or in stage WHO-4. (table 3a and 3b).

Clinical Stage		Immunological severity level §		
		SEVERE (< 200 CD4/µl)	INTERMEDIATE (200-349 CD4/µl)	MODERATE (≥ 350 CD4/ µl)
Stage I	194 (54.8%)	30	55	107
Stage II	121 (34.2%)	44	35	41
Stage III	36 (10.2%)	22	9	4
Stage IV	3 (0.8%)	3	0	0
TOTAL	**354**	**99**	**99**	**152**

§ data not available for 4 patients

Table 3a. Clinical and immunological staging of HIV-infected pregnant women

Clinical stage		Immunological severity level ¥		
		SEVERE (< 200 CD4/µl)	INTERMEDIATE (200-349 CD4/µl)	MODERATE (≥ 350 CD4/µl)
Stage I	15 (41.7%)	2	6	6
Stage II	10 (27.8%)	5	2	3
Stage III	11 (30.6%)	7	2	1
Stage IV	0	0	0	0
TOTAL	**36**	**14**	**10**	**10**

¥ data not available for 2 patients

Table 3b. Clinical and immunological staging of HIV-infected partners

Altogether, the mean CD4+ value in the adult sample is 350.5 CD4+/µl (range 1 - 1769 CD4+/µl), higher in women (361.6 ± σ 253.7) than in men (281.3 ± σ 188), although this difference is not statistically significant (p=0.067).

As many as 113/384 (29.4%) patients (99 women and 14 partners) had a CD4+ cell count below 200 cells/μl at recruitment, immediately meeting the 2006 WHO guidelines eligibility criteria to start HAART. As a matter of fact, 95/113 patients started HAART within 6 months while 5/113 (all in clinical stage WHO-1) started HAART at a later time and 13/113 never started treatment because they were lost to follow-up or died soon after recruitment.

4. Discussion

Since the results of the HIVNET-012 (Guay et al, 1999) and other PMTCT clinical trials (Dabis et al., 1999; Shaffer et al., 1999) were made available, the adoption of single-dose NVP at delivery as preventive strategy to reduce mother to child HIV transmission rate has avoided many neonatal infections in Developing Countries, allowing at the same time to detect - and cure - a high number of HIV-infected women.

However, the early emergence of HIV nevirapine-resistant strains urged to identify alternative strategies (Johnson et al, 2005).

To face these limits, WHO guidelines for PMTCT were reviewed in order to avoid the risk of viral resistances (WHO, 2006). Moreover, WHO approved MTCT-plus strategy in 2003, suggesting the adoption of a program of comprehensive care for the HIV-positive woman and for all the members of her family.

These treatments include health care, social and psychological support, reproductive health and family planning services, education and nutritional support. With this initiative, the international community has recognized the centrality of the family's role and the great contribution that women offer to the fight against AIDS (Rabkin et al., 2003).

Our study assesses the effectiveness of the MCTC-plus routine implementation in real life condition in an urban area of a resource-limited Sub-Saharian African country (Burkina Faso) to detect HIV+ family members of HIV-infected pregnant women.

In 2002, the national PMTCT program started in Burkina Faso, in three different pilot sites, including St. Camille Medical Center. The number of PTMCT centers in Burkina Faso has progressively and rapidly expanded to 803 in 2008, with a complete coverage of all Health Districts in the Country (CNLS Data, 2009).

This decentralized approach is in line with the most recent recommendations for the progressive increase of antiretroviral coverage as close as possible to the patients' households (Ferradini et al., 2006).

MTCT-plus program activities are in fact considered as the most important tool to detect HIV-infected people as early as possible.

The effectiveness of MTCT-plus program depends, first of all, on the VCT acceptance rate, the real entry point into the program. Actually, wide variations in the VCT acceptance rate were recorded in different geographic environment especially because of different cultural and organizational factors (Perez et al., 2004; Pignatelli et al., 2006; Tonwe-Gold et al., 2009).

The high number of pregnancies (more than 3,000/year) and of the ante-natal visits did not allowed our staff to provide an individual counselling and obliged us to adopt the opt-in strategy. This may explain the low VCT acceptance rate observed in our centre (20.1%) compared to 80% acceptance rate recorded in other centres in Burkina Faso where the opt-out strategy is adopted (MSFL, 2006).

Nevertheless we did not observe any relevant loss in the follow-up, proving that women that accept opt-in VCT are highly motivated and willing to follow the program. In our experience the availability of antiretroviral drugs is not a relevant determinant for the acceptance of VCT. In fact, we did not observe any increase in the VCT acceptance rate linked to the increasing HAART availability over time. This observation suggests that cultural factors (partner's consensus, stigmatisation, illness perception, level of education) still play a very important role. An indirect confirmation comes from the higher educational level of our sample compared to that of the general female population attending the centre, 71% of which is illiterate (UNDP report 2009). Education is one of the most important factors facilitating VCT acceptance, together with obstetric history (Pignatelli et al., 2006; Perez et al., 2006).

The recorded HIV prevalence rate at St. Camille Medical Center is then significantly higher than in the general population of Ouagadougou (about 4%) and than the national statistics (1.8%): this suggests not only a predisposition of the women in our urban environment to undergo the test, but a further selection of the population for the PMTCT.

In fact, until the end of 2005, the SCMC in Ouagadougou was the only existing centre in Burkina Faso that implemented the MTCT-plus program. Pregnant seropositive women, followed by other centres, were often reported to SCMC just for the PMTCT before returning to their original center for follow-up.

The choice to implement the MTCT-plus program at the St Camille Medical Center compared to other centers, is due to the possibility to have access to many services that are not available in other centers, such as free formula milk, free laboratory follow up (test for children) and the possibility to have access to a Paediatrics unit and to the only neonatology unit existing in the Country. These facts also explain why many HIV-infected women (472/826; 57.1% of those women tested HIV-infected in our study) chose to deliver at the SCMC and to return for continuous follow-up at the original living area once the delivery has taken place.

The repeated offer to test the woman's family members in the period before and after childbirth and during the counselling meetings gave good results in our study as already reported. In particular, the involvement of the male partner in the VCT and the couple counselling was a very important element in order to increase the number of people taking part in the preventive programs (Katz et al., 2009).

On average, the immune status of the HIV-positive male partners was more compromised than the one of the pregnant females, suggesting the presence of an older infection. This fact, even if not statistically significant, matches with other report in the country (Saleri et al., 2009).

The number of HIV-negative male patients is not negligible (67/182, 36.5% of the tested partners). This is in line with data showing that in Burkina Faso about two thirds of HIV-infected couples are sero-discordant (de Walque, 2007). This shows the usefulness of the MTCT-plus protocol as a unique opportunity to promote preventive measure for negative partners.

The average number of living children is low (1.8/woman), especially if compared to the high fertility rate in Burkina Faso (6.2/woman) (CIA, 2009). This is probably due to the high foetal and infant mortality rate in mothers infected at St. Camille Medical Center (Pignatelli et al., 2006). In fact as many as 249 previously dead children were reported in our sample (249/896; 27.8%).

The lower fertility rate in HIV+ women, especially in the advanced stages of the illness, could be another possible reason (Le Coeur et al., 2005), and this reinforce the need to link HIV treatment and reproductive health services in the framework of the MTCT-plus initiative.
The screening of the children born from previous pregnancies was probably hampered by the fear of the parents to verify the status of the infection in their children for whom PMTCT protocols was not adopted and by the fear that elder children may reveal the secret in the community.
As expected, HIV infected pregnant women that entered the PMTCT program were almost all asymptomatic. However, CD4+ lymphocyte count is essential in order to identify those HIV-infected women that are eligible for the HAART. The mother to child HIV transmission rate (4.3%) is due to the failure of the nevirapine mono-prophylaxis and to the limited access to the HAART for those who needed it before 2006.
The relative older age of the women in our sample compared to the average of the age of the pregnant women at the SCMC is probably due to the fact that the older women are more free to autonomously accept the VCT proposal and can be more worried about the previous and "unexplainable" loss of a child (Pignatelli et al., 2006).
The decreasing trend recorded in the sero-prevalence rate among the younger pregnant women in Burkina Faso can be due to the campaigns focused on the education to health (UNAIDS/OMS/UNICEF/UE, 2006). This effort needs to be strengthened at every level.
The progressive increase of HAART availability in resource limited Countries underlines the role of MTCT-plus programs as a possible tool capable to identify motivated people in a sufficiently initial stage of the illness in order to benefit from the antiretroviral treatment.
In our study, the following socio-cultural factors have limited the effectiveness of the program: (i) refusal of the male partner to undergo the test (ii) refusal of the parents to test the children from previous pregnancies (iii) refusal of the pregnant woman to inform the partner about her serostatus. These reasons possibly find their explanation in the social stigma that HIV still cause in Western Africa.

5. Conclusion

The MTCT-plus approach might be an important tool to increase the early detection of HIV infected patients in the household of the infected pregnant women, allowing for beneficial early treatment. Furthermore detection of discordant couples offers possibilities to prevent infection. However, its effectiveness in the real-life condition of Western Africa is hampered by cultural factors that act at different levels (VCT uptake, notification to the partner, testing of previous children) and it requires new and innovative approaches in order to expand the adoption of HIV testing in Developing Countries.
The positive impact that HAART has on the lives of those affected may further increase acceptance of VCT and reduce stigma, thus allowing to save ever more people.

6. ESTHER-Brescia study group

Dpt for Infectious Diseases, Spedali Civili General Hospital (Dr Lina R. Tomasoni, Dr M. Gulletta, Dr Silvio Caligaris, Dr Eugenia Quiros); **Dpt of Neonatology, Spedali Civili**

General Hospital (Dr P. Villani, Dr D. Cattarelli); **St Camille Medical Center (**Brother Luise, Brother Sébastien Rouamba, Dr Dabogo Sia, Father Marc Zombré, Father François Sedogo, Father Dr Paul Ouedraogo, Dr Ghislaine Sawadogo, Dr Korotimi Sanogo, Dr Jedida Simpore, M.me Agnes Thombiano, M.me Josephine Ouedraogo, M.me Therese Ouba), **National Committee against AIDS and STDs, Burkina Faso** (Dr André Joseph Tiendrebeogo, Dr Marie Joseph Sanou, Dr. Genevieve Onadja, Dr Francine Ouedraogo), **National Institute of Health, Rome, Italy** (Dr Stefano Vella), **Post-Graduate Specialty School in Infectious Diseases, University of Brescia, Italy** (Dr Chiara Baiguera, Dr Daniele Bella, Dr Barbara Cadeo, Dr Chiara Cattaneo, Dr Silvia Lorenzotti, Dr Chiara Pezzoli, Dr Katiela Prestini, Dr Cristina Uccelli, Dr Laura Soavi, Dr Giuseppe Lapadula, Dr. Emanuele Focà, Dr Viviana Bergamaschi, Dr Manuela Rosina, Dr Antonella Ricci), **Post-Graduate Specialty School in Tropical Medicine, University of Brescia, Italy** (Dr Giuseppina De Iaco, Dr Maria Manfrin, Dr Cecilia Pizzocolo, Dr Nuccia Saleri, Dr Susanna Capone, Dr Alessandro Pini, Dr Veronica Del Punta, Dr Sara Bigoni, Dr Silvia Odolini, Dr Lucia Urbinati), **Post-Graduate Specialty School in Pediatrics, University of Brescia, Italy** (Dr Sara Aliprandi, Dr Veronica Bennato, Dr Elisa Bertoni, Dr Sara Boccacci, Dr Federica Bruni, Dr Marco Cattalini, Dr Gemma Cattaneo, Dr Valeria Consolati, Dr Donatella De Martiis, Dr Rosaria Fausti, Dr Monica Filisetti, Dr Chiara Gualeni, Dr Sarah Guarisco, Dr Livia Grazzani, Dr Elisa Marniga, Dr Roberto Marzollo, Dr Moira Pinotti, Dr Chiara Ravelli, Dr Francesca Ricci, Dr Elena Soncini, Dr Mariateresa Sinelli, Dr Elena Spinelli, Dr Laura Morali, Dr Chiara Monfredini), **PhD in Methodologies and Appropriate Technologies in International Co-operation for Development** (Dr Fabio Buelli, Dr Beatrice Autino, Dr Marianna Bettinzoli); **Medicus Mundi Italy** (Mr Massimo Chiappa, Mr Giovanni Zoppi, Mrs Cinzia Ferrante, Mrs Marina Martinetto, Mrs Patrizia Marcotti, Dr Alessia Melzani, Dr Arianna Andreoli)

7. Acknowledgement

The project was made possible thanks to the agreement between the Spedali Civili General Hospital of Brescia and the Camillian health structures in Burkina Faso and the technical-scientific support assured by the University of Brescia and the University of Ouagadougou.

Trainees doctors in Tropical Medicine, Infectious Diseases and in Pediatrics at the University of Brescia, acting on the behalf of the NGO Medicus Mundi Italy (grant from the Italian Ministry of Foreign Affairs) work together with the local medical staff from Burkina.

Many national and international organization participated to the realization of the study: the ESTHER project, the World Bank through TAP (Treatment Acceleration Program), the Global Fund against HIV, Tuberculosis and Malaria, UNICEF, the Italian Ministry of Foreign Affairs, the Italian High Institute of Health, the Lombardy Region, the province of Brescia, the Municipality of Brescia, the CARIPLO Foundation.

Special thanks to the strong and indispensable collaboration of the Ministry of Health of Burkina Faso and the Program for the Application and the Decentralization of the Burkinan Health System, the Burkina National Committee against AIDS and Sexually Transmitted Infections, the World Health Organization (WHO), the offices of the World Bank, UNICEF in Burkina Faso, and the Local Technical Unit of the Italian Embassy in Burkina Faso.

8. References

Berer M: *Reducing perinatal HIV transmission in developing countries through antenatal and delivery care, and breastfeeding: supporting infant survival by supporting mother's survival.* Bull. World Health Org., 1999; 77: 871-877.

Brahmbhatt H, Kigozi G, Wabwire-Mangen F, Serwadda D, Lutalo T, Nalugoda F, Sewankambo N, Kiduggavu M, Wawer M, Gray R: *Mortality in HIV-infected and uninfected children of HIV-infected and uninfected mothers in rural Uganda.* JAIDS, 2006; 41: 504-508.

CIA *World Factbook Demographic Statistics*, 2009.

CNLS Burkina Faso: *Données de la PTME en 2009* ; www.cnls.bf; 2009.

Dabis F, Msellati P, Meda N, Welffens-Ekra C, You B, Manigart O, Leroy V, Simonon A, Cartoux M, Combe P, Ouangré A, Ramon R, Ky-Zerbo O, Montcho C, Salamon R, Rouzioux C, Van de Perre P, Mandelbrot L: *6-months efficacy, tolerance and acceptability of a short regimen of oral zidovudine to reduce vertical transmission of HIV in breastfed children in Côte d'Ivoire and Burkina Faso: a double blind placebo-controlled multicentre trial.* Lancet, 1999; 353:781-785.

de Walque D: *Sero-discordant couples in five African countries: implications for prevention strategies.* Population and Development Review, 2007, 33(3):501-523.

Ferradini L, Jeannin A, Pinoges L, Izopet J, Odhiambo D, Mankhambo L, Karungi G, Szumilin E, Balandine S, Fedida G, Carrieri MP, Spire B, Ford N, Tassie JM, Guerin PJ, Brasher C: *Scaling up of highly active antiretroviral therapy in a rural distrct of Malawi: an effectiveness assessement.* Lancet, 2006; 367: 1335-1369.

Guay LA, Musoke P, Fleming T, Bagenda D, Allen M, Nakabiito C, Sherman J, Bakaki P, Ducar C, Deseyve M, Emel L, Mirochnick M, Fowler MG, Mofenson L, Miotti P, Dransfield K, Bray D, Mmiro F, Jackson JB: *Intrapartum and neonatal single-dose nevirapine compared with zidovudine for prevention of mother-to-child transmission of HIV-1 in Kampala, Uganda: HIVNET 012 randomised trial.* Lancet 1999; 354: 795-804.

Johnson JA, Li JF, Morris L, Martinson N, Gray G, McIntyre J, Heneine W : *Emergence of drug-resistant HIV-1 after intrapartum administration of single-dose nevirapine is substantially underestimated.* J. Infect. Dis., 2005; 192: 16-23.

Katz DA, Kiarie JN, John-Stewart GC, Richardson BA, John FN, Farquhar C: *Male perspectives on incorporating men into antenatal HIV counselling and testing.* PLoS One. 2009 Nov 2;4(11):e7602.

Koblavi-Dème S, Maurice C, Yavo D, Sibailly TS, N'guessan K, Kamelan-Tano Y, Wiktor SZ, Roels TH, Chorba T, Nkengasong JN: *Sensitivity and Specificity of Human Immunodeficiency Virus Rapid Serologic Assays and Testing Algorithms in an Antenatal Clinic in Abidjan, Ivory Coast.* J. Clin. Microbiol. 2001; 39 (5) : 1808–1812.

Le Coeur S, Khlat M, Halembokaka G, Augereau-Vacher C, Batala-M'Pondo G, Baty G, Ronsmans C: *HIV and the magnitude of pregnancy-related mortality in Point Noir, Congo.* AIDS, 2005 ; 19 : 69-75.

Medecins sans Frontières Luxembourg (MSFL). *Prise en charge des PVVIH/SIDA dans le district sanitaire de Pissy.* Rapport. annuel. 2005. [msfl-ouaga@luxembourg.msf.org]

Perez F, Orne-Gliemann J, Mukotekwa T, Miller A, Glenshaw M, Mahomva A, Dabis F: *Prevention of mother to child transmission of HIV: evaluation of a pilot programme in a district hospital in rural Zimbabwe*. Brit. Med. J., 2004; 329: 1147-1150.

Perez F, Zvandaziva C, Engelsmann B, Dabis F: *Acceptability of routine HIV testing ("opt-out") in antenatal services in two rural districts in Zimbabwe*. JAIDS, 2006; 41: 514-520.

Pignatelli S, Simpore J, Pietra V, Ouedraogo L, Conombo G, Saleri N, Pizzocolo C, De Iaco G, Tall F, Ouiminga A, Carosi G, Castelli F: *Factors predicting uptake of Voluntary Counselling and Testing (VCT) in a real-life setting in a mother-to-child Centre in Ouagadougou (Burkina Faso)*. Trop. Med. Int. Health, 2006; 11:350-357.

Rabkin M, El-Sadr WM: *Saving mothers, saving families. The MCTC-plus initiative. WHO perspective and practice in antiretroviral treatment. Case Study* , Geneva, WHO, 2003.

Saleri N, Capone S, Pietra V, De Iaco G, Del Punta V, Rizzi M, Levi M, Rouamba S, Somé E, Simporé J, Patroni A, Carosi G, Castelli F: *Outcome and predictive factors of mortality in hospitalized HIV-patients in Burkina Faso*. Infection. 2009 Apr;37(2):142-7.

Shaffer N, Chuachoowong R, Mock PA, Bhadrakom C, Siriwasin W, Young NL, Chotpitayasunondh T, Chearskul S, Roongpisuthipong A, Chinayon P, Karon J, Mastro TD, Simonds RJ: *Short-course zidovudine for perinatal HIV-1 transmission in Bangkok,Thailand: a randomised controlled trial*. Lancet. 1999; 353:773-780.

Simporé J, Pietra V, Savadogo A, Pignatelli S, Nikiema JB, Nadembega WMC., Yara J, Zoungrana N, Bakouan D, Colizzi V, Castelli F, Musumeci S: *Reduction of mother-to-child transmission of HIV (MTCT-HIV) at Saint Camille Medical Center (SCMC) in Ouagadougou, Burkina Faso*. J. Med. Virol., 2006; 78:148-152.

Simporé J, Pietra V, Pignatelli S, Karou D, Nadembega WM, Ilboudo D, Ceccherini-Silberstein F, Ghilat-Avoid-Belem WN, Bellocchi MC, Saleri N, Sanou MJ, Ouedraogo CM, Nikiema JB, Colizzi V, Perno CF, Castelli F, Musumeci S: *Effective program against mother-to-child transmission of HIV at Saint Camille Medical Centre in Burkina Faso*. J. Med. Virol. 2007 Jul;79(7):873-9.

Tonwe-Gold B, Ekouevi DK, Bosse CA, Toure S, Koné M, Becquet R, Leroy V, Toro P, Dabis F, El Sadr WM, Abrams EJ: *Implementing family-focused HIV care treatment: the first 2 years' experience of the mother-to-child transmission-plus program in Abidjan, Cote d'Ivoire*. Trop. Med. Int. Health, February 2009; 14:204-212.

UNAIDS. *Report on the global AIDS epidemic*. Geneva, 2006.

UNAIDS/WHO/UNICEF/EU. *Burkina Faso. Epidemiological Fact Sheet*, August 2006.

United Nations Development Program report 2009, [http://hdrstats.undp.org/en/indicators/99.html]

World Health Organization (WHO): *Prevention of mother-to-child transmission of HIV : selection and use of nevirapine*. Technical Notes. Geneva, 2001.

World Health Organization (WHO): *HIV and Infant Feeding. Framework for priority action*. Geneva, 2003a.

World Health Organisation (WHO): *Scaling up antiretroviral therapy in resource-limited settings – Guidelines for a public health approach*. Geneva, 2003b.

World Health Organization (WHO): *Saving mothers, saving families : the MTCT-PLUS Initiative. Perspectives and practice in antiretroviral treatment*. Case study. Geneva, 2003c.

World Health Organization (WHO): *Antiretroviral drugs and the prevention of mother-to-child transmission of HIV infection in resource-constrained settings. Recommendations for use.* 2004 revision Report of a Technical Consultation, Geneva, 5–6 February 2004 .

World Health Organization (WHO). *Antiretroviral drugs for treating pregnant women and preventing HIV infection in infants in resource-limited settings. Towards universal access.* Geneva, 2006.

7

Nikavir in Chemoprevention Regimens of Vertical HIV Transmission

Elvira Ivanova[1], Nadezhda Shmagel[1] and Natalia Vorobeva[2]
[1]*Perm Regional AIDS Center*
[2]*Vagner Perm State Academy of Medicine*
Russian Federation

1. Introduction

The first cases of HIV infection in the Russian Federation were identified in 1987. Between 1987 and 1996 over 90% of individuals acquired infection via homosexual contacts (Segeda, 2006; Berrous, 2000).

Since 1996 there has been a dramatic growth of incidence rate due to the parenteral use of psychoactive drugs (Montgomery, 2000; UNAIDS, 2001; Des Jarlais, 2001). Since then, in the Russian Federation a narcodependent type of epidemic process has formed. It is characterized by high intensity and a rapid growth of the incidence rate (Adabekov & Mamaev, 2005; Rakhmanova, 2004).

Due to a large share of women of the active reproductive age among the HIV-infected individuals and the tendency for its further growth as well as the increasing percentage of HIV distribution through sexual transmission (Terentyeva, 2006), there is a current annual growth of pregnancy and delivery rates among women infected with HIV (Terentyeva, 2006). Compared with 2000, in 2010 the absolute number of deliveries has increased 15 times. By 2010 deliveries by HIV-infected women accounted to 0.4% of the total number of deliveries in the Russian Federation.

The actual increase in the share of women among the newly identified cases of HIV infection may be regarded as an indirect evidence of activation of heterosexual transmission of HIV. 62% of HIV-positive pregnant women identified in 2010 were infected through sexual contacts. Along with the growth of heterosexual route of infection an associated risk of mother-to-child transmission of HIV has increased as well.

The mortality rate among children born from HIV-positive mothers is high. 25% of HIV-positive and 12% of HIV-negative children die before the age of five (Rogers, 1984; Rakhmanova, 2006).

By the end 2010, 12000 individuals with HIV infection were registered in Permsky Krai, over one third of them (35%) being females. Between 1999 and 2010 1634 children were born from HIV-infected mothers. 40 of them died and 73 have got HIV infection. Every 192nd delivery is in a woman infected with HIV (in the Russian Federation the ratio is 1 per 250).

Thus, a current high intensity of epidemic process of HIV infection has emphasized the necessity for HIV prevention among the newborns. Considering an unprecedented growth of the incidence rate and low birth rate in the Russian Federation this issue is a priority.

Mother-to-child transmission of HIV occurs during pregnancy, delivery and during the postpartum period while breast-feeding. In 1994 the US Center for Disease Control (CDC) recommended a three-stage chemoprevention with zidovudine (Retrovir) for mothers during pregnancy, delivery and postnatally for children (Barlett & Gallant, 1964; Friis, 2001). Along with the rejection of breast-feeding those measures decreased the risk of infection by 2% (Connor, 1994; European Collaborative Study, 2005; Jasseron, 2008; Townsend, 2008). The earliest recommendations on the vertical chemoprophylaxis of HIV were provided by Rakhmanova in 1997 and later by V.Pokrovsky and O.Yurin (2000-2001). Currently, there are American (CDC, 2008) and European (FACS, 2008) Guidelines. Nevertheless the number of antiretroviral agents available for prevention of vertical HIV transmission is rather small. Moreover, their recognized toxicological manifestations considerably restrict the possibility of HIV chemoprevention. Therefore the search, development and clinical implementation of the new low-toxic anti HIV agents with prolonged action are all of immense importance.

2. History of creation of Nikavir

In the middle of the 1980s academician A. Krayevsky initiated investigations of the anti-HIV activity of a group of nucleoside containing compounds, newly synthesized at the laboratory of the Engelhardt Institute of Molecular Biology of the Russian Academy of Sciences, which including a modified phosphate group in 5′-position. 5′-H-phosphonat 3′-azido-3′-desoxythymidine in the form of sodium salt appeared to be a highly active substance with the best cytotoxic properties. It was named phosphazide; its brand name is Nikavir (Fig. 1).

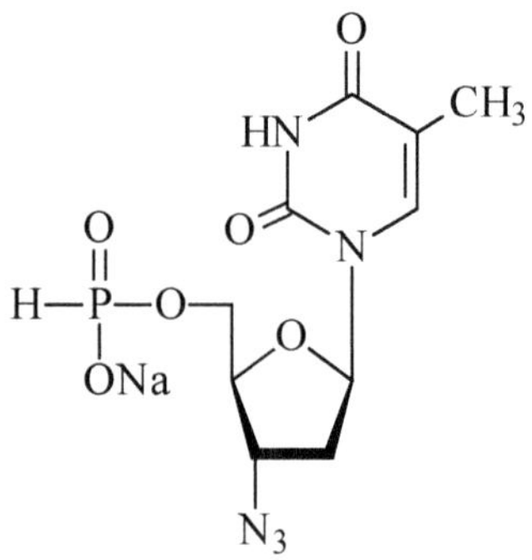

Fig. 1. Formula of Nikavir (phosphazide).

In 1986 Nikavir was identified as a drug that possesses a high level of anti-HIV efficiency in respect to HIV reproduction in H9, MOLT and MT-4 lymphoblastic cell cultures (Galegov, 1988).

Comparative studies of cytotoxic activity of Nikavir and zidovudine were performed at the Ivanovsky Institute of Virology of the Russian Academy of Medical Sciences. It vividly showed that Nikavir concentrations in the range of 0.25-15 μM considerably decreased the number of viral antigen expressing cells while the number of live cells considerably increased compared to the control sample (infected with the culture virus and not treated with the drug). In the control sample the number of live cells decreased from 97% to 18%, the number of virus antigen expressing cells was 69%. With addition of Nikavir the number of live cells increased to 72% and the number of virus antigen expressing cells dropped to 20%. Similar results were obtained with the addition of zidovudine but compared to Nikavir it proved its considerably higher level of toxicity. The selectivity index of Nikavir was twice the number than that of zidovudine (Tarussova, 1990).

Later, a group of researchers from Canada proved a considerably lower toxicity of Nikavir with lymphoblastoid cell lines compared to zidovudine. Nikavir and zidovudine showed a marked efficiency with experimental HIV-1 infection in cord blood mononuclear cells. However, cytotoxic effect of zidovudine appeared by 33 times higher than that of Nikavir. Selectivity index of Nikavir was by 13.6 times higher than that of zidovudine (Machado, 1999).

It is known that in response to each antiretroviral agent drug resistant HIV-1 mutants are developed. It is the result of structural changes of HIV-1 genome due to substitution of one or several nucleic bases. It was found that HIV-1 resistance to Nikavir formed significantly slower than to zidovudine (Selimova, 1999). Resistance to Nikavir develops within a 72 days passivation of the virus (10 infectious cycles) whereas resistance to zidovudine occurs within 26 days (6 infectious cycles). The fact that extensive selection with Nikavir yielded only a single D67N substitution, also associated with resistance to zidovudine, rather than other zidovudine-resistance associated mutations as well, may also be a positive indication in regard to the potential of Nikavir to combat HIV disease (Machado, 1999).

Preclinical toxicological and pharmacokinetic studies of Nikavir were performed at the Institute of Experimental Cardiology of Russian Cardiological Scientific Production Complex. It was established that Nikavir belongs to the category of low-toxic drugs. LD_{50} (average lethal dose) for mice of BABL/c line given in a single intragastric introduction was equal to 8200-8830 mg/kg, that for intra-abdominal introduction – 2260-2390 mg/kg. Zidovudine proved to be far more toxic: in intragastric intake its LD_{50} was 2380-2730 mg/kg and 1320-1660 mg/kg in intra-abdominal introduction. During rat testing Nikavir LD_{50} in intragastric and intra-abdominal introduction were 12200-12950 mg/kg and 2490-2510 mg/kg respectively. No damaging effect was established in the investigation of chronic toxicity in daily (90 days) intragastric introduction of Nikavir to rats (Khandazhinskaya, 2010).

Chronic toxicity was studied in dogs following 2-month oral dosing (tablets 0.2 g), 400 mg/kg during the first month and 200 mg/kg body weight during the second. It was found that tablets (400 mg/kg, 20-fold human dose) taken by dogs for a month caused some reduction of appetite and motor activity. Reduction of the doses to 200 mg/kg did not result in toxic effects in chronic experiments. Toxicity was also not observed in pathological experiments after the completion of the chronic testing. It showed that Nikavir was well assumed and did not affect hematological (granulocytopenia and anemia) or biochemical parameters of liver, kidney and pancreas functioning and metabolic reactions (Khandazhinskaya, 2010).

Basic methods (predominant lethality identification and the Ames test) did not show any mutagenic action as well as the DNA-damaging and allergic effects. Experimental studies on pregnant rats demonstrated a sufficiently lower embriotoxic and teratogenic action of Nikavir compared with zidovudine (Khandazhinskaya, 2010).

Nikavir is a prodrug: after its per oral introduction to dogs only zidovudine can be identified in their blood. However 40-50 minutes after intragastric introduction to mice of tritium-labeled Nikavir both Nikavir and zidovudine were found in blood plasma. The peak radioactivity level of zidovudine was considerably higher than of Nikavir (Skoblov, 2004).

The pharmacokinetic studies established that Nikavir is characterized by a smoother pharmacokinetic curve compared to zidovudine (Galegov, 2004; Khandazhinskaya, 2010). The half-life time of Nikavir from blood plasma surpasses zidovudine by 4 times and this allows to recommend fewer daily intakes.

Thus, due to its high anti-HIV efficiency *in vitro*, low cytotoxicity, favorable pharmacokinetic indices and low toxicity in laboratory animals Nikavir was recommended for clinical evaluation studies.

The first phase of clinical investigation (safety and tolerance) was conducted in 1997. It showed that Nikavir was well-tolerated by all patients. There were no main side-effects observed in zidovudine administration (anemia, neutropenia) as well as less frequent untoward gastrointestinal manifestations, headache and insomnia (Yurin, 1998). It should be noted that not a single case of anemia known to the major side-effect of zidovudine was observed.

Further clinical trial (therapeutic efficiency) was conducted as a multicenter clinical trial under coordination of the Russian Federal AIDS Center, Moscow. The local participating centers were Republican Clinical Infection Hospital in Izhora settlement (St. Pertersburg), Regional AIDS Centers in Tver, Nizhny Novgorod and Tyumen (Yurin, 2001).

At the first stage Nikavir was used as a monotherapy. The trial included 103 patients (75 males and 28 females, average age 26 years). According to HIV-infection classification (USA, CDC, 1987) 69.9% were diagnosed A2 stage, 23.3% had A1 stage and 6.8% had B1 and B2 stages. The therapy course lasted 12 weeks. Patients received daily doses ranging from 400 mg to 1200 mg Nikavir. Its therapeutic efficiency was assessed by such clinical criteria as disease progression or its absence; immunological criteria included changes CD4+ T-lymphocytes count per 1 mm^3 of blood; virological criteria included changes of HIV RNA levels per 1 ml of plasma. CD4 lymphocytes were counted with flow cytometry method using Fac Scan apparatus (Becton Dickenson, USA) and monoclonal antibodies (Becton Dickenson, USA). HIV RNA levels were measured with PCR method (Amplicor Roche HIV-1 Monitor, Hoffmann-La Roch, Switzerland).

During treatment no cases of HIV progress were noted. The pretreatment baseline mean CD4 lymphocytes count was 350 cells/mm^3. After 4 weeks of treatment the mean CD4 lymphocyte index increased by 20 cells and by 80 cells following 12 weeks ($p<0.05$). A reliable decrease of HIV RNA levels was observed starting with the second week of therapy (-0.53 lg copies/ml, $p<0.05$), which remained unchanged after 4 and 12 weeks of therapy (-0.53 and -0.44 lg copies/ml respectively).

The most frequent negative Nikavir-related effects were mild nausea and malaise registered in 30% of patients receiving maximal daily dosage of 1200 mg. No essential changes in hematological indices were revealed. For 1% of patients therapy was temporary stopped due to a moderate granulocytopenia. In 5.8% of cases Nikavir therapy was initiated in spite of grade 1-2 toxicity thrombocytopenia. In all cases the on-going therapy was associated with notable increase of thrombocyte count and disappearing signs of toxicity. During the trial no worth considering changes in biochemical blood values were registered.

The conducted trial demonstrated good efficiency and tolerability of Nikavir monotherapy and allowed to recommend a regimen of 400 mg twice daily (Yurin, 2001).

The next stage was aimed at investigation of possible outcomes following change of zidovudine to Nikavir regimens due to the development of untoward events of grade 2-4 toxicity. In 47 patients zidovudine was substituted by Nikavir because of nausea and vomiting (40.4% of cases), anemia (46.8%) and granulocytopenia (12.8% of cases) whereas

44.7% of patients received Nikavir as monotherapy and 55.3% as a component of highly active antiretroviral therapy (HAART). No cases of Nikavir-associated untoward events were observed and there were no cases of discontinued therapy. Mild nausea was noted in 6.4% of cases and 2.1% had grade 1 toxic anemia. Besides, 36-48 weeks following substitution of zidovudine by Nikavir a considerable growth of CD4 lymphocytes by 70-100 cells/mm^3 was found (Yurin, 2000).
Since 1999 Nikavir was approved for clinical application in the chemotherapy of HIV-infected patients. Currently it is manufactured in the tablet form of 200 mg N 20 and is used for treatment of HIV and AIDS in Russian Federation.

3. Comparative studies of embriotoxic and teratogenic properties of zidovudine and Nikavir

In terms of anemia, significantly fewer Nikavir-associated hemopoetic impairments make it a more perspective drug for therapeutic application for HIV-infected pregnant women than zidovudine. Because of this, evidence-based findings obtained in the comparative studies of embriotoxic and teratogenic properties of zidovudine and Nikavir performed in 2005 at the laboratory of drug toxicology of Institute of Experimental Cardiology under the guidance of professor E. Arzamastsev are of a considerably interest.
Tests were performed among 80 pregnant rats of Wistar line divided into 4 equal groups. Group 1 included animals for control, group 2 received zidovudine (dose of 100mg/kg of body weight once a day), group 3 received Nikavir (dose of 100mg/kg of body weight once a day). As the period of zidovudine half-excretion is less than that of Nikavir group 4 received zidovudine in the total daily dosage of 100 mg/kg in 2 doses (50 mg/kg at 9 a.m. and 5 p.m.).
The tested doses corresponded to a 12.5 multiple of the maximum daily doses of 600 mg/individual or 8 mg/kg approved for pregnant women with HIV.
Intragastric introduction of zidovudine and Nikavir to pregnant rats in the tested doses of 100 mg/kg provided the significant ($p<0.05$) evidence of the body mass retardation in pregnant rats compared with the controls on the 3rd week, while the less marked body mass retardation was observed in Nikavir administration and a two-dose introduction of zidovudine (Table 1).
No statistically significant difference was established in such parameters evaluated for embriotoxicity of zidovudine and Nikavir as the duration of pregnancy, numbers of alive fetuses, implantation places, yellow bodies, fetal body mass, cranioclaudal size in the pregnant rats receiving preparations in the dose of 100 mg/kg and the controls. Likewise data of preimplantation and postimplantation death in experimental groups did not significantly differ from those in the controls as well (Table 2).

Observation periods	Animal groups			
	Controls	Zidovudine 100 mg/kg	Zidovudine 50+50 mg/kg	Nikavir 100 mg/kg
1st week	110±1.6	107±1.6	107±1.1	109±1.4
2nd week	121±1.7	116±1.8	120±1.4	119±1.3
3rd week	135±3.0	121±2.4	130±2.6	124±1.7

Table 1. Body mass dynamics in pregnant rats (% ratio of baseline parameters) in intragastric introduction of zidovudine and Nikavir.

Parameters	Animal groups			
	Controls	Zidovudine 100 mg/kg	Zidovudine 50+50 mg/kg	Nikavir 100 mg/kg
Duration of pregnancy, days	22.9±0.4	22.4±0.5	22.5±0.4	22.7±0.4
Number of fetuses per 1 rat	8.0±0.9	7.6±1.1	7.6±1.1	8.1±1.2
Number of implantation places per rat	8.2±0.6	8.0±2.1	7.9±1.0	8.4±1.4
Number of yellow bodies per rat	8.7±0.7	8.6±0.7	8.4±0.8	8.9±0.8
Preimplantation death, %	5.8	7.0	5.9	5.6
Postimplantation death, %	2.4	5.0	3.8	3.6
Craniocaudal fetal size, cm	2.7±0.2	2.5±0.1	2.5±0,2	2.6±0.1
Fetal body mass, g	3.1±0.1	3.1±0.2	3.3±0,1	3.2±0.1

Table 2. Embriotoxicity indices of zidovudine and Nikavir administered in the intragastric dose of 100 mg/kg introduced to rats within 1-19 days of gestation.

Microscopy and microanatomical examination (standard Wilson-Dyiban dissection) of fetuses perinatally exposed to zidovudine and Nikavir in tested doses did not reveal any malformations or defects of the visceral development. The incidence rate of malformations in the experimental groups did not significantly differ from the controls.

Development of the skeletal system in rat fetuses treated perinatally with zidovudine and Nikavir in the tested dose of 100 mg/kg was studied. The analysis of the alizarin stained total samples from the experimental groups showed the reduction in the number of ossification centers in the 2nd and 4th metacarpal bones, the 3rd and the 4th metatarsal bones, sublingual and pubic bones. These changes were more evident in the zidovudine group on a daily dose of 100 mg/kg. (Table 3).

Absence of ossification centers in fetal skeletons	Animal groups			
	Controls	Zidovudine 100 mg/kg	Zidovudine 50+50 mg/kg	Nikavir 100 mg/kg
Sternum, absolute number per brood	2.6	2.7	2.4	2.5
Sublingual bone, %	2.4	6.6	4.3	4.8
Forefeet, %				
2nd metacarpal bone	13.5	20.9	15.1	14.2
3rd metacarpal bone	3.6	4.2	4.1	3.2
4th metacarpal bone	4.8	8.9	5.3	3.3
Hind limbs, %				
2nd metatarsal bones	7.0	12.0	12.1	11.2
3rd metatarsal bones	8.3	8.0	7.8	7.0
4th metatarsal bones	7.0	14.2	8.6	8.1
Bones of the trunk, %				
ischiadic	0	0	0	0
iliac	0	0	0	0
pubic	4.0	6.6	5.8	5.2

Table 3. Fetal skeletal development on the 20th day of prenatal development.

It was established that an intragastric once-daily dose of 100 mg/kg and a 50+50 mg/kg dose of zidovudine as well as Nikavir daily dose of 100 mg/kg given within 1-19 days of gestation did not cause any change in the number of the offspring born.

Body mass dynamics and offspring postnatal mortality indices in the experimental zidovudine and Nikavir groups treated perinatally did not significantly differ compared with the controls (Table 4).

Parameters	Animal groups			
	Controls	Zidovudine 100 mg/kg	Zidovudine 50+50 mg/kg	Nikavir 100 mg/kg
Number of born offspring	8.8±1.4	8.1±0.9	8.5±1.2	8.3±1.5
Postnatal mortality, %	3.6	4.2	3.9	3.8
Body mass, g				
At birth	7.6±0.2	7.3±0.6	7.4±0.5	7.3±0.7
7th day of life	20.3±1.3	18.3±1.8	20.1±1.1	19.1±1.6
14th day of life	37.3±3.5	35.5±1.6	36.4±1.5	35.6±1.7
2nd day of life	43.8±3.1	47.7±2.0	45.9±1.8	46.0±1.5
28th day of life	56.3±2.5	58.1±2.6	56.7±2.5	57.5±2.1

Table 4. Postnatal development in the group receiving 100 mg/kg of zidovudine and Nikavir doses in the prenatal period (1-19 days of gestation).

Other parameters of the offspring development observed (hair covering, incisor eruption, opening of eyes, helix detachment, vagina opening, testicle descending, time of reflex maturation, etc.) were within the normal term limits for this animal species.

In conclusion it should be noted that daily intragastric administration of zidovudine and Nikavir in a once-daily dose of 100 mg/kg (a 12.5 multiple of the maximum daily doses for pregnant women) to pregnant rats from within 1-19 days of gestation was found to retard their body mass gain in the third trimester. A twice-daily dose of zidovudine (50+50 mg/kg) at 9 a.m. and 5 p.m. partly moderates its negative effect on the body mass gain.

A once-daily dose intragastric introduction of zidovudine and Nikavir as well as a twice-daily dose zidovudine (50+50 mg/kg) do not influence such embryotoxicity criteria as the duration of pregnancy, number of yellow bodies, number of alive fetuses, number of implantation places, embryo body mass, cranioclaudal size, as well as preimplantation and postimplantation death rate.

A single-dose intragastric 100 mg/kg zidovudine and Nikavir given within 1-19 days of gestation did not cause any malformations and developmental defects in the offspring. However, in the introduction of theses preparations in a daily intragastric dose of 100 mg/kg within 1-19 days of gestation both the decrease in the number of ossification centers and retardation of embryonic skeletal ossification were observed.

It was due to the effect of zidovudine and Nikavir that there were no ossification centers in the 2nd and 4th metacarpal bones, the 3rd and the 4th metatarsal bones, sublingual and pubic bones of the embryos. The noted changes were more marked in the embryos of the experimental group which received a once-daily dose of 100 mg/kg zidovudine in the perinatal period. Adverse effects reduced in a twice-daily dose introduction of zidovudine (50+50 mg/kg) and a once-daily intragastric 100 mg/kg dose of Nikavir.

During the observation period no further adverse influence of the tested agents on the following offspring development was noted. It was not accompanied by any term deviations and was within the normal time limits natural for the normal physiological development of this animal species.

Thus, studies on animal models have provided reliable evidence that compared to zidovudine Nikavir possesses a less damaging impact on fetal development and thus may be a more preferable choice for ART in HIV-infected pregnant women.

4. Experience of Nikavir use in various regiments of vertical HIV transmission chemoprophylaxis

The first experience of Nikavir use in different regiments of vertical HIV chemoprophylaxis was obtained by the staff workers of the Russian Federal AIDS Center (Detkova, 2003).

Three groups of 96 HIV-infected pregnant women were observed. Groups 1 and 2 received Nikavir in the dose of 200 mg/kg 3 times a day after 14 gestation weeks (within 16 to 36 weeks of gestation, the average time 25-27 weeks of gestation). Group 1 of 27 women were administered intravenous zidovudine in labour. Newborns were given oral zidovudine syrup (Retrovir) in the dose of 2 mg/kg body mass every 6 hours for 6 weeks. Group 2 (17 women) were given a single dose of 200 mg Viramun at the onset of labour. Newborns were given Viramun suspension in the dose of 2 mg/kg body mass once daily for 3 days. Group 3 included 52 women who did not receive chemoprevention. The only preventive measure was exclusion of breastfeeding.

A total of the women under observation delivered alive babied (27 newborns in group 1, 17 newborns in group 2 and 52 newborns in group 3). Body weight parameters of newborns given chemoprevention slightly surpassed those in group 3 though the difference was not significant (3022±223 and 2731±558 g respectively, $p=0.196$). The children were followed-up during 72 weeks. By 72 weeks 34.6% of group 3 were diagnosed HIV-infection (stable positive serological evidence HIV DNA in PCR). Children in group 1 were born healthy. Only one newborn in group 2 was diagnosed HIV which was possibly due to the continuous drug addiction of his mother and her inappropriate following the Nikavir regimen during pregnancy (adherence to preventive therapy was <60%).

Application of Nikavir in pregnancy showed its good tolerability. The major therapy-associated side-effect was a mild gastric syndrome found in 25% of women. Application of Nikavir aimed at prevention during pregnancy was not found to affect either the pregnancy course in HIV-infected pregnant women or maturation and vital capacity of newborns. No significant association between application of Nikavir as intrapartum prevention and both the pregnancy course in HIV-infected pregnant women and maturation and vital capacity of newborns was established.

A further clinical trial of efficiency and safety of chemoprevention with Nikavir in pregnant HIV-infected women was carried out at the Republican Clinical Infection Hospital (Izhora settlement, St. Petersburg) (unpublished data) as well as at Regional AIDS Centers in St. Petersburg (Zakharova, 2008) and Perm (Ivanova, 2010).

The clinical trial conducted at the Republican Clinical Infection Hospital in 2005-2006 involved 20 pregnant women aged 20-31 at 26-28 weeks of gestation with normal laboratory values.

Group 1 (10 women) was given 200 mg Nikavir 3 times daily. Their viral load <3000 copies/ml. Group 2 (10 women) was given 200 mg Nikavir 3 times daily + Epivir in conventional dosage. Their baseline viral load was 3000-30000 copies/ml.

Assessment of therapy was based on registration of clinical and laboratory indicators of HIV progress.

Nikavir therapy demonstrated good tolerance (100% of patients have finished research). No severe adverse events were observed. There were only 2 associated with therapy registered cases of moderate abdominal pain which did not require its cessation. No deviations in laboratory findings were noted.

The end of Nikavir therapy was followed by elevation of the mean CD4 lymphocyte counts. Of note, before delivery 50% of women were referred to a higher immunological category. Such elevation tendency persisted until the end of the investigation.

There was a marked reduction of viral load noted in the process of therapy. In 4 weeks of treatment the level of viral load reduced below the level of detection in 60% of women in both groups and in 90% before the delivery but it was less than 1000 copies/ml.

No cases of perinatal HIV transmission were registered.

Thus Nikavir appears to be a highly efficient agent for treatment of HIV-infected pregnant women as its effect has been confirmed by the obtained clinical and immunological evidence.

A clinical Nikavir trial at St. Petersburg Regional AIDS Center involved 30 pregnant women aged 20-35 years (mean age 26 years) at 14-34 weeks of gestation and infection term from 1 to 6 years. 36.6% of examined women presented with a history of drug addiction and 50% chronic hepatitis C. A total of patients did not receive anti-retroviral preparations.

In accordance with the baseline viral load 23 patients were administered Nikavir as a monotherapy and 7 patients received dual therapy.

In a monotherapy schedule Nikavir was given in a dosage of 200 mg in 3 doses. In combined dual therapy Nikavir was supplemented with Epivir in a daily dosage of 150 mg in 2 doses. In accordance with the Russian Federation standards at the onset of labour the women were given intravenous zidovudine. Newborns received an extended therapy with zidovudine in syrup (Retrovir) for 6 weeks following the delivery.

The pretreatment viral load in the majority of women (67%) did not exceed 10000 copies/ml. By the 4th week the total of the group demonstrated a significant reduction of viral load indices ($p<0.05$). At 28 weeks of gestation the total number of patients with undetectable optimal level of viral load was 33%. At 36 weeks the reduction tendency was stable. In the following postpartum period HIV RNA levels did not exceed the baseline indices (Table 5).

Observation time	Viral load levels				
	<400 copies/ml	400-1000 copies/ml	1000-10000 copies/ml	10000-50000 copies/ml	>50000 copies/ml
Pretreatment, patients	3 (10%)	1 (3%)	19 (67%)	3 (10%)	3 (10%)
After 4 weeks of therapy, patients	9 (37%)	3 (13%)	9 (37%)	2 (9%)	0
28 weeks of gestation, patients	8 (35%)	2 (9%)	11 (47%)	2 (9%)	0
36 weeks of gestation, patients	7 (37%)	4 (21%)	8 (42%)	0	0
1 month postpartum, patients	2 (11%)	0	13 (68%)	4 (21%)	0
3 months postpartum, patients	2 (10%)	4 (20%)	13 (65%)	0	1 (5%)
6 months postpartum, patients	3 (16%)	2 (11%)	10 (52%)	4 (21%)	0

Table 5. The intra-treatment dynamics of viral load in pregnant women.

Patients with viral load over 10000 copies/ml received the dual therapy (Nikavir+Epivir). Already by the 4th week of therapy the viral load in half of the patients reduced to the undetectable level and remained at that level till 36 weeks of gestation. The same was true about the patient who was transferred from the monotherapy group due to the increase of her viral load above 10000 copies/ml.

Starting with the 4th week of treatment an overall significant increase of the mean values of the percentile CD4 lymphocytes indices irrespective of the drug intake regimen was noted. After discontinuation of treatment CD4 lymphocytes indices returned to the baseline.

The mean Hb values did not exceed the norms before initiation of therapy (117 g/l). It was noted that mean Hb values decreased during chemoprophylaxis. Hb decrease lower 100 g/l was improved with administration of iron-containing preparations. By 36 weeks of gestation mean Hb values were not different from baseline (Table 6).

Hemoglobin	Observation time			
	Pretreatment	Post 4 weeks of treatment	28 week of gestation	36 week of gestation
Mean value, g/liter	116.5±9.2	106.3±8.5	107.9±7.3	114.9±8.1
Minimal value, g/liter	89	91	86	96
Maximal value, g/liter	150	130	128	140
< 100 g/liter, patients	3 (10%)	12 (40%)	6 (20%)	2 (7%)
>100 g/liter, patients	27 (90%)	18 (60%)	24 (80%)	26 (93%)

Table 6. Hb level in Nikavir treatment of pregnant women.

The controllable biochemical blood serum values did not correlate with the therapeutic regimen and did not deviate from the normal during the whole observation time.

Proper adherence to therapy was associated with good tolerance of the applied regimens.

In the majority of patients the labour course and the delivery methods did not differ from those in the average population.

Viral load monitoring findings in children provided by the attending pediatricians confirmed the absence of HIV-1 virus in 100% of newborns at three examinations during a 6 months period.

Thus, the obtained findings allow considering Nikavir one of the most perspective agents for the practice of perinatal prophylaxis of vertical transmission of HIV-1 virus. However, a continuous monitoring of Hb levels and viral load for the prompt correction of the switch regimen from monotherapy to combination (dual) therapy as well as an additional administration of iron-containing preparations is necessary.

The clinical trial conducted at Perm Regional AIDS Center involved 38 HIV infected and their 38 newborns. Group 1 (20 women, aged 18-30) was given Nikavir+Epivir therapy. Group 2 (18 women aged 19-32) was given one the HAART regimens (Nikavir+Epivir+Viramun or Kaletra). The total of patients on chemoprevention schedule did not take the agents previously. The therapy was started at 23-32 weeks of gestation depending on the time of their first visit.

During the first hour of labor a dose of 2 mg/kg/h of zidovudine was given intravenously followed by 1 mg/kg/h until the end of the labor. Starting with the 8th hour of life the newborns were given of zidovudine in syrup (Retrovir) in an oral dose of 2 mg/kg every 6 hours during 6 weeks.

45% women in group 1 and 44% women in group 2 had transvaginal delivery. Pre-term delivery was registered in 2 women - 1 from each group at 32 and 34 weeks of gestation respectively. There were no cases of intrapartum complications and breast-feeding.
Prior to chemoprophylaxis a total of group 1 women were clinically diagnosed the stage A1 HIV infection. Half of group 2 women were diagnosed the stage B1 HIV infection associated with oral candidiasis and grade 1 anemia. On clinical examination of both groups performed 1.5 months after delivery no progression of HIV was revealed. The structure of associated diseases included viral hepatitis C in 45% and 60% of women from group 1 and group 2 respectively. Chlamydial infection was identified in 5% of women in group 1.
Prior chemoprophylaxis the baseline viral load in group 1 women ranged from 500 to 382000 copies/ml (mean 8280); 4 weeks after the start of chemoprevention it dropped by 6 times to 886; it was undetectable at 36 weeks of gestation (<500 copies/ml). The pretreatment baseline mean CD4 lymphocytes count was 478 cells/mm^3 and 545 cells/mm^3 before delivery (Fig. 2).
The baseline viral load in group 2 women was >200 000 copies/ml, 4 weeks after the start of chemoprevention it dropped by about 300 times. Prepartum viral load was undetectable (<500 copies/ml) and 1.5 months after delivery with discontinuation of treatment it increased to over 20000 copies/ml. The pretreatment baseline mean CD4 lymphocytes count was twice lower compared with group 1; after 4 weeks of HAART and before delivery it increased and insignificantly lowered 1.5 month postpartum when treatment was discontinued. Therefore, following the discontinuation of HAART in group 2 viral load parameters increased while CD4 lymphocytes count decreased.

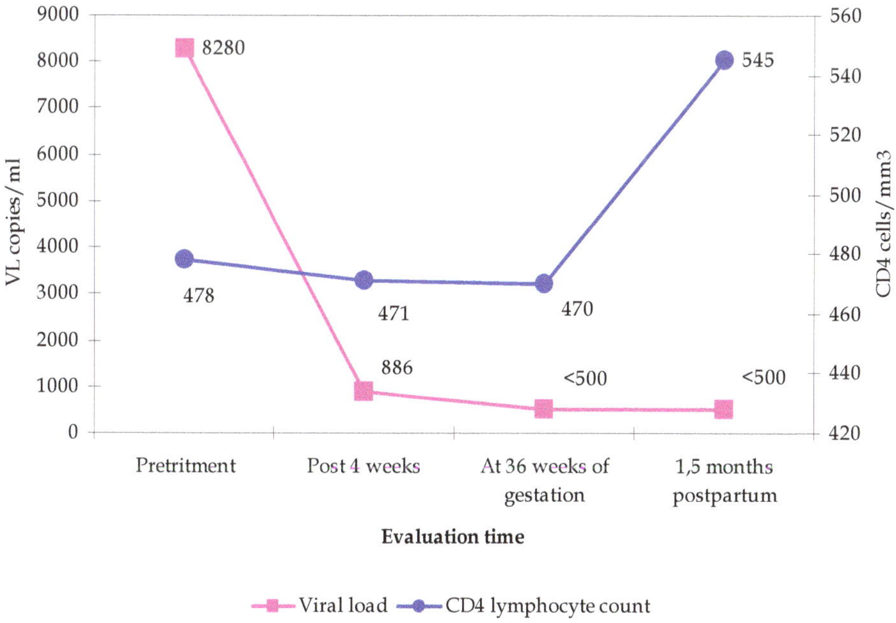

Fig. 2. Parameters of viral load and CD4 lymphocytes at various terms of examination of women administered Nikavir+Epivir.

The total of children born to HIV-infected mothers was referred to the category of risk with diagnosed perinatal HIV infection contact and was examined for the presence of HIV-1 DNA. The obtained results were negative.

The agents proved an appropriate tolerance in both therapeutic regimens. No significant side effects and adverse events associated with the tested agents were noted. The parameters of vital capacity were in compliance with the normal natural course of pregnancy. The haemogram analysis was performed to predict the possible side effects of chemoprevention. In this connection it was found that at the time of conception both red blood cell counts and white blood cell counts were normal. In both groups the Hb level was insignificantly decreased: 101 g/l in group 1 and 106 g/l in 17% of group 2 respectively. 4 weeks after the start of therapy and at 36 weeks of gestation no changes in the parameters of peripheral blood were noted ($p>0.05$). The total of women received the preventive therapy of anemia including the diet and iron-containing preparations in conventional doses. By 36 weeks of gestation a tendency of thrombocyte count elevation was observed - 297.9 and 271.8 g/l respectively. At different terms the findings of the functional liver tests (ALT, AST, bilirubin) were within the normal limits in both groups.

Thus, absence of HIV-1 infection in children born to HIV-infected pregnant women testifies high efficiency of both chemoprevention regimens with Nikavir both in combination with Epivir and in HAART. An evident positive outcome of this therapy is confirmed by the significant decrease of viral load to undetectable level of viral RNA during therapy starting with the 4th week of gestation up to delivery. Simultaneous elevation of CD4 lymphocytes is undoubtedly an evidence of beneficial effect of both regimens of chemoprevention on the immune status of HIV-infected pregnant women. Excellent adherence to chemoprevention therapy (100%) was associated with good tolerance of the employed agents. The safety of Nikavir application both in combination with Epivir and in HAART schedule was proved by the absence of toxic effect on biochemical blood values at various gestation terms. An insignificant elevation of thrombocyte count by 36 weeks of gestation in both groups may be regarded as a physiological factor preparing the organism of a woman to delivery.

The obtained results allow to regard Nikavir to be one of the most potent perspective agents used in the schedules of chemoprevention of vertical transmission of HIV-1infection.

5. Comparative characteristics of methods of perinatal chemoprophylaxis with Nikavir

5.1 Actuality

Currently, the choice of available antiretroviral agents for chemoprevention of perinatal infection is not extensive. The standard schedules of HAART are widely used. A number of various prevention patterns based on the expert opinion, theoretical research and evidence of preclinical animal studies has been suggested. However, substantiation of choice of methods of chemoprevention of perinatal HIV infection, efficiency and safety of different preparations and their side-effect estimation have not been sufficiently investigated.

Thus, method of chemoprophylaxis of vertical transmission of HIV-1 with Nikavir+Epivir in HAART schedule which is known to produce less side-effects compared to the analogue schedules with Combivir is becoming actual.

The present investigation was performed in June 2007 - October 2008 in the setting of Perm Regional AIDS Center and is based on the analysis of epidemiology data as well as the evidence from clinical and laboratory studies.

5.2 Adherence to HAART for perinatal prevention in HIV infected pregnant women

An important factor of the prevention of the perinatal transmission of HIV virus is the formation of an adherence to persistent intake of antiretroviral preparations.

With the aim of the analysis of the adherence to chemoprevention two groups of patients with the past history of intravenous psycho-active agents were suggested a self-completed questionnaire. The group 1 included 31 women who had not been administered chemoprevention therapy due to the early gestation term. The group 2 contained 23 women undergoing HAART. The age in both groups was 18-25 years.

The answers to the question on the time of registration their pregnancy at the women consultation center were as follows: 45.2% in the group 1 and 30.4% in the group 2 were registered at the term before 12 weeks of gestation. Thus, the majority of the respondents delayed their visit to their gynecologist for registration of their pregnancy for later than 12 weeks of gestation (54.8% and 69.4% respectively).Their attendance of gynecological check-ups was self-assessed as neither regular nor frequent by 22.6% of respondents in group 1 and 17.4% in group 2. 77.4% attended gynecologist at the women consultation center but only 64.5% attended the HIV/AIDS Prevention Center.

It is worth noting the fact that before starting chemoprophylaxis almost 30% of woman did not visit gynecologist regularly and 9% missed such visits during the antiviral therapy.

A considerable part of pregnant women (80.6% and 73.9% respectively) strictly followed the administrations of their doctors while the others neglected the professional advice. Thus, 3% of women in group 1 and 6% in group 2 have taken responsibility to decide themselves which of the doctor's recommendations they are to follow. And 16.2% noted that prior chemoprophylaxis they underwent only those examinations which considered being necessary. However, with the beginning of antiretroviral therapy women become more responsible and underwent all the administered examinations.

The majority of women in both groups consider the ultimate goal of chemotherapy to be the birth of a healthy child (83.6% and 95.6% respectively).

45.3% of women did not express apprehension of chemoprevention and revealed an adequately positive attitude to it. The investigation analyzed persistent detrimental habits in pregnant HIV infected women which they could not abandon even being pregnant. About half of them smoked (45.1% and 43.5% respectively) and 3.2% women of group 1 took alcohol. 2 patients of group 1 (6.4%) gave a negative answer to the question about the influence of irregular and incorrect intake of antiretroviral preparations on the therapeutic effect.

A considerable number of pregnant women strictly followed recommendations of their doctors (80.6% and 73.9% respectively) while others neglect certain administrations on diet (34.7% and 54.6% respectively).

In summary, investigation of adherence to perinatal chemoprevention in HIV infected pregnant women demonstrated high level of motivation aimed at birth of a healthy child. However, along with following the therapeutic regimen their specialist check-up visiting was neither regular nor timely. The majority of women kept to their harmful habits (smocking) and did not follow recommendations on their diet which was possibly due to their low social status. Consequently, every third pregnant woman before administration of chemoprevention and every second woman during chemoprevention did not attend their obstetricians and gynecologists regularly. In this connection one should note the necessity of organization of School of Adherence to Chemoprevention which can provide social-psychological counseling aimed at formation of positive motivation to doctor's recommendations, following the daily regimen and regular intake of antiretroviral preparations as well as refuse of detrimental habits which is of a particular importance for pregnant drug-addicts.

5.3 Purpose

- to study efficiency of Nikavir in combination with Epivir and Kaletra in chemoprophylaxis of perinatal transmission of HIV-1 infection on the basis of the RNA HIV-1 plasma parameters and the estimated number of children with negative quality PCR reaction for DNA HIV-1 at the age of 1.5 months and 3 months;
- to provide a comparative evaluation of safety and tolerability of Nikavir and Combivir in the HAART chemoprevention schedule in HIV infected pregnant women.

5.4 Materials

The start of antiretroviral prevention was determined by the time of the first appointment with a gynecologist for pregnancy diagnosis. Chemoprevention of vertical HIV mother-to-child virus transmission with various agents was performed in 36 women with A1 (62%) and B2 (38%) HIV stage (USA, CDC, 1987) at 23-32 gestation weeks as well as their 36 newborns. B2 stage manifested with moderate symptoms of oral mucosa candidiasis. 65% of observation group were diagnosed anemia mild to moderate degrees. No intrapartum complications occurred. There were no cases of breast-feeding.

The group 1 included 18 pregnant HIV infected women aged 19-32 (mean age 24 years) receiving Nikavir+Epivir+Kaletra chemoprevention. The group 2 included 18 women aged 19-28 (mean age 23.5 years) receiving Combivir+Kaletra chemoprevention. From the 28th week of gestation until the delivery they received Nikavir administered in the dosage of 600 vg for 3 intakes daily. Combivir and Kaletra were given in standard schedule.

During the first hour of labor 2 mg/kg/h of zidovudine were given intravenously followed by 1 mg/kg/h until the end of the labor.

Starting with the 8th hour of life the newborn babies were given a 6 weeks course of zidovudine in syrup (Retrovir) in the dosage of 2 mg/kg every 6 hours.

Epidemiological analysis of the routes of infection revealed the leading share of sexual HIV-1 transmission: 83% of pregnant women in Nikavir chemoprevention schedule group 1 and 89% in group 2. Parenteral route was revealed in 17% and 11% of cases respectively. Thus, there was a mixed type of epidemic process, the sexual transmission rate 5-8 times surpassing the parenteral one (cases of intravenous drugs).

5.5 Methods

The evaluation of the results of the investigation was based on analysis of the clinical, epidemiological and laboratory monitoring of HIV infection course in pregnant women and their newborns.

Manifestations of HIV epidemic process were studied according to the following criteria:

- identification of the routes of HIV infection of pregnant women;
- estimination of the HIV infection risk factors for newborn children (analysis of delivery methods, chemoprevention schedules, cases of breast feeding).

Clinical assessment included evaluation of HIV manifestations in pregnant women before chemoprevention, 4 weeks after its start, before delivery at 36 weeks of gestation and 1.5

month after delivery. At the same terms the patients were examined by different specialists to register HIV associated diseases and adverse effects of therapy. Women were examined by infectionists, gynecologists, obstetricians, immunologists, etc. and the newborns by neonatologists, infectionists, pediatricians and other specialists according to indications.

The HIV diagnosis in women was based on enzyme immunoassay (EIA) detecting HIV antibodies ("Jenscreen Ulra HIV Ag/At") and immunoblot analysis (IMB) ("Blot-HIV") for HIV-1 virus specific proteins antibodies. HIV diagnosis in newborns was excluded on the basis of EIA and IMB monitoring during the period of observation starting at birth and thereafter at the age of 1.5 and 3 months.

Laboratory examination included leucocyte and thrombocyte counts performed with MEK-7222 hemoanalyzer and standard urinalyses. Biochemical blood values were identified with Conelab, 20 automated analyzer supplied with ion selection section for evaluation of the functional state of the liver and kidneys. The studied parameters were compared with the standards established for Perm.

The associated diseases of HIV infected pregnant women were revealed with serological IMB tests for HBsAg, hepatitis C virus, herpes simplex, cytomegalovirus, toxoplasmosis, chlamydia and Wassermann test.

Instrumental methods included ECG, ultrasonic examination abdominal and pelvic organs if indicated.

Cellular immunity in pregnant HIV infected women was assessed by the absolute and percentage levels of CD4 lymphocyte subpopulation with monoclonal antibodies ("Beston Diskinzon" USA) at "FACS Caliber" cytofluorimeter by flow cytometer method. The obtained findings were compared with the norms established by the Russian Federal AIDS Center (Pokrovsky, 2001).

Molecule-biological diagnosis in pregnant HIV infected women receiving chemoprevention was based on the detection of HIV-1 RNA plasma levels with polymerase chain reaction (PCR) and "Amplisensy HIV-monitor FRT" test-systems ("Interlabservice") before antiretroviral therapy, 4 weeks after it was started, 4 weeks before the supposed delivery term and 1.5 month after delivery.

For the early diagnosis of HIV in newborns detection of HIV-1 DNA plasma levels with PCR and "Amplisense DNA HIV-96" test-systems ("Interlabservice") was carried out. They were performed two tests at the age of 1.5 and 3 months.

Adherence to antiretroviral perinatal prevention regimen in pregnant HIV infected women was studied with the questionnaire method assessing their social profile, clinical and laboratory examinations, intake of preparations and attitude to chemoprevention.

From 28 week of gestation until the delivery they received Nikavir administered in the dosage of 600 mg for 3 intakes daily. Combivir and Kaletra were given in conventional doses. During the first hour of labor 2 mg/kg/h of zidovudine were given intravenously followed by 1 mg/kg/h within the labor.

Starting with their eighth hour of life the newborn babies were given a 6 weeks course of zidovudine in syrup (Retrovir) orally in the dose of 2 mg/kg every 6 hours.

5.6 Statistical analysis

The overall data of pregnant HIV infected women receiving the targeted agents in therapeutic doses have been statistically assessed. Descriptive and frequency ratio analyses of the total adverse events revealed within the investigation period have been performed.

In considering antiretroviral efficiency the data of the number (index) of women with RNA HIV-1 levels lower than 500 cells/ml blood serum (test-system sensitivity rate) were analyzed.
The number of DNA HIV-1 negative children aged 1.5 and 3 months has been assumed to be the paramount index of antiretroviral efficiency. Safety was assessed using the mean indices of clinical and laboratory control.

5.7 Results

5.7.1 Clinical examination; evaluation of side effects

Tolerance of therapeutic schedules proved to be satisfactory. No marked therapy-related side effects and adverse events were revealed. Vital indices corresponded to physiological course of pregnancy.
No signs of HIV progress were noted on the clinical evaluation of women in both groups performed 1.5 month after delivery.
Parameters of side effects of chemoprevention were analyzed within the on-going clinical observation considering hemoglobin levels, erythrocyte, thrombocyte and leucocyte count values at the established terms.
Pregnancy in group 1 women was associated with the concurrent anemia grade 1-2 (mean Hb 101 g/l) while women in group 2 had normal red blood values (mean Hb 114 g/l). Following a 4 week intake of preparations hemoglobin level decreased to 109 g/l (Fig. 3).

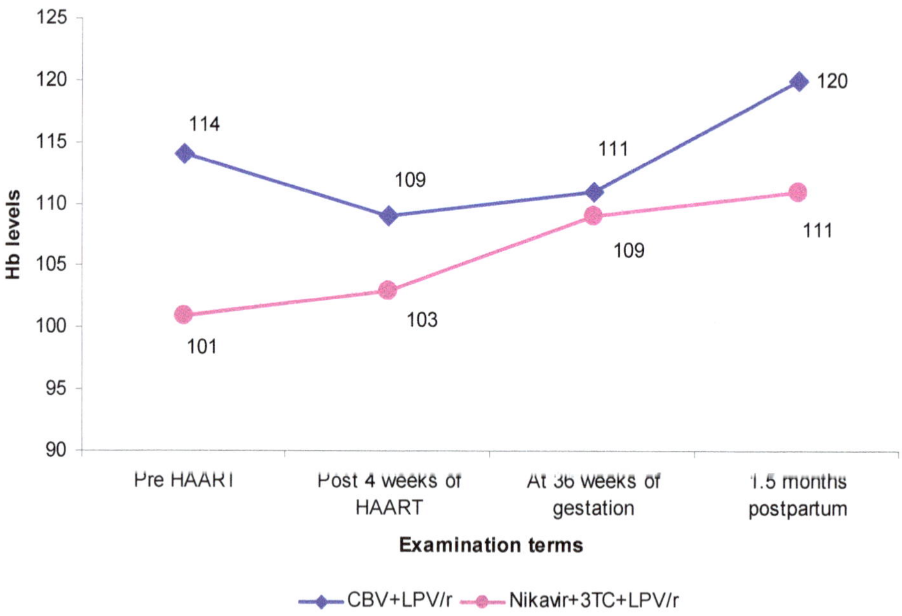

Fig. 3. Dynamics of Hb levels in pregnant HIV-infected women.

Erythrocyte count level parameters prior chemoprevention was $3.5x10^{12}/l$ and $3.9x10^{12}/l$ in group 1 and 2 respectively. After 4 weeks of therapy and at 36 weeks of gestation a certain decrease of this parameter in group 2 women was noted (Fig. 4).

In both groups no thrombopenia was noted before initiation, during and after chemoprevention (Fig. 5).
During pregnancy the leucocyte formula values were within the normal limits in women of both groups (Fig. 6).
Thus, 4 weeks after the start of therapy and at 36 weeks of gestation there was no significant decrease in the peripheral blood parameters. The total of women underwent anemia preventive treatment with diet and preparations of iron in the standard daily dosing schedule.
In both groups no statistically significant difference in functional liver test values (ALT, AST, bilirubin) at different terms of pregnancy was found.

5.7.2 Immunological and virological evaluation of chemoprevention schedules efficiency

Assessment of chemoprevention efficiency t was based on HIV-1 RNA viral load level and the CD4 lymphocyte count before antiretroviral therapy, 4 weeks after its start, at 36 weeks of gestation and 1.5 month after delivery.
At the beginning of treatment CD4 lymphocytes values were 1.5 times lower in group 1 patients (259 and 376 cells/mm^3 consequently). With the concurrent chemoprevention there was an almost double increase in group 1 prepartum CD4 lymphocytes levels (by 1.93 times) and that by 1.3 times in group 2 compared to the baseline values. After interruption of therapy in group 1 (1.5 month after deliver) CD4 lymphocytes count decreased to 321 cells/mm^3 (Fig. 7).

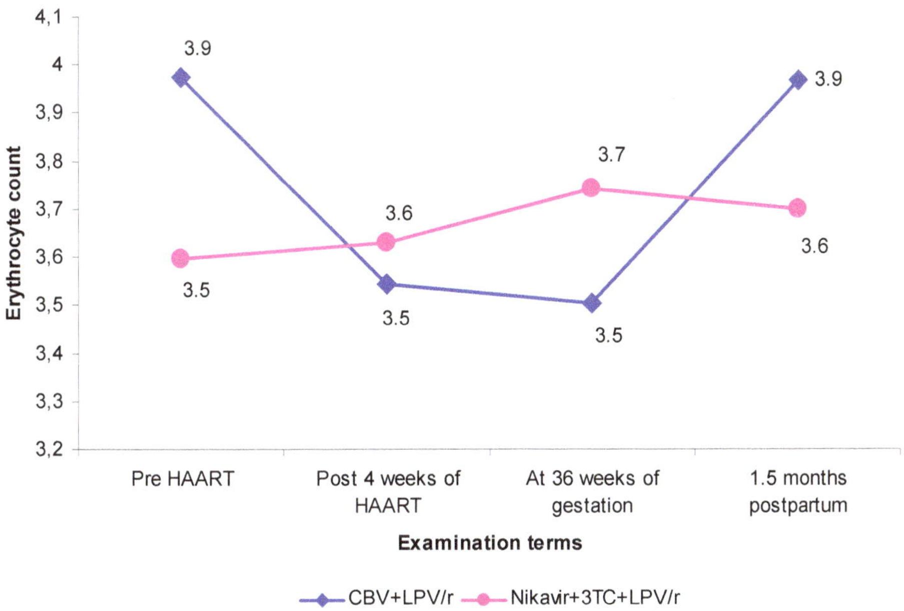

Fig. 4. Erythrocyte values in pregnant HIV-infected women.

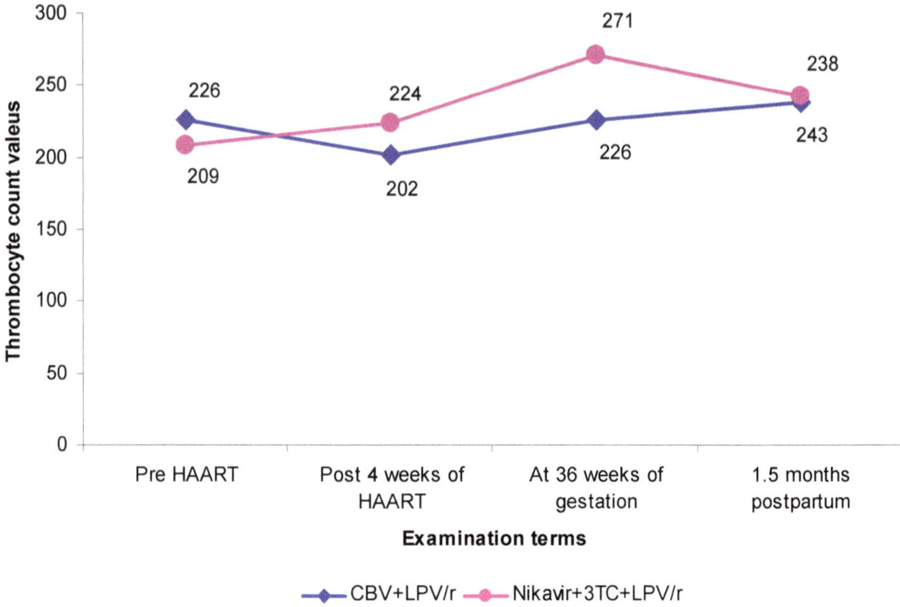

Fig. 5. Thrombocyte count values in pregnant women.

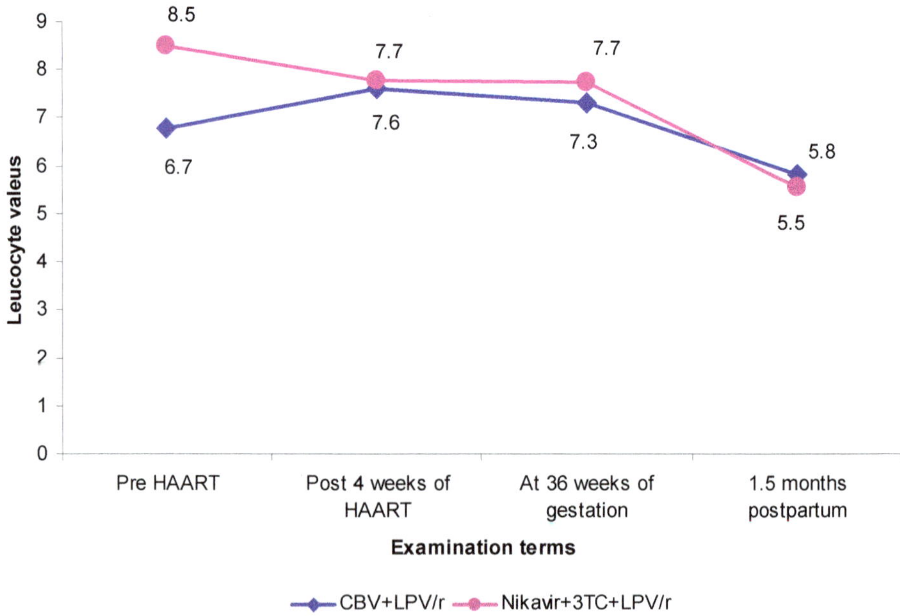

Fig. 6. Leucocyte values in pregnant HIV-infected women.

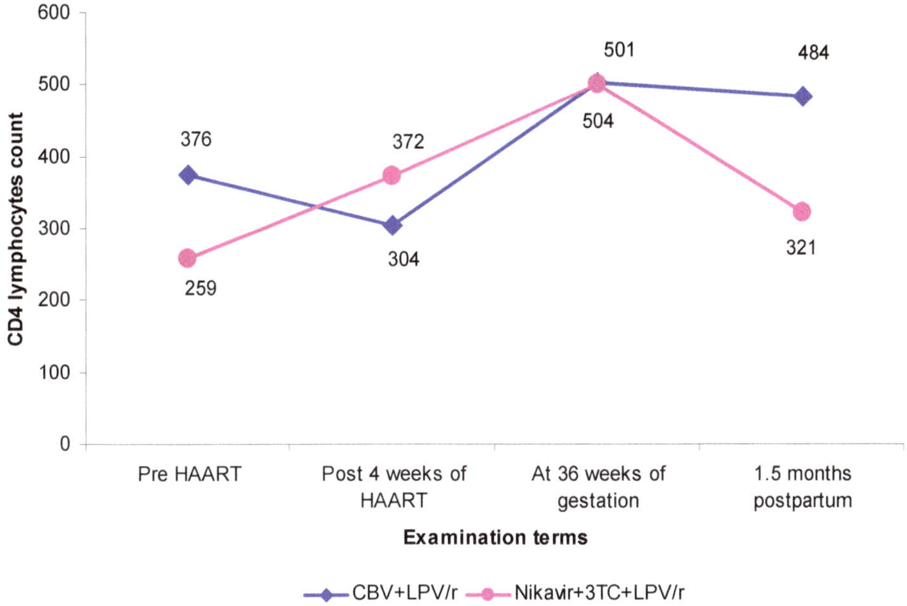

Fig. 7. CD4 lymphocytes profile in pregnant women.

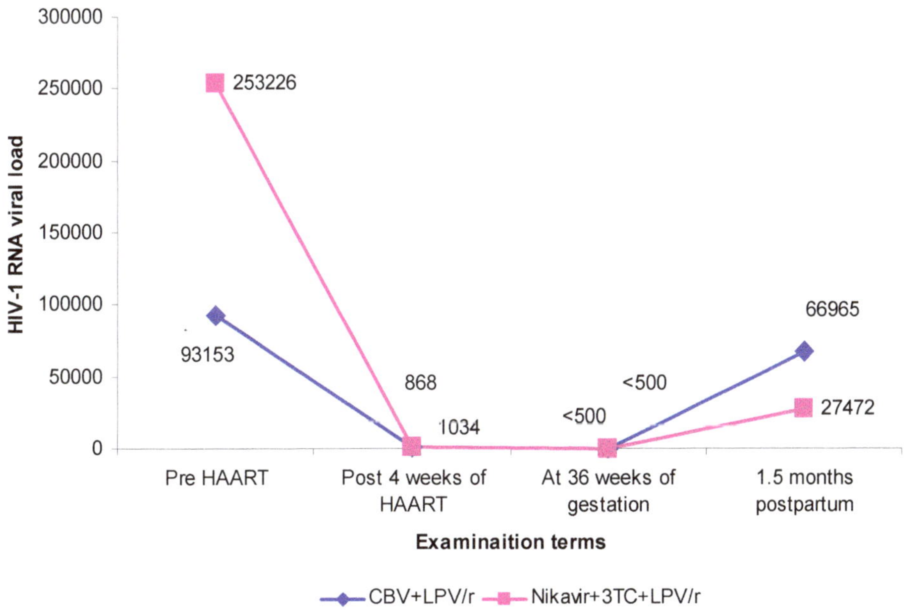

Fig. 8. Viral load profile in pregnant women.

The baseline HIV-1 RNA viral load in group 1 was 253226 copies/ml of blood; 4 weeks after the start of chemoprevention it dropped by 293 times (3 lg_{10}); it was undetectable before delivery while 1.5 month after interruption it increased to 27472 copies. At the beginning of chemoprevention HIV-1 RNA viral load in group 2 ranged between 8010 and 1 930000 copies/ml (mean 93153), it dropped to undetectable level before delivery (<500 copies/ml) and remained unchanged till delivery (Fig. 8).

5.7.3 Assessment of HIVchemoprophylaxis efficiency in newborns

Efficiency assessment of chemoprevention of mother-to-child transmission of HIV infection in both groups was based on exclusion of HIV in newborns with perinatal HIV contact aged 1.5 and 3 months. All children of HIV-infected mothers were assigned to the risk category with the diagnosis of perinatal HIV contact and were examined for the presence of HIV-1 DNA using PCR at the above mentioned terms. There were no positive results.

According to the current regulations children of HIV-infected mothers are to be followed-up till the age of 18 months. At present they are under the on-going observation.

5.8 Summary

Negative HIV-1 test in 100% of 3 months children born from HIV mothers is a reliable proof of a high efficiency of applied HAART schedules aimed at perinatal chemoprevention.

Efficiency of HAART schedules in vertical HIV transmission both with Nikavir+Epivir+Kaletra and combivir+Kaletra was confirmed by a significant stable decrease of viral load from the 4th week of gestation until delivery.

Increase of CD4 lymphocyte parameters in the time of chemoprevention is the evidence of the positive effect of such therapy schedules on the immune status of pregnant HIV-infected women.

A considerably high degree of adherence to chemoprevention was associated with good tolerability of the applied schedules.

Safety of HAART schedules was proved by the absence of toxic outcomes in biochemical indices in pregnant HIV-infected women at different terms of pregnancy.

However, application of Combivir+Kaletra schedule revealed the tendency to the decrease of red blood parameters (hemoglobin and erythrocytes) and thrombocytes at the 4th week of therapy and before delivery.

In HAART schedule with Nikavir+Epivir+Kaletra no decrease of hemoglobin, erythrocytes and thrombocytes counts at the fourth week of therapy and before delivery was revealed.

6. Conclusion

Despite the rapid development of chemoprophylaxis of HIV infection for as many as almost 30 years the range of ART preparations used currently is limited. The most widely applied agent is zidovudine though its major recognized side effect is still hemotoxicity (in the first place anemia). As in this respect Nikavir appears to be a considerably more advantageous component of chemoprophylaxis of HIV vertical transmission comparing to zidovudine its application seems to be extremely beneficial. The above mentioned positive data on successful replacement of zidovudine in cases of its intolerance (namely, anemia cases) with Nikavir makes it the preparation of choice. Besides, there is a reported evidence from the previous comparative Nikavir - zidovudine studies of a better tolerance of Nikavir in prevention of parenteral transmission of HIV (Ivanova, 2007).

Low toxicity and good tolerance of Nikavir open up new perspectives for its therapeutic application in HIV patients suffering from chronic liver diseases (Kvartchenko, 2006).
Finally, some recent studies have reported on the successful application of Nikavir in the treatment of coinfections: HIV+ hepatitis C (Gankina, 2010), HIV + tuberculosis (Panteleyev, 2010). Treatment of such categories of patients is an extremely challenging task of paramount importance. At present several on-going intensive studies continue to investigate potentials of Nikavir in the treatment of coinfections.

7. Acknowledgements

We would like to express our gratitude to the head doctor of Perm Regional AIDS Center, merited doctor of the Russian Federation K. Khafizov for providing an opportunity to conduct our research on the basis of his center.
We would also thank pediatricians, obstetricians, gynecologists and all our colleagues who contributed to our research.
We express our gratitude to the head of the diagnostic laboratory of Perm Center for Eradication and Prevention of AIDS and Infectious Diseases S. Zverev.
Also we are grateful to Alexander Kononov (the General Director of Joint-Stock Company «Association AZT») for the presented materials on stories of creation of a preparation of Nikavir and results of comparative studying embryotoxicity and teratogenicity Nikavir and zidovudine.

8. References

Detkova N. (2003). Chemoprevention of mother-to-child HIV transmission. *Authorized reference work of dissertation of candidate of medical sciences*, Moscow.

Detkova N., Sokolova E., Bobkova M., et al. (2003). Nevirapin (viramun) - an agent for prevention of mother-to-child transmission of HIV. *Epidemiology and Infectious Diseases*, N 6, p. 55-57.

Galegov G. (2004). Nikavir (phosphazide) as an antiretroviral agent: antiHIV efficiency, toxicology, pharmacology and certain perspectives of its clinical application. *Atibiotics and Chemotherapy*, v. 49, N7, p. 3-8.

Galegov G., Korneeva M., Nosyik D., et al. (1988).Azidothymidine and some of its analogues as inhibitors of HIV production. *Molecular Biology*, v. 2, p. 802-806.

Gankina N., Kravchenko A., Kuimova U., et al. (2010).Nucleoside inhibitors in ART schedules of HIV and chronic hepatitis C. *Infectious Diseases*, N 1, p. 14-18.

Ivanova E., et al. (2006). Clinical and immunological features of HIV infection in pregnant women. The 7th Russia Congress of Infectionists on New technologies in diagnosis and prevention of infectious diseases, Abstract Book, Nizhny Novgorod, p. 115.

Ivanova E., Vorobeva N. (2009). Nikavir in perinatal chemoprophylaxis. The IV (XIII) International Scientific Conference Oncology - the 21st century, Hoschimin, Viet-Nam, p. 88-91.

Ivanova E., Vorobeva N., Krasnopyerova N., et al. (2007). Prevention of HIV infection in medical personnel. Scientific Session, Perm, p. 110-112.

Ivanova E., Shapiro A., Martsenyuk M., et al. (2007). Adherence to chemoprophylaxis in pregnant HIV-infected women. AIDS, *Cancer and Public Health Russia Journal*, v. 11, N1, p. 65-67.

Ivanova E., Shmagel N., Vorobeva N., et al. (2009). Efficiency and safety of nikavir in the HIV vertical transmission. The III Conference on HIV/AIDS in the East Europe and Central Asia, Abstract Book, Moscow, v. 1, p. 59-60.

Ivanova E., Shmagel N., Vorobeva N., et al. (2010). Application of nikavir in perinatal chemoprophylaxis. The XII Russia National Congress. *Man and Medicine*, Moscow, p. 341.

Ivanova E., Shmagel N., Vorobeva N., et al. (2010). Nikavir in the chemoprevention regiment of vertical HIV transmission. *Virology Issues* , v. 55., N 2, p. 31-34.

Ivanova E., Shmagel N., Vorobeva N., et al. (2010). Phosphazide as an agent of combined therapy in perinatal HIV chemoprophylaxis. *Russia Immunology Journal*, v. 4 (13), N 4, p. 433.

Khandazhinskaya A., Matyugina E., Shirokova E. (2010). Anti-HIV therapy with AZT prodrugs: AZT phosphonate derivatives, current state and prospects, Expert Opin. *Drug Metab. Toxicol.*, Vol. 6, p. 1-14.

Kravchenko A. (2004). Application of nikavir in ART. Department of Medicine, N2 (10), pp.90-92, 166-172.

Kravchenko A., Gankina N. (2006). Efficiency and safely of phosphazide in circuit oh HAART in HIV-infected treatment-naïve patient, 8 International Congress on drug therapy in HIV-infection, Glasgow, UK, Abstr. P395.

Kravchenko A., Salamov G., Bogoslovskaya E., et al. (2001). A triple combined antiretroviral therapy with the use of HIV reverse transcriptase inhibitors. Epidemiology and Infectious diseases, № 4, p. 32-35.

Kravchenko A., Sitdyikova U., Serebrovskaya L., et al. (2003). Combined antiretroviral therapy of HIV-infected patients with the use of "strengthened" HIV protease inhibitors. *Infectious Diseases*, v. 1, N 1, p. 14-19.

Krayevsky A., Tarussova N., Zhu Q., et al. (1992). 5′-Hydrogenphosphonates and 5′-methylphosphonates of sugar modified pyrimidine nucleosides as potential anti-HIV-1 agents. *Nucleosides & Nucleotides*, Vol. 11(2-4), p. 177-196.

Machado J., Tsoukas C., Salomon H., et al. (1999). Antiviral activity and resistance profile of phosphazid - a novel prodrug of AZT, 6th Conference on Retrovirus and Opportunistic Infections, Chicago, USA.

On the approval of the instructing regulations on prevention of mother-to-child HIV transmission and the form of written informed concent for HIV chemoprevention. Order of RF Ministry for Public Health N 606 from 19.12.2003.

Pantelyeev A., Goliusova M., Kabanova V. (2010). Results of phosphazide (Nikavir) application in HIV patients with tuberculosis. *HIV and Immunosuppression*, N 2, p. 75-79.

Pokrovsky V.,Yurin O., Belyaeva V., et al. (2001). Clinical diagnosis and treatment of HIV infection. Practical quid for students, interns, residents and doctors of all specialties.Moscow, RF Ministry for Public Health Higher Education Scientific Medical Center, p.92.

Segeda S., Turbina G., Sokolova O. (2006). Prevention of the intrauterine fetal infection with agents of opportunistic infections in HIV patients. Conference on HIV/AIDS in the Eastern Europe and Central Asia, Moscow, p.137.

Selimova L., Krayevsky A., Galegov G. (1999). Recombination of phosphazide and kriksivan inhibits HIV-1 strain replication resistant to azidotimidin. *Academy of Sciences Reports*, v. 369, N 6, p. 847-849.

Skoblov Y., Karpenko I., Shirokova E., et al. (2004). Intracellular metabolism and pharmacokinetics of 5′-hydrogenphosphonate of 3′-azido-2′,3′-dideoxythymidine. *Antiviral Research*, Vol. 63(2), p. 107-113.

Tarusova N., Krayevsky A., Korneeva M., et al. (1989). Reduction of HIV reproduction in cell culture with 5′-phosphonates of 3′-azido-2′,3′-dideoxynucleosides. *Molecular Biology*, v. 23, p.1716-1723.

Tarussova N., Krayevsky A., Korneyeva M., et al. (1990). New phosphonate derivatives of nucleosides analogues as anti-HIV agents. *Coll. Czech. Chem. Commun.*, Vol. 55, p. 133-136.

Tarussova N., Kukhanova M., Krayevsky A., et al. (1991). Inhibition of Human Immunodeficiency Virus (HIV) production by 5′-hydrogenphosphonates of 3′-azido-2′,3′-dideoxynucleosides. *Nucleosides & Nucleotides*, Vol. 10 (1-3), p. 351-354.

Terentyeva Zh., Voronin E. (2006). Perinatal prevention of HIV on the territory of the Russia Federation in 2005. *AIDS.Sex.Health*, N58, p. 32

Tsoukas C., Hatzaxis G., Pokrovsky V., et al. (1999). A dose range study of the antiretroviral activity of phosphonovir. Submitted to the International Symposium on HIV. *Leukemia and Opportunistic Cancers*, Marrakech, Morocco.

Tsoukas C., Pokrovsky V., Krayevsky A. (1998). A phase I study of PZT (3′-azido-2′,3′-dideoxythymidine-5′-H-phosphonate) in patients with HIV infection. International Conference on the Discovery and Clinical Development of Antiretroviral Therapies St. Thomas, West Indies, US Virgin Islands.

Vorobeva N., Ivanova E., Shmagel N. (2009). Evaluation of nikavir+epivir efficiency in chemoprevetion of vertical HIV transmission. The 14th Russia National Congress Man and Medicine, Moscow, p. 379.

Wainberg M., Gotte, M., Salomon, H. et al. (1998). Development of drug resistance following nucleoside treatment of HIV disease, XIII International Round Table Nucleosides. *Nucleotides and Their Biological Applications*, Montpellier, France.

Yasko M., Shipitsin A., Khandazhinskaya A., et al. (2006). New alkil- and aminocarbonil-phosphonic acid derivatives containing 3′- azido-3-desoxythymidine. *Biorganic Chemistry*, v. 32, N 6, p. 603-608.

Yurin O., Kravchenko A., Afonina L., et al. (2000). Treatment of the patients with intolerance to AZT by phosphazid, 5 International Congress on drug therapy in HIV-infection, Glasgow, UK, AIDS, Vol. 14, Suppl. 4, Abstr., p. 13.

Yurin O., Kravchenko A., Golokhvastova E. (1997). A phaze 1 clinical study of nikavir. Scientific practical conference on Topical issues of HIV infection, St Petersburg, p. 154-155.

Yurin O., Kravchenko A., Kanestri V., et al. (2000). First experience of the application of phosphazid the new nucleotide analogue in HAART, 13 International AIDS Conference, Durban, South Africa, Abstract book, Vol. 1, Abstr. TuPeB3205.

Yurin O., Kravchenko A., Serebrovskaya L., et al. (1998). The phase 1 of the clinical trial of "Phosphazid", the new reverse transcriptase inhibitor, 4 International Congress on drug therapy in HIV-infection, Glasgow, UK, AIDS, Vol. 12, Suppl. 4, Abstr., p. 240.

Yurin O., Kravchenko A., Afonina L., et al. (2001). Nikavir - a novel domestic antiretroviral agent. Epidemiology and Infectious diseases, № 1, p. 43-45.

Zakharova N., Kuptsov D., Mishustina Y., et al. (2008). Experience of nikavir (phosphazide) application in chemoprevetion of the vertical HIV transmission. *Infectious Diseases*, Anthology, St.Petersburg, 2007, p. 93-98.

8

Exosomes Decrease *In Vitro* Infectivity of HIV-1 Preparations: Implication for CD4+T Lymphocyte Depletion *In Vivo*

Subra Caroline, Burelout Chantal, Proulx Sophie, Simard Sébastien and Gilbert Caroline

Centre de Recherche en Rhumatologie et Immunologie (CRRI), Département de Médecine, Faculté de Médecine, Université Laval, Québec, Canada

1. Introduction

1.1 Nature and role of exosomes

Since their identification by Johnstone et al (Johnstone et al., 1987), exosomes have gained importance in understanding many biological processes. Exosomes are vesicles expelled by cells into the extracellular milieu. They originate from internal endocytic compartments called multivesicular bodies (MVB) and are released following fusion of MVB with the plasma membrane (Stoorvogel et al., 2002). Numerous cell types, including tumour, foetal, epithelial and haematopoietic cells share the characteristics of releasing exosomes upon activation by cytokines (Abusamra et al., 2005; Ahn and Johnstone, 1993; Altieri, Khan, and Tomasi, 2004; Peche et al., 2006; Segura, Amigorena, and Thery, 2005; Taylor, Akyol, and Gercel-Taylor, 2006; van Niel and Heyman, 2002). Initially associated with the elimination of obsolete proteins during reticulocyte maturation, exosomes are now known to play several roles in intercellular communication (for reviews, (Chaput and Thery, 2010) and (Record et al., 2011)). Based on the presence of various molecules within the vesicle membrane or lumen, it has been proposed that exosomes are particularly involved in regulation of the immune response, for example tolerance induction (Admyre et al., 2006; Frangsmyr et al., 2005; Kapsogeorgou et al., 2005; Karlsson et al., 2001; Kim, Morse, and Choi, 2006; Larregina et al., 2004; Mallegol, van Niel, and Heyman, 2005; Ostman, Taube, and Telemo, 2005; Peche et al., 2003; Peche et al., 2006; Quah and O'Neill, 2005a; Segura, Amigorena, and Thery, 2005; Taylor, Akyol, and Gercel-Taylor, 2006; Van Niel et al., 2003), antigen presentation (Andre et al., 2004; Chaput et al., 2004; Clayton et al., 2003; Kleijmeer et al., 2001; Peche et al., 2003; Raposo et al., 1996; Thery et al., 2002), cancer immunotherapy (Amigorena, 2000; Andre et al., 2001; Mignot et al., 2006; Quah and O'Neill, 2000; Zitvogel et al., 1998), control of receptor expression (Ahn and Johnstone, 1993; Hawari et al., 2004; Levine, 2004), mechanisms involved in cell death (Abusamra et al., 2005; Farsad, 2002; Iero et al., 2008; Lenassi et al., 2010; Zhang et al., 2006) and control of inflammation (Abusamra et al., 2005; Kim et al., 2006; Levine, 2004). Exosomes may also contain functional miRNA (Pegtel et al., 2010) or deliver bioactive lipids (Esser et al., 2010; Subra et al., 2010). Depending on the function and on the activation state of the secreting cells, exosomes thus regulate multiple pathways in neighbouring cells in autocrine, paracrine and juxtacrine fashion.

The mechanism by which molecules are sorted in exosomes involves a recycling process that is influenced by molecular lateral mobility within lipid domains (de Gassart et al., 2003; de Gassart et al., 2004). MHC-II, co-stimulatory molecules, enzymes (Alonso et al., 2007; Baynes et al., 1991) and heat-shock proteins (HSP) (Lancaster and Febbraio, 2005) are among the proteins associated with exosomes (Segura, Amigorena, and Thery, 2005; Segura et al., 2005; Skokos et al., 2001).

Exosomes are similar to retroviruses not only in terms of size but also the molecules they incorporate and their ability to activate immune cells. Exosomes are slightly smaller and more heterogeneous in size (30-100 nm) than HIV-1 particles (100 nm). The most obvious similarity between these two types of particles is the presence of molecules of host origin. For example, incorporation of MHC-I and MHC-II by virions and by exosomes has been described (Cantin, Fortin, and Tremblay, 1996; Cantin, Martin, and Tremblay, 2001; Gansuvd et al., 2003; Raposo et al., 2002; Vincent-Schneider et al., 2002). In addition, several cell-surface molecules such as LFA-1 integrins (CD11a, CD18), co-stimulatory molecules (CD28, CD54) and complement-neutralizing molecules (CD55, CD59) are associated with both particles (Cantin, Methot, and Tremblay, 2005; Nguyen et al., 2003; Thery et al., 2001; Thery et al., 1999). Finally, the buoyant density of exosomes ranges from 1.13 to 1.21 g/l, while that of HIV-1 particles ranges from 1.16 to 1.18 g/l (Thery et al., 2001; Wang et al., 1999). Similar protein and lipid composition as well as buoyant densities render the separation of exosomes from virions quite difficult using standard techniques such as density-gradient centrifugation. These problems prompted us to use an Optiprep™-based velocity gradient method (Cantin et al., 2008), which has allowed us to show clearly that exosomes can be separated completely from viruses, based on detection of exosome marker (acetylcholinesterase) and HIV-1 marker (capsid protein p24).

The relationship between exosome biogenesis and retrovirus assembly has not yet been described in satisfactory detail. Although considerable evidence points to the takeover of the intracellular machinery responsible for MVB biogenesis (located at the cytoplasmic membrane) in the case of HIV-1 budding from $CD4^+$ T lymphocytes (CD4TL), virions are found in endosomes of macrophages and dendritic cells (DCs), suggesting an internal budding process (Booth et al., 2006; Gould, Hildreth, and Booth, 2004; Morita and Sundquist, 2004; Nguyen et al., 2003). Comparative studies of exosomes and HIV-1 particle production pathways (Nguyen et al., 2003) based on observations of similar viral budding (Derse et al., 1987) and uptake by cells (Izquierdo-Useros et al., 2010) indicate that retroviruses evolved by exploiting the exosome release pathway.

The highly varied exosome composition and content suggest crucial roles for these vesicles in intercellular communication (Thery, Zitvogel, and Amigorena, 2002), transport of genetic material (mRNA or microRNA) (Valadi et al., 2007) and exchange of proteins (Andre et al., 2004; Thery, Zitvogel, and Amigorena, 2002), or in inflammation by carrying bioactive lipids (Esser et al.; Subra et al., 2010). Numerous studies indicate more efficient T cell activation by exosomes released from mature (mDCs) than from immature DCs (iDCs) (Admyre et al., 2006; Chaput and Thery, 2010; Segura, Amigorena, and Thery, 2005). In other studies, an inhibitory role for exosomes in the immune response has been described and particularly in the induction of T cell death via either FasL or galactin-9 by tumour-derived exosomes (Abusamra et al., 2005; Alonso et al., 2007; Chaput and Thery, 2010; Klibi et al., 2009; Ren et al.; Xie et al., 2010) (Andreola et al., 2002; Monleon et al., 2001). Compelling evidence for a role of the HIV-1 protein Nef (released in association with exosomes) in inducing apoptosis of bystander CD4TL has been published recently (Lenassi et al., 2010). All of these data have led us to examine the involvement of exosomes in CD4TL depletion during HIV-1 infection.

1.2 Rapid depletion of CD4TL during primary infection

HIV-1-caused disease is characterized by a state of chronic immune activation due to sustained inflammation and immune hyperactivation that persists even under antiretroviral therapy (HAART) (Imami et al., 2001). Several observations from non-pathogenic *simian immunodeficiency virus* (SIV) infection, HIV-1 infected "elite controllers", "elite suppressors" or long-term non-progressors reveal a good correlation between low level of activation of the immune system and absence of clinical signs of AIDS (Bailey et al., 2008; Fontaine et al., 2011; Milush et al., 2007; Shacklett, 2010; Silvestri et al., 2003). In contrast, strongly increased immune activation characterized by dysregulated neutrophil and macrophage functions (Roilides et al., 1990; Torre et al., 2002), polyclonal B cell activation (Aberg et al., 2005), increased T cell turnover (Aberg et al., 2005), increased numbers of T cells with an activated phenotype (Aberg et al., 2005) and increased levels of pro-inflammatory molecules are hallmarks of disease progression in pathogenic infections by primate (HIV/SIV) lentiviruses (Ascher and Sheppard, 1988), (Giorgi et al., 1999; Liu et al., 1997). More significant is that a major rapid loss of mucosal CD4TL occurs in the gut-associated lymphoid tissues quite early in HIV-1 infection (Brenchley, Price, and Douek, 2006; Brenchley et al., 2004; Mehandru et al., 2004). At this stage, both mucosal lymph node destruction (which initiates immune dysfunction) and loss of integrity of the gut epithelium allow microbial products to cross the intestinal barrier. This translocation phenomenon produces high levels of circulating bacterial lipopolysaccharides (Brenchley, Price, and Douek, 2006) and thus contributes to the maintenance of the inflammatory state and systemic immune activation observed in chronic HIV-1-infected patients (Brenchley, Price, and Douek, 2006; Marchetti et al., 2008). These studies all point to early events in HIV-1 infection as decisive determinants of the irreversible damage inflicted on immune cells. It is well established that dendritic cells (DCs) are involved early in HIV-1 transmission (Granelli-Piperno et al., 1998; Manel et al., 2010; Tsunetsugu-Yokota et al., 1997). It is also known that CD4TL, more particularly the Th17 mucosal subset (Cecchinato and Franchini, 2010; Cecchinato et al., 2008; Elhed and Unutmaz, 2010; Favre et al., 2009; Milush et al., 2011; Paiardini, 2010) are dysregulated (Elbim et al., 2009; Hofman et al., 1999; Okada, Takei, and Tashiro, 1997; Okada, Takei, and Tashiro, 1998; Pitrak et al., 1996; Roilides et al., 1993; Roilides et al., 1990; Szelc et al., 1992; Thorsen, Busch-Sorensen, and Sondergaard, 1989) in pathogenic HIV-1/SIV infection (Brenchley et al., 2008; Elbim et al., 2009; Elbim et al., 2008; Favre et al., 2009).

A rapid decrease thus occurs in the numbers of both infected and uninfected CD4TL within the very first weeks of infection. CD4TL are known to play a pivotal role in orchestrating the immune response as well as in the development, maturation and maintenance of cytotoxic T cells (Matloubian, Concepcion, and Ahmed, 1994; Zajac et al., 1998), the development of a humoral response and B cell antibody class switching (Tsuji et al., 1994), control of the bactericidal activity of macrophages and induction of HIV-1-specific CD4 and CD8 T cell responses. In fact, HIV-1 infection and the specific immune response to it depend largely on CD4TL functionnality and depletion of these cells during primary infection constitutes major interference, perhaps explaining the long-term inability of the host immune response to control the infection. Different mechanisms have been proposed to explain the significant depletion of CD4TL in the gut-associated lymphatic tissues. Among these, direct infection of CD4TL by the virus (Arnoult et al., 2003), cytotoxic activity of CD8 T cells against infected cells (Sewell et al., 2000) and cytopathic effects on bystander cells or abortive infection (Doitsh et al., 2010) are the most plausible. However, additional factors, including HIV-1 proteins such as Vpr, Tat, Nef, VpU, proteases and gp120 (Varbanov, Espert, and Biard-Piechaczyk, 2006; Wan and Chen, 2010), mechanisms such as activation-induced cell death (AICD) mediated by Fas, TNF and TRAIL/APO2 (Lichtner et al., 2004) or dysregulation of cytokine/chemokine production (Saelens et al., 2004) can contribute to CD4TL death. Moreover, the detection of Nef in exosomes and the known involvement of this viral protein in apoptosis add support to the potential role of exosomes in bystander cell viability (Lenassi et al., 2010). We therefore propose another mechanism involving the release, from HIV-1-loaded iDCs, of exosomes that can induce functional defects in CD4TL and contribute to their elimination.

1.3 The role of dendritic cells in HIV-1 primary infection

The weakening of the immune system begins soon after the virus enters the body, which it does principally via the mucosal tissues. Following transmission of HIV-1, the virus crosses the mucosal barrier and is met by DCs, which are among the first cells to encounter the virus (Hladik and McElrath, 2008). A major immune system cell type involved in capturing and internalizing HIV-1 is the iDCs, which then migrates principally to the lymph nodes of the gastrointestinal tract, a site of HIV-1 replication during acute infection. Despite the progress that has been made in understanding iDC/HIV-1 interactions as well as virion sequestration and transmission to CD4TL, several fundamental questions surrounding the near total depletion of memory CD4TL observed during the acute infection (Brenchley et al., 2004; Guadalupe et al., 2003; Li et al., 2005; Mattapallil et al., 2005; Mehandru et al., 2004) remain unanswered. It is well known that both cells play a pivotal role in the dissemination of HIV-1, in the establishment of infection and also in anti-HIV-1 immunity.

It is now well established that HIV-1 entry into CD4TL is mediated by cellular chemokine receptors such as CCR5 or CXCR4. However, we, along with others, have found that additional factors, such as the DC-SIGN and DCIR lectins can mediate virus attachment to DCs and its subsequent endocytosis (Cambi et al., 2009; Geijtenbeek et al., 2000; Lambert et al., 2008; Permanyer, Ballana, and Este, 2010). Indeed, several recent studies have shown virions concentrated in late endocytic compartments also called multivesicular bodies (MVBs) or MHC class II compartments in mature DCs (Garcia et al., 2005; Izquierdo-Useros et al., 2009; Kwon et al., 2002), where they are sheltered both from the action of antiviral drugs and the immune response. Mature DCs are capable of stocking viral particles and migrating via the lymphatic network to lymph nodes and thus constitute reservoirs of virions. At this stage, it is thought that mDCs can transmit virions to T cells through two sequential routes: an early route known as trans-infection, via passive transfer through late endosomes, or a later route called cis-infection following productive infection (Turville et al., 2004). Fusion of late endosomes with the DC plasma membrane releases large numbers of virions into intercellular space called the virological synapse, which can infect nearby target cells (Moir, Chun, and Fauci, 2010; Piguet and Steinman, 2007). Endosomes contain the intraluminal vesicles that become exosomes when delivered into this space at the same time as the viral particles contained in HIV-1-loaded DCs. Exosomes and virions thus pass via the late endosome across the cell to be exchanged with other cells (Izquierdo-Useros et al., 2010).

After their migration to the lymph nodes, iDCs likely transfer HIV-1 to CD4TL with great efficiency and simultaneously release exosomes. The ability of exosomes to activate CD4TL, thereby enhancing HIV-1 replication, or to induce T cell apoptosis directly, could contribute

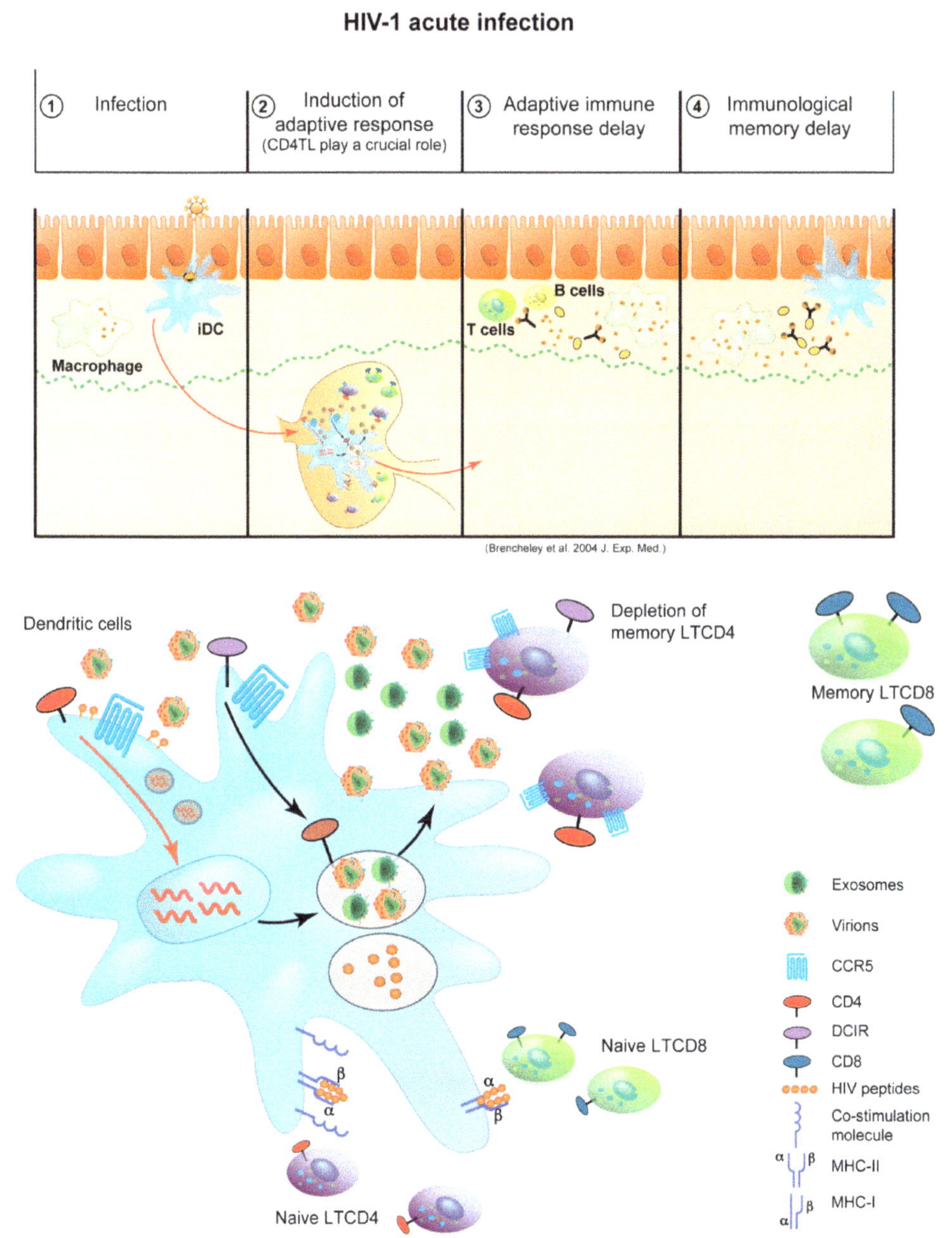

Fig. 1. Potential Role of exosomes in HIV-1 infection

to the massive depletion of CD4TL. Indeed, our preliminary observations show that HIV-1 increases exosome release from iDCs. Some studies have shown that exosomes can activate T cells and consequently are involved in the regulation of the immune response (Admyre et al., 2006; Segura et al., 2005; Thery et al., 2002). Furthermore, the Fas-ligand on exosomes can also induce apoptosis of both CD4 and CD8 T cells (Abusamra et al., 2005; Alonso et al., 2007; Alonso et al., 2005; Segura, Amigorena, and Thery, 2005). It should be noted that the capacity of exosomes to regulate the viability of CD4 T cell sub-populations has not yet been fully investigated in the context of HIV-1 infection. In order to answer this important fundamental question, new methods are needed for separating mixtures of exosomes and HIV-1 to purity.

HIV-1 is a retrovirus that causes a slow but sustained depletion of CD4TL during the chronic stage of infection, leading to progressive failure of the immune system. The principal immune cell type that captures and internalizes HIV-1 is the iDC. HIV-1-loaded iDCs migrate to the lymph nodes of the gastrointestinal tract, a major site of HIV-1 replication during acute infection. Given that CD4TL play a pivotal role in the orchestration of the immune response, the rapid and sustained disappearance of mucosal CD4TL (within the first 15 days) compromises the development of both the cellular and humoral responses to HIV-1 infection. Exosomes release by DCs or CD4TL can contribute to elimination of CD4TL as well as other cell deregulations characterizing this crucial phase.

2. Protocol to study the role of exosomes in CD4TL viability in the context of HIV-1 infection

2.1 Cell purification

Experiments were performed using human primary cells, DCs and CD4TL. Cells were isolated from peripheral blood mononuclear cells (PBMCs) obtained from anonymous and healthy volunteer donors. PBMCs were prepared by centrifugation on a lymphocyte separation medium from Wisent Inc. (St Bruno, QC, Canada). $CD14^+$ cells were then isolated using a monocyte positive selection kit according to the manufacturer's instructions (Stemsep Human CD14 positive selection Kit, STEMCell Technologies, Vancouver, BC, Canada) using an AutoMacs (Miltenyl Biotech, Auburn, CA, USA) and a previously established procedure (Bounou et al., 2004; Gilbert et al., 2007a; Gilbert et al., 2007b). $CD14^+$ cells were cultured in six-well plates at a concentration of 1 X 10^6 cells/ml. To generate iDCs, purified monocytes were cultured in complete culture medium supplemented every two days with granulocyte-macrophage colony-stimulating factor (1,000 U/ml) from Genscript (Cedarlane Laboratories, Burlington, ON, Canada) and IL-4 (200 U/ml) from R&D Systems (Minneapolis, MN, USA) for 6 to 7 days. Expression of CD3 and CD19 was measured to assess contamination with T and B cells respectively. Expression of HLA-DR, CD86, DC-SIGN, CD83 and CD14 was monitored to verify the immature phenotypes of DCs. In the immature state, DCs express a high level of DC-SIGN and low level of CD83, whereas mature DCs express CD83 and high levels of ICAM-1, HLA-DR and CD86.

CD4TL were isolated using a negative selection kit according to the manufacturer's instructions (Stemsep Human CD4 T cell enrichment kit, STEMCell Technologies). In some experiments, these cells were activated with phytohemagglutinin-L (1 µg/ml) to obtain mitogen-stimulated cells and maintained at a density of 2 x 10^6 cells/ml in RPMI supplemented with IL-2 (30 U/ml) obtained through the AIDS Repository Reagent Program

(Germantown, MD, USA). Experiments were performed with cell preparations that were devoid of contamination (i.e. DC purity > 95%; CD4TL purity > 98%). In all culture media, bovine exosomes from foetal bovine serum (FBS) were eliminated by O/N ultracentrifugation at 100,000*xg*. Complete RPMI 1640 culture medium contains FBS, penicillin G, streptomycin, glutamine from Wisent and primocin and plasmocin from Invivogen (San Diego, CA, USA).

2.2 Virus production and purification

Virions were produced by transient transfection in human embryonic kidney 293T cells (HEK293T) as previously described (Cantin et al., 1997). Plasmids used include pJR-CSF (R5-tropic), pNLAD8 (R5-tropic), pNL4-3balenv (R5-tropic) and pNL4-3 (X4-tropic). The pNL4-3balenv vector (provided by R. Pomerantz, Thomas Jefferson University, Philadelphia, PA, USA) was generated by replacing the *env* gene of the T-tropic HIV-1 strain, NL4-3, with that of the macrophage-tropic HIV-1 Bal strain, thus resulting in an infectious molecular clone with R5-tropic properties (Dornadula et al., 1999). Other plasmids were obtained from the AIDS Repository Reagent Program (Germantown, MD, USA). Several viral preparations were obtained from primary cells. Peripheral blood from healthy donors was centrifuged on lymphocyte separation medium (Wisent) to obtain PBMCs. NL4-3Balenv virions were propagated by acute infection of PBMCs (1.5×10^7 cells/ml) with virus (500 ng/ml) for six days.

2.3 Separation of exosomes and virions by velocity gradient

Exosomes, microvesicles and virions contained in cell-free supernatants were passed through a 0.22 μm filter or centrifuged, 10 min at 10,000*xg* to eliminate micro-particles. Filtered virus and/or exosomes from 293T cells or PBMCs were concentrated by ultracentrifugation in an Optima L-90K Beckman Coulter centrifuge (Fullerton, CA) for 45 min at 31,500 rpm (100,000*xg*) in a 70 Ti rotor. The pellet containing virions and microvesicles/exosomes was re-suspended in 500 μl of PBS. HIV-1 viral particles were then centrifuged through a 6-18% Optiprep™ (60% iodixanol) separation gradient from Sigma Aldrich® (Winston Park, CA, USA) as previously described (Dettenhofer and Yu, 1999). The densities of each gradient fraction were below 1.13 g/ml, as shown in Figure 2. The virus preparations were then centrifuged using the Optima L-90K centrifuge for 75 min at 52,000 rpm (250,000*xg*) in a NVT65 rotor. Gradient fractions were collected from the top. Optiprep™ separation medium possesses intrinsic properties such as neutral pH and physiological osmolarity (Dettenhofer and Yu, 1999; Ford, Graham, and Rickwood, 1994; Van Veldhoven, Baumgart, and Mannaerts, 1996) that make it highly suitable for efficient separation of viral entities from cellular debris and microvesicles (Dettenhofer and Yu, 1999; Hermens et al., 1999; Moller-Larsen and Christensen, 1998; Zolotukhin et al., 1999). This technique, identical to the velocity gradient adapted by Dettenhofer (Dettenhofer and Yu, 1999) for HIV-1 separation, is also very efficient for separating microvesicle contaminants from HIV-1 preparations. The results depicted in Figure 3A (black rectangles) express the separation efficiency in terms of quantity of viral $p24^{gag}$ protein, which is concentrated in fraction 15.6. Electron microscopy, performed at the Armand Frappier Institute Microscopy Laboratory using standard protocol (Alain et al., 1987; Hammond et al., 1981), confirmed that fractions 15.6 and 16.8 contain concentrated and homogenous viral particles (10^{11} per ml). Virion contents were normalized by means of an in-house sensitive double-antibody sandwich enzyme-linked immunosorbent assay (ELISA) specific for the viral $p24^{gag}$ protein (Bounou, Leclerc, and Tremblay, 2002).

The distribution of fractions containing exosomes along the gradient was evaluated by measuring acetylcholinesterase (AChE) activity, which is a commonly used specific exosome marker (Fig. 3A, open rectangles) (Gastpar et al., 2005; Rieu et al., 2000). This enzyme activity was measured following a procedure previously described (Cantin et al., 2008). Briefly, 30 µl of standard or sample were mixed with PBS pH 8 containing acetylthiocholine and PBS pH 7 containing 5,5-dithio-*bis*-(2-nitrobenzoic acid) to obtain final reagent concentrations of respectively 1.25 mM and 0.1 mM in a volume of 200 µl and held at room temperature. Changes in absorption at 450 nm were monitored for 10 min with a plate reader spectrophotometer (ELX808, BIO-TEK instruments, Winooski, VT, USA). Glycosylphosphatidylinositol-anchored AChE as well as other GPI proteins are localized in the MVB and are part of the exosome membrane (Gastpar et al., 2005; Johnstone et al., 1987). The results illustrated in Figure 3 show that AChE activity is concentrated in fractions 8.4 to 12 and microscopic observations showed that 10^8 particles/ml are present in these fractions. To confirm the efficiency of this velocity gradient method for separating HIV-1 from exosomes, we also checked for the presence of infectious particles in each gradient fraction (i.e. infectivity on TZM-bl cells (Cantin et al., 2008) or measure of spliced TAT on CD4TL). Infectivity assays using the TZM-bl indicator cell line showed that fractions 14.4 to 16.8 contained fully infectious virus while fractions 8.4 to 12 contained insignificant amounts. These results thus clearly indicate that our procedures can isolate exosomes and HIV-1 particles differentially and independently. We are satisfied that fractions 8.4 to 12 of the Optiprep™ gradients contained exosomes exclusively, while fractions 14.4 to 16.8 contained infectious viruses.

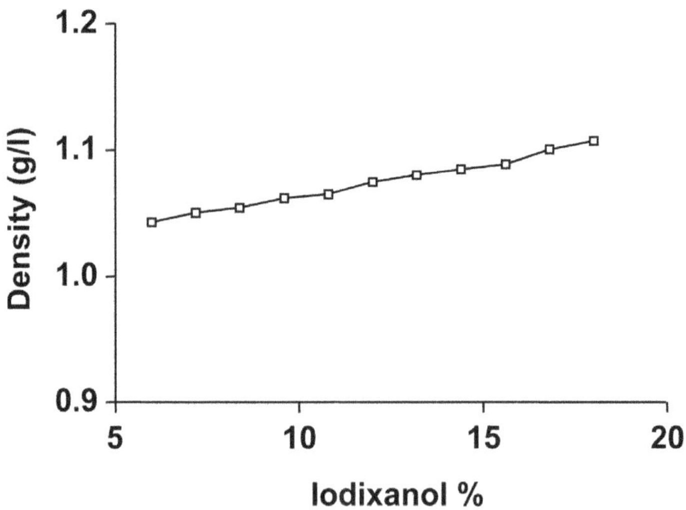

Fig. 2. Density of gradient fractions

The particularity of velocity gradient separation resides in its capacity to isolate particles of similar density. The density range of 6 to 18 % of Optiprep™ is 1.03 to 1.13 g/l.

2.4 Rapid purification of exosomes

A quick alternative procedure for eliminating exosomes prior to contacting the cells with HIV-1 preparation consisted of immuno-depleting AChE-bearing vesicles directly from 100,000*xg* pellet (starting material) as shown in Figure 3B. Briefly, ultracentrifuged cells supernatants were diluted in PBS and incubated with protein A/G beads pre-coated with anti-AChE (AE-1 from ATCC) or with isotypic control antibodies (IgG1). The beads (exosomes) and final supernatants (infectious viruses without exosomes) were kept for viral Titer determination (data not shown) and AChE assay (Fig. 3B). The results show that 95% of the AChE activity was recovered using the anti-AChE beads after the first round of precipitation. Exosomes can be eluted from the beads in two minutes using 50 µl of 0.2M glycine in 0.1M KH_2PO_4 pH 3. Acidic pH was then neutralized by adding 100 µl of 0.1M K_2HPO_4 (pH 8.8). It should be noted that this treatment does not affect AChE activity.

2.5 Analysis of protein contained in each gradient fraction

Several proteins including LFA-1 are known to be present on both particles and were quantified in exosome/HIV-1 preparations by means of an in-house enzymatic sandwich-type immunoassay. Plates were initially coated with anti-LFA-1 (MEM-25) (50 µg/ml) in carbonate buffer. After three washes with PBS/0.1% Tween 20, the non-specific sites were blocked with PBS/0.1% Tween 20/1% BSA for 1 hr at RT. The plates were washed and 75 µl of each gradient fraction mixed with 0.5% Triton X-100 to cause lysis were added and the plates were then held overnight at 4°C. The plates were then washed three times and biotinylated anti-LFA-1 (TSI/22) (0.5 µg/ml) was added in blocking solution for 1 hr at RT. After three more washings, streptavidin-peroxidase conjugate was added for 30 min at RT. The plates were washed and the detection was performed by the addition of the TMB-S substrate followed by the addition of H_3PO_4. Absorbance at 450 nm was read to quantify LFA-1 in each fraction. Figure 3C shows that LFA-1 is present on both vesicles (exosomes and fully infectious virions) and also in uncharacterized particles from fractions 13.2 and 14.4.

Both methods (Optiprep™ gradient and immunodepletion) were used to purify exosomes. These methods were employed to eliminate exosomes from all viral or mock preparations before contact with cells and results depicted in Figure 3D show that depletion of exosomes from the HIV-1 preparation increased cell viability.

2.6 Electron microscopy procedure and examination of negative-stain specimens

The protocol described by Hammond et al. and Alain et al was performed with each analytical fraction (Alain et al., 1987; Hammond et al., 1981). Briefly, microvesicle preparation was fixed with an equal volume of 2% paraformaldehyde and 50–200 µL in a micro-ultracentrifuge tube with a formvar-coated electron microscopy grid at the bottom were concentrated for 5 minutes at 120,000*xg* (20 psig) using an Airfuge ultracentrifuge (Beckman, Palo Alto, CA, USA). The grids were dried on bibulous paper and stained for 1 min with a drop of 3% phosphotungstic acid (pH 6.0). The concentration, shape and overall appearance of the microvesicles were examined with a Hitachi 7100 (Hitachi, Japan) transmission electron microscope (see Fig. 3A).

2.7 Virus infection assays

Indicator cell line TZM-bl, which carries a stably integrated luciferase reporter gene under the control of the HIV-1 regulatory element known as the long terminal repeat (Thibault et

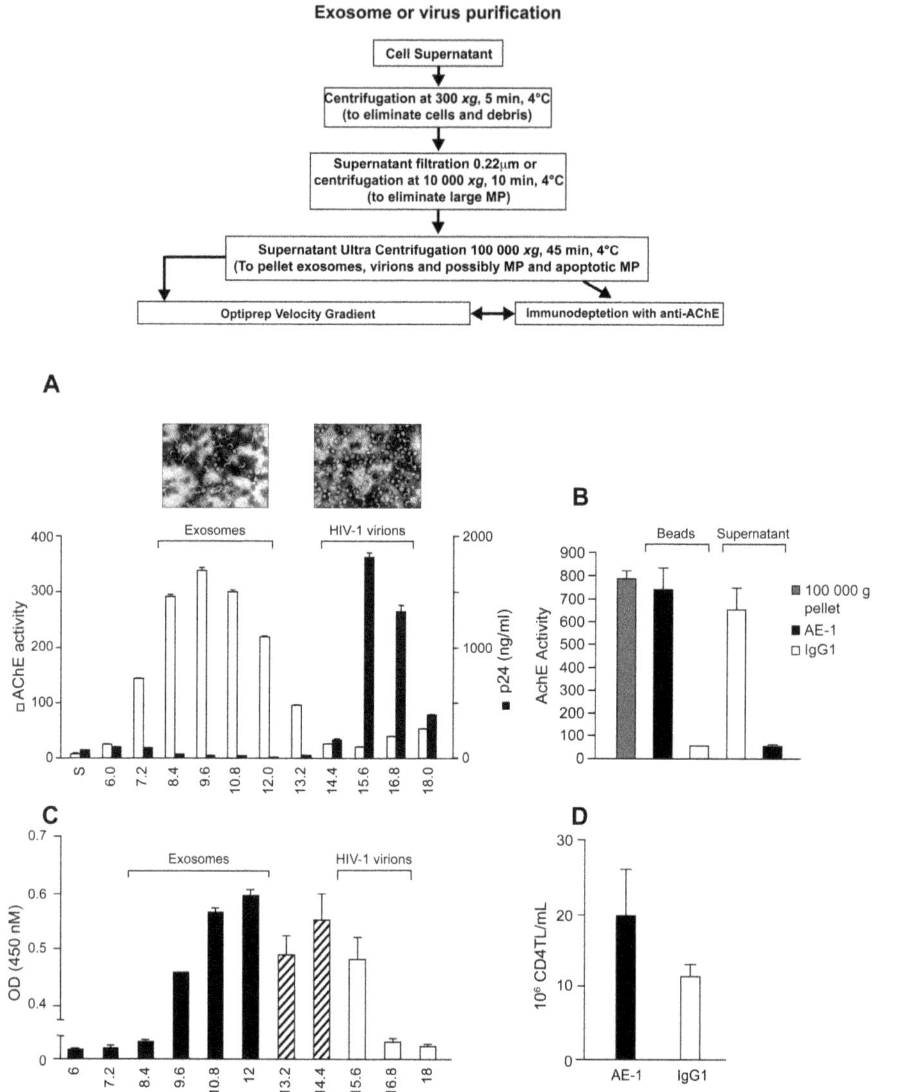

Fig. 3. Exosome and virus purification
The upper panel illustrates the purification protocols based on Optiprep™ velocity gradient and on immunocapture. Panel A shows velocity gradient purification of NL4-3balenv virions produced on HEK293T cells by transient transfection. Gradients were overlaid with 100,000*xg* centrifugal pellet. Viral protein $p24^{gag}$ (black rectangles) was measured by ELISA. AChE activity (x10^6 OD/min, open rectangles) was evaluated in each fraction by colorimetry. Each fraction was examined by electron microscopy for particle quality and quantity. Panel B represents the results obtained by immunocapture with AChE. Panel C shows the presence of LFA-1 in each gradient fraction. Finally, panel D shows that depletion of exosomes increased cell viability. These results show that we are able to separate exosomes from HIV-1 particles.

al., 2007; Wei et al., 2002; Zhao et al., 2005), was used to quantify infectious viral particles after exosomes depletion. Each well contained 1.5 x 10^4 cells plus 100 µl of fraction in a final volume of 200 µl. Plates were incubated for 48 hrs. All experimental points were done in triplicate. Luciferase activity was determined following a modified version of a known protocol (Barbeau et al., 1997; Berube et al., 1996). Briefly, cell-free supernatant (100 µl) withdrawn from each well and mixed with solution containing 25 mM Tris phosphate pH 7.8, 2 mM dithiothreitol, 1% Triton X-100 and 10% glycerol (25 µl) to cause vesicle lysis was held at room temperature for 30 min. A 20-µl aliquot of this mixture was then mixed with 100 µl of luciferase assay buffer (20 mM Tricine, 1.07 mM $(MgCO_3)_4 \cdot Mg(OH)_2 \cdot 5\ H_2O$, 2.67 mM $MgSO_4$, 0.1 mM EDTA, 270 µM coenzyme A, 470 µM luciferin, 530 µM ATP and 33.3 mM dithiothreitol) and the luciferase reaction was monitored on a Dynex MLX microplate luminometer for 20s/well after a 2-5s delay.

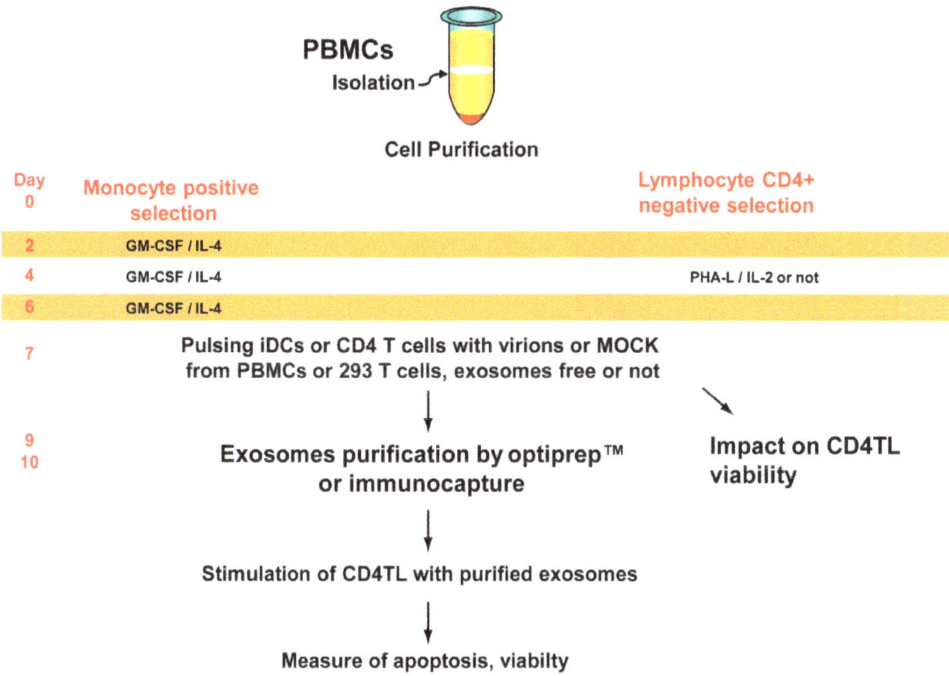

Fig. 4. Experimental set-up
This figure illustrates the experimental set-up used to test the impact of exosomes on cell viability.

3. Results

3.1 Loading of DCs or CD4TL with HIV-1 induces the release of large amounts of exosomes into the extracellular medium

Exosomes contain several molecules that can either eliminate or activate CD4TL (Quah and O'Neill, 2005b; Segura et al., 2005; Thery et al., 2002). Moreover, exosome-like vesicles found in plasma induce apoptosis in a FasL-like manner (Ren et al., 2010). Although exosomes release by DCs have been studied extensively (Chaput et al., 2006; Izquierdo-Useros et al., 2009; Thery et al., 2001; Thery et al., 1999), the release mechanism and the nature of the exosomes produced by HIV-1-loaded cells (DCs or CD4TL) have not been thoroughly investigated. To begin to answer this question, the experimental set up proposed in Figure 4 and methods presented in Figure 3 were used.

DCs and CD4TL pulsed with NL4-3balenv and washed several times were cultured for respectively 2 or 5 days. Exosomes and virions were isolated initially by differential centrifugation and exosome levels were determined by measuring exosomal AChE activity (Cantin et al., 2008). These results, presented in Figure 5, confirmed higher levels of exosomes secreted by iDCs and CD4TL pulsed with purified HIV-1 (1.4 fold and 1.9 respectively, Fig. 5A, B). Using Optiprep™ velocity gradients to separate exosomes and HIV-1, we processed the pellet obtained following sedimentation centrifugation. As

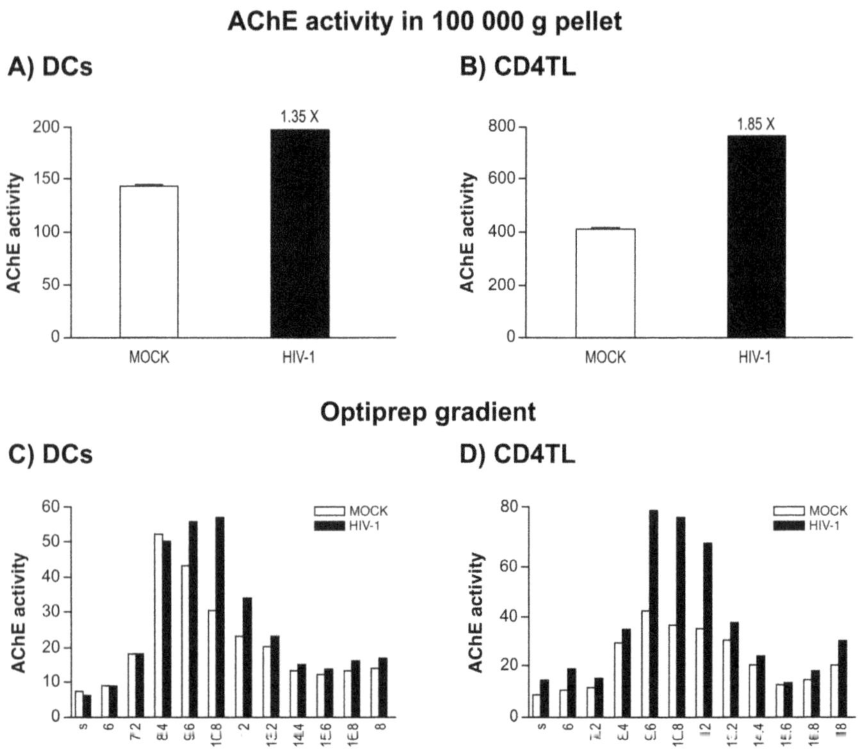

Fig. 5. Exosomes released by DCs and CD4TL after pulsing with HIV-1

I DCs **(A, C)** or CD4TL **(B, D)** were incubated for 2h with exosome-free NL4-3balenv HIV-1 virus or mock preparation and cultured for an additional 72h. Cell-free supernatants were obtained by centrifugation and exosomes in the pellets were quantified by measuring AChE activity (x10^6 DO/min). Exosomes were then separated from HIV-1 on an Optiprep gradient and the exosome content (based on AchE activity) of each fraction was determined. Data are representative of five independent donors. These results show that HIV-1 induced exosome release (in fractions 9.6 through 12) by both cell types (mean increases of 1.4-fold for DCs and 1.9-fold for CD4TL, based on at least 5 independent experiments).

expected, exosomes were concentrated in iodixanol fractions 8.4-12.0% on the Optiprep™ gradient (Fig. 5C, D). Large amounts of exosomes produced by HIV-1-loaded cells accumulated in fractions starting at 9.6% iodixanol (in comparison to the control condition, open bar). The velocity method thus allows efficient separation of exosomes which accumulate in iodixanol fractions 8.4 to 12 % as illustrated in Figure 3. Immature DCs release exosomes and are highly relevant to HIV-1 primary infection since they are involved in the capture of HIV-1 in mucosal tissues and play a crucial role in the subsequent transmission of the virus to CD4TL in the lymph nodes (Gilbert et al., 2007a; Gilbert et al., 2007b; Turville et al., 2004) as illustrated in Figure 1.

3.2 Impact of exosome depletion on CD4TL p24 production and infectivity

The large increase in exosome release by HIV-1-pulsed cells, combined with the results showing that exosomes from these cells induced apoptosis, is particularly relevant in the context of HIV-1 infection for several reasons. These results could explain in part the severe depletion of mucosal CD4TL, a cell type very susceptible to HIV-1. In addition, these cells play a pivotal role in orchestrating immune response and their decline during the early phase of infection undoubtedly delays the specific response to HIV-1. Furthermore, most laboratory preparations of HIV-1 contain exosomes, which may explain in vitro observations such as cytokine release, apoptosis, atypical gene expression, infectivity and so on. Since it became clear that exosomes play a major role in several aspects of the immune response to HIV-1, we sought to evaluate their impact on HIV-1 p24 production and infectivity. NL4-3balenv produced by transfection of 293T cells was made free of exosomes by immunocapture with anti-AE-1. Activated CD4TL were pre-incubated for 2h at 37°C with either exosome-free or exosome-containing HIV-1 preparation washed and then incubated for up to 5 days. ELISA was used to determine viral protein p24 in culture supernatants. Figure 6A shows that infection in the presence of exosomes is transient and less efficient

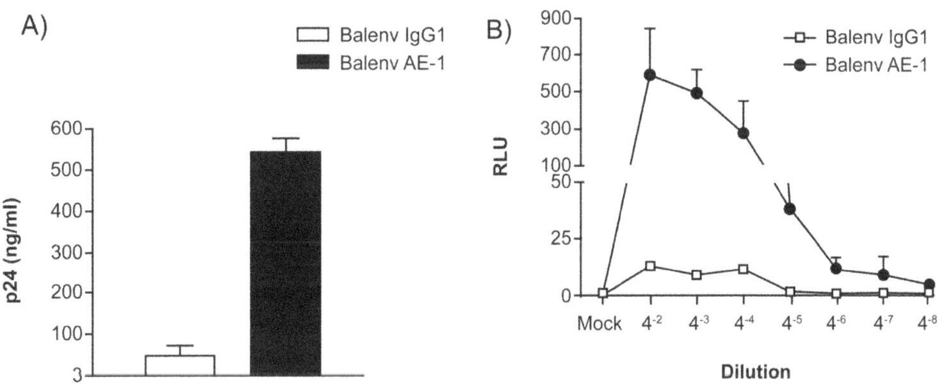

Fig. 6. Impact of exosomes on p24 production and HIV-1 infectivity
Panel A) P24 production was evaluated in the supernatants of CD4TL cultured for up to 5 days after pulsing with NL4-3balenv preparation either free of exosomes (Balenv AE-1) or not (Balenv IgG1). Panel B) TZM-bl cells were incubated with several dilutions of HIV-1 preparation either immunodepleted (Balenv AE-1) or not (Balenv IgG1) and maintained in culture for 48 hrs before lysis. Results are representative of two independent experiments.

than in their absence (solid bar). To evaluate virion infectivity, indicator cell line TZM-bl was incubated with several dilutions of HIV-1 preparation either exosome-depleted or not. Panel B of Figure 6 shows that the exosome-depleted preparation is more infectious than the non-depleted preparation. All these results provide additional evidence that exosomes derived from HIV-1-pulsed cells influence cell viability (figure 3D) and indirectly p24 production and infectivity. They suggest that the presence of exosomes in culture supernatants of HIV-1-stimulated cells should be considered in all laboratory experiments with HIV-1.

4. Conclusion

Exosome biogenesis and the HIV-1 virion assembly pathway converge in a common intracellular compartment. Moreover, both types of vesicle can be released during the trans-infection process in DCs (Izquierdo-Useros et al., 2009). However, exosome secretion in the context of HIV-1 infection has not been properly investigated, due primarily to lack of effective methods of separating the two types of vesicles. Their separation using antibodies directed against specific membrane antigens is often suboptimal since exosomes and HIV-1 display approximately the same antigen expression pattern in addition to several other surface molecules. This is why flow cytometry, ELISA or bead capture techniques based on specific markers are not sufficiently discriminating for the separation of exosomes, extraneous micro-particles and HIV-1. Alternatively, immunocapture with anti-CD45 (Chertova et al., 2006; Trubey et al., 2003), used to separate only micro-particles derived from leucocyte plasma membranes, does not eliminate exosomes originating from the endosomal membrane and cannot be used to separate exosomes from HIV-1. We have shown that AChE appears essentially excluded from the HIV-1 fraction, since the major portion of its activity is recovered in the early Optiprep™ fractions (8.4 to 12), in which no virus is detected (Cantin et al., 2008). Based on this observation, depletion of 100,000*xg* pellets with protein-A/G-bound anti-AChE on agarose beads appears to provide excellent means of rapidly purifying virions or capturing exosomes (Cantin et al., 2008). Using these methods, we have observed that HIV-1 contact with DCs or CD4TL enhances extracellular exosome release and that these exosomes can affect the viability of nearby cells such as CD4TL. These results are in agreement with observations concerning the pro-apoptotic role of Nef accessory proteins. Using Optiprep™ gradients, recent work has shown that the viral protein Nef is enclosed in exosomes, conferring to it the capacity to trigger apoptosis of uninfected bystander T cells (Lenassi et al., 2010).

In summary, the results of the present study show that relatively simple methods of purifying both exosomes and HIV-1 contained in the same cell supernatant are now available. Achieving very highly purified exosomes from HIV-1 preparations is a definite advantage in studying the respective roles of both vesicles as well as the links between them. These methods could also provide the opportunity for specific isolation of exosomes secreted by a variety of cell types and could prove useful in experiments that require highly purified exosome preparations to study their roles in various biological processes. Indeed, these purification steps are crucial in studies involving mixtures of exosomes and HIV-1 (or for that matter, other retroviruses) as starting material. We may anticipate that these methods will constitute a significant contribution to the use of exosomes for vaccination or gene therapy. In addition, we strongly believe that an improved and standardized method of exosome purification should lead to more comparable results among different laboratories and lessen discrepancies such as those seen among several studies in recent years as well as facilitate the interpretation of new results to be published in this subject area.

5. Acknowledgments

The authors wish to thank Dr Lahlou Hadji for his technical assistance in editing this manuscript and for constructive comments. We also thank Dr. Stephen Davids for proofreading. We are also grateful to M. Robert Alain for his assistance with the electron microscopy analyses and to Odette Simard for excellent technical contributions. This work was supported by start-up funds to CG from the Centre Hospitalier Universitaire de Québec and an operating grant to CG from the Canadian Institutes of Health Research (CIHR) (MOP-188726). CG is recipient of a level-1 junior researcher award from the Fonds de la Recherche en Santé du Québec and a New Investigator Award from CIHR. C.S. is the recipient of a fellowship award from the Canadian Institutes of Health Research HIV/AIDS Research Program.

6. References

Aberg, J. A., Zackin, R. A., Brobst, S. W., Evans, S. R., Alston, B. L., Henry, W. K., Glesby, M. J., Torriani, F. J., Yang, Y., Owens, S. I., and Fichtenbaum, C. J. (2005). A randomized trial of the efficacy and safety of fenofibrate versus pravastatin in HIV-infected subjects with lipid abnormalities: AIDS Clinical Trials Group Study 5087. *AIDS Res Hum Retroviruses* 21(9), 757-67.

Abusamra, A. J., Zhong, Z., Zheng, X., Li, M., Ichim, T. E., Chin, J. L., and Min, W. P. (2005). Tumor exosomes expressing Fas ligand mediate CD8+ T-cell apoptosis. *Blood Cells Mol Dis* 35(2), 169-73.

Admyre, C., Johansson, S. M., Paulie, S., and Gabrielsson, S. (2006). Direct exosome stimulation of peripheral human T cells detected by ELISPOT. *Eur J Immunol* 36(7), 1772-81.

Ahn, J., and Johnstone, R. M. (1993). Origin of a soluble truncated transferrin receptor. *Blood* 81(9), 2442-51.

Alain, R., Nadon, F., Seguin, C., Payment, P., and Trudel, M. (1987). Rapid virus subunit visualization by direct sedimentation of samples on electron microscope grids. *J Virol Methods* 16(3), 209-16.

Alonso, R., Mazzeo, C., Merida, I., and Izquierdo, M. (2007). A new role of diacylglycerol kinase alpha on the secretion of lethal exosomes bearing Fas ligand during activation-induced cell death of T lymphocytes. *Biochimie* 89(2), 213-21.

Alonso, R., Rodriguez, M. C., Pindado, J., Merino, E., Merida, I., and Izquierdo, M. (2005). Diacylglycerol kinase alpha regulates the secretion of lethal exosomes bearing Fas ligand during activation-induced cell death of T lymphocytes. *J Biol Chem* 280(31), 28439-50.

Altieri, S. L., Khan, A. N., and Tomasi, T. B. (2004). Exosomes from plasmacytoma cells as a tumor vaccine. *J Immunother* 27(4), 282-8.

Amigorena, S. (2000). Cancer immunotherapy using dendritic cell-derived exosomes. *Medicina (B Aires)* 60 Suppl 2, 51-4.

Andre, F., Andersen, M., Wolfers, J., Lozier, A., Raposo, G., Serra, V., Ruegg, C., Flament, C., Angevin, E., Amigorena, S., and Zitvogel, L. (2001). Exosomes in cancer immunotherapy: preclinical data. *Adv Exp Med Biol* 495, 349-54.

Andre, F., Chaput, N., Schartz, N. E., Flament, C., Aubert, N., Bernard, J., Lemonnier, F., Raposo, G., Escudier, B., Hsu, D. H., Tursz, T., Amigorena, S., Angevin, E., and Zitvogel, L. (2004). Exosomes as potent cell-free peptide-based vaccine. I. Dendritic cell-derived exosomes transfer functional MHC class I/peptide complexes to dendritic cells. *J Immunol* 172(4), 2126-36.

Andreola, G., Rivoltini, L., Castelli, C., Huber, V., Perego, P., Deho, P., Squarcina, P., Accornero, P., Lozupone, F., Lugini, L., Stringaro, A., Molinari, A., Arancia, G., Gentile, M., Parmiani, G., and Fais, S. (2002). Induction of lymphocyte apoptosis by tumor cell secretion of FasL-bearing microvesicles. *J Exp Med* 195(10), 1303-16.

Arnoult, D., Petit, F., Lelievre, J. D., and Estaquier, J. (2003). Mitochondria in HIV-1-induced apoptosis. *Biochem Biophys Res Commun* 304(3), 561-74.

Ascher, M. S., and Sheppard, H. W. (1988). AIDS as immune system activation: a model for pathogenesis. *Clin Exp Immunol* 73(2), 165-7.

Bailey, J. R., O'Connell, K., Yang, H. C., Han, Y., Xu, J., Jilek, B., Williams, T. M., Ray, S. C., Siliciano, R. F., and Blankson, J. N. (2008). Transmission of human immunodeficiency virus type 1 from a patient who developed AIDS to an elite suppressor. *J Virol* 82(15), 7395-410.

Barbeau, B., Bernier, R., Dumais, N., Briand, G., Olivier, M., Faure, R., Posner, B. I., and Tremblay, M. (1997). Activation of HIV-1 long terminal repeat transcription and virus replication via NF-kappaB-dependent and -independent pathways by potent phosphotyrosine phosphatase inhibitors, the peroxovanadium compounds. *J Biol Chem* 272(20), 12968-77.

Baynes, R. D., Shih, Y. J., Hudson, B. G., and Cook, J. D. (1991). Characterization of transferrin receptor released by K562 erythroleukemia cells. *Proc Soc Exp Biol Med* 197(4), 416-23.

Berube, P., Barbeau, B., Cantin, R., Sekaly, R. P., and Tremblay, M. (1996). Repression of human immunodeficiency virus type 1 long terminal repeat-driven gene expression by binding of the virus to its primary cellular receptor, the CD4 molecule. *J Virol* 70(6), 4009-16.

Booth, A. M., Fang, Y., Fallon, J. K., Yang, J. M., Hildreth, J. E., and Gould, S. J. (2006). Exosomes and HIV Gag bud from endosome-like domains of the T cell plasma membrane. *J Cell Biol* 172(6), 923-35.

Bounou, S., Giguere, J. F., Cantin, R., Gilbert, C., Imbeault, M., Martin, G., and Tremblay, M. J. (2004). The importance of virus-associated host ICAM-1 in human immunodeficiency virus type 1 dissemination depends on the cellular context. *Faseb J* 18(11), 1294-6.

Bounou, S., Leclerc, J. E., and Tremblay, M. J. (2002). Presence of host ICAM-1 in laboratory and clinical strains of human immunodeficiency virus type 1 increases virus infectivity and CD4(+)-T-cell depletion in human lymphoid tissue, a major site of replication in vivo. *J Virol* 76(3), 1004-14.

Brenchley, J. M., Paiardini, M., Knox, K. S., Asher, A. I., Cervasi, B., Asher, T. E., Scheinberg, P., Price, D. A., Hage, C. A., Kholi, L. M., Khoruts, A., Frank, I., Else, J., Schacker, T.,

Silvestri, G., and Douek, D. C. (2008). Differential Th17 CD4 T-cell depletion in pathogenic and nonpathogenic lentiviral infections. *Blood* 112(7), 2826-35.
Brenchley, J. M., Price, D. A., and Douek, D. C. (2006). HIV disease: fallout from a mucosal catastrophe? *Nat Immunol* 7(3), 235-9.
Brenchley, J. M., Schacker, T. W., Ruff, L. E., Price, D. A., Taylor, J. H., Beilman, G. J., Nguyen, P. L., Khoruts, A., Larson, M., Haase, A. T., and Douek, D. C. (2004). CD4+ T cell depletion during all stages of HIV disease occurs predominantly in the gastrointestinal tract. *J Exp Med* 200(6), 749-59.
Cambi, A., Beeren, I., Joosten, B., Fransen, J. A., and Figdor, C. G. (2009). The C-type lectin DC-SIGN internalizes soluble antigens and HIV-1 virions via a clathrin-dependent mechanism. *Eur J Immunol* 39(7), 1923-8.
Cantin, R., Diou, J., Belanger, D., Tremblay, A. M., and Gilbert, C. (2008). Discrimination between exosomes and HIV-1: purification of both vesicles from cell-free supernatants. *J Immunol Methods* 338(1-2), 21-30.
Cantin, R., Fortin, J. F., Lamontagne, G., and Tremblay, M. (1997). The acquisition of host-derived major histocompatibility complex class II glycoproteins by human immunodeficiency virus type 1 accelerates the process of virus entry and infection in human T-lymphoid cells. *Blood* 90(3), 1091-100.
Cantin, R., Fortin, J. F., and Tremblay, M. (1996). The amount of host HLA-DR proteins acquired by HIV-1 is virus strain- and cell type-specific. *Virology* 218(2), 372-81.
Cantin, R., Martin, G., and Tremblay, M. J. (2001). A novel virus capture assay reveals a differential acquisition of host HLA-DR by clinical isolates of human immunodeficiency virus type 1 expanded in primary human cells depending on the nature of producing cells and the donor source. *J Gen Virol* 82(Pt 12), 2979-87.
Cantin, R., Methot, S., and Tremblay, M. J. (2005). Plunder and stowaways: incorporation of cellular proteins by enveloped viruses. *J Virol* 79(11), 6577-87.
Cecchinato, V., and Franchini, G. (2010). Th17 cells in pathogenic simian immunodeficiency virus infection of macaques. *Curr Opin HIV AIDS* 5(2), 141-5.
Cecchinato, V., Trindade, C. J., Laurence, A., Heraud, J. M., Brenchley, J. M., Ferrari, M. G., Zaffiri, L., Tryniszewska, E., Tsai, W. P., Vaccari, M., Parks, R. W., Venzon, D., Douek, D. C., O'Shea, J. J., and Franchini, G. (2008). Altered balance between Th17 and Th1 cells at mucosal sites predicts AIDS progression in simian immunodeficiency virus-infected macaques. *Mucosal Immunol* 1(4), 279-88.
Chaput, N., Flament, C., Viaud, S., Taieb, J., Roux, S., Spatz, A., Andre, F., LePecq, J. B., Boussac, M., Garin, J., Amigorena, S., Thery, C., and Zitvogel, L. (2006). Dendritic cell derived-exosomes: biology and clinical implementations. *J Leukoc Biol* 80(3), 471-8.
Chaput, N., Taieb, J., Schartz, N. E., Andre, F., Angevin, E., and Zitvogel, L. (2004). Exosome-based immunotherapy. *Cancer Immunol Immunother* 53(3), 234-9.
Chaput, N., and Thery, C. (2010). Exosomes: immune properties and potential clinical implementations. *Semin Immunopathol.*
Chertova, E., Chertov, O., Coren, L. V., Roser, J. D., Trubey, C. M., Bess, J. W., Jr., Sowder, R. C., 2nd, Barsov, E., Hood, B. L., Fisher, R. J., Nagashima, K., Conrads, T. P., Veenstra, T. D., Lifson, J. D., and Ott, D. E. (2006). Proteomic and biochemical analysis of purified human immunodeficiency virus type 1 produced from infected monocyte-derived macrophages. *J Virol* 80(18), 9039-52.

Clayton, A., Harris, C. L., Court, J., Mason, M. D., and Morgan, B. P. (2003). Antigen-presenting cell exosomes are protected from complement-mediated lysis by expression of CD55 and CD59. *Eur J Immunol* 33(2), 522-31.

de Gassart, A., Geminard, C., Fevrier, B., Raposo, G., and Vidal, M. (2003). Lipid raft-associated protein sorting in exosomes. *Blood* 102(13), 4336-44.

de Gassart, A., Geminard, C., Hoekstra, D., and Vidal, M. (2004). Exosome secretion: the art of reutilizing nonrecycled proteins? *Traffic* 5(11), 896-903.

Derse, D., Dorn, P. L., Levy, L., Stephens, R. M., Rice, N. R., and Casey, J. W. (1987). Characterization of equine infectious anemia virus long terminal repeat. *J Virol* 61(3), 743-7.

Dettenhofer, M., and Yu, X. F. (1999). Highly purified human immunodeficiency virus type 1 reveals a virtual absence of Vif in virions. *J Virol* 73(2), 1460-7.

Doitsh, G., Cavrois, M., Lassen, K. G., Zepeda, O., Yang, Z., Santiago, M. L., Hebbeler, A. M., and Greene, W. C. (2010). Abortive HIV infection mediates CD4 T cell depletion and inflammation in human lymphoid tissue. *Cell* 143(5), 789-801.

Dornadula, G., Zhang, H., Shetty, S., and Pomerantz, R. J. (1999). HIV-1 virions produced from replicating peripheral blood lymphocytes are more infectious than those from nonproliferating macrophages due to higher levels of intravirion reverse transcripts: implications for pathogenesis and transmission. *Virology* 253(1), 10-6.

Elbim, C., Monceaux, V., Francois, S., Hurtrel, B., Gougerot-Pocidalo, M. A., and Estaquier, J. (2009). Increased neutrophil apoptosis in chronically SIV-infected macaques. *Retrovirology* 6, 29.

Elbim, C., Monceaux, V., Mueller, Y. M., Lewis, M. G., Francois, S., Diop, O., Akarid, K., Hurtrel, B., Gougerot-Pocidalo, M. A., Levy, Y., Katsikis, P. D., and Estaquier, J. (2008). Early divergence in neutrophil apoptosis between pathogenic and nonpathogenic simian immunodeficiency virus infections of nonhuman primates. *J Immunol* 181(12), 8613-23.

Elhed, A., and Unutmaz, D. (2010). Th17 cells and HIV infection. *Curr Opin HIV AIDS* 5(2), 146-50.

Esser, J., Gehrmann, U., D'Alexandri, F. L., Hidalgo-Estevez, A. M., Wheelock, C. E., Scheynius, A., Gabrielsson, S., and Radmark, O. Exosomes from human macrophages and dendritic cells contain enzymes for leukotriene biosynthesis and promote granulocyte migration. *J Allergy Clin Immunol* 126(5), 1032-40, 1040 e1-4.

Esser, J., Gehrmann, U., D'Alexandri, F. L., Hidalgo-Estevez, A. M., Wheelock, C. E., Scheynius, A., Gabrielsson, S., and Radmark, O. (2010). Exosomes from human macrophages and dendritic cells contain enzymes for leukotriene biosynthesis and promote granulocyte migration. *J Allergy Clin Immunol* 126(5), 1032-40, 1040 e1-4.

Farsad, K. (2002). Exosomes: novel organelles implicated in immunomodulation and apoptosis. *Yale J Biol Med* 75(2), 95-101.

Favre, D., Lederer, S., Kanwar, B., Ma, Z. M., Proll, S., Kasakow, Z., Mold, J., Swainson, L., Barbour, J. D., Baskin, C. R., Palermo, R., Pandrea, I., Miller, C. J., Katze, M. G., and McCune, J. M. (2009). Critical loss of the balance between Th17 and T regulatory cell populations in pathogenic SIV infection. *PLoS Pathog* 5(2), e1000295.

Fontaine, J., Chagnon-Choquet, J., Valcke, H. S., Poudrier, J., and Roger, M. (2011). High expression levels of B lymphocyte stimulator (BLyS) by dendritic cells correlate with HIV-related B-cell disease progression in humans. *Blood* 117(1), 145-55.

Ford, T., Graham, J., and Rickwood, D. (1994). Iodixanol: a nonionic iso-osmotic centrifugation medium for the formation of self-generated gradients. *Anal Biochem* 220(2), 360-6.

Frangsmyr, L., Baranov, V., Nagaeva, O., Stendahl, U., Kjellberg, L., and Mincheva-Nilsson, L. (2005). Cytoplasmic microvesicular form of Fas ligand in human early placenta: switching the tissue immune privilege hypothesis from cellular to vesicular level. *Mol Hum Reprod* 11(1), 35-41.

Gansuvd, B., Hagihara, M., Higuchi, A., Ueda, Y., Tazume, K., Tsuchiya, T., Munkhtuvshin, N., Kato, S., and Hotta, T. (2003). Umbilical cord blood dendritic cells are a rich source of soluble HLA-DR: synergistic effect of exosomes and dendritic cells on autologous or allogeneic T-Cell proliferation. *Hum Immunol* 64(4), 427-39.

Garcia, E., Pion, M., Pelchen-Matthews, A., Collinson, L., Arrighi, J. F., Blot, G., Leuba, F., Escola, J. M., Demaurex, N., Marsh, M., and Piguet, V. (2005). HIV-1 trafficking to the dendritic cell-T-cell infectious synapse uses a pathway of tetraspanin sorting to the immunological synapse. *Traffic* 6(6), 488-501.

Gastpar, R., Gehrmann, M., Bausero, M. A., Asea, A., Gross, C., Schroeder, J. A., and Multhoff, G. (2005). Heat shock protein 70 surface-positive tumor exosomes stimulate migratory and cytolytic activity of natural killer cells. *Cancer Res* 65(12), 5238-47.

Geijtenbeek, T. B., Kwon, D. S., Torensma, R., van Vliet, S. J., van Duijnhoven, G. C., Middel, J., Cornelissen, I. L., Nottet, H. S., KewalRamani, V. N., Littman, D. R., Figdor, C. G., and van Kooyk, Y. (2000). DC-SIGN, a dendritic cell-specific HIV-1-binding protein that enhances trans-infection of T cells. *Cell* 100(5), 587-97.

Gilbert, C., Barat, C., Cantin, R., and Tremblay, M. J. (2007a). Involvement of Src and Syk Tyrosine Kinases in HIV-1 Transfer from Dendritic Cells to CD4+ T Lymphocytes. *J Immunol* 178(5), 2862-2871.

Gilbert, C., Cantin, R., Barat, C., and Tremblay, M. J. (2007b). Human Immunodeficiency Virus Type 1 Replication in Dendritic Cell-T-Cell Cocultures Is Increased upon Incorporation of Host LFA-1 due to Higher Levels of Virus Production in Immature Dendritic Cells. *J Virol* 81(14), 7672-82.

Giorgi, J. V., Hultin, L. E., McKeating, J. A., Johnson, T. D., Owens, B., Jacobson, L. P., Shih, R., Lewis, J., Wiley, D. J., Phair, J. P., Wolinsky, S. M., and Detels, R. (1999). Shorter survival in advanced human immunodeficiency virus type 1 infection is more closely associated with T lymphocyte activation than with plasma virus burden or virus chemokine coreceptor usage. *J Infect Dis* 179(4), 859-70.

Gould, S. J., Hildreth, J. E., and Booth, A. M. (2004). The evolution of alloimmunity and the genesis of adaptive immunity. *Q Rev Biol* 79(4), 359-82.

Granelli-Piperno, A., Delgado, E., Finkel, V., Paxton, W., and Steinman, R. M. (1998). Immature dendritic cells selectively replicate macrophagetropic (M-tropic) human immunodeficiency virus type 1, while mature cells efficiently transmit both M- and T-tropic virus to T cells. *J Virol* 72(4), 2733-7.

Guadalupe, M., Reay, E., Sankaran, S., Prindiville, T., Flamm, J., McNeil, A., and Dandekar, S. (2003). Severe CD4+ T-cell depletion in gut lymphoid tissue during primary human immunodeficiency virus type 1 infection and substantial delay in restoration following highly active antiretroviral therapy. *J Virol* 77(21), 11708-17.

Hammond, G. W., Hazelton, P. R., Chuang, I., and Klisko, B. (1981). Improved detection of viruses by electron microscopy after direct ultracentrifuge preparation of specimens. *J Clin Microbiol* 14(2), 210-21.

Hawari, F. I., Rouhani, F. N., Cui, X., Yu, Z. X., Buckley, C., Kaler, M., and Levine, S. J. (2004). Release of full-length 55-kDa TNF receptor 1 in exosome-like vesicles: a mechanism for generation of soluble cytokine receptors. *Proc Natl Acad Sci U S A* 101(5), 1297-302.

Hermens, W. T., ter Brake, O., Dijkhuizen, P. A., Sonnemans, M. A., Grimm, D., Kleinschmidt, J. A., and Verhaagen, J. (1999). Purification of recombinant adeno-associated virus by iodixanol gradient ultracentrifugation allows rapid and reproducible preparation of vector stocks for gene transfer in the nervous system. *Hum Gene Ther* 10(11), 1885-91.

Hladik, F., and McElrath, M. J. (2008). Setting the stage: host invasion by HIV. *Nat Rev Immunol* 8(6), 447-57.

Hofman, P., Fischer, F., Far, D. F., Selva, E., Battaglione, V., Bayle, J., and Rossi, B. (1999). Impairment of HIV polymorphonuclear leukocyte transmigration across T84 cell monolayers: an alternative mechanisms for increased intestinal bacterial infections in AIDS? *Eur Cytokine Netw* 10(3), 373-82.

Iero, M., Valenti, R., Huber, V., Filipazzi, P., Parmiani, G., Fais, S., and Rivoltini, L. (2008). Tumour-released exosomes and their implications in cancer immunity. *Cell Death Differ* 15(1), 80-8.

Imami, N., Hardy, G., Burton, C., Pires, A., Pido-Lopez, J., Moss, R., Gazzard, B., and Gotch, F. (2001). Immune responses and reconstitution in HIV-1 infected individuals: impact of anti-retroviral therapy, cytokines and therapeutic vaccination. *Immunol Lett* 79(1-2), 63-76.

Izquierdo-Useros, N., Naranjo-Gomez, M., Archer, J., Hatch, S. C., Erkizia, I., Blanco, J., Borras, F. E., Puertas, M. C., Connor, J. H., Fernandez-Figueras, M. T., Moore, L., Clotet, B., Gummuluru, S., and Martinez-Picado, J. (2009). Capture and transfer of HIV-1 particles by mature dendritic cells converges with the exosome-dissemination pathway. *Blood* 113(12), 2732-41.

Izquierdo-Useros, N., Naranjo-Gomez, M., Erkizia, I., Puertas, M. C., Borras, F. E., Blanco, J., and Martinez-Picado, J. (2010). HIV and mature dendritic cells: Trojan exosomes riding the Trojan horse? *PLoS Pathog* 6(3), e1000740.

Johnstone, R. M., Adam, M., Hammond, J. R., Orr, L., and Turbide, C. (1987). Vesicle formation during reticulocyte maturation. Association of plasma membrane activities with released vesicles (exosomes). *J Biol Chem* 262(19), 9412-20.

Kapsogeorgou, E. K., Abu-Helu, R. F., Moutsopoulos, H. M., and Manoussakis, M. N. (2005). Salivary gland epithelial cell exosomes: A source of autoantigenic ribonucleoproteins. *Arthritis Rheum* 52(5), 1517-21.

Karlsson, M., Lundin, S., Dahlgren, U., Kahu, H., Pettersson, I., and Telemo, E. (2001). "Tolerosomes" are produced by intestinal epithelial cells. *Eur J Immunol* 31(10), 2892-900.

Kim, H. P., Morse, D., and Choi, A. M. (2006). Heat-shock proteins: new keys to the development of cytoprotective therapies. *Expert Opin Ther Targets* 10(5), 759-69.

Kim, S. H., Bianco, N., Menon, R., Lechman, E. R., Shufesky, W. J., Morelli, A. E., and Robbins, P. D. (2006). Exosomes derived from genetically modified DC expressing FasL are anti-inflammatory and immunosuppressive. *Mol Ther* 13(2), 289-300.

Kleijmeer, M. J., Escola, J. M., UytdeHaag, F. G., Jakobson, E., Griffith, J. M., Osterhaus, A. D., Stoorvogel, W., Melief, C. J., Rabouille, C., and Geuze, H. J. (2001). Antigen loading of MHC class I molecules in the endocytic tract. *Traffic* 2(2), 124-37.

Klibi, J., Niki, T., Riedel, A., Pioche-Durieu, C., Souquere, S., Rubinstein, E., Le Moulec, S., Guigay, J., Hirashima, M., Guemira, F., Adhikary, D., Mautner, J., and Busson, P. (2009). Blood diffusion and Th1-suppressive effects of galectin-9-containing exosomes released by Epstein-Barr virus-infected nasopharyngeal carcinoma cells. *Blood* 113(9), 1957-66.

Kwon, D. S., Gregorio, G., Bitton, N., Hendrickson, W. A., and Littman, D. R. (2002). DC-SIGN-mediated internalization of HIV is required for trans-enhancement of T cell infection. *Immunity* 16(1), 135-44.

Lambert, A. A., Gilbert, C., Richard, M., Beaulieu, A. D., and Tremblay, M. J. (2008). The C-type lectin surface receptor DCIR acts as a new attachment factor for HIV-1 in dendritic cells and contributes to trans- and cis-infection pathways. *Blood* 112(4), 1299-307.

Lancaster, G. I., and Febbraio, M. A. (2005). Exosome-dependent trafficking of HSP70: a novel secretory pathway for cellular stress proteins. *J Biol Chem* 280(24), 23349-55.

Larregina, A. T., Morelli, A. E., Tkacheva, O., Erdos, G., Donahue, C., Watkins, S. C., Thomson, A. W., and Falo, L. D., Jr. (2004). Highly efficient expression of transgenic proteins by naked DNA-transfected dendritic cells through terminal differentiation. *Blood* 103(3), 811-9.

Lenassi, M., Cagney, G., Liao, M., Vaupotic, T., Bartholomeeusen, K., Cheng, Y., Krogan, N. J., Plemenitas, A., and Peterlin, B. M. (2010). HIV Nef is secreted in exosomes and triggers apoptosis in bystander CD4+ T cells. *Traffic* 11(1), 110-22.

Levine, S. J. (2004). Mechanisms of soluble cytokine receptor generation. *J Immunol* 173(9), 5343-8.

Li, Q., Duan, L., Estes, J. D., Ma, Z. M., Rourke, T., Wang, Y., Reilly, C., Carlis, J., Miller, C. J., and Haase, A. T. (2005). Peak SIV replication in resting memory CD4+ T cells depletes gut lamina propria CD4+ T cells. *Nature* 434(7037), 1148-52.

Lichtner, M., Maranon, C., Vidalain, P. O., Azocar, O., Hanau, D., Lebon, P., Burgard, M., Rouzioux, C., Vullo, V., Yagita, H., Rabourdin-Combe, C., Servet, C., and Hosmalin, A. (2004). HIV type 1-infected dendritic cells induce apoptotic death in infected and uninfected primary CD4 T lymphocytes. *AIDS Res Hum Retroviruses* 20(2), 175-82.

Liu, Z., Cumberland, W. G., Hultin, L. E., Prince, H. E., Detels, R., and Giorgi, J. V. (1997). Elevated CD38 antigen expression on CD8+ T cells is a stronger marker for the risk of chronic HIV disease progression to AIDS and death in the Multicenter AIDS Cohort Study than CD4+ cell count, soluble immune activation markers, or combinations of HLA-DR and CD38 expression. *J Acquir Immune Defic Syndr Hum Retrovirol* 16(2), 83-92.

Mallegol, J., van Niel, G., and Heyman, M. (2005). Phenotypic and functional characterization of intestinal epithelial exosomes. *Blood Cells Mol Dis* 35(1), 11-6.

Manel, N., Hogstad, B., Wang, Y., Levy, D. E., Unutmaz, D., and Littman, D. R. (2010). A cryptic sensor for HIV-1 activates antiviral innate immunity in dendritic cells. *Nature* 467(7312), 214-7.

Marchetti, G., Bellistri, G. M., Borghi, E., Tincati, C., Ferramosca, S., La Francesca, M., Morace, G., Gori, A., and Monforte, A. D. (2008). Microbial translocation is associated with sustained failure in CD4+ T-cell reconstitution in HIV-infected patients on long-term highly active antiretroviral therapy. *AIDS* 22(15), 2035-8.

Matloubian, M., Concepcion, R. J., and Ahmed, R. (1994). CD4+ T cells are required to sustain CD8+ cytotoxic T-cell responses during chronic viral infection. *J Virol* 68(12), 8056-63.

Mattapallil, J. J., Douek, D. C., Hill, B., Nishimura, Y., Martin, M., and Roederer, M. (2005). Massive infection and loss of memory CD4+ T cells in multiple tissues during acute SIV infection. *Nature* 434(7037), 1093-7.

Mehandru, S., Poles, M. A., Tenner-Racz, K., Horowitz, A., Hurley, A., Hogan, C., Boden, D., Racz, P., and Markowitz, M. (2004). Primary HIV-1 infection is associated with preferential depletion of CD4+ T lymphocytes from effector sites in the gastrointestinal tract. *J Exp Med* 200(6), 761-70.

Mignot, G., Roux, S., Thery, C., Segura, E., and Zitvogel, L. (2006). Prospects for exosomes in immunotherapy of cancer. *J Cell Mol Med* 10(2), 376-88.

Milush, J. M., Mir, K. D., Sundaravaradan, V., Gordon, S. N., Engram, J., Cano, C. A., Reeves, J. D., Anton, E., O'Neill, E., Butler, E., Hancock, K., Cole, K. S., Brenchley, J. M., Else, J. G., Silvestri, G., and Sodora, D. L. (2011). Lack of clinical AIDS in SIV-infected sooty mangabeys with significant CD4+ T cell loss is associated with double-negative T cells. *J Clin Invest.*

Milush, J. M., Reeves, J. D., Gordon, S. N., Zhou, D., Muthukumar, A., Kosub, D. A., Chacko, E., Giavedoni, L. D., Ibegbu, C. C., Cole, K. S., Miamidian, J. L., Paiardini, M., Barry, A. P., Staprans, S. I., Silvestri, G., and Sodora, D. L. (2007). Virally induced CD4+ T cell depletion is not sufficient to induce AIDS in a natural host. *J Immunol* 179(5), 3047-56.

Moir, S., Chun, T. W., and Fauci, A. S. (2010). Pathogenic Mechanisms of HIV Disease. *Annu Rev Pathol.*

Moller-Larsen, A., and Christensen, T. (1998). Isolation of a retrovirus from multiple sclerosis patients in self-generated Iodixanol gradients. *J Virol Methods* 73(2), 151-61.

Monleon, I., Martinez-Lorenzo, M. J., Monteagudo, L., Lasierra, P., Taules, M., Iturralde, M., Pineiro, A., Larrad, L., Alava, M. A., Naval, J., and Anel, A. (2001). Differential secretion of Fas ligand- or APO2 ligand/TNF-related apoptosis-inducing ligand-carrying microvesicles during activation-induced death of human T cells. *J Immunol* 167(12), 6736-44.

Morita, E., and Sundquist, W. I. (2004). Retrovirus budding. *Annu Rev Cell Dev Biol* 20, 395-425.

Nguyen, D. G., Booth, A., Gould, S. J., and Hildreth, J. E. (2003). Evidence that HIV budding in primary macrophages occurs through the exosome release pathway. *J Biol Chem* 278(52), 52347-54.

Okada, H., Takei, R., and Tashiro, M. (1997). HIV-1 Nef protein-induced apoptotic cytolysis of a broad spectrum of uninfected human blood cells independently of CD95(Fas). *FEBS Lett* 414(3), 603-6.

Okada, H., Takei, R., and Tashiro, M. (1998). Inhibition of HIV-1 Nef-induced apoptosis of uninfected human blood cells by serine/threonine protein kinase inhibitors, fasudil hydrochloride and M3. *FEBS Lett* 422(3), 363-7.

Ostman, S., Taube, M., and Telemo, E. (2005). Tolerosome-induced oral tolerance is MHC dependent. *Immunology* 116(4), 464-76.

Paiardini, M. (2010). Th17 cells in natural SIV hosts. *Curr Opin HIV AIDS* 5(2), 166-72.

Peche, H., Heslan, M., Usal, C., Amigorena, S., and Cuturi, M. C. (2003). Presentation of donor major histocompatibility complex antigens by bone marrow dendritic cell-derived exosomes modulates allograft rejection. *Transplantation* 76(10), 1503-10.

Peche, H., Renaudin, K., Beriou, G., Merieau, E., Amigorena, S., and Cuturi, M. C. (2006). Induction of tolerance by exosomes and short-term immunosuppression in a fully MHC-mismatched rat cardiac allograft model. *Am J Transplant* 6(7), 1541-50.

Pegtel, D. M., Cosmopoulos, K., Thorley-Lawson, D. A., van Eijndhoven, M. A., Hopmans, E. S., Lindenberg, J. L., de Gruijl, T. D., Wurdinger, T., and Middeldorp, J. M. (2010). Functional delivery of viral miRNAs via exosomes. *Proc Natl Acad Sci U S A* 107(14), 6328-33.

Permanyer, M., Ballana, E., and Este, J. A. (2010). Endocytosis of HIV: anything goes. *Trends Microbiol* 18(12), 543-51.

Piguet, V., and Steinman, R. M. (2007). The interaction of HIV with dendritic cells: outcomes and pathways. *Trends Immunol* 28(11), 503-10.

Pitrak, D. L., Tsai, H. C., Mullane, K. M., Sutton, S. H., and Stevens, P. (1996). Accelerated neutrophil apoptosis in the acquired immunodeficiency syndrome. *J Clin Invest* 98(12), 2714-9.

Quah, B., and O'Neill, H. C. (2000). Review: the application of dendritic cell-derived exosomes in tumour immunotherapy. *Cancer Biother Radiopharm* 15(2), 185-94.

Quah, B. J., and O'Neill, H. C. (2005a). The immunogenicity of dendritic cell-derived exosomes. *Blood Cells Mol Dis* 35(2), 94-110.

Quah, B. J., and O'Neill, H. C. (2005b). Maturation of function in dendritic cells for tolerance and immunity. *J Cell Mol Med* 9(3), 643-54.

Raposo, G., Moore, M., Innes, D., Leijendekker, R., Leigh-Brown, A., Benaroch, P., and Geuze, H. (2002). Human macrophages accumulate HIV-1 particles in MHC II compartments. *Traffic* 3(10), 718-29.

Raposo, G., Nijman, H. W., Stoorvogel, W., Liejendekker, R., Harding, C. V., Melief, C. J., and Geuze, H. J. (1996). B lymphocytes secrete antigen-presenting vesicles. *J Exp Med* 183(3), 1161-72.

Record, M., Subra, C., Silvente-Poirot, S., and Poirot, M. (2011). Exosomes as intercellular signalosomes and pharmacological effectors. *Biochem Pharmacol.*

Ren, Y., Yang, J., Xie, R., Gao, L., Yang, Y., Fan, H., and Qian, K. Exosomal-like vesicles with immune-modulatory features are present in human plasma and can induce CD4+ T-cell apoptosis in vitro. *Transfusion.*

Ren, Y., Yang, J., Xie, R., Gao, L., Yang, Y., Fan, H., and Qian, K. (2010). Exosomal-like vesicles with immune-modulatory features are present in human plasma and can induce CD4+ T-cell apoptosis in vitro. *Transfusion.*

Rieu, S., Geminard, C., Rabesandratana, H., Sainte-Marie, J., and Vidal, M. (2000). Exosomes released during reticulocyte maturation bind to fibronectin via integrin alpha4beta1. *Eur J Biochem* 267(2), 583-90.

Roilides, E., Holmes, A., Blake, C., Pizzo, P. A., and Walsh, T. J. (1993). Impairment of neutrophil antifungal activity against hyphae of Aspergillus fumigatus in children infected with human immunodeficiency virus. *J Infect Dis* 167(4), 905-11.

Roilides, E., Mertins, S., Eddy, J., Walsh, T. J., Pizzo, P. A., and Rubin, M. (1990). Impairment of neutrophil chemotactic and bactericidal function in children infected with human immunodeficiency virus type 1 and partial reversal after in vitro exposure to granulocyte-macrophage colony-stimulating factor. *J Pediatr* 117(4), 531-40.

Saelens, X., Festjens, N., Vande Walle, L., van Gurp, M., van Loo, G., and Vandenabeele, P. (2004). Toxic proteins released from mitochondria in cell death. *Oncogene* 23(16), 2861-74.

Segura, E., Amigorena, S., and Thery, C. (2005). Mature dendritic cells secrete exosomes with strong ability to induce antigen-specific effector immune responses. *Blood Cells Mol Dis* 35(2), 89-93.

Segura, E., Nicco, C., Lombard, B., Veron, P., Raposo, G., Batteux, F., Amigorena, S., and Thery, C. (2005). ICAM-1 on exosomes from mature dendritic cells is critical for efficient naive T-cell priming. *Blood* 106(1), 216-23.

Sewell, A. K., Price, D. A., Oxenius, A., Kelleher, A. D., and Phillips, R. E. (2000). Cytotoxic T lymphocyte responses to human immunodeficiency virus: control and escape. *Stem Cells* 18(4), 230-44.

Shacklett, B. L. (2010). Immune responses to HIV and SIV in mucosal tissues: 'location, location, location'. *Curr Opin HIV AIDS* 5(2), 128-34.

Silvestri, G., Sodora, D. L., Koup, R. A., Paiardini, M., O'Neil, S. P., McClure, H. M., Staprans, S. I., and Feinberg, M. B. (2003). Nonpathogenic SIV infection of sooty mangabeys is characterized by limited bystander immunopathology despite chronic high-level viremia. *Immunity* 18(3), 441-52.

Skokos, D., Le Panse, S., Villa, I., Rousselle, J. C., Peronet, R., Namane, A., David, B., and Mecheri, S. (2001). Nonspecific B and T cell-stimulatory activity mediated by mast cells is associated with exosomes. *Int Arch Allergy Immunol* 124(1-3), 133-6.

Stoorvogel, W., Kleijmeer, M. J., Geuze, H. J., and Raposo, G. (2002). The biogenesis and functions of exosomes. *Traffic* 3(5), 321-30.

Subra, C., Grand, D., Laulagnier, K., Stella, A., Lambeau, G., Paillasse, M., De Medina, P., Monsarrat, B., Perret, B., Silvente-Poirot, S., Poirot, M., and Record, M. (2010). Exosomes account for vesicle-mediated transcellular transport of activatable phospholipases and prostaglandins. *J Lipid Res* 51(8), 2105-20.

Szelc, C. M., Mitcheltree, C., Roberts, R. L., and Stiehm, E. R. (1992). Deficient polymorphonuclear cell and mononuclear cell antibody-dependent cellular cytotoxicity in pediatric and adult human immunodeficiency virus infection. *J Infect Dis* 166(3), 486-93.

Taylor, D. D., Akyol, S., and Gercel-Taylor, C. (2006). Pregnancy-associated exosomes and their modulation of T cell signaling. *J Immunol* 176(3), 1534-42.

Thery, C., Boussac, M., Veron, P., Ricciardi-Castagnoli, P., Raposo, G., Garin, J., and Amigorena, S. (2001). Proteomic analysis of dendritic cell-derived exosomes: a secreted subcellular compartment distinct from apoptotic vesicles. *J Immunol* 166(12), 7309-18.

Thery, C., Duban, L., Segura, E., Veron, P., Lantz, O., and Amigorena, S. (2002). Indirect activation of naive CD4+ T cells by dendritic cell-derived exosomes. *Nat Immunol* 3(12), 1156-62.

Thery, C., Regnault, A., Garin, J., Wolfers, J., Zitvogel, L., Ricciardi-Castagnoli, P., Raposo, G., and Amigorena, S. (1999). Molecular characterization of dendritic cell-derived exosomes. Selective accumulation of the heat shock protein hsc73. *J Cell Biol* 147(3), 599-610.

Thery, C., Zitvogel, L., and Amigorena, S. (2002). Exosomes: composition, biogenesis and function. *Nat Rev Immunol* 2(8), 569-79.

Thibault, S., Tardif, M. R., Barat, C., and Tremblay, M. J. (2007). TLR2 signaling renders quiescent naive and memory CD4+ T cells more susceptible to productive infection with X4 and R5 HIV-type 1. *J Immunol* 179(7), 4357-66.

Thorsen, S., Busch-Sorensen, M., and Sondergaard, J. (1989). Reduced neutrophil production of leukotriene B4 associated with AIDS. *Aids* 3(10), 651-3.

Torre, D., Gennero, L., Baccino, F. M., Speranza, F., Biondi, G., and Pugliese, A. (2002). Impaired macrophage phagocytosis of apoptotic neutrophils in patients with human immunodeficiency virus type 1 infection. *Clin Diagn Lab Immunol* 9(5), 983-6.

Trubey, C. M., Chertova, E., Coren, L. V., Hilburn, J. M., Hixson, C. V., Nagashima, K., Lifson, J. D., and Ott, D. E. (2003). Quantitation of HLA class II protein incorporated into human immunodeficiency type 1 virions purified by anti-CD45 immunoaffinity depletion of microvesicles. *J Virol* 77(23), 12699-709.

Tsuji, T., Nibu, R., Iwai, K., Kanegane, H., Yachie, A., Seki, H., Miyawaki, T., and Taniguchi, N. (1994). Efficient induction of immunoglobulin production in neonatal naive B cells by memory CD4+ T cell subset expressing homing receptor L-selectin. *J Immunol* 152(9), 4417-24.

Tsunetsugu-Yokota, Y., Yasuda, S., Sugimoto, A., Yagi, T., Azuma, M., Yagita, H., Akagawa, K., and Takemori, T. (1997). Efficient virus transmission from dendritic cells to CD4+ T cells in response to antigen depends on close contact through adhesion molecules. *Virology* 239(2), 259-68.

Turville, S. G., Santos, J. J., Frank, I., Cameron, P. U., Wilkinson, J., Miranda-Saksena, M., Dable, J., Stossel, H., Romani, N., Piatak, M., Jr., Lifson, J. D., Pope, M., and Cunningham, A. L. (2004). Immunodeficiency virus uptake, turnover, and 2-phase transfer in human dendritic cells. *Blood* 103(6), 2170-9.

Valadi, H., Ekstrom, K., Bossios, A., Sjostrand, M., Lee, J. J., and Lotvall, J. O. (2007). Exosome-mediated transfer of mRNAs and microRNAs is a novel mechanism of genetic exchange between cells. *Nat Cell Biol* 9(6), 654-9.

van Niel, G., and Heyman, M. (2002). The epithelial cell cytoskeleton and intracellular trafficking. II. Intestinal epithelial cell exosomes: perspectives on their structure and function. *Am J Physiol Gastrointest Liver Physiol* 283(2), G251-5.

Van Niel, G., Mallegol, J., Bevilacqua, C., Candalh, C., Brugiere, S., Tomaskovic-Crook, E., Heath, J. K., Cerf-Bensussan, N., and Heyman, M. (2003). Intestinal epithelial exosomes carry MHC class II/peptides able to inform the immune system in mice. *Gut* 52(12), 1690-7.

Van Veldhoven, P. P., Baumgart, E., and Mannaerts, G. P. (1996). Iodixanol (Optiprep), an improved density gradient medium for the iso-osmotic isolation of rat liver peroxisomes. *Anal Biochem* 237(1), 17-23.

Varbanov, M., Espert, L., and Biard-Piechaczyk, M. (2006). Mechanisms of CD4 T-cell depletion triggered by HIV-1 viral proteins. *AIDS Rev* 8(4), 221-36.

Vincent-Schneider, H., Stumptner-Cuvelette, P., Lankar, D., Pain, S., Raposo, G., Benaroch, P., and Bonnerot, C. (2002). Exosomes bearing HLA-DR1 molecules need dendritic cells to efficiently stimulate specific T cells. *Int Immunol* 14(7), 713-22.

Wan, Z. T., and Chen, X. L. (2010). Mechanisms of HIV envelope-induced T lymphocyte apoptosis. *Virol Sin* 25(5), 307-15.

Wang, J. J., Horton, R., Varthakavi, V., Spearman, P., and Ratner, L. (1999). Formation and release of virus-like particles by HIV-1 matrix protein. *AIDS* 13(2), 281-3.

Wei, X., Decker, J. M., Liu, H., Zhang, Z., Arani, R. B., Kilby, J. M., Saag, M. S., Wu, X., Shaw, G. M., and Kappes, J. C. (2002). Emergence of resistant human immunodeficiency virus type 1 in patients receiving fusion inhibitor (T-20) monotherapy. *Antimicrob Agents Chemother* 46(6), 1896-905.

Xie, Y., Zhang, H., Li, W., Deng, Y., Munegowda, M. A., Chibbar, R., Qureshi, M., and Xiang, J. (2010). Dendritic cells recruit T cell exosomes via exosomal LFA-1 leading to inhibition of CD8+ CTL responses through downregulation of peptide/MHC class I and Fas ligand-mediated cytotoxicity. *J Immunol* 185(9), 5268-78.

Zajac, A. J., Blattman, J. N., Murali-Krishna, K., Sourdive, D. J., Suresh, M., Altman, J. D., and Ahmed, R. (1998). Viral immune evasion due to persistence of activated T cells without effector function. *J Exp Med* 188(12), 2205-13.

Zhang, H. G., Liu, C., Su, K., Yu, S., Zhang, L., Zhang, S., Wang, J., Cao, X., Grizzle, W., and Kimberly, R. P. (2006). A membrane form of TNF-alpha presented by exosomes delays T cell activation-induced cell death. *J Immunol* 176(12), 7385-93.

Zhao, C., Cantin, R., Breton, M., Papadopoulou, B., and Tremblay, M. J. (2005). DC-SIGN-mediated transfer of HIV-1 is compromised by the ability of Leishmania infantum to exploit DC-SIGN as a ligand. *J Infect Dis* 191(10), 1665-9.

Zitvogel, L., Regnault, A., Lozier, A., Wolfers, J., Flament, C., Tenza, D., Ricciardi-Castagnoli, P., Raposo, G., and Amigorena, S. (1998). Eradication of established murine tumors using a novel cell-free vaccine: dendritic cell-derived exosomes. *Nat Med* 4(5), 594-600.

Zolotukhin, S., Byrne, B. J., Mason, E., Zolotukhin, I., Potter, M., Chesnut, K., Summerford, C., Samulski, R. J., and Muzyczka, N. (1999). Recombinant adeno-associated virus purification using novel methods improves infectious titer and yield. *Gene Ther* 6(6), 973-85.

Part 3

Understanding Immunological Aspects of HIV in an Infected Person

9

RNAi-Based Gene Expression Strategies to Combat HIV

Fiona T. van den Berg and Marc S. Weinberg
Antiviral Gene Therapy Research Unit (AGTRU), University of the Witwatersrand South Africa

1. Introduction

Antiretroviral drugs have made a significant impact on HIV/AIDS disease progression and have significantly extended the life expectancy of HIV-infected individuals, particularly when used in combination therapies such as HAART (highly active antiretroviral therapy). However, despite this success, recent reports indicate that HIV morbidity and mortality remain at epidemic proportions. It is estimated that over 33 million people are currently infected with the virus worldwide, while sub-Saharan Africa accounted for approximately 70% of all infected individuals and AIDS-related deaths in 2009 (UNAIDS, 2010). Issues of drug resistance, drug toxicity, correct patient compliance and the inability to remove latent reservoirs of infection remain significant problems to overcome. The need to develop novel and improved therapeutic strategies against HIV therefore remains an important medical objective. Gene-based therapies hold much promise as alternative treatment strategies for HIV/AIDS. Anti-viral gene therapies aim to provide a once-off, long-lasting treatment against the virus and thereby address some of the shortcomings associated with current antiretroviral therapies.

A gene therapy against HIV offers several unique advantages, including the sustained inhibition of viral replication and the removal of virus from cellular reservoirs. Moreover, by improving specificity, the common toxic side effects associated with current antiretrovial regimens can be diminished. A number of different RNA-based and protein-based gene therapy strategies have been explored and some have reached phase 1 and 2 clinical trials. Our research focuses on the development of RNA-based antiviral strategies and in particular, those that utilise gene expression strategies based on RNA interference (RNAi). In this chapter, we examine basic concepts and review recent advances in the development of expressed RNAi-based systems against HIV, with a focus on progress in construct and target design. We also discuss topics related to the use of RNAi-based strategies, including appropriate construct expression, target specificity, viral escape mutations and effective construct delivery. We aim to identify desirable properties of an RNAi-based anti-HIV therapy and highlight the future developments that are required to make this approach a reality.

2. RNA interference

RNA interference (RNAi) is a gene silencing phenomenon in which RNA molecules act to silence the expression of particular genes at a post-transcriptional level in the cell. RNAi has become a popular tool in the development of antiviral therapeutics as the potent silencing mechanism can be redirected against viral genes to inhibit viral replication. RNAi was first described by Fire *et. al.* (Fire *et al.*, 1998) and has since been demonstrated in a number of different organisms including yeast, plants and animals. The mediators of RNAi are short 21- and 22- nucleotide (nt) RNAs known as small interfering RNAs (siRNAs) or microRNAs (miRNAs) and are derived from longer double stranded (ds) RNAs. SiRNAs/miRNAs direct the silencing of complementary gene transcripts in a sequence-specific manner. RNAi was first described in mammalian cells in 2001 (Elbashir *et al.*, 2001a) and subsequent research has moved swiftly to reveal a number of pathway components and mechanisms. Mammalian RNAi is now emerging as a complex network with several alternative RNA forms and levels of regulatory interactions (Breving and Esquela-Kerscher, 2009); (Ding *et al.*, 2009). RNAi-based therapeutics, however, still make use of the central RNAi pathway involved in miRNA biogenesis (Figure 1). Our discussion of RNAi-based strategies begins here with a description of this major RNAi pathway and how it can be redirected to inhibit viral replication.

The mammalian RNAi pathway mediates gene silencing through the generation of miRNAs. MiRNA regulation of genes is both essential and ubiquitous and has been implicated in the regulation of developmental timing, cellular differentiation, apoptosis, cell proliferation and organ development (Bartel, 2004). MiRNAs are expressed from non-protein-coding genes in intergenic or intronic regions as single or polycistronic transcripts by RNA polymerase II (Lee *et al.*, 2004); (Cullen, 2004). MiRNA transcripts are usually several kilobases long and fold back upon themselves to form characteristic hairpin structures known as primary-microRNAs (pri-miRNAs) with flanking sequences, a partially duplexed stem and a terminal loop. Pri-miRNAs are processed in the RNAi pathway in two successive enzymatic steps (Lee *et al.*, 2002b) to produce mature miRNAs from the double-stranded stem region.

The first processing step occurs in the nucleus where the pri-miRNA is cleaved asymmetrically by the "microprocessor" complex to produce a shorter ~ 70 nt hairpin known as a precursor-microRNA (pre-miRNA) with a 2 nt overhang at the 3′ hydroxyl end. The microprocessor complex includes two essential proteins, namely, the RNAse III enzyme Drosha and the DGCR8 (DiGeorge critical region 8) protein (Han *et al.*, 2004). The pre-miRNA is exported from the nucleus to the cytoplasm by the nuclear karyopherin Exportin-5 (Exp-5) in a Ran-GTP-dependant manner (Yi *et al.*, 2003); (Lund *et al.*, 2004). In the second processing step, the pre-miRNA is cleaved asymmetrically by another RNase III enzyme, Dicer (Paddison *et al.*, 2002) to produce staggered ~22 base pair (bp) miRNA/miRNA* duplex with 2 nt overhangs at each 3′ hydroxyl end. Dicer is thought to form a complex with TRBP (TAR RNA-binding protein) (Chendrimada *et al.*, 2005) and PACT (protein activator of protein kinase PKR) (Lee *et al.*, 2006).

One strand of the miRNA/miRNA* duplex is selected as the mature miRNA or guide strand and loaded into the RNA-induced silencing complex (RISC) (Martinez *et al.*, 2002a). The guide strand (miRNA) is typically selected from the duplex as a result of weaker 5′ end pairing, while the remaining passenger strand (miRNA*) is degraded (Khvorova *et al.*, 2003); (Schwarz *et al.*, 2003). In certain cases, both strands of the duplex may be capable of RISC incorporation. RISC facilitates sequence-specific gene silencing and is directed by the guide sequence to complementary regions in the 3′ untranslated regions of target messenger RNAs. RISC-targeting results in the cleavage, degradation or translational suppression of a gene transcript, depending on the level of total complementation between the miRNA and

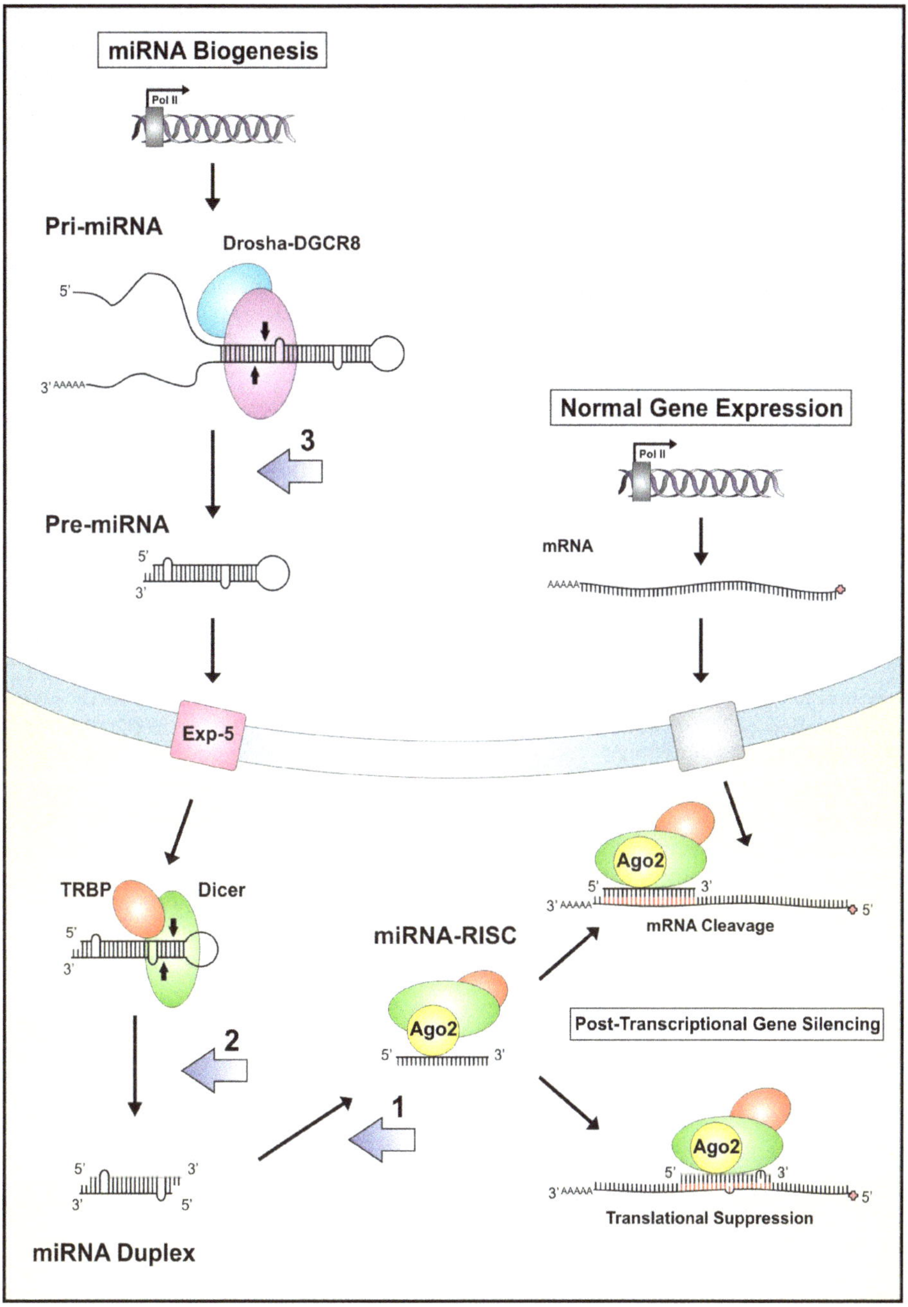

Fig. 1. The mammalian microRNA biogenesis pathway which mediates RNAi. Artificial antiviral constructs can be introduced at points 1, 2 and 3 of the pathway and processed to inhibit viral replication.

target sequence (Hutvagner and Zamore, 2002); (Zeng *et al.*, 2003). Guide strands with near-perfect complementation tend to mediate cleavage of the target by activating the core catalytic Argonaute-2 (Ago-2) protein of RISC. Target cleavage is also a typical characteristic of siRNA-mediated gene silencing. Most miRNAs exhibit incomplete complementation, resulting in translational suppression. Complete complementation, however, is still required for the seed region of the miRNA (5′ position 2-7) for effective target knockdown (Brennecke *et al.*, 2005) and a single mismatch in this region can prevent silencing (Elbashir *et al.*, 2001b).

To redirect the RNAi silencing pathway to silence viral genes, artificial anti-viral siRNAs and miRNAs can be introduced into the cell to enter different points of the RNAi pathway (Figure 1: 1, 2, 3). Antiviral guide sequences are designed to be complementary to viral transcripts and can be incorporated into various forms of artificial RNAi intermediates including pri-miRNAs, pre-miRNAs, and miRNAs. Once in the pathway, these anti-viral intermediates are processed to give therapeutic guide sequences which act to suppress viral gene expression and inhibit viral replication. RNAi strategies have been used against incoming viral RNA to prevent integration, but it appears as if the strength of RNAi remains in its role in post-transcriptionl gene silencing (PTGS). Incoming viral RNA appears to be unsuitable for targeting as it is bound by several proteins and transcribed within a short time frame, which may limit its susceptibility to RNAi. A number of different antiviral constructs and targeting and delivery strategies have been investigated against HIV with varying success and are discussed in the following sections.

3. Antiviral RNAi constructs

The potential application of RNAi for the treatment of HIV was recognised shortly after the first application of RNAi modalities in mammalian cells (Capodici *et al.*, 2002; Coburn and Cullen, 2002; Jacque *et al.*, 2002; Lee *et al.*, 2002a; Martinez *et al.*, 2002b). However, it soon became apparent that RNAi therapies fall into two broad groups: those that are expressed in the cell and those that are not. The basic forms of antiviral RNAi constructs are shown in Figure 2. There are specific advantages and drawbacks associated with both synthetic and expressed constructs with regard to delivery, duration of inhibition and dose control (Table 1), but which type of anti-viral construct is best suited for the treatment of HIV?

3.1 Non-expressed, synthetic RNAi constructs

Small interfering RNAs (siRNAs) are the most common form of non-expressed RNAi constructs. Initial studies of RNAi induction in mammalian cells showed that siRNAs can be used as powerful tools for artificial gene silencing. Despite the relative potency of siRNAs, their use in a permanent therapeutic application is limited by the lack of continued expression (Tuschl and Borkhardt, 2002). Although, this feature can be useful for particular applications where topical administration is possible and doses can be more easily controlled. An siRNA (ALN-RSV01) against nucleocapsid expression of Respiratory Syncytial Virus (RSV) was successfully delivered to healthy individuals in the form of a nasal spray in a randomized, double-blind, placebo-controlled clinical trial (Devincenzo *et al.*, 2010). The treatment was shown to decrease the number of infected subjects by 38%, independently of other factors like pre-existing RSV antibody and intranasal pro-inflammatory cytokines. While siRNAs may not be suitable for once-off gene therapies, this example demonstrates how novel delivery methods can enable successful siRNA use in a therapeutic setting.

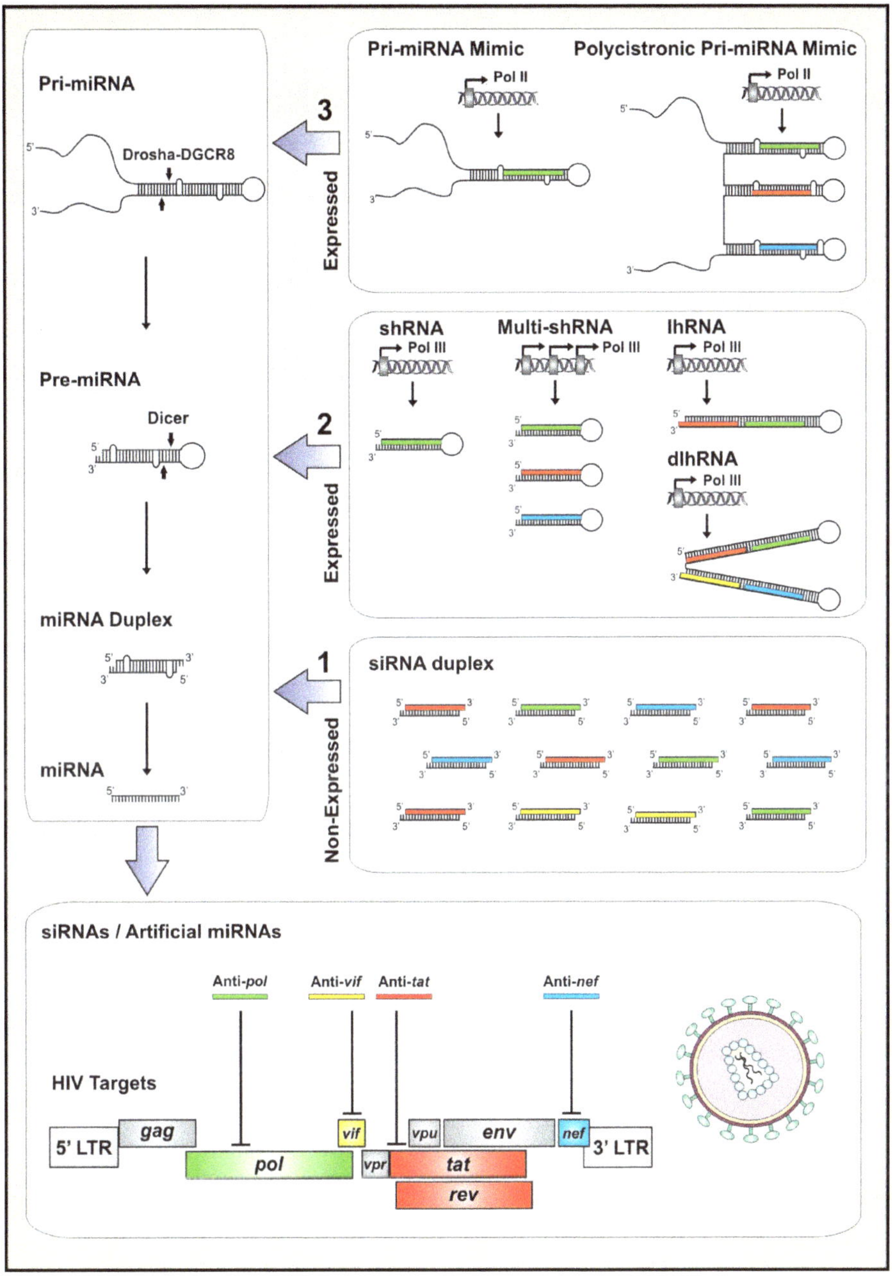

Fig. 2. Various forms of therapeutic constructs used to trigger antiviral RNAi. Each construct generates antiviral siRNA or miRNA guide sequences (green, yellow, red and blue) which initiate silencing of complementary viral targets. Constructs may be non-expressed or expressed in a singular or multiple format (combinatorial-RNAi).

	Non-Expressed Constructs	Expressed Constructs
Singular forms	Small interfering RNAs (siRNAs)	Short hairpin RNAs (shRNAs) Primary microRNA mimics (shRNA-miRs)
Combinatorial forms	Multiple siRNAs	Multiple shRNA cassettes Extended short hairpins (e-shRNAs) Long hairpin RNAs (lhRNAs, dlhRNAs) Polycistronic microRNA mimics
Potential as a once-off treatment?	No. Therapeutic effects are transient. Multiple or continuous treatments are required.	Yes. Auto-expression sustains the supply of anti-viral effectors.
Regulated cellular production?	No. SiRNAs are chemically synthesised.	Yes, but this is dependent on the type of promoter selected. Cell-specific or inducible promoters are favourable.
Dicer/ Drosha processing?	No. SiRNAs are suitable substrates for direct association with RISC.	Yes. Anti-viral siRNA/miRNA guides must be processed from RNA precursors by Drosha and/or Dicer.
Saturation of the RNAi pathway?	Less likely as processing and export enzymes are not utilised.	A serious concern related to over-expression of artificial constructs. Choice of expression system is critical.
Dose	Doses can be more easily predicted and controlled as construct expression is not a factor.	Exact expression levels under specific promoters can only be determined empirically and may vary with time and genetic background.
Delivery	SiRNAs can be administered directly. Chemical modifications can be included for enhanced absorption or targeting to a specific tissue.	More complex. Viral vectors are often used for transduction, but issues with safety and efficacy persist. Cell-based delivery systems appear promising.

Table 1. A comparison of non-expressed and expressed antiviral RNAi constructs.

3.1.1 siRNAs

SiRNA duplexes have been shown to effectively silence a number of HIV target genes. SiRNAs against mRNAs of the Gag protein and CD4 cellular receptor have been shown to inhibit post-integrative expression events with a four-fold reduction in viral entry and a 47 % decrease in p24 expression in HIV cell culture challenge assays (Novina *et al.*, 2002). SiRNAs against *tat* and *rev* transcripts specifically inhibited protein function and viral replication in human T cell lines and primary lymphocytes (Coburn and Cullen, 2002). SiRNA duplexes against the long terminal repeat (LTR) and accessory genes *vif* and *nef* were shown to be effective at inhibiting viral production from infectious molecular clones by 30 to 50 fold in 24 hours (Jacque *et al.*, 2002).

Exogenous siRNAs in the form of duplexes were found to be the most effective at redirecting the silencing mechanism against both endogenous and transfected genes (Elbashir *et al.*, 2001a), while the characteristic 2 nt overhangs at both the 5′ and 3′ ends are an essential feature (Caplen *et al.*, 2001). Artificial siRNAs are selected for RISC incorporation more directly and there is no need for Drosha or Dicer processing (Figure 1, point 1). This can prevent saturation of the RNAi pathway components and interference with the essential miRNA biogenesis. The use of short siRNA duplexes is preferable over longer dsRNAs which were previously used, as interferon responses in the cell can be avoided. The most effective synthetic siRNA duplexes are designed to be about 19 - 21 nts in length with 3′ overhangs, but it has also been shown that shorter siRNAs of only 16 nts may trigger more potent RNAi as a result of higher RISC-loading capacity(Chu and Rana, 2008).

The chemical synthesis of siRNA duplexes is conceptually simple, as are the methods of electroporation, microinjection and liposome-mediated transfections for siRNA introduction into cells. The continuous need for these methods in large-scale siRNA use, however, can become labour-intensive. Coupled with the transient nature of siRNA-induced gene silencing (maximum ~ 1 week), the advantages of an expressed siRNA construct in therapeutic applications are clear. Nevertheless, novel delivery mechanisms for synthetic siRNAs have been developed for HIV. Specifically, studies in humanized mouse models of HIV using anti-gp120 aptamer-siRNA chimeras have demonstrated their potential as specific antiviral agents (Neff *et al.*, 2011); (MacRae *et al.*, 2008); (Zhou and Rossi, 2010). Similarly, siRNAs conjugated to single-chained monoclonal antibody fragments targeted to T-cell or lymphocyte-specific receptors have shown promise *in vivo* (Kim *et al.*, 2010; Kumar *et al.*, 2008). However, these methods are in the earlier stages of development and there are still several delivery and potency hurdles which must be overcome. The focus of this review will be on expressed RNAi modalities, where siRNA duplexes are expressed from plasmid DNA vectors with lasting effects on gene silencing.

3.2 Expressed RNAi constructs

SiRNAs that are generated from expression cassettes have the advantage of sustained production which makes them suitable for long-term, once-off therapeutic applications. Recent developments in construct design and delivery methods have shown much promise for the advancement of siRNA expression systems against HIV. In earlier siRNA expression studies, linear cassettes were constructed to code for both sense and antisense sequences of the siRNA duplex under the control of separate promoters and termination signals (Lee *et al.*, 2002a); (Miyagishi and Taira, 2002). Expressed siRNAs then associate post-transcriptionally to form a duplex with 2 - 4 nt uridine overhangs. This system was found to be effective against HIV-1 sequences and siRNAs targeting a highly-accessible region of the *rev* transcript were found to inhibit viral transcript expression (Lee *et al.*, 2002a). However, the reliability of correct siRNA duplex association *in vivo* is questionable. Most siRNA expression constructs are now designed to generate mimics of RNAi intermediates in the form of siRNA or miRNA hairpin precursors which are processed by Drosha and/or Dicer enzyme complexes (Figure 2). This is preferable for more reliable siRNA processing in a manner that is regulated by the RNAi pathway, but inappropriate expression levels can lead to saturation of critical RNAi components.

The choice of promoter is therefore critical in achieving suitable levels of construct expression. Polymerase III (pol III) promoter sequences, like human U6 snRNA (small nuclear RNA U6) or H1 (human RNAse P H1), are commonly used to drive efficient expression of short downstream sequences and often feature in short hairpin expression cassettes. They have been well characterised in earlier ribozyme expression studies (Good *et al.*, 1997) and are suitable to drive nuclear expression in a wide range of human cell types (Paul *et al.*, 2002). However, the high level of constitutive expression from pol III promoters can be undesired in a long-term therapeutic treatment. Polymerase II (pol II) promoters, like the human cytomegalovirus (CMV) promoter, are now being favoured for lower and potentially regulatable expression of pri- and pre-mRNA mimics. They allow for safer tissue-specific expression of constructs with tighter *in vivo* regulation (Cullen, 2005); (Giering *et al.*, 2008). Other types of inducible promoters have also been investigated for regulated expression in the presence of an activator molecule (Jacque *et al.*, 2002), which would satisfy the need for greater control of construct expression in therapeutic applications.

3.2.1 Short hairpin RNAs

Short hairpin RNAs (shRNAs) were developed for the expression of siRNA duplexes (Paul *et al.*, 2002). ShRNAs are essentially mimics of precursor-miRNAs that are processed by Dicer to produce staggered siRNA duplexes. ShRNAs typically have short, completely complementary stem regions of about 19 -29 base pairs (bp), a 2 nt 3′ overhang and one of several commonly used terminal loops. Synthetic shRNAs have been shown to trigger more effective gene silencing than siRNA duplexes with the same guide sequences (Siolas *et al.*, 2005). The association of shRNAs with Dicer may result in more effective loading of guide sequences onto RISC, as Dicer forms part of the RISC-loading complex (RLC) (MacRae *et al.*, 2008).

A variety of different guide sequences can be expressed from shRNAs. Sequence composition of individual guides can affect the processing efficiency, but common shRNA formats generally give high levels of expression. An shRNA against the HIV-1 transactivator (Tat) protein gene was incorporated into an H1-driven expression cassette and delivered to cells through the use of a recombinant AAV (adeno-associated virus) DNA vector (Boden *et al.*, 2003). In a cell culture challenge assay with the infectious molecular clone HIV-1NL$_{4.3}$, HIV-1 p24 antigen levels were decreased by 97% 48 hours post-transfection in cells expressing the sh*tat* compared to control cells. The high mutability of HIV, however, severely hinders the potency of silencing by a single shRNA in a long-term application. In cells stably expressing sh*tat*, HIV-1 replication was reduced by 95% in the first three weeks, but had again risen by day 25 as a result of a nonsynonymous mutation in the targeted region.

The silencing efficacy of an shRNA mostly depends on the level of conservation of the HIV target sequence and shRNAs with equal processing do not necessarily result in the same level of HIV inhibition. ShRNAs against the viral integrase sequence (shIN) and the U3 region of the viral genome required for integration (shU3) showed a more potent inhibitory effect on HIV-1 replication than sh*tat* in shRNA-transduced MT-4 or primary CD4_ T cells (Nishitsuji *et al.*, 2006). In p24 viral replication assays, sh*int* produced a ~ 4 fold reduction in p24 production, while sh*tat* resulted in a ~2.5 fold reduction four days post-infection. In contrast, a similar hairpin against the U5 region of the viral genome resulted in weak inhibition, possibly due to high GC content. At 10 days postinfection, viral replication was again detected in the shTat-transformed MT-4 cells, while HIV-1 replication was undetectable for up to 1 month postinfection, in cells that received shIN or shU3. While this is an improvement, the use of single shRNAs is still unsuitable for long-term HIV suppression.

The choice of stem and loop structures must also be carefully considered in shRNA design. A completely duplexed stem assists in preserving shRNA structure and can be useful for the prevention of 3′ - 5′ exonuclease attack (Paul *et al.*, 2002), but is not a necessity and the high level of duplex stability may also interfere with strand selection. While typical stem lengths of about 19 bp are effective, longer 29 bp stems can be more potent triggers of RNAi with more effective processing, suggesting that Dicer requires a minimum stem length for efficient cleavage (Siolas *et al.*, 2005). Loop sizes are more variable and can be anywhere between 3 and 9 nts in size. A recent investigation has confirmed that loop sequences are indeed critical in determining shRNA function against HIV-1 sequences (Schopman *et al.*, 2010). ShRNAs with sub-optimal loop sequences (Brummelkamp *et al.*, 2002) can be slightly altered to increase RNA activity by up to 7 fold. The size of optimal loops appears to be between 7 and 10 nts, while decreasing loops to 5 nts or less appears to be detrimental to RNAi activity. Particular loop structures, especially those derived from pri-miRNAs, can enhance processing of weak shRNAs. The importance of loop structure may be attributed to Dicer co-factors, like the KH-type splicing regulatory protein (KSRP), which binds to the terminal loop and affects processing (Vermeulen *et al.*, 2005); (Trabucchi *et al.*, 2009) .

Pol III promoters like U6 or H1 are well suited for the constitutive expression of shRNAs in a range of cell types. The pol III termination signal consists of a short stretch of uridine residues which are cleaved at the termination site after two residues. This is ideal for the generation of a 3′ UU overhang in the hairpin, which is important for the efficiency and the specificity of siRNA processing by Dicer. Robust shRNA expression from pol III promoters can be detrimental for a therapeutic application. High levels of sustained expression can lead to cytotoxicity and even to a lethal saturation of the RNAi pathway. The long-term effects of robust shRNA expression were investigated in the livers of adult mice and found to cause liver injury, organ failure and death within one month (Grimm *et al.*, 2006). Morbidity was associated with the downregulation of natural liver miRNAs, which suggested that competition exists for components of the RNAi pathway such as Exportin-5. In a more recent publication, Ago-2 (Slicer) was identified as the primary rate-limiting determinant of both *in vitro* and *in vivo* RNAi efficacy, toxicity, and persistence (Grimm *et al.*, 2010). Ago/shRNA coexpression studies have shown that increased Ago-2 and Exp-5 expression can rescue long-term U6-driven shRNA expression in adult mice with enhanced silencing of exogenous and endogenous hepatic targets, reduced hepatotoxicity, and extended RNAi stability of more than 3 months. The benefits of using a weaker promoter were demonstrated in this study where *in vivo* toxicity was alleviated, allowing for sustained target silencing of over a year. Overall, shRNAs are very potent gene-silencing moieties, but their safe and effective use in anti-HIV gene therapies is dependent on appropriate promoter and target selection.

3.2.2 Mimics of microRNA precursors

There seem to be several advantages in creating antiviral constructs with properties that are similar to endogenous miRNA precursors. This includes the incorporation of mismatches into the stem region, the use of longer stems and different terminal loops. Enhanced silencing has been observed for siRNAs derived from hairpins based on precursor-miRNAs (pre-miRNAs). SiRNAs against the HIV-1 *tat* gene were placed into the natural pre-miR-30 backbone and found to be 80% more effective at reducing HIV replication than the same guide expressed from a conventional shRNA (Boden *et al.*, 2004). Hairpins based on primary-microRNAs (pri-miRNAs) with pol II promoters have also been shown to induce potent, stable and regulatable gene silencing *in vivo*, even when present as a single copy in the genome (Dickins *et al.*, 2005). These pri-miR mimics have been described as second-generation shRNAs and termed shRNA-miRs (Silva *et al.*, 2005).

Artificial miRNAs not only show a greater inhibitory efficacy against HIV targets when compared to conventional shRNAs (Liu *et al.*, 2008), but may also be better at suppressing imperfect HIV-1 targets (Liu *et al.*, 2009a). This enhanced silencing ability has been attributed to more efficient processing in the RNAi pathway by both Drosha and Dicer enzyme complexes. Pri-miRNA mimics may also be subjected to regulatory mechanisms and other important components of the RNAi pathway, unlike substrate mimics introduced further on in the pathway (Obernosterer *et al.*, 2006). In addition, there may be functional differences between RISC-siRNA and RISC-miRNA with respect to Ago protein association.

As might be implied from nature, it is necessary to maintain several key elements of natural pri-miRNA structures for effective processing of artificial miRNAs. It has been suggested that a large terminal loop (≥ 10 nts), a stem between 26 and 40 bp and at least 40 nts of non-structured flanking RNA sequences are required for efficient processing by Drosha (Zeng *et al.*, 2005). Single-stranded flanking sequences may form part of the Drosha-RNA interface (Zeng and Cullen, 2005) and it seems logical to preserve the natural flanking sequences in the use of miRNA precursors as scaffolds. Preservation of natural loop sequences also appears to be desirable and has been shown to rescue the inhibitory potential of weakly functioning shRNAs (Schopman *et al.*, 2010).

In comparisons of the silencing ability of shRNA and artificial microRNA constructs with similar guide strands, shRNAs were generally found to produce a more potent silencing effect (Boudreau *et al.*, 2008). This has, however, been attributed to a higher level of expression both *in vivo* and *in vitro*. As already discussed, higher expression of shRNAs is undesirable in a therapeutic setting. Artificial miRNAs with a lower expression are processed more efficiently in the RNAi pathway and cause less of a bottleneck which can lead to saturation toxicity. SiRNAs expressed from a microRNA backbone do not appear to show the same level of inhibitory competition for nuclear export by Exportin-5 and incorporation into RISC (Castanotto *et al.*, 2007). Pri-miRNA mimics therefore appear to be safer option for therapeutic use and show less disruption of natural microRNA biogenesis (Boudreau *et al.*, 2009). Pri-miRNAs, however, do not show consistent processing over a range of different guide sequences, as can be observed for shRNAs. Pri-miRNAs therefore appear to be a more favourable expression format for siRNAs, but sufficient processing of guide sequences must be assessed empirically.

3.3 Combinatorial RNAi constructs

Despite the potency of RNAi against HIV targets in short term studies, the sustained inhibition of viral replication is not possible with a single siRNA construct. Viral escape mutations arise readily in response to the strong selective pressure of effective RNAi constructs. SiRNAs directed against the viral *nef* gene and introduced into human T cells by retroviral transduction successfully inhibit viral replication at first, but after several weeks of culture RNAi-resistant viruses developed (Gregory *et al.*, 2004). Viral mutations included nucleotide substitutions or deletions in the Nef gene that modified or deleted the siRNA-Nef target sequence. Similarly, expressed shRNAs targeting the HIV-1 *tat* gene soon give rise to a viral quasispecies harbouring a point mutation in the shRNA target region which abolishes antiviral activity of tat shRNA (Boden *et al.*, 2003). Silent mutations in protein-coding sequences can also occur. Viral escape mutations are, however, not limited to point mutations in the siRNA target sequences. Mutations can occur in other regions of the genome that alter the local RNA secondary structure of the target site and diminish siRNA binding (Westerhout *et al.*, 2005).

The key to successful HIV inhibition lies in the targeting of several highly conserved regions simultaneously in a combinatorial approach (co-RNAi). This strategy has been used in a number of conventional drug regimens and aims to reduce the emergence of viral escape mutants by inhibiting multiple HIV targets. Expressed shRNA and shRNA-miR constructs can be adapted to produce multiple siRNAs and combined in single plasmid vectors. RNAi constructs can also be more easily adapted than small molecules in response to viral evolution. Several studies have investigated viral mutation pathways in response to particular therapeutic stimuli in order to identify and block anticipated escape paths. Interestingly, viral escape paths against shRNA therapy differ to those triggered by drug therapy (Applegate *et al.*, 2010).

3.3.1 Multiple short hairpin RNAs

Multiple short hairpins can be used against HIV simply through the use of multiple vectors or through the design of consecutive shRNA constructs. The simultaneous use of two separate hairpins against the CCR5 and CXCR4 cellular receptors has been shown to protect transduced primary macrophages against HIV infection (Lee *et al.*, 2003). The consistent delivery and expression of two separate shRNAs in an equal ratio is not precise using a simultaneous approach and multiple shRNA constructs are preferable for more controlled expression levels. A bi-specific construct containing a U6-driven shRNA against CXCR4 and an H1-driven shRNA against the CCR5 has been shown to effectively downregulate both targets simultaneously (Anderson and Akkina, 2005). When the siRNA expressing transduced cells were challenged with X4 and R5 tropic HIV-1, they demonstrated marked viral resistance. Targeting of three different HIV regions is even more favourable for effective coRNAi and has been demonstrated using a multi-shRNA construct. Three H1-driven shRNAs against two *pol* and one *gag* sequence were successfully used to create an additive inhibition of viral production and delay viral escape (ter Brake *et al.*, 2006).

Combining multiple shRNAs with the same construct structure can be problematic. The use of repeated promoter sequences can lead to rearrangements and deletions of whole transcriptional units as a result of recombination in lentiviral delivery vectors. To prevent this, non-identical pol III promoters U6, H1, and 7SK and the polymerase II U1 promoter can be used to drive simultaneous expression in a multi-shRNA cassette which can inhibit HIV without viral escape (ter Brake *et al.*, 2008). However, equivalent expression of each siRNA is not guaranteed and high expression levels of several anti-viral guides still occurs which can lead to even more serious saturation toxicity (McIntyre *et al.*, 2009). ShRNAs, even in a multiple format, are therefore not necessarily the most preferable expression systems for therapeutic applications.

3.3.2 Long hairpin RNAs

To avoid issues associated with the toxicity of multiple promoter-driven constructs, several adjacent siRNA sequences can be incorporated into single long hairpin constructs (lhRNAs) under the control of one promoter. Consecutive Dicer cleavage is required along the length of the hairpin to release individual siRNA duplexes (Paddison *et al.*, 2002). A modified long hairpin against a 50 nt region of the integrase gene effectively suppressed both wild-type and sh*int*-resistant viral strains (Nishitsuji *et al.*, 2006). A U6-driven long hairpin RNA spanning a possible 60 bp of a 5′LTR target region has shown silencing of respective target sequences and inhibition of HIV replication (Barichievy *et al.*, 2007). The greatest silencing in this format was observed for the target corresponding to the base of the hairpin stem.

In a more pre-meditated approach, several well-characterised shRNA sequences can be concatenated into a single long or extended shRNA (e-shRNA). E-shRNAs were designed with two siRNAs against *nef* and *pol* HIV-1 sequences which were efficiently processed and showed viral inhibition (Liu *et al.*, 2007). The position of the two siRNAs was found to be critical for the generation of functional siRNAs. In a further step, the generation of three siRNAs from a single U6-driven hairpin was investigated against *tat, rev* and *vif* (Saayman *et al.*, 2008). All sequences were capable of target silencing depending on their position within the hairpin and processing efficiency decreased from the stem of the hairpin towards the terminal loop. Spacing between the siRNA sequences within the duplex stem region can also affect processing efficiency. E-shRNAs can be extended to include a maximum of 3 siRNAs with an optimal length of 66 bp. Further stem extension results in a loss of RNAi activity (Liu *et al.*, 2009a). A size limit of 80 bp has also been suggested and the incorporation of G:U wobbles may have several advantages related to hairpin expression (Sano *et al.*, 2008).

A further advancement which circumvents the length limitation of lhRNAs is the use of a long hairpin concatenation. A recent study has shown that four functional anti-HIV siRNAs can be derived from a single Pol III-generated transcript comprising two adjacent long hairpin RNA precursors (Saayman *et al.*, 2010). Two active anti-HIV siRNAs were engineered into each of two lhRNAs, which were arranged in tandem to create a double long hairpin (dlhRNA) expression cassette. Each hairpin component was found to generate two of four unique siRNA sequences (*tat, nef,* LTR and *int*) and thereby mediate dual-targeting. Processing of the individual siRNAs was found to be affected by both internal ordering and spacing between siRNAs. An inverse correlation between siRNA silencing potency and increased spacing was observed, while processing at the 3′ position of each lhRNA was more variable. Optimal siRNA processing was found to occur when only one mismatched base pair was placed between each siRNA in accordance with predicted Dicer cleavage intervals. Effective multiple processing was achieved by manipulating the order of the siRNA-encoding sequences to create an optimized combinatorial dlhRNA expression cassette. Despite the use of a pol III promoter, expression potency of the individual guides is diluted and therefore less likely to cause toxic saturation. This work has highlighted the versatility of dlhRNAs and shown that they are a promising construct form for effective silencing of multiple HIV targets.

3.3.3 Polycistronic primary microRNA mimics

Safe and controlled expression of siRNAs is a particular concern in coRNAi. Once again, a logical way of doing this is to mimic mammalian microRNA expression systems. MiRNAs are often expressed as pol II-driven polycistronic units in the cell and multiple siRNAs can be expressed in a similar fashion. In some systems, effective singular miRNA mimics, like those based on the pri-miR30 backbone, were simply incorporated in tandem under the control of a single pol II promoter to express two or three artificial guides (Han *et al.*, 2006)

(Ely *et al.*, 2009). Different pri-miRNA backbones have different expression aptitudes for individual sequences and the ordering of pri-miRNA expression units can affect both expression and silencing abilities. The preservation of natural pri-miRNA structural elements is still required in multiple constructs with a minimum of 22 nt of natural flanking sequence required at the 5′ arm and at least 15 nt at the 3′ arm (Zeng and Cullen, 2005). In addition to this, extra restriction sequences must often be included to create the tandem format. This can be very useful for creating modular pri-miRNA units that can be exchanged as required. On the other hand, extra artificial and repetitive natural flanking sequences in the expressed transcript can interact in an unexpected fashion to form undesirable secondary structures which prevent or alter processing of the intended guide sequences.

Multiple guide sequences can be incorporated into other natural miRNA precursor forms. In an earlier example, the BIC non-coding RNA with its embedded miR-155 miRNA precursor was used as a scaffold for construction of the SIBR vector (Chung *et al.*, 2006). Synthetic miRNA sequences were incorporated into a modified miR-155 stem-loop, along with flanking sequences from the third exon of the BIC transcript, which proved to be sufficient for the expression of miR-155. It was found that two artificial miRNAs could be expressed from a single polycistronic transcript to give effective inhibition of targets without a decrease in the efficacy of individual target suppression. Alternatively, up to 8 tandem copies of the same artificial miRNA can be expressed from the SIBR vector in tandem for enhanced expression, but this is not a favourable option for HIV inhibition where strong silencing of a single target should be avoided.

A simpler approach for polycistronic design is to mimic entire naturally occurring polycistronic pri-miRNA units. Multiple effective siRNAs can be inserted into a naturally occurring polycistronic scaffold and expressed from a single promoter sequence. The mir-17-92 polycistron has been successfully used as a scaffold for four siRNAs against *rev/tat*, *gag*, *pol* and leader HIV sequences (Liu *et al.*, 2008). In this example, each siRNA sequence was initially incorporated into an individual pri-miRNA structure with about 40 nts of flanking sequences and assessed. In doing so, the passenger strand was altered with the use of predictive secondary structure software to maintain all mismatches, bulges and thermodynamic stability as far as possible. Positioning of guide sequences in each pri-miRNA hairpin was found to be crucial for optimal processing. Individual hairpins showed moderate anti-HIV activity, but co-expression of two or more hairpins in a polycistronic format gave greatly enhanced silencing from each individual pri-miRNA component. Antiviral siRNAs have also been engineered into the tri-cistronic miR-106b cluster (Aagaard *et al.*, 2008) to produce 3 siRNAs against *tat/rev*, *tat* and *rev*. In both of these examples, polycistronic expression systems appear to have an intrinsic inhibitory activity greater than that of conventional shRNA constructs or individual hairpins.

In all examples of mimic design, it appears that the preservation of key structural elements is crucial for effective processing and inhibitory function. Although the predictive software for this purpose is of a very high standard, folded structures and sequence interactions *in vivo* can never be guaranteed. This is of particular concern when modular pri-miRNA units are being combined in a novel way. Guide sequence expression from pri-miRNA mimics is also variable and can depend on both the anti-viral sequence and backbone used. Transposition of 19 nt siRNAs from shRNA expression systems into pri-miRNA units can be tricky as miRNA sequences can be up to 24 nts in length. Only one guide can be used per pri-miRNA hairpin, which means that combinatorial constructs will inevitably contain quite a lot of extra, non-guide sequence. Construct size can be a limiting factor for insertion into viral vectors, but polycistronic pri-miRNA units are still generally within an acceptable size range. In general, the use of pri-miRNA mimics requires more planning and testing of individual components, while the final construct behaviour can only really be observed experimentally. This makes polycistronic miRNA expression systems more labour intensive, but thorough testing should be part of any therapeutic strategy. The extra input may be well worthwhile if the potential advantages of combined HIV targeting at an appropriate expression level with regulated and efficient processing can be realised.

3.3.4 Therapeutic constructs

Overall, it appears as if dlhRNAs or polycistronic mimics appear to possess the best combinations of desirable properties for a therapeutic RNAi application. Developments are, however, still required before these constructs can be implemented in a clinical setting. Expression systems can be further optimised to give restricted expression in target cell populations and therefore reduce the risk of unwanted off target effects (OTEs). More specific expression can be achieved through the use of a haematopoietic or T-cell-specific promoter (Liu *et al.*, 2008). The WAS promoter, for example, is active in human hematopoietic precursor cells (CD34+), T lymphocytes, B cells and dendritic cells, but not in non-haematopoietic cells and may be an excellent candidate (Charrier *et al.*, 2007). Expression could ideally be further restricted to HIV infected cells by using the HIV-1 LTR promoter to express the miRNA polycistron only in the presence of the viral Tat protein (Unwalla *et al.*, 2004). Furthermore, RNAi activators are probably best used in combination with other types of RNA- or protein-based anti-HIV constructs in a therapeutic application to mediate an even more potent viral inhibition that does not rely on a single genetic mechanism. A polycistronic miRNA mimic, for example, can be combined with a TAR decoy for enhanced viral inhibition. ShRNAs can also be applied therapeutically in combination with other RNA-based constructs, for example, an anti-CCR5 ribozyme and a TAR decoy for greater protection against from HIV-1 challenge (Wilson *et al.*, 2003). It therefore seems that the best therapeutic approaches involve the use of combinations of both RNAi triggers and different types of inhibitory mechanisms, while maintaining natural RNAi processing and overall cellular function as far as possible.

4. RNAi target selection

A critical factor in the success of any RNAi-inducing therapeutic strategy is the choice of target sequence. Highly effective therapeutic effectors can be rendered ineffective in a clinical setting if careful consideration is not given to the long-term targeting strategy. SiRNAs have been designed against most regions of HIV-encoded RNAs, including *tat, rev, gag, pol, nef, vif, env, vpr,* and the long terminal repeat (Figure 2). However, there is no single Achilles heel in the HIV genome and targeting of several highly conserved regions across multiple viral strains is a requirement for a clinically relevant RNAi-based therapy. *In silico* approaches for target identification are therefore crucial, although targeting strategies must still be experimentally validated.

Highly conserved HIV sequences are rare. In an extensive study of siRNA target prediction for optimal design of siRNAs, highly conserved sequences were analysed from the Los Alamos HIV Sequence Database covering 495 divergent strains of subtype M (Naito *et al.*, 2007). Of the 4 million potential 21-mer siRNA target sites, only 5.2 % showed a level of conservation greater than 50%. Highly conserved (> 80%) siRNA target sequences are very rare (< 1 %) and only about 14 % of these rare potential sites correspond to functional siRNA predictions. This finding has called for serious reconsideration of the clinical potential of numerous previous studies which generally target regions outside of this highly conserved category.

Highly conserved target sites are essential in a therapeutic application to successfully inhibit mixed and fluctuating viral populations. Ideal target regions of the HIV genome include essential regulatory regions of viral gene expression. Among these are the primer activation signal (PAS), primer binding site (PBS), packaging signal (ψ), central polypurine tract (cPPT), central termination sequence (CTS) and 3′ polypurine tract (3′ PPT). These regions are conserved at the nucleotide sequence level, presumably to conserve secondary RNA structures which are important for viral fitness. Other highly conserved potential siRNA target sites include the packaging signal, TAR/polyA and regions in protease and integrase protein codes. It does not seem possible for a single siRNA to target all known HIV-strains, but this work by Naito *et. al.* suggests that it is theoretically possible to target >99% of circulating subtype M strains with escape resistance by combining only two siRNAs against highly conserved viral sequences.

In other previous studies, it has been suggested that four conserved sequences will be sufficient to inhibit several hundred circulating viral stains (Leonard and Schaffer, 2005). It is, however, unlikely that sequences across several viral strains will harbour sufficient sequence identity to be effectively targeted by the same set of four shRNAs. It has since been proposed that more than four shRNAs should be utilised in therapeutic design such that each viral strain will be effectively targeted by at least four shRNAs (McIntyre *et al.*, 2011). ShRNA combinations of seven H1-driven expression units were found to provide up to 87% coverage for all known HI V strains and 100% coverage of clade B subtypes. Position within a specific (1 - 7) multi-shRNA cassette generally had little effect on the suppressive activity of individual shRNAs when expressed in isolation, but when shRNA expression was simultaneous, expression decreased for shRNAs in position 3 - 7. The effective and equal expression of 6 or 7 tandem shRNAs is a challenge and the use of so many pol III promoter units poses a substantially higher risk of toxic saturation of the endogenous RNAi pathway. However, the possibility of inhibiting multiple viral strains simultaneously is a tempting motivation for further development of both multi-shRNA and larger polycistronic mimic expression systems.

As an alternative to highly mutable viral sequences, host dependency factors (HDFs) encoded by the cell can also be targeted to further inhibit viral replication. The CD4 receptor required for viral entry is an obvious choice, but is also present on other host cells in which silencing of CD4 may result in undesirable side-effects. The CCR5 and CXCR4 co-receptors are more attractive targets for silencing and have been investigated (Novina *et al.*, 2002, Song *et al.*, 2003). There are however many other host factors involved in HIV replication, such as those required for Tat binding to TAR (cyclin T1 and CDK9) and those that bind to the LTR to control gene expression (NF-κB, SP1, LBP, and LEF). SiRNAs against the NF-κB p65 subunit resulted in decreased viral replication (Surabhi and Gaynor, 2002). Large screen studies have also revealed numerous other potential targets (Brass *et al.*, 2008). Cellular targeting is promising, but must be used with caution as the inhibition of cellular proteins can have widespread effects on cellular function with undesirable side effects.

5. Safety & toxicity of RNAi activators

A primary concern with the use of RNAi-based strategies is that of safety and the specificity of the inhibitory effect *in vivo*. The presence of double stranded RNA (dsRNA) can activate cellular defence mechanisms which lead to a non-specific halt in translation and cell death. DsRNA induces an interferon type 1 (IFN-1) response in the cell which in turn activates the transcription of other immune effector molecules, IFN stimulated genes (ISGs) and Dicer-related pathways (de Veer *et al.*, 2005); (Karpala *et al.*, 2005). DsRNA can also activate the retinoic-acid inducible gene-I (RIG-I) and members of the oligoadenylate synthetase (OAS) receptor family which catalyze the synthesis of 2′-5′ oligoadenylates to activate a latent cellular endoribonuclease (RNASEL), which in turn cleaves cellular and viral mRNAs. A key effector molecule is the dsRNA-responsive protein kinase receptor (PKR) which functions to block translation of both viral and cellular proteins. PKR activation is typically induced by long dsRNA molecules (>30 nts), but can also be induced by exogenously introduced short 19–29 nt dsRNAs. SiRNAs and shRNAs can induce an IFN response in cells through toll-like receptors (TLRs), particularly TLR3 (Kariko *et al.*, 2004). Ironically, these immune responses play a role in viral defense systems of the cell, but can create issues for the introduction of artificial anti-viral constructs. However, siRNA sequences tend to be only weak inducers of the IFN response and the use of siRNA expression systems can be effective in avoiding an immune response (Robbins *et al.*, 2006).

Another major concern with RNAi activators is the unintentional suppression of cellular transcripts with partial sequence complementation described as off-target effects (OTEs). As the seed region (position 2-7 nt) is the most crucial determinant of target specificity, it seems probable that several cellular transcripts will be susceptible to such a short region of sequence complementation. Some microarray studies have shown that even targets with one or two base pair mismatches with an siRNA can be affected (Jackson *et al.*, 2003). The use of multiple guide sequences is required for effective long-term viral inhibition, but this increases the number of potential OTEs. In a number of studies, cellular toxicity has not been observed, suggesting that OTEs may not necessarily have a significant impact on cellular function (Liu *et al.*, 2008). Nonetheless, extensive attempts should be made to predict potential OTEs before clinical application.

Saturation of the endogenous RNAi pathway with highly expressed RNAi-activators, like pol III-driven shRNAs, can have potentially lethal toxic side effects (Grimm *et al.*, 2006). As already mentioned, polycistronic pri-miRNA mimics can be useful in avoiding competition with the components of the pathway through reduced expression levels and more regulated processing of guide sequences. The natural properties of these mimics may also be useful in avoiding immune stimulation and careful target selection may reduce unwanted OTEs. Although, the complete reduction of OTEs is unlikely and extensive screening of *in vivo* cell expression patterns may be the only real way to assess the extent of undesirable effects.

6. RNAi towards the clinic

A number of RNAi-based effectors have reached clinical trials, but safe and effective expression and delivery of RNAi constructs remains an obstacle for most therapeutic approaches. Recent developments have shown much promise in addressing common delivery issues. Novel nanotechnologies have been used for the delivery of exogenous siRNAs (Davis *et al.*, 2010), while lentiviral vectors that are stably transduced with an extended hairpin expression cassette have been shown to durably inhibit HIV-1 in T-cells (Liu *et al.*, 2009b). Finer details of lentiviral optimisation are now being elucidated and it seems that unique strategies are required for shRNA and miRNA expressing vectors (Schopman *et al.*, 2010).

Cell-based delivery appears to be the most promising approach for the development of a realistic therapeutic strategy (Figure 3). Essentially, haematopoietic stem cells (HSCs) are collected from suitable donor candidates and transduced *ex vivo* with anti-HIV expression constructs. Lentiviral vectors are preferable for this purpose as they can mediate integration of therapeutic constructs into the cellular genome even in non-dividing cells for long-term construct expression (Naldini *et al.*, 1996). Transduced HSCs are then infused into an HIV-infected patient where they can give rise to HIV-resistant cell populations. This method allows for controlled transduction of target cell populations where aberrant integrative events may be detected and eliminated *ex vivo*.

Cell-based delivery may involve allogeneic or autologous cell transplantation. In a pivotal allogeneic study, replicating HIV remained undetected in a recipient patient 20 months after transplantation and termination of HAART (Hutter *et al.*, 2009). In this case, HSCs were obtained from a donor homozygous for a naturally occurring HIV-resistant phenotype and successfully transplanted into an HIV-infected patient with acute myeloid leukemia following myeloablative therapy. Cells with the Δ32CCR5 mutation harbour a 32 bp deletion in the gene for chemokine receptor 5 and are protected from infection by R5-tropic viral subtypes. This strategy proved to be effective for treating leukaemia and preventing viral replication. Notorious HIV-reservoirs, like the intestinal lamina propria, remained HIV free 159 days after transplantation. While this approach seems ideal for effective HIV inhibition *in vivo*, homozygous donors for the CCR5 mutation are rare, occurring in only ~ 1% of the white population. Nonetheless, this promising strategy can be adapted for the delivery of HSCs with an artificial HIV-resistant genotype.

Autologous cell-based approaches do not require matching of HLA genotypes and avoid the host-versus-graft complications. In a recent RNA-based example, a ribozyme (OZ1) against the *tat-vpr* region of the HIV genome was delivered to patients through transduced autologous CD34+ hematopoietic progenitor cells (Mitsuyasu, 2009). Progenitor cells were transduced with a murine retroviral vector encoding the OZ1 ribozyme. The cell-delivery method was assessed through a randomised, double-blind, placebo-controlled phase 2 gene transfer clinical trial with 74 HIV-1 infected individuals. The OZ1 group showed significantly lower viral loads after 40 weeks and significantly higher CD4+ lymphocyte counts through 100 weeks. This study demonstrated that cell-delivered gene transfer can be both a safe and effective therapeutic strategy.

In a more recent clinical trial, three RNA-based anti-HIV constructs were introduced into patients undergoing transplantation for AIDs-related lymphoma (DiGiusto *et al.*, 2010). HIV-infected individuals represent a unique and ethically-sound research group where marrow ablation can be performed prior to transplantation. A *tat/rev* short hairpin, TAR decoy and CCR5 ribozyme combination construct was used to modify the patient's own CD34+ cells through lentiviral transduction. Transduced cells showed no difference in haematopoietic potential compared to non-transduced cells in *in vitro* analysis and were successfully engrafted in four patients. Expression of the anti-HIV moieties was initially as high as 22 %, but declined to ~1% over four weeks of cell culture. Persistent siRNA expression was observed at low levels for up to 24 months in multiple lineages. No short-term toxicity was associated with the infusion of the genetically modified cells, and observed toxicities were instead related to the standard autologous hematopoietic cell transplantation (HCT) procedure.

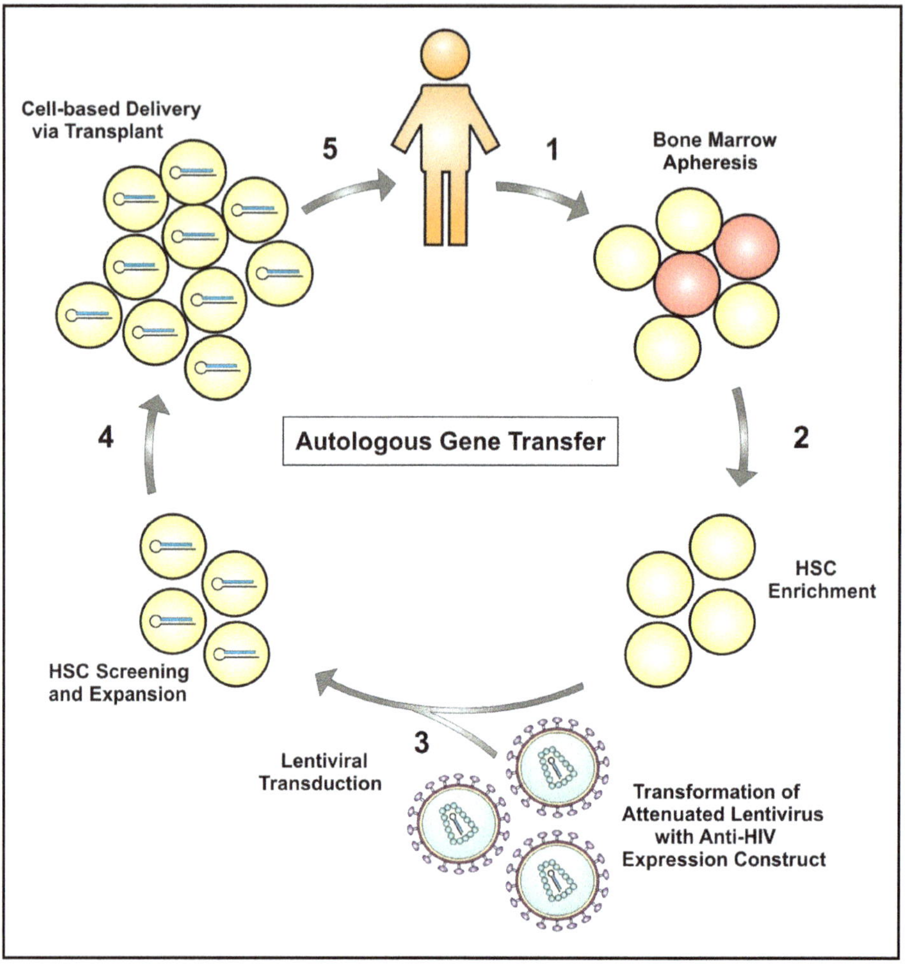

Fig. 3. An overall scheme for an RNAi-based therapy against HIV. SiRNAs or expressed RNAi constructs are delivered to infected cells by direct or vector-mediated methods

This study has demonstrated a viable approach for effective therapeutic expression of RNAi-based constructs against HIV-1. Persistent, constitutive shRNA expression over 24 months was not found to be toxic to peripheral blood cells and there was no evidence for lineage-specific toxicity. An artificial, anti-HIV expression vector can therefore be stably expressed in human blood cells without significant toxic side effects. The method of *ex vivo* lentiviral transduction and autologous cell-based gene transfer has been demonstrated as a safe and effective means of construct expression. The long term inhibitory effect on viral replication and evolution in the absence of anti-retroviral drugs remains to be seen. The demonstration of sustained anti-viral siRNA expression, however, has moved us one step closer to the realisation of a clinically applicable once-off treatment against HIV-1 infection. Further improvements in transduction and transplantation procedures are likely to yield even more favourable results for the therapeutic application of RNAi.

7. Conclusion

A genetic approach using expressed RNAi modalities offers the possibility of a once-off treatment against HIV with permanent and sustained viral inhibition and without common toxic side effects associated with current drug regimens. In this chapter, we have discussed the pros and cons of several RNAi-inducers that can be used to inhibit HIV replication. To summarise, an ideal RNAi-based gene therapy against HIV will make use of a combination of effective siRNA sequences in a single expression vector against at least four, but preferably six or seven, highly conserved viral target sequences or host dependency factors. This will provide potent silencing of target sequences across all known viral strains and prevent the emergence of viral escape mutants. Each siRNA sequence needs to be expressed at an equivalent and appropriate level under the control of a regulatable or HIV-inducible pol II promoter to avoid biased targeting and prevent the toxic and potentially lethal competition-based saturation of the natural RNAi pathway. The use of polycistronic pri-miRNA mimic expression systems appears most favourable and the preservation of natural structural motifs appears to enhance processing and silencing capabilities, as well as avoid activation of the innate immune system, which may otherwise occur with the introduction of exogenous constructs. Off-target effects should be modelled as far as possible before therapeutic testing and should be limited to non-significant effects. The most suitable delivery method to date appears to be through autologous cell-based gene transfer transplantation in a myeloablated recipient background with *ex vivo* lentiviral transduction of the patient's own haematopoietic progenitor cells. This is quite a comprehensive list of desirable properties for an ideal RNAi-based therapy against HIV and is the result of intensive research over the past decade. Further developments are necessary for the realisation of a safe and effective genetic therapy against HIV, but in light of the research presented here, we are moving closer.

8. Acknowledgments

This work was supported by the South African National Research Foundation, Medical Research Council and the Poliomyelitis Research Foundation. FvdB is a recipient of a scholarship from the Mellon Postgraduate Mentoring Programme.

9. References

Aagaard, L. A., Zhang, J., von Eije, K. J., Li, H., Sætrom, P., Amarzguioui, M., and Rossi, J. J. (2008). Engineering and optimization of the miR-106b cluster for ectopic expression of multiplexed anti-HIV RNAs. *Gene Therapy*, 1 - 14.

Anderson, J., and Akkina, R. (2005). HIV-1 resistance conferred by siRNA cosuppression of CXCR4 and CCR5 coreceptors by a bispecific lentiviral vector. *AIDS Res Ther 2*, 1-12.

Applegate, T. L., Birkett, D. J., McIntyre, G. J., Jaramillo, A. B., Symonds, G., and Murray, J. M. (2010). In silico modeling indicates the development of HIV-1 resistance to multiple shRNA gene therapy differs to standard antiretroviral therapy. *Retrovirology 7*, 83.

Barichievy, S., Saayman, S., Von Eije, K. J., Morris, K. V., Arbuthnot, P., and Weinberg, M. S. (2007). The Inhibitory Efficacy of RNA POL III-Expressed Long Hairpin RNAs Targeted to Untranslated Regions of the HIV-1 5_ Long Terminal Repeat. *Oligonucleotides 17*, 419-431.

Bartel, D., P. (2004). MicroRNAs: Genomics, Biogenesis, Mechanism, and Function. *Cell 116*, 281-297.

Boden, D., Pusch, O., Lee, F., Tucker, L., and Ramratnam, B. (2003). Human immunodeficiency virus type 1 escape from RNA interference. *J Virol 77*, 11531-11535.

Boden, D., Pusch, O., Silbermann, R., Lee, F., Tucker, L., and Ramratnam, B. (2004). Enhanced gene silencing of HIV-1 specific siRNA using microRNA designed hairpins. *Nucleic Acids Research 32*, 1154-1158.

Boudreau, R. L., Martins, I., and Davidson, B. L. (2009). Artificial MicroRNAs as siRNA Shuttles: Improved Safety as Compared to shRNAs In vitro and In vivo. *Molecular Therapy 17*, 169-175.

Boudreau, R. L., Monteys, A. M., and Davidson, B. L. (2008). Minimizing variables among hairpin-based RNAi vectors reveals the potency of shRNAs. *RNA 14*, 1834-1844.

Brass, A. L., Dykxhoorn, D. M., Benita, Y., Yan, N., Engelman, A., Xavier, R. J., Lieberman, J., and Elledge, S. J. (2008). Identification of host proteins required for HIV infection through a functional genomic screen. *Science 319*, 921-926.

Brennecke, J., Stark, A., Russell, R. B., and Cohen, S. M. (2005). Principles of microRNA-target recognition. *PLoS Biol 3*, e85.

Breving, K., and Esquela-Kerscher, A. (2009). The complexities of microRNA regulation: mirandering around the rules. *The International Journal of Biochemistry & Cell Biology.*

Brummelkamp, T. R., Bernards, R., and Agami, R. (2002). A system for stable expression of short interfering RNAs in mammalian cells. *Science 296*, 550-553.

Caplen, N. J., Parrish, S., Imani, F., Fire, A., and Morgan, R. A. (2001). Specific inhibition of gene expression by small double-stranded RNAs in invertebrate and vertebrate systems. *Proc Natl Acad Sci U S A 98*, 9742-9747.

Capodici, J., Kariko, K., and Weissman, D. (2002). Inhibition of HIV-1 infection by small interfering RNA-mediated RNA interference. *J Immunol 169*, 5196-5201.

Castanotto, D., Sakurai, K., Lingeman, R., Li, H., Shively, L., Aagaard, L., Soifer, H., Gatignol, A., Riggs, A., and Rossi, J. J. (2007). Combinatorial delivery of small interfering RNAs reduces RNAi efficacy by selective incorporation into RISC. *Nucleic Acids Research 35*, 5154-5164.

Charrier, S., Dupre, L., Scaramuzza, S., Jeanson-Leh, L., Blundell, M. P., Danos, O., Cattaneo, F., Aiuti, A., Eckenberg, R., Thrasher, A. J., *et al.* (2007). Lentiviral vectors targeting WASp expression to hematopoietic cells, efficiently transduce and correct cells from WAS patients. *Gene Ther 14*, 415-428.

Chendrimada, T. P., Gregory, R. I., Kumaraswamy, E., N., J., Cooch, N., Nishikura, K., and Shiekhatter, R. (2005). TRBP recruits the Dicer complex to AGO2 for microRNA processing and gene silencing. *Nature 436*, 740-744.

Chu, C.-Y., and Rana, T. M. (2008). Potent RNAi by short RNA triggers. *RNA 14*, 1714-1719.

Chung, K. H., Hart, C. C., Al-Bassam, S., Avery, A., Taylor, J., Patel, P. D., Vojtek, A. B., and Turner, D. L. (2006). Polycistronic RNA polymerase II expression vectors for RNA interference based on BIC/miR-155. *Nucleic Acids Res 34*, e53.

Coburn, G. A., and Cullen, B. R. (2002). Potent and specific inhibition of human immunodeficiency virus type 1 replication by RNA interference. *J Virol 76*, 9225-9231.

Cullen, B. R. (2004). Transcription and Processing of Human microRNA Precursors. *Molecular Cell 16*, 861-865.

Cullen, B. R. (2005). Human immunodeficiency virus: nuclear RNA export unwound. *Nature 433*, 26-27.

Davis, M. E., Zuckerman, J. E., Choi, C. H., Seligson, D., Tolcher, A., Alabi, C. A., Yen, Y., Heidel, J. D., and Ribas, A. (2010). Evidence of RNAi in humans from systemically administered siRNA via targeted nanoparticles. *Nature 464*, 1067-1070.

de Veer, M. J., Sledz, C. A., and Williams, B. R. (2005). Detection of foreign RNA: implications for RNAi. *Immunol Cell Biol 83*, 224-228.

Devincenzo, J., Lambkin-Williams, R., Wilkinson, T., Cehelsky, J., Nochur, S., Walsh, E., Meyers, R., Gollob, J., and Vaishnaw, A. (2010). A randomized, double-blind, placebo-controlled study of an RNAi-based therapy directed against respiratory syncytial virus. *Proc Natl Acad Sci U S A.*

Dickins, R. A., Hemann, M. T., Zilfou, J. T., Simpson, D. R., Ibarra, I., Hannon, G. J., and Lowe, S. W. (2005). Probing tumor phenotypes using stable and regulated synthetic microRNA precursors. *Nat Genet 37*, 1289-1295.

DiGiusto, D. L., Krishnan, A., Li, L., Li, H., Li, S., Rao, A., Mi, S., Yam, P., Stinson, S., Kalos, M., *et al.* (2010). RNA-based gene therapy for HIV with lentiviral vector-modified CD34(+) cells in patients undergoing transplantation for AIDS-related lymphoma. *Sci Transl Med 2*, 36ra43.

Ding, X. C., Weiler, J., and Grosshans, H. (2009). Regulating the regulators: mechanisms controlling the maturation of microRNAs. *Trends Biotechnol 27*, 27-36.

Elbashir, S. M., Harborth, J., Lendeckel, W., Yalcin, A., Weber, K., and Tuschl, T. (2001a). Duplexes of 21-nucleotide RNAs mediate RNA interference in cultured mammalian cells. *Nature 411*, 494-498.

Elbashir, S. M., Lendeckel, W., and Tuschl, T. (2001b). RNA interference is mediated by 21- and 22-nucleotide RNAs. *Genes & Development 15*, 188-200.

Ely, A., Naidoo, T., and Arbuthnot, P. (2009). Efficient silencing of gene expression with modular trimeric Pol II expression cassettes comprising microRNA shuttles. *Nucleic Acids Res 37*, e91.

Fire, A., Xu, S., Montgomery, M. K., Kostas, S. A., Driver, S. E., and Mello, C. C. (1998). Potent and specific genetic interference by double-strandedRNAin Caenorhabditis elegans. *Nature 391*, 806-811.

Giering, J. C., Grimm, D., Storm, T. A., and Kay, M. A. (2008). Expression of shRNA from a tissue-specific pol II promoter is an effective and safe RNAi therapeutic. *Mol Ther 16*, 1630-1636.

Good, P. D., Krikos, A. J., Li, S. X., Bertrand, E., Lee, N. S., Giver, L., Ellington, A., Zaia, J. A., Rossi, J. J., and Engelke, D. R. (1997). Expression of small, therapeutic RNAs in human cell nuclei. *Gene Ther 4*, 45-54.

Gregory, R. I., Yan, K.-p., Amuthan, G., Chendrimada, T., Doratotaj, B., Cooch, N., and Shiekhattar, R. (2004). The Microprocessor complex mediates the genesis of microRNAs. *Nature 432*.

Grimm, D., Streetz, K. L., Jopling, C. L., Storm, T. A., Pandey, K., Davis, C. R., Marion, P., Salazar, F., and Kay, M. A. (2006). Fatality in mice due to oversaturation of cellular microRNA/short hairpin RNA pathways. *Nature 441*, 537-541.

Grimm, D., Wang, L., Lee, J. S., Schurmann, N., Gu, S., Borner, K., Storm, T. A., and Kay, M. A. (2010). Argonaute proteins are key determinants of RNAi efficacy, toxicity, and persistence in the adult mouse liver. *J Clin Invest 120*, 3106-3119.

Han, J., Lee, Y., Yeom, K.-H., Kim, Y. K., Jin, H., and Kim, V. N. (2004). The Drosha-DGCR8 complex in primary miRNA processing. *Genes & Development 18*, 3016-3027.

Han, J., Lee, Y., Yeom, K.-H., Nam, J.-W., Heo, I., Rhee, J.-K., Sohn, S. Y., Cho, Y., Zhang, B.-T., and Kim, V. N. (2006). Molecular Basis for the Recognition of Primary microRNAs by the Drosha-DGCR8 Complex. *Cell 125*, 887-901.

Hutter, G., Nowak, D., Mossner, M., Ganepola, S., Mussig, A., Allers, K., Schneider, T., Hofmann, J., Kucherer, C., Blau, O., *et al.* (2009). Long-term control of HIV by CCR5 Delta32/Delta32 stem-cell transplantation. *N Engl J Med 360*, 692-698.

Hutvagner, G., and Zamore, P. D. (2002). A microRNA in a multiple-turnover RNAi enzyme complex. *Science 297*, 2056-2060.

Jackson, A. L., Bartz, S. R., Schelter, J., Kobayashi, S. V., Burchard, J., Mao, M., Li, B., Cavet, G., and Linsley, P. S. (2003). Expression profiling reveals off-target gene regulation by RNAi. *Nat Biotechnol 21*, 635-637.

Jacque, J. M., Triques, K., and Stevenson, M. (2002). Modulation of HIV-1 replication by RNA interference. *Nature 418*, 435-438.

Kariko, K., Bhuyan, P., Capodici, J., and Weissman, D. (2004). Small interfering RNAs mediate sequence-independent gene suppression and induce immune activation by signaling through toll-like receptor 3. *J Immunol 172*, 6545-6549.

Karpala, A. J., Doran, T. J., and Bean, A. G. (2005). Immune responses to dsRNA: implications for gene silencing technologies. *Immunol Cell Biol 83*, 211-216.

Khvorova, A., Reynolds, A., and Jayasena, S. D. (2003). Functional siRNAs and miRNAs exhibit strand bias. *Cell 115*, 209-216.

Kim, S. S., Peer, D., Kumar, P., Subramanya, S., Wu, H., Asthana, D., Habiro, K., Yang, Y. G., Manjunath, N., Shimaoka, M., and Shankar, P. (2010). RNAi-mediated CCR5 silencing by LFA-1-targeted nanoparticles prevents HIV infection in BLT mice. *Mol Ther 18*, 370-376.

Kumar, P., Ban, H. S., Kim, S. S., Wu, H., Pearson, T., Greiner, D. L., Laouar, A., Yao, J., Haridas, V., Habiro, K., *et al.* (2008). T cell-specific siRNA delivery suppresses HIV-1 infection in humanized mice. *Cell 134*, 577-586.

Lee, M. T., Coburn, G. A., McClure, M. O., and Cullen, B. R. (2003). Inhibition of human immunodeficiency virus type 1 replication in primary macrophages by using Tat-

or CCR5-specific small interfering RNAs expressed from a lentivirus vector. *J Virol 77*, 11964-11972.

Lee, N. S., Dohjima, T., Bauer, G., Li, H., Li, M.-J., Ehsani, A., Salvaterra, P., and Rossi, J. (2002a). Expression of small interfering RNAs targeted against HIV-1 rev transcripts in human cells. *Nature Biotechnology 19*, 500-505.

Lee, Y., Hur, I., Park, S. Y., Kim, Y. K., Suh, M. R., and Kim, V. N. (2006). The role of PACT in the RNA silencing pathway. *The EMBO Journal 25*, 522-532.

Lee, Y., Jeon, K., Lee, J.-T., Kim, S., and Kim, V. N. (2002b). MicroRNA maturation: stepwise processing and subcellular localization. *The EMBO Journal 21*, 4663-4670.

Lee, Y., Kim, M., Han, J., Yeom, K. H., Lee, S., Baek, S. H., and Kim, V. N. (2004). MicroRNA genes are transcribed by RNA polymerase II. *The EMBO Journal 23*, 4051-4060.

Leonard, J. N., and Schaffer, D. V. (2005). Computational design of antiviral RNA interference strategies that resist human immunodeficiency virus escape. *J Virol 79*, 1645-1654.

Liu, Y. P., Gruber, J., Haasnoot, J., Konstantinova, P., and Berkhout, B. (2009a). RNAi-mediated inhibition of HIV-1 by targeting partially complementary viral sequences. *Nucleic Acids Res 37*, 6194-6204.

Liu, Y. P., Haasnoot, J., and Berkhout, B. (2007). Design of extended short hairpin RNAs for HIV-1 inhibition. *Nucleic Acids Res 35*, 5683-5693.

Liu, Y. P., Haasnoot, J., ter Brake, O., Berkhout, B., and Konstantinova, P. (2008). Inhibition of HIV-1 by multiple siRNAs expressed from a single microRNA polycistron. *Nulceic Acids Research 36*, 2811-2824.

Liu, Y. P., von Eije, K. J., Schopman, N. C., Westerink, J. T., ter Brake, O., Haasnoot, J., and Berkhout, B. (2009b). Combinatorial RNAi against HIV-1 using extended short hairpin RNAs. *Mol Ther 17*, 1712-1723.

Lund, E., Guttinger, S., Calado, A., Dahlberg, J. E., and Kutay, U. (2004). Nuclear export of microRNA precursors. *Science 303*, 95-98.

MacRae, I. J., Ma, E., Zhou, M., Robinson, C. V., and Doudna, J. A. (2008). In vitro reconstitution of the human RISC-loading complex. *PNAS 105*, 512-517.

Martinez, J., Patkaniowska, A., Urlaub, H., Luhrmann, R., and Tuschl, T. (2002a). Sinlge-stranded antisense siRNAs guide target RNA cleavage in RNAi. Cell *110*, 563-574.

Martinez, M. A., Clotet, B., and Este, J. A. (2002b). RNA interference of HIV replication. *Trends Immunol 23*, 559-561.

McIntyre, G. J., Groneman, J. L., Yu, Y. H., Jaramillo, A., Shen, S., and Applegate, T. L. (2009). 96 shRNAs designed for maximal coverage of HIV-1 variants. *Retrovirology 6*, 55.

McIntyre, G. J., Groneman, J. L., Yu, Y. H., Tran, A., and Applegate, T. L. (2011). Multiple shRNA combinations for near-complete coverage of all HIV-1 strains. *AIDS Res Ther 8*, 1.

Mitsuyasu, e. a. (2009). Phase 2 gene therapy trials of an anti-HIV ribozyme in autologous CD34+ cells. *Nature medicine 15*.

Miyagishi, M., and Taira, K. (2002). U6 promoter-driven siRNAs with four uridine 3' overhangs efficiently suppress targeted gene expression in mammalian cells. *Nat Biotechnol 20*, 497-500.

Naito, Y., Nohtomi, K., Onogi, T., Uenishi, R., Ui-Tei, K., Saigo, K., and Takebe, Y. (2007). Optimal design and validation of antiviral siRNA for targeting HIV-1. *Retrovirology 4*, 80.

Naldini, L., Blomer, U., Gallay, P., Ory, D., Mulligan, R., Gage, F. H., Verma, I. M., and Trono, D. (1996). In vivo gene delivery and stable transduction of nondividing cells by a lentiviral vector. *Science 272*, 263-267.

Neff, C. P., Zhou, J., Remling, L., Kuruvilla, J., Zhang, J., Li, H., Smith, D. D., Swiderski, P., Rossi, J. J., and Akkina, R. (2011). An aptamer-siRNA chimera suppresses HIV-1 viral loads and protects from helper CD4(+) T cell decline in humanized mice. *Sci Transl Med 3*, 66ra66.

Nishitsuji, H., Kohara, M., Kannagi, M., and Masuda, T. (2006). Effective Suppression of Human Immunodeficiency Virus Type 1 through a Combination of Short- or Long-Hairpin RNAs Targeting Essential Sequences for Retroviral Integration. *Journal of Virology 80*, 7658-7666.

Novina, C. D., Murray, M. F., Dykxhoorn, D. M., Beresford, P. J., Riess, J., Lee, S. K., Collman, R. G., Lieberman, J., Shankar, P., and Sharp, P. A. (2002). siRNA-directed inhibition of HIV-1 infection. *Nat Med 8*, 681-686.

Obernosterer, G., Leuschner, P. J., Alenius, M., and Martinez, J. (2006). Post-transcriptional regulation of microRNA expression. *Rna 12*, 1161-1167.

Paddison, P. J., Caudy, A. A., and Hannon, G. J. (2002). Stable suppression of gene expression by RNAi in mammalian cells. *Proc Natl Acad Sci U S A 99*, 1443-1448.

Paul, C. P., Good, P. D., Winer, I., and Engelke, D. R. (2002). Effective expression of small interfering RNA in human cells. *Nat Biotechnol 20*, 505-508.

Robbins, M. A., Li, M., Leung, I., Li, H., Boyer, D. V., Song, Y., Behlke, M. A., and Rossi, J. J. (2006). Stable expression of shRNAs in human CD34+ progenitor cells can avoid induction of interferon responses to siRNAs in vitro. *Nat Biotechnol 24*, 566-571.

Saayman, S., Arbuthnot, P., and Weinberg, M. S. (2010). Deriving four functional anti-HIV siRNAs from a single Pol III-generated transcript comprising two adjacent long hairpin RNA precursors. *Nucleic Acids Res 38*, 6652-6663.

Saayman, S., Barichievy, S., Capovilla, A., Morris, K. V., Arbuthnot, P., and Weinberg, M. S. (2008). The Efficacy of Generating Three Independent Anti-HIV-1 siRNAs from a Single U6 RNA Pol III-Expressed Long Hairpin RNA. *PLoS ONE 3*, e2602.

Sano, M., Li, H., Nakanishi, M., and Rossi, J. J. (2008). Expression of long anti-HIV-1 hairpin RNAs for the generation of multiple siRNAs: advantages and limitations. *Mol Ther 16*, 170-177.

Schopman, N. C., Liu, Y. P., Konstantinova, P., ter Brake, O., and Berkhout, B. (2010). Optimization of shRNA inhibitors by variation of the terminal loop sequence. *Antiviral Res 86*, 204-211.

Schwarz, D. S., Hutvagner, G., Du, T., Xu, Z., A., N., and Zamore, P. D. (2003). Asymmetry in the assembly of the RNAi enzyme complex. *Cell 115*, 199-208.

Silva, J. M., Li, M. Z., Chang, K., Ge, W., C., G. M., Rickles, R. J., Siolas, D., Hu, G., Paddison, P. J., Schlabach, M. R., *et al.* (2005). Second-generation shRNA libraries covering the mouse and human genomes. *Nature Genetics 37*, 1281-1288.

Siolas, D., Lerner, C., Burchard, J., Ge, W., Linsley, P. S., Paddison, P. J., Hannon, G. J., and Cleary, M. A. (2005). Synthetic shRNAs as potent RNAi triggers. *Nature Biotechnology 23*, 227-231.

Song, E., Lee, S. K., Dykxhoorn, D. M., Novina, C., Zhang, D., Crawford, K., Cerny, J., Sharp, P. A., Lieberman, J., Manjunath, N., and Shankar, P. (2003). Sustained small interfering RNA-mediated human immunodeficiency virus type 1 inhibition in primary macrophages. *J Virol 77*, 7174-7181.

Surabhi, R. M., and Gaynor, R. B. (2002). RNA interference directed against viral and cellular targets inhibits human immunodeficiency Virus Type 1 replication. *J Virol 76*, 12963-12973.

ter Brake, O., Konstantinova, P., Ceylan, M., and Berkhout, B. (2006). Silencing of HIV-1 with RNA Interference: A Multiple shRNA Approach. *Molecular Therapy 14*, 883-892.

ter Brake, O., t Hooft, K., Liu, Y. P., Centlivre, M., von Eije, K. J., and Berkhout, B. (2008). Lentiviral vector design for multiple shRNA expression and durable HIV-1 inhibition. *Mol Ther 16*, 557-564.

Trabucchi, M., Briata, P., Garcia-Mayoral, M., Haase, A. D., Filipowicz, W., Ramos, A., Gherzi, R., and Rosenfeld, M. G. (2009). The RNA-binding protein KSRP promotes the biogenesis of a subset of microRNAs. *Nature 459*, 1010-1014.

Tuschl, T., and Borkhardt, A. (2002). Small interfering RNAs: a revolutionary tool for the analysis of gene function and gene therapy. *Molecular Interventions 2*, 158- 167.

UNAIDS (2010). UN Report on the Global AIDS Epidemic, pp. 1 - 364.

Unwalla, H. J., Li, M. J., Kim, J. D., Li, H. T., Ehsani, A., Alluin, J., and Rossi, J. J. (2004). Negative feedback inhibition of HIV-1 by TAT-inducible expression of siRNA. *Nat Biotechnol 22*, 1573-1578.

Vermeulen, A., Behlen, L., Reynolds, A., Wolfson, A., Marshall, W. S., Karpilow, J., and Khvorova, A. (2005). The contributions of dsRNA structure to Dicer specificity and efficiency. *RNA 11*, 674-682.

Westerhout, E. M., Ooms, M., Vink, M., Das, A. T., and Berkhout, B. (2005). HIV-1 can escape from RNA interference by evolving an alternative structure in its RNA genome. *Nucleic Acids Res 33*, 796-804.

Wilson, J. A., Jayasena, S., Khvorova, A., Sabatinos, S., Rodrigue-Gervais, I. G., Arya, S., Sarangi, F., Harris-Brandts, M., Beaulieu, S., and Richardson, C. D. (2003). RNA interference blocks gene expression and RNA synthesis from hepatitis C replicons propagated in human liver cells. *PNAS 100*, 2783-2788.

Yi, R., Qin, Y., Macara, I. G., and Cullen, B. R. (2003). Exportin-5 mediates the nuclear export of pre-microRNAs and short hairpin RNAs. Genes & *Development 17*, 3011-3016.

Zeng, Y., and Cullen, B. R. (2005). Efficient Processing of Primary microRNA Hairpins by Drosha Requires Flanking Nonstructured RNA Sequences. *The Journal of Biological Chemistry 280*, 27595-27603.

Zeng, Y., Yi, R., and Cullen, B. R. (2003). MicroRNAs and small interfering RNAs can inhibit mRNA expression by similar mechanisms. *PNAS 100*, 9779-9784.

Zeng, Y., Yi, R., and Cullen, B. R. (2005). Recognition and cleavage of primary microRNA precursors by the nuclear processing enzyme Drosha. *The EMBO Journal 24*, 138-148.

Zhou, J., and Rossi, J. J. (2010). Aptamer-targeted cell-specific RNA interference. *Silence 1*, 4.

10

Natural Catalytic Antibodies in Norm and in HIV-Infected Patients

Georgy A. Nevinsky
Institute of Chemical Biology and Fundamental Medicine of SD of RAS
Russia

1. Introduction

Antibodies (Abs) have been first characterized as proteins which are produced by the immune system and have a sole function of binding other molecules, called antigens, with the goal of eliciting an immune response. In this classical conception, Abs act similarly to enzymes in specific binding other molecules. However, in contrast to enzymes they do not have the ability to catalyze chemical conversions of their bound partners. For the vast majority of Abs, this observation is correct. However, in a 1946 consideration of enzyme function, Linus Pauling first hypothesized that the active center of an enzyme is closely juxtaposed to a "strained configuration" of its substrate (that is, targeted against the structure of the transition state) rather than to the native conformation of the substrate molecule (Pauling, 1946). This idea led Jencks in 1969 to propose that Abs generated in an anti-hapten immune response against chemically stable analogs of the transition-state of a reaction of interest could potentially display an enzymatic activity (Jencks, 1969).

In 1985, a general method for generating catalytic monoclonal Abzs against transition state analogs, and a way to use those Abs to accelerate chemical reactions, was first described (Schochetman & Massey, 1985). One year later two groups were able to produce the first monoclonal Abs with catalytic properties, which were generated against hapten analogs of the transition states for *p*-nitrophenylphosphorylcholine (Pollack et al., 1986) or for monoaryl phosphonate esters (Tramontano et al., 1986[a], 1986[b]). The artificial monoclonal anti-hapten catalytic Abs were termed abzymes (derived from **antib**ody en**zyme**).

The evolution of the technology of artificial Abzs during the last ~two decades has led not only to the rapid development of direct approaches for the generation of Abs with specified properties, but also to the creation of strategies to revise the targeting specificity of individual Abzs. Such modifications of antigen binding specificity can be achieved genetically *in vitro*, by application of the site directed mutagenesis, or genetic selection or screening (using approaches such as phage display). Alternatively, modification can be induced directly on purified antibody, *via* selective chemical modification by direct introduction of catalytic groups into the Ab combining site. Some studies describing these approaches include (Keinan, 2005, and refs therein). The employment of the approaches have demonstrated that the substrate specificity (and/or the specific activity) of some artificial Abzs is comparable to or even higher than that of enzymes with the same catalytic activity (Barbas et al., 1997; Janda et al., 1997; Keinan, 2005, and refs therein).

Artificial Abzs against transition chemical states of different reactions have been studied intensively (Thayer et al., 1999). Mechanistic basis for the activity of such Abzs is becoming well understood (Janda et al., 1997; Thayer et al., 1999; Keinan, 2005, and refs therein). The field of artificial Abzs has been amply reviewed recently (Martin & Schultz, 1999; Suzuki, 1994; Keinan, 2005, and refs therein), for more detailed description of the relevant reactions.

During last two decades it has become clear that auto-Abs from the sera of patients with different autoimmune (AI) diseases can possess enzymic activities (Suzuki, 1994; Keinan, 2005; Nevinsky et al., 2002[a], 2002[b], 2003, 2005, 2010[a], 2010[b], and refs therein). The first example of a natural Abz was an IgG found in bronchial asthma patients, which hydrolyzes intestinal vasoactive peptide (VIP) (Paul et al., 1989), the second was an IgG with DNase activity in SLE (Shuster, et al., 1992), and the third was an IgG with RNase activity in SLE (Buneva et al., 1994). Later, different natural catalytic IgG and/or IgA, IgM hydrolyzing oligopeptides, proteins, DNA, RNA, nucleotides, and polysaccharides were detected in the sera of patients with several autoimmune (AI) and viral pathologies, and Abzs with these and other different activities were discovered in healthy human milk (for review see Nevinsky et al., 2002[a], 2002[b], 2003, 2005, 2010[a], 2010[b]).

The phenomenon of catalysis by auto-Abzs is extremely interesting and potentially applicable in many different fields including new types of efficient catalysts, new generation of drugs, evaluation of the functional roles of Abzs in innate and adaptive immunity, and understanding of certain aspects of self-tolerance and of the destructive or positive responses in AI diseases. The field of monoclonal Abzs with immunotherapeutic potential has recently been reviewed (Wentworth et al., 1998; Tellier, 2002; Zhou et al., 2002; Nishi, 2003; Stockwin and Holmes, 2003; Hanson et al., 2005; Gabibov et al., 2006; Planque et al., 2008; Wójcik & Kieć-Kononowicz, 2008). Some general possibilities of present and future therapeutic Abs and Abzs application were discussed in (Stockwin & Holmes, 2003). Abs and Abzs can be used to neutralize pathogens, toxins and endogenous mediators of pathology. As cell-targeting reagents, Abs can be used to modulate cytoplasmic cascades or to tag specific cells for complement- or effector-mediated lysis. Abs can also be modified to deliver toxic or modulatory payloads (small molecules, radionuclides and enzymes) and engineered to bind multiple epitopes or even to have novel catalytic activity. The modular structure of Igs and the availability of Ab fragment libraries also make it possible to produce variable-domain therapeutics (Fab, single-chain and domain of Abs). Although exhibiting less favorable kinetics *in vivo*, these fragments are straightforward to express and easily penetrate tissues, making them especially useful as neutralizing or delivery agents. The number of approved Abzs is expected to increase in the near term, as the platform is adopted as a viable alternative to small molecule discovery (Stockwin & Holmes, 2003). The Abzs strategy can be employed for new methods of drug synthesis, as well as for in vivo therapies. Catalytic antibodies seem to be a promising tool for therapeutic purposes, because of their specificity and stereoselectivity. For instance, cocaine-hydrolyzing Abzs have been developed, and may provide a novel approach to the problems of drug addiction (Hanson et al., 2005). Possible application of Abzs for prodrug activation and their potential utility in clinical oncology was also discussed (Nishi, 2003). Abzs have two distinct advantages over canonical enzymes: first, they can be selected to perform reactions not catalyzed by endogenous enzymes, and second, they can be humanized to minimize their immunogenicity (Stockwin & Holmes, 2003).

2. Features of the immune status of patients with AIDS, bacterial, and autoimmune diseases

HIV-1 is the etiologic agent of an extremely dangerous human disease, AIDS (Fauci et al., 2008, and refs therein). The association of immune dysfunction in patients with HIV infection and AIDS and the development of AI diseases are very interesting. At this moment the spectrum of reported autoimmune phenomena in AIDS patients is increasing (for review see Zandman-Goddard & Shoenfeld, 2002). A special feature of ADs is high concentrations of auto-Abs (Abs to many different endogenous antigens) (Zouali, 2001; Pisetsky, 2001). The development of AI diseases is characterized by spontaneous generation of primary Abs to proteins, nucleic acids and their complexes, polysaccharides, nucleotides etc. (Earnshaw & Rothfield, 1985; Raptis & Menard, 1980). Later the secondary idiotypic and then antiidiotypic Abs to the primary ones are usually generated, etc. Immunization of animals with DNA or RNA and especially their complexes with proteins leads to the production of anti-DNA and anti-RNA Abs (Gottieb & Shwartz, 1972; Mitsuhashi et al., 1978).

During frank loss of immunocompetence, AI diseases that are predominantly T cell subtype CD8 driven predominate. There is evidence for B cell stimulation and many auto-Abs are reported in HIV patients. HIV-dependent activation of B lymphocytes leads to the production of auto-Abs not only to different viral proteins including HIV reverse transcriptase (RT) and integrase (IN), but also to human cell components, and various immune complexes including anti-cardiolipin, anti-beta2 GPI, anti-DNA, anti-small nuclear ribonucleoproteins, anti-thyroglobulin, anti-thyroid peroxidase, anti-myosin, and anti-erythropoietin and possibly other human cell and blood components (Fauci et al., 2008; Zandman-Goddard & Shoenfeld, 2002). The list of reported autoimmune diseases in HIV/AIDS includes SLE, anti-phospholipid syndrome, vasculitis, primary biliary cirrhosis, polymyosits, Graves' disease, and idiopathic thrombocytopenic purpura (Zandman-Goddard & Shoenfeld, 2002). The presence of AI phenomena and production of auto-Abs in chronic bacterial and viral infections including HIV could be related to molecular mimicry between microbial or viral and host antigens (Zandman-Goddard & Shoenfeld, 2002; Hentati et al., 1994; Ternynck et al., 1991), altered self, abnormal expression of immunoregulatory molecules, and the anti-idiotypic network (Barzilai et al., 2008).

Interestingly, some other viral infections similarly to ADs can also demonstrate AI reactions leading to the formation of Abs to various human and viral antigens. Compared with healthy donors, concentrations of DNA and anti-DNA Abs are higher not only in patients with SLE (36% of SLE patients), but also in multiple sclerosis (17-18%), primary Sjogren's syndrome (18%), Hashimoto's thyroiditis (23%), myasthenia gravis (6%), rheumatoid arthritis (7%), autoimmune hepatitis (Shoenfeld et al., 1988, 1989), and also in lymphoproliferative (Kozyr et al., 1998) and some viral diseases including viral hepatitis, AIDS (Gololobov et al., 1994), and TBE (Garmashova et al., 2004). In the sera of patients with several AI diseases, RNA and anti-RNA Abs were also detected (Blanco et al., 1991; Sato et al., 1994; Hirokawa et al., 2002; Ikeda et al., 2003).

AIDS, TBE, and hepatitis demonstrating strong reorganization of immune system have some similarities with typical AI diseases such as SLE (HT, and others) which is a systemic AI polyetiologic diffuse disease that is characterized by disorganization of conjunctive tissues with the paramount damage to skin and visceral capillaries (Hhachn, 1996). All known AI and viral diseases like AIDS, viral hepatitis, and TBE are characterized by significant disturb the immune status of the patients accompanied by humoral and cellular

AI reactions, with detectable tissue-specific and organ-nonspecific Abs (Bigazzi, 1983; Sugiama & Yamamota, 1996; Nevinsky, 2010[b]). At the same time, microbial and viral infections expose the human organism to different components from the parasite's cells and viral particles, including protein, DNA, RNA, lipids, and polysaccharides. The sera of mice infected with different microbe's bacterial pathogens contain a variety of Abs to the parasite's antigens and to human lipids, proteins, and nuclear components, including anti-DNA Abs (Ternynck et al., 1991; Unterkircher et al., 1993; Matsiota-Bernard et al., 1993, 1996; Hentati et al., 1994; Boekel et al., 1997; Wun et al., 2001). The origin of anti-DNA Abs in the infections remains speculative; some of them may arise inadvertently in the course of a normal immune response due to the induction by Abs that bear structures (mimotopes) mimicking DNA (Wun et al., 2001). The immunoregulatory effect of the infection seems to be related, at least partially, to the increase in a particular population of Abs, the polyreactive Abs (Matsiota-Bernard et al., 1996). It has been proposed that bacterial and viral infectious agents can act in some cases through the mechanism of molecular mimicry and stimulate development of different AI diseases. For instance, the agents responsible for molecular mimicry in multiple sclerosis include measles, hepatitis B, herpes simplex, influenza, papilloma, and Epstein-Bar viruses (Steinman, 2001). Thus, AI reactions in different AI, viral and bacterial infection diseases are very similar and may be strongly associated.

3. The origin of artificial and natural abzymes

Artificial Abzs can be obtained by immunization of animals with chemically stable analogs of transition states of chemical reactions (reviewed in Martin & Schultz, 1999; Nevinsky et al., 2000[a]; Tanaka, 2002; Tanaka and Barbas, 2002; Dias et al., 2002; Keinan, 2005). On the other hand, artificial antiidiotypic Abs can also possess catalytic activity (Barbas et al., 1997; Wentworth et al., 1998). Building on earlier observations on the existence of idiotypic determinants related to the antigen, Jerne proposed that the immune system is self-regulated by a network of idiotype–anti-idiotype interactions (Jerne, 1974). The simplified model of this network may be schematically presented as follows:

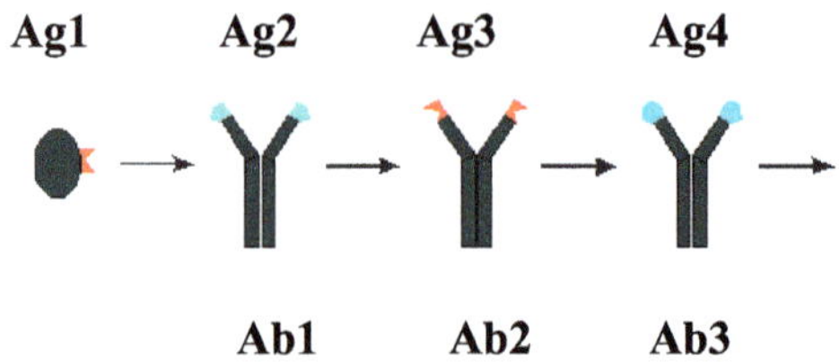

Antibodies 1 and 2 are termed idiotype and anti-idiotype, respectively, etc. There is convincing evidence that such idiotype–anti-idiotype networks are actually present in the body. The presence of blood serum Ab4 (in the notation shown in the scheme) has been confirmed in experimental animals (Jerne, 1974).

If the active site of an enzyme plays the role of antigen triggering this anti-idiotypic chain, it is logical to suggest that the secondary anti-idiotypic Ab2 may possess the structure, a part of which represents an "internal image" or "mould" of the active site of this enzyme, and, consequently, these Abs may possess some properties of this enzyme. This remarkable property of idiotypic mimicry has been exploited to raise monoclonal antiidiotypic Abzs with several different catalytic activities (reviewed in Keinan, 2005; Nevinsky et al., 2005).

The origin of natural Abzs in different AI, viral and bacterial diseases may be complex. Similarly to artificial Abzs against analogs of transition states of catalytic reactions, naturally occurring Abzs with DNase and RNase activities may be Abs raised directly against free DNA and RNA or these nucleic acids acting as haptens bound to different proteins and resembling transition states of catalytic reactions (Nevinsky et al., 2003, 2005, 2010[a], 2010[b], and refs therein). Immunization of rabbits with pure DNA and RNA generated Abs interacting with DNA and possessing weak DNase and RNase activities (Krasnorutskii et al., 2008[a], 2008[b]). Many SLE anti-DNA Abs are directed against histone-DNA nucleosomal complexes appearing as a result of internucleosomal cleavage during apoptosis (Founel & Muller, 2002). Apoptotic cells are the primary source of antigens and immunogens in SLE, and certain features in recognition, processing, and/or presentation of apoptotic auto-antigens by antigen-presenting cells can trigger AI processes (Founel & Muller, 2002). Anti-DNA-protein and anti-RNA-protein complexes and other antinuclear antibodies were found in the sera of patients with multisystem connective tissue disease (Gottieb & Shwartz, 1972). Therefore, we have emulated such natural complexes using complexes of DNA and RNA with methylated bovine serum albumin (mBSA). Immunization of rabbits with complex of DNA and RNA with mBSA elicited production of 10-50-fold more active DNase and RNase IgGs, while pIgGs from animals immunized with mBSA were catalytically inactive (Krasnorutskii et al., 2008[a], 2008[b]). Immunization of healthy rabbits with DNase I, DNase II, and pancreatic RNase A also produced anti-idiotypic IgGs with intrinsic DNase and RNase activities (Krasnorutskii et al., 2008[c], 2008[d], 2009). Thus, DNase and RNase Abzs in different AI diseases may be a cocktail of Abs against complexes of DNA and RNA with proteins and antiidiotypic Abzs to very different DNA- and RNA-hydrolyzing enzymes.

Healthy humans and patients with many diseases with insignificant AI reactions usually lack Abzs or develop Abzs with very low catalytic activities, often on a borderline of the sensitivity of detection methods (Nevinsky et al., 2002[a], 2002[b], 2003, 2005, 2010[a], 2010[b], and refs therein). Natural Abzs hydrolyzing DNA and RNA are described from the sera of patients with several AI (SLE; Shuster, et al., 1992; Buneva et al., 1994; Andrievskaya et al., 2000, 2002; Vlassov et al., 1998), Hashimoto's thyroiditis and polyarthritis (Vlasov et al., 1998), multiple sclerosis (MS) (Baranovskii et., 1998, 2001; Nevinsky et al., 2001), asthma (Galvita et al., 2007), and viral and bacterial diseases: viral hepatitis (Baranovskii et al., 1997; Vlasov et al., 1999), tick bone encephalitis (TBE; Parkhomenko et al., 2010), AIDS (Odintsova et al., 2006[a]), and several diseases caused by different bacterial infections (Parkhomenko et al., 2009). It was shown, that like in the case of AI-patients, IgGs with DNase activity from autoimmune mice are the earliest and statistically significant markers of pathology and these activities are detectable at the pre-disease stage, when there are no visible markers of SLE pathology or significant proteinuria, and anti-DNA titres are within the typical ranges of these indicators for healthy mice (Dubrovskaya et al., 2003; Andryushkova et al., 2007; Kuznetsova et al., 2007).

Using different approaches convincing evidence was provided that, similarly to Abzs from SLE and MS patients (Savel'ev et al., 2003; Ivanen et al., 2002, 2004), amylase activity is intrinsic to autoimmune mouse polyclonal IgGs (Andryushkova et al., 2006, 2007). It was shown that the relative activities of IgGs from MRL-lpr/lpr mice in the hydrolysis of DNA, ATP, and polysaccharides correlate very well with some visible (pink spots, baldness of the head and parts of the back, general health deterioration, etc.) and biochemical (proteinuria, Ab titers to native and denatured DNA) markers of AI pathologies during various stages of mouse SLE (Andryushkova et al., 2006, 2007, 2009). Similarly to Abzs with DNase and RNase activities, catalytic Abs with polysaccharide-hydrolysing activity can be Abs directly against polysaccharides and their complexes with proteins and enzymes and second antiidiotypic Igs against different enzymes hydrolyzing polysaccharides (Andryushkova et al., 2006, 2007, 2009; Nevinsky et al., 2005, 2010[a], 2010[b]).

IgGs and/or IgMs and IgAs hydrolyzing different peptides and proteins were also found in AI and other diseases: vasoactive intestinal peptide (VIP) in asthma (Paul et al., 1989), thyroglobulin in HT and rheumatoid arthritis (Li et al., 1995; Kalaga et al., 1995), prothrombin in multiple myeloma (Thiagarajan et al., 2000), protein factor VIII in haemophilia A (Lacroix-Desmazes et al., 1999), and myelin basic protein (MBP) in MS (Polosukhina et al., 2004, 2005, 2006, 2006; Legostaeva et al., 2010). Some healthy humans produce Abzs with low VIP- (Paul et al., 1989), and thyroglobulin-hydrolyzing activities (Kalaga et al., 1995), but usually healthy volunteers and patients with many diseases with insignificant autoimmune reactions lack Abzs with proteolytic activity (Nevinsky et al., 2002[a], 2002[b], 2003, 2005, 2010[a], 2010[b], and refs therein). Since immunization of AI mice results in a dramatically higher incidence of Abzs with a higher activity than in conventionally used normal mouse strains (Tawfik et al., 2002; Nishi, 2002), the formation of Abzs in AI and some viral diseases may be much more profuse. The question is why autoimmunization of AI patients and mice results in a dramatically higher incidence of catalytically inactive Abs and Abzs with enzyme properties as compared with healthy humans and animals.

MRL-lpr/lpr mice spontaneously developing a SLE-like disorder are a very promising model to study the mechanisms of natural Abzs generation and their role in the pathogenesis of pronounced AI disturbances. A mutation in the *lpr* gene of these mice leads to a deficit in functional Fas ligand and dysregulation of apoptosis in homozygotes (Watanabe-Fukunada et al., 1992; Nagata & Suda, 1995). As a result, the mice develop SLE-like phenotype, including accumulation of double-negative T cells ($CD4^-$ $CD8^-$ $B220^+$ TCR^+) in the peripheral lymphoid organs.

Recently we have carried out the first analysis of possible correlations between the relative activities (RAs) of mouse IgGs in the hydrolysis of DNA, ATP, and polysaccharides with several clinical and biochemical markers of AI pathologies (proteinuria, Ab titers to native and denatured DNA) at various stages of mouse SLE (Andryushkova et al., 2006, 2007, 2009). An ever-growing number of observations suggested that AI diseases may originate from defects in hematopoietic stem cells (Ikehara et al., 1990). Therefore, lymphocyte proliferation and apoptosis at different stages of the AI disorder development in MRL-lpr/lpr mice were also studied. It was shown that IgGs from the sera of 2-7 month-old control non-autoimmune (CBAxC57BL)F1 and BALB/c mice and 2-3 months-old MRL-lpr/lpr mice (conditionally healthy mice) are catalytically inactive (Andryushkova et al., 2006, 2007, 2009). During spontaneous development of deep SLE-like pathology a specific reorganization of immune system of these mice leads to conditions associated with a production of IgGs hydrolyzing DNA, ATP, and polysaccharides with low catalytic activities (conditionally pre-diseased mice) (Andryushkova et al., 2006, 2007, 2009). First significant changes in differentiation and proliferation of mice bone marrow hematopoietic stem cells (HSC; granulocytic-macrophagic colony-forming unit; erythroid burst-forming unit, and granulocytic-erythroid-megacaryocytic-macrophagic colony-forming unit) in pre-diseased in comparison with healthy mice are most likely only temporary, since a transition from the pre-diseased to diseased mice is associated not only with an increase in the RAs of different Abzs and proteinuria, but also with a significant additional change in the profile of HSC differentiation. This change seems to be the most important factor in the irreversible switching of the mouse immune system to an AI mode, since the changes in cell proliferation and apoptosis in different organs occur mainly on transition from healthy to pre-diseased mice and the observed differences in these indices between pre-diseased and diseased mice are insignificant (Andryushkova et al., 2006, 2007, 2009). Immunization of healthy young AI mice leads to the highest increase in urine protein, titers of anti-DNA Abs as well as DNase, amylase and ATPase Abz activities, occurring in parallel with a significant decrease in apoptosis, especially in bone marrow, thymus and spleen. However, the profile of HSC differentiation in immunized mice is quite different from the pre-diseased and spontaneously diseased mice, but comparable with that for young healthy animals. It was shown, that in contrast to spontaneously diseased AI mice, immunization with DNA does not remarkably affect bone marrow stem cells; the increased levels of anti-DNA Abs and Abzs in immunized mice may be mainly provided by an activation of lymphocyte differentiation and proliferation in different organs, first of all in the spleen, with a concomitant decrease in apoptosis. A significant decrease in apoptosis in the immunized mice may be an important factor providing the increased number of specific lymphocytes producing auto-Abs and Abzs, which are normally eliminated. Very high urine protein concentration and visible markers of SLE demonstrated by the immunized mice may be a result of kidney and spleen dysfunction (Andryushkova et al., 2006, 2007, 2009). Overall, in contrast to immunization of healthy mice an appearance of Abzs and increase in their activity is associated with changes in differentiation and proliferation of mice bone marrow HSC. At the onset of AI diseases (pre-disease condition), Abs are usually contain catalytic Abzs produced by a single clone, or at least a relatively narrow repertoire of Abzs with relatively low relative activities. In the course of chronic AI pathology development, the repertoire of Abzs constantly widens and Abs with significantly higher RAs can be found. In addition, the number of Abzs with high RAs usually increases during exacerbation of AI pathologies (Nevinsky et al., 2003, 2005, 2010[a], 2010[b], and refs therein). It should be mentioned, that the detection of Abzs was shown to be the earliest and statistically significant indicator of development of different autoimmune diseases in humans (Nevinsky et al., 2003, 2005, 2010[a], 2010[b], and refs therein) and animals (Andryushkova et al., 2006, 2007, 2009).

4. Catalytic antibodies of HIV-infected patients

4.1 Purification of natural abzymes

Natural Abzs from sera of patients are usually polyclonal in origin and are products of different immuno-competent cells (Nevinsky et al., 2000[b], 2002[a], 2002[b], 2003, 2005, 2010[a], 2010[b], and refs therein). Natural Abz purification is one of the most complicated aspects of their study; it was discussed in detail in review (Nevinsky et al., 2000[b]).

In study Abzs from the sera of HIV-infected patients, electrophoretically and immunologically homogeneous AIDS Ab fraction (pIgG+pIgM+pIgA) was first purified by chromatography of the serum proteins on Protein A-Sepharose under conditions that remove non-specifically bound proteins (Odintsova et al., 2006[a], 2006[b]; Baranova et al., 2009, 2010). pIgMs were separated from pIgAs and pIgGs by FPLC gel filtration of the total Ab fraction on a Superdex 200 (Baranova et al., 2009, 2010). The homogeneity of the 150 kDa IgG was confirmed by SDS-PAGE with silver staining, which showed a single band under nonreducing conditions and two bands corresponding to the H and L chains after reduction

(Fig. 1). Since IgM has a very high molecular mass (~970 kDa), it cannot enter SDS-PAGE gels under nonreducing conditions (Fig. 1A, lane 2). Two bands corresponding to the H and L chains of pIgMs were evident after Ab reduction (Fig. 1B, lane 1). The absence of any protein bands in the gel corresponding to pIgMs under nonreducing conditions (Fig. 1A, lane 2) and the presence of only two bands corresponding to the heavy and light chains under reducing conditions (Fig. 1B, lane 1) demonstrates the absence of protein contaminations in the pIgM preparations.

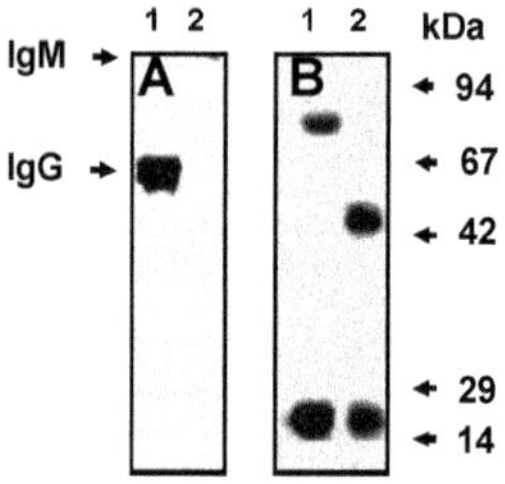

Fig. 1. SDS-PAGE in a nonreducing 4–15% gradient gel followed by silver staining of control pIgGs (lane 1) and pIgMs (lane 2) after affinity chromatography on protein A-Sepharose and FPLC gel filtration on a Superdex 200 column (A). SDS-PAGE of pIgGs (lane 2) and pIgMs (lane 1) in a reducing 12% gel (B).

4.2 Criteria to establish that catalytic activity is intrinsic to antibodies

The application of rigid criteria allowed the authors of the first article concerning natural Abzs (Paul et al., 1989) to conclude that VIP-hydrolyzing activity is an intrinsic property of Abs from the sera of patients with asthma. Later several additional criteria were proposed (for review see Nevinsky et al., 2000[a], 2002[a], 2002[b], 2003, 2005).

It was shown that non-fractionated on affinity sorbents bearing immobilized DNA or specific protein substrates, pIgGs and pIgMs from HIV infected patients effectively hydrolyze DNA (Odintsova et. al., 2006[a]), HIV-1 RT, human casein, human serum albumin (HAS; Odintsova et. al., 2006[b]), and HIV-1 IN (Baranova et. al., 2009, 2010) but not many other tested proteins. We applied a set of strict criteria worked out previously (Paul et al., 1989, Nevinsky et al., 2000[a], 2002[a]) for an analysis of DNase and proteolytic activity as an intrinsic property of AIDS IgGs and/or IgMs. The most important of these are: i) electrophoretic homogeneity of pIgGs and pIgMs (Fig. 1); ii) the complete absorption of AIDS IgGs and IgMs with the DNase or proteolytic activities by Sepharose bearing immobilized anti-light chain of human Abs leading to a disappearance of the activity from the solution and recover following its elution with an acidic buffer (pH 2.6), iii) FPLC gel filtration of IgGs using an acidic buffer (pH 2.6) did not lead to a disappearance of the activity, which tracked exactly with IgGs or IgMs. The fulfilment of these criteria was observed for Abzs with all activities mentioned above (Odintsova et. al., 2006[a], 2006[b]; Baranova et. al., 2009, 2010).

To exclude possible artefacts due to hypothetical traces of contaminating enzymes, pIgGs were subjected to SDS-PAGE in a gel co-polymerized with calf thymus DNA, and their DNase activity was detected by incubating the gel in the standard reaction buffer (Fig. 2). Ethidium bromide staining of the gels after the electrophoresis and refolding of IgGs revealed sharp dark bands against a fluorescent background of DNA. Fig. 2B demonstrates a typical example for AIDS IgGs (lane 1); there was no hydrolysis of DNA by control Abs from healthy donors (lane 2). Control human urine (lane 3) and bovine pancreatic DNase I (lane 4) also cleaved DNA, but produced bands in the position well below (33–36 kDa) the intact pIgGs (150 kDa). Since SDS dissociates all protein complexes, the detection of the DNase activity in the gel zone corresponding only to intact IgGs together with the absence of any other activity band or protein band (Fig. 2B), provides direct evidence that AIDS pIgGs hydrolyze DNA and are not contaminated by canonical DNases. In addition, after incubation of IgGs with DTT only light chains of AIDS IgGs demonstrated DNase activity (Fig. 2C).

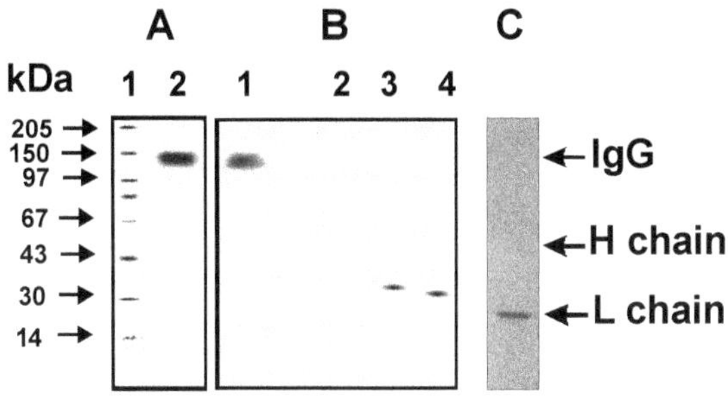

Fig. 2. *In situ* SDS-PAGE analysis of DNase activity of AIDS intact IgGs (lane 1), healthy humans (lane 2) (B); human urine (lane 3) and bovine pancreatic DNase I (lane 4, B) in nonreducing conditions. IgGs were analyzed in reducing conditions after Abs incubation with DTT (C). After electrophoresis, the gel containing 3 μg/ml thymus DNA (B and C) was incubated under special conditions for protein refolding and hydrolysis of nucleic acids; the nuclease activity was visualized by ethidium bromide staining of the gels (B and C). The longitudinal slices of the same gel were used for Coomassie R250 staining to reveal the positions of IgG bands (lane 2, A) and protein molecular mass markers (lane 1, A).

AIDS IgGs and IgMs were separated by SDS-PAGE respectively under nonreducing and reducing conditions and their proteolytic activity was detected after the extraction of proteins from excised gel slices (Baranova et. al., 2009, 2010). The detection of IN-hydrolyzing activity in the gel region corresponding only to IgG, together with the absence of any other bands of the activity or protein, provided direct evidence that IgG possesses IN-hydrolyzing activity. Similar results were obtained for AIDS IgGs hydrolyzing HIV RT, HSA, and human casein (Odintsova et. al., 2006b).

As mentioned above, pIgMs cannot enter the gel. The absence of IN-hydrolyzing activity from all gel zones corresponding to the intact pIgMs under nonreducing conditions (data not shown), together with hydrolysis of IN only with separated heavy and light chains of IgMs under reducing conditions and the absence of any other bands of the activity (Fig. 3) provides a direct evidence that IgM possesses IN-hydrolyzing activity.

It was shown (Odintsova et. al., 2006b), that in contrast to known different nonspecific proteases hydrolyzing many proteins, AIDS pIgGs non-fractionated by affinity chromatography on Sepharoses bearing specific immobilized proteins efficiently hydrolyze only: human casein > HIV-1 RT > HSA but not many other tested proteins. Later it was shown that AIDS IgGs and IgMs also hydrolyze HIV-1 integrase (for example, Fig. 4) (Baranova et. al., 2009, 2010).

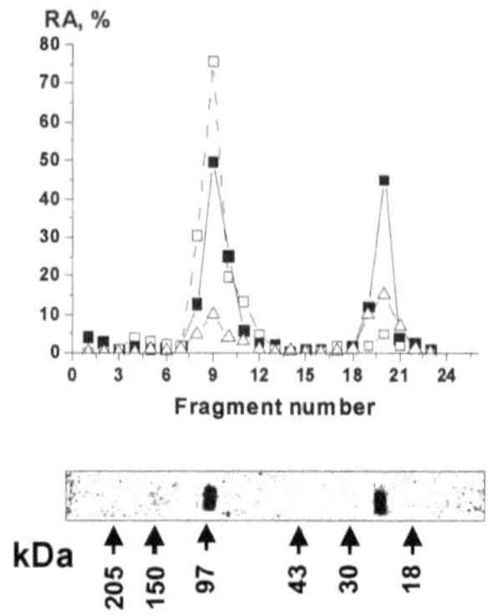

Fig. 3. SDS-PAGE analysis of IN-hydrolyzing activity of AIDS IgMs. After reducing SDS-PAGE of purified AIDS IgMs the gel was incubated under special conditions for renaturation of Abs. The relative IN-hydrolyzing activity (RA, %) was quantified using the extracts of fragments (2-3-mm each) of one longitudinal slice of the gel corresponding to 3 individual IgMs: (■), IgM1; (□), IgM2; (Δ), IgM3.

It was shown that immunogenic VIP (Paul et al., 1989), human MBP (Ponomarenko et al., 2006; Legostaseva at al., 2010), human milk casein (Odintsova et al., 2011), stimulate formation of Abzs which in contrast to canonical proteases efficiently hydrolyze only antigen-proteins, but not many other proteins tested. To analyze the "average" proteolytic activity of AIDS Abzs, two mixtures of equal amounts of electrophoretically homogeneous pIgGs ($pIgG_{mix}$) and pIgMs ($pIgM_{mix}$) with different relatively high and average activities from the sera of seven patients were prepared. After purification of anti-IN Abs on IN-Sepharose these Abzs hydrolyzed only IN and cannot hydrolyze other proteins including viral RT (Fig. 4). In addition, it was shown that AIDS pIgGs and pIgMs after their purification on sorbents bearing immobilized HIV RT (Fig. 4), human casein or HSA specifically hydrolyzed only cognate protein, but not many other proteins including HIV IN

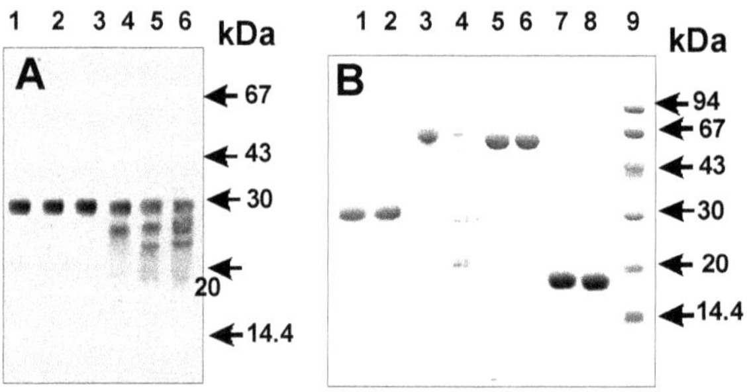

Fig. 4. SDS-PAGE analysis of protein hydrolysis by AIDS IgGs and IgMs. A, HIV-1 IN was incubated for alone (1) or in the presence of pIgGs from two healthy donors (2 and 3) and pIgGs from two different AIDS patients (4 and 5), or with AIDS IgGs purified on IN-Sepharose (6). B, AIDS IgMs purified on RT-Sepharose were incubated with different proteins without (odd numbers) and with Abs (even numbers): HIV-1 IN (1 and 2); p66 HIV RT (3 and 4); HSA (5 and 6); myelin basic protein (7 and 8). Lane 9 corresponds to mixture of standard protein markers with known molecular masses.

(Odintsova et al., 2006[b]). It means that within pools of AIDs pIgGs and pIgMs only specific anti-IN Abzs are able to hydrolyze intact globular molecules of viral integrase (Baranoba et al., 2009, 2010), while specific anti-HSA, anti-casein, and anti-RT IgGs hydrolyze their specific target proteins (Odintsova et. al., 2006[b]).

4.3 Comparison of the relative catalytic activity of Abs from different AIDS patients

Sera of ten healthy donors, 110 HIV-infected patients (18–40-years-old; men and women) including 65 at the stage of pre-AIDS and 45 at the stage of generalized lymphadenopathy (GL) according to the classification of the Center of Disease Control and Prevention were used to analyze the catalytic activities of IgGs and IgMs (Odintsova et al., 2006[a], 2006[b]; Baranova et al., 2009, 2010). Patients with pre-AIDS stage were characterized by a decrease in their body mass up to 10%, fungal, bacterial and viral lesions of skin and mucosal surfaces, shingles, repeating pharyngitis, sinusitis, otitis, and frequent acute respiratory infection.

Polyclonal IgGs from 10 healthy controls were inactive in DNA hydrolysis (Odintsova et al., 2006[a]). Similar results were obtained earlier for several groups of 10-20 healthy humans used as controls in the studies of DNase Abs from the sera of patients with AI diseases (Nevinsky *et al.*, 2003, 2005, 2010[a], 2010[b] and refs therein).The type of plasmid supercoiled (sc) DNA hydrolysis by AIDS pIgGs did not depend on the Ab concentration and the rate of the hydrolysis linearly increased with the increase in IgG concentration and time of incubation (Odintsova et al., 2006[a]). Fig. 5 illustrates a cleavage of plasmid DNA (14 μg/ml) by Abs (0.3 mg/ml) from several AIDS patients after 4 h of incubation. One can see that in this period some Abs cause only single breaks in one strand of supercoiled DNA (lanes 1-3), whereas others cause multiple breaks and as a result the formation of linear DNA (lanes 4-6). The most active Abs hydrolyze DNA into short and medium length ODNs (lanes 7-10). It should be mentioned that Fig. 5 in principle illustrates a range of possible changes of the relative DNase activities for patients with not only AIDS but also with different AI diseases and viral pathologies previously analyzed (Nevinsky *et al.*, 2000[a], 2003, 2005, 2010[a], 2010[b] and refs therein). When passing from one pathology to another only the values of a relative percent of patients with low, middle and high DNase activities is usually changed.

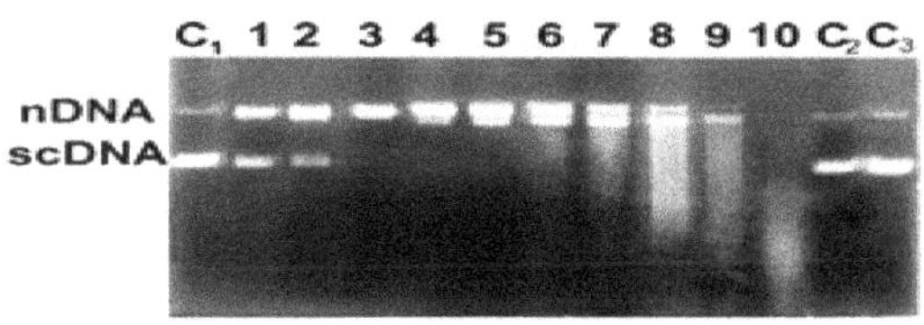

Fig. 5. DNase activities of catalytic AIDS IgGs from different patients in the cleavage of supercoiled (sc) and nicked (n) plasmid DNA (14 μg/ml). Lanes 1–10, IgGs (0.3 mg/ml; incubation for 4 h) from the sera of 10 different patients; C_1, scDNA incubated alone; C_2 and C_3, scDNA incubated with Ab from the sera of two healthy donors.

The efficiency of DNA cleavage was calculated from the increase of DNA in the band of scDNA (10-40 % of initial DNA hydrolysis); the measured RAs (%) for IgGs were normalized to standard conditions (0.1 mg/ml Abs, 2 h) and a complete transition of scDNA to its relaxed form was taken for 100%. While four AIDS IgG preparations were completely inactive, the remaining 106 IgG samples (96 %) demonstrated the RAs from 5 to 100% of scDNA hydrolysis (Table 1).

On the fist step we have analyzed the RAs of proteolytic activity of AIDS pIgGs in the hydrolysis of many different proteins including HIV RT, HSA, and human β-casein (Odintsova et al., 2006[b]). It was shown that among all proteins used, IgGs from different HIV-infected patients with detectable or high rate hydrolyze only HIV-1 reverse transcriptase (RT), human serum albumin (HSA), and human β-casein. Interestingly, the highest rate of the hydrolysis was observed for β-casein (Odintsova et al., 2006[b]). Therefore, the RA of 110 AIDS IgGs in the hydrolysis of casein was analyzed. The efficiency of casein cleavage was analysed by SDS-PAGE and calculated from the decrease in the band of non-hydrolyzed casein taking into account the control reaction incubated in the absence of IgGs.

Relative activity, % of scDNA hydrolysis	Number of IgG preparations with DNase activity**	Number of IgG preparations with casein-hydrolyzing activity***
0	4 (4 %)*	5 (5 %)
5 - 20	21 (19 %)	11 (10 %)
21 - 40	33 (30 %)	24 (21.4 %)
41 - 60	18 (16.4 %)	25 (22.7 %)
61 - 80	7 (6.4 %)	20 (18.2 %)
81 - 100	17 (15.5 %)	25 (22.7 %)
Number of preparations and stage of disease	Average DNase RA	Average protease RA
Generalized lymphadenopathy (45)	40.2 % ± 26.3 %	53.6 % ± 22.6 %
pre-AIDS (65)	44.7 % ± 21.3 %	51.5 % ± 25.9 %

*Percent of total number of patients (110) is given in parenthesis.
**A complete transition of 14 μg/ml scDNA to its relaxed form (0.1 mg/ml IgGs, 2 h) was taken for 100%.
***A complete hydrolysis of 0.1 mg/ml human β-casein (0.1 mg/ml IgGs, 2 h) was taken for 100%.

Table 1. The relative catalytic activities of AIDS IgGs in the hydrolysis of scDNA and β-casein in the case of total group and patients with different stages of diseases development.

Purified pIgGs from ten healthy donors were unable to catalyze casein hydrolysis, whereas 105 of 110 IgGs (95 %) demonstrated high or detectable casein-hydrolyzing activity (Table 1). With the development of the disease at the stage of pre-AIDS, IgGs from some patients demonstrated a high DNase activity (≥80 % of DNA hydrolysis) but the average RA was 44.7 % ± 21.3 % (Table 1). At the stage of generalized lymphadenopathy, IgGs from 4 of 45 patients (8.8 %) did not possess detectable DNase activity. However, the average RA value of DNase activity for this group of patients (40.2 % ± 26.3 %) was comparable with that for the pre-AIDS group. At the same time, the number of IgG preparations with very high activities (≥80 % of DNA hydrolysis) was significantly lower in the GL group. At the GL stage, 5 of 45 (11 %) Abs were completely inactive, while several IgGs demonstrated high RA in the hydrolysis of casein (up to 86.7%); the average RA for all 45 patients was 53.6 % ± 22.6 % (Table 1). All 65 IgGs from patients with pre-AIDS were catalytically active, but the average RA (51.5 % ± 25.9 %) was comparable with that for IgGs from patients with GL (Table 1). Each group of patients corresponding to GL and pre-AIDS stage was divided into two subgroups with either rapid or slow progression of the disease. According to the recommendations of the Center of Disease Control and Prevention, the transition time from GL to pre-AIDS stage (≤ 2 and > 2 years, respectively) was used as the measure of the disease rate of progression. The number of GL patients demonstrating a detectable proteolytic activity was comparable in the case of rapid (41.7 %) and slow (47.8%) progression, while DNase activity was observed in 41.3 % of the patients with rapid progression and only in 29.5% of the patients with slow progression. In the pre-AIDS group, the number of IgGs with DNase and proteolytic activity was slightly higher in patients with rapid progression (55.8 and 58.1 %, respectively) than in patients with slow (50.7 and 51.8 %) progression of the disease.

On first glance, high activity of IgGs from the blood of AIDS patients in hydrolysis of β-casein (which is not a typical component of human blood) is unexpected. However, it was recently shown by 2D electrophoresis that six of nine sera from AIDS patients contained Abs against casein, and five against human milk lactalbumin (Goldfarb, 2001). Thereby, the activation of β-casein synthesis in AIDS patients driven by not yet understood factor can not be excluded. It is interesting that mRNA corresponding to the gene encoding for β-casein is produced in mouse T-killer cells (also for unknown reason) (Grusby et al., 1990). In this way, it can not be excluded that genes, encoding for β-casein, as well as this protein itself, can play a special (but not yet known) role in the HIV virus life cycle, its replication, or development of AI reactions in AIDS patients.

At the same time, so far Abzs hydrolyzing HSA were found only in AIDS patients. A possible reason of production of HSA-hydrolyzing Abs in AIDS patients is also not known.

Later the RAs of AIDS IgGs (Baranova et al., 2009) and IgMs (Baranova et al., 2010) in the hydrolysis of IN were analyzed. Sera of 19 HIV-infected patients (18-40 yr old; men and women) including 13 at the stage of pre-AIDS and 6 at the stage of GL were used to study IN-hydrolyzing activity of IgGs, while 18 Ab preparations corresponding to pre-AIDS stage and 8 preparations to GL were used to analyze RAs of IgMs.

pIgGs and pIgMs from ten control healthy donors were unable to catalyze IN hydrolysis. Interestingly, 11 of 13 IgGs from patients with pre-AIDS (84.6 %) and 6 of 6 (100 %) with GL demonstrated detectable of high IN-hydrolyzing activity (Baranova et al., 2009). There was no statistically significant difference in the IgG RAs between the two groups of patients; average values of IgG IN-hydrolyzing RAs were 1.99 ± 1.68 for pre-AIDS and 3.4 ± 1.31 (μM IN/1h)/mg of Abs for GL patients. All 16 IgMs purified from patients with pre-AIDS (100%) and 6 of 8 IgMs (75%) from patients with GL demonstrated high or detectable IN-hydrolyzing activity (Baranova et al., 2010). There was no statistically significant difference ($p = 0.71$) in the IgM RAs between the two groups of patients; the average values of IgM IN-hydrolyzing RAs were 3.8 ± 2.2 μM IN per hour per mg of Abs (range 0.3–7.3 μM IN per hour per mg of Abs) for pre-AIDS and 3.3 ± 2.6 μM IN per hour per mg of Abs (range 0–8.1 μM IN per hour per mg of Abs) for GL.

Overall, in the case of Abs with DNase, casein-, and IN-hydrolyzing activity we have found only a negligible difference in the RAs of Abs from HIV-infected patients at the GL and pre-AIDS stages. However, it is not surprising and agrees with the published data that a detection of Abzs is the earliest indicator of the development of many AI diseases in humans and animals (Andryushkova et al., 2006, 2007, 2009; Nevinsky et al., 2005, 2010[a], 2010[b], and refs therein). According to our data, various catalytic activities of Abzs are usually very easily detectable at the onset of AI diseases when the total concentrations of non-catalytic

Abs to specific auto-antigens have not yet increased significantly and correspond to their ranges for healthy donors. At the early stages of AI diseases, the repertoire of Abzs is usually relatively small but it greatly increases with the progress of the disease, leading to the generation of catalytically diverse abzymes with different activities and functions (Nevinsky *et al.*, 2003, 2005, 2010[a], 2010[b] and refs therein). In addition, AI reactions in the case of some viral diseases including AIDS patients are in some extent similar to AI diseases. At the same time, immunization of AI mice produces an unexpectedly high increase in the number of clones secreting various auto-Abs, including Abzs, in comparison with normal mice (Nishi, 2002; Tawfik et al., 2002).

HIV-1 RT- and IN-hydrolzying pIgGs and IgMs from HIV-infected patients were the first examples of catalytic Abzs produced in humans against viral proteins after a viral infection (Odintsova et al., 2006[b]; Baranova et al., 2009, 2010). In addition, it was shown for the first time that HIV infection stimulates autoimmune reactions leading to the formation of Abzs that hydrolyze at least two human proteins, HSA and casein. It is known that HIV infection stimulates the development of many AI diseases (Zandman-Goddard et al., 2002). One can suppose that in some other viral and bacterial infections may induce similar processes to some extent.

During many infections, the human organism is exposed to different bacterial components including protein, DNA, RNA, and polysaccharides (Ternynck et al., 1991; Unterkircher et al., 1993; Matsiota-Bernard et al., 1993, 1996; Hentati et al., 1994; Boekel et al., 1997; Wun et al., 2001). Because of their ability to bind a variety of exogenous antigens, including bacterial and viral ones, natural Abs play a major role in the primary line of defense against infections. Some results suggest that the synthesis of auto-Abs and Abs directed against bacterial antigens at least partially follow distinct pathways, but with the existing experimental data it is impossible to determine unambiguously whether these two Ab populations are produced by the same or distinct B-cell subpopulations (Matsiota-Bernard et al., 1993). Recently, DNase activity in the patients with diseases caused by several bacterial infections has been analyzed (Parkhomenko et al., 2008). The catalytic activities were significantly lower than in patients with different AI pathologies and increased in the following order: streptococcal infection (erysipelas) < urogenital chlamydiosis associated with arthritis (Reiter's disease) < meningococcal meningitis < shigellosis < suppurative surgical infections caused by *Staphylococcus aureus* < suppurative surgical infections caused by epidermal staphylococci < urogenital ureaplasmosis associated with reactive arthritis.

In addition, DNA-hydrolyzing IgGs was found in the sera of patients with hepatitis (Baranovskii et al., 1997) and tick bone encephalitis (Parkhomenko et al., 2010-11). Interestingly, TBE like HIV infection of humans stimulate formation of Abzs with several proteolytic activities (Parkhomenko T., personal communication). The RAs of IgGs in the hydrolysis of DNA increased in the following order: diabetes ≤ bacterial infections ≤ viral hepatitis < polyarthritis < Hashimoto's thyroiditis < AIDS ≤ MS < SLE (Nevinsky *et al.*, 2003, 2005, 2010[a], 2010[b] and refs therein).

Taking these observations together, we suggest that the specific activity of polyclonal Abs from the sera of patients with diseases caused by bacterial infections are usually lower than those for typical AI diseases and most probably they can differ in their biological functions. It was shown that the specific reorganization of immune system during the spontaneous development of a profound SLE-like pathology in MRL-lpr/lpr mice is associated with changes in the differentiation profile and the level of proliferation of bone marrow hematopoietic stem cells and with production of DNase, ATPase, and amylase Abzs

(Andryushkova et al., 2006, 2007, 2009). Immunization of healthy mice with DNA also leads to production of DNase Abzs; however, it is associated only with increased lymphocyte proliferation and suppression of apoptosis of lymphocytes in different organs (especially spleen), but not with a change in differentiation of the bone marrow cells. Immune processes after immunization of mammals with bacterial DNA, proteins, polysaccharides during many infectious diseases may be considered similar to those after immunization of healthy mice with DNA, different proteins and enzymes. According to theoretical analysis, the adaptive improvement of the catalytic turnover is limited by the rate of B cell receptor signal transduction, as rapid release of antigen fragments from catalytic B cell receptors aborts clonal selection, but production of catalysts can occur at increased levels under conditions of rapid B cell signaling in AI disease (Paul et al., 2006). In addition, the RAs of DNase Abs increased with the progress of the AI pathology, while the time course of immunization associated with some infections is usually not so long as compared with AI diseases, which can have chronic character. In contrast to AI diseases, treatment and recovery of patients with bacterial infections usually eliminates Abzs with various activities. In addition, Abzs may have protective functions in patients with bacterial infections. It was shown that the presence of IgG endowed with serine protease-like activity in the plasma of patients with sepsis strongly correlates with their survival (Lacroix-Desmazes et al., 2005).

In contrast to DNase abzymes, the polysaccharide-hydrolyzing Abs are usually present even in the sera of healthy humans and their activity remarkably increases in the sera of patients and animals with different AI diseases (Andryushkova et al., 2006; 2007) and especially with pathologies caused by viral infections (Buneva V.N., personal communication). Formation of specific Abs against DNA and other components of bacteria and some viruses during infections of healthy mammals suggests that the specific catalytic Abs can mostly hydrolyze these bacterial and viral components.

It is possible that co-action of Abzs with proteolytic and polysaccharide-hydrolyzing activities can at least partially degrade bacterial cell walls and viral particles and facilitate the entry of Abzs into the bacterial cells and hydrolysis of bacterial DNA, proteins and other components. This cooperative action of abzymes with different catalytic activities may have a protective effect against diseases caused by bacterial and viral infections. At the same time, in contrast to many viral and bacterial infections, HIV-infection stimulates AI reactions. Therefore, at the first stage of AIDS development catalytic Abzs against different viral components can protect humans, similarly to the situation in bacterial and viral infections that do not stimulate AI reactions. Later, due to molecular mimicry between viral and host antigens, viral antigens can affect hematopoietic stem cells and trigger the development of AI processes.

5. Extreme diversity of AIDS abzymes

5.1 Structural diversity of AIDS abzymes

DNase, RNase, ATPase, amylase, and protease Abzs may show very different contributions of variable domains of H- and L-chains to their active centers. Chromatographically separated light chains of IgGs from the sera of asthma patients were found to be active in the hydrolysis of VIP (Sun et al., 1994; 1997). The light chain of the VIP Abz was expressed in bacteria, purified, and found to possess an intrinsic catalytic activity (Tyutyulkova et al., 1996). The Abz-dependent hydrolysis of DNA and RNA by isolated light chains of IgGs from SLE, MS, asthma, and other AI patients, as well as from MRL-lpr/lpr mice, is more efficient than by intact Abs (Dubrovskaya et al., 2003; Galvita et al., 2007; Andrievskaya et al., 2000, 2002; Baranovskii et al., 2001; Nevinsky et al., 2005, 2010[a], 2010[b]). A similar situation was observed for human milk IgGs and sIgAs with DNase and RNase activities (Kanyshkova et al., 1997; Nevinsky et al., 2000[a]). In addition, both H and L-chains of sIgAs had affinity to DNA-cellulose but only L-subunits hydrolyzed DNA and RNA (Nevinsky et al., 2000[c]). At the same time, it was demonstrated that the catalytic center of recombinant variable fragment (scFv) of DNase IgGs from AI-prone MRL-lpr/lpr mice may be located at the interface between the light and heavy chains and that after separation both of these chains are able to hydrolyze DNA (Kim et al., 2006).

It was shown that only separated light chains of AIDS IgGs hydrolyze DNA, while heavy chains is catalytically inactive (Odintsova et al., 2006[a]). On the contrary, both light and heavy chains of mouse IgGs after separation were active in the ATP hydrolysis (Andryushkova et al., 2009). Intact rat pIgGs and their separated H- and L-chains possess both peroxidase and oxidoreductase catalytic activity (Nevinsky et al., 2010[a]). The observed IN-hydrolyzing activity of AIDS pIgM L- and H-chains separated by SDS-PAGE (Fig. 3) may have different underlying causes. First, it is possible that these pIgMs contain a mixture of Abzs with only light or only heavy chains being catalytically active. However, similarly to mouse monoclonal DNase (Kim et al., 2006), catalytic centers of AIDS IgMs hydrolyzing IN may be located at the interface between the light and heavy chains, with both separated chains capable of hydrolysis of IN.

From the crystal structure of a catalytic Ab with esterase-like activity, it was concluded that the ligand *p*-nitrophenyl acetate interacts with amino acid residues of both light and heavy chains of Abzs and that both types of subunits are required for catalysis (Golinelli-Pimpaneau et al., 1994). Taken together, it is obvious that light and heavy chains of different Abzs including AIDS Abs can contribute to the active sites of Abzs in different ways.

The next question concerning the structural diversity of AIDS Abzs relates to the type of the proteolytic activity of their catalytic sites. Proteolytic IgGs from the sera of patients with asthma hydrolyzing VIP (Paul et al., 1989), Hashimoto thyroiditis and rheumatoid arthritis hydrolyzing thyroglobulin (Li eta l., 1995; Kalaga et al., 1995) are serine-like proteases, and their activity is most strongly reduced after incubation with specific serine protease inhibitors PMSF or AEBSF. It was shown that casein-hydrolyzing sIgAs from human milk (Odintsova et al., 2006; 2011) and hMBP-hydrolyzing IgGs and IgMs from the sera of patients with MS (Polosukhina et al., 2004, 2005, 2006) contain not only Ab subfractions with serine-like, but also specific subfractions with metal-dependent activity.

We have analyzed the type of proteolytic activity of AIDS pIgGs and pIgMs in the hydrolysis of IN and β-casein. It was shown, that in contrast to milk sIgAs (Odintsova et al., 2006; 2011) and similarly to several other proteolytic Abzs, only specific inhibitor of serine protease AEBSF significantly suppress AIDS pIgG-dependent hydrolysis of β-casein, while EDTA has no significant effect.

We have analyzed the type of IN-hydrolyzing activity of ten AIDS pIgGs; several typical examples are given in Fig. 6 (Baranova et al., 2009). Leupeptin, an inhibitor of many different proteases, demonstrated significant inhibition of proteolytic activity of only 2 of 10 individual AIDS IgGs (Table 2). A similar situation was observed for a specific inhibitor of acidic proteases, pepstatin A, which significantly inhibited IN-hydrolyzing activity of only two IgGs. Surprisingly, a significant inhibition of serine protease-like activity was also found only for 2 of 10 AIDS IgGs (Table 2). Proteolytic activity of five of ten AIDS IgGs was inhibited by 40-96 % after incubating the IgGs with EDTA. An incubation of IgGs with iodoacetamide (a specific inhibitor of thiol proteases) usually has no remarkable effect on their proteolytic activity (Paul et al., 1989; Li et al., 1995; Kalaga et al., 1995; Odintsova et al., 2006; 2011; Polosukhina et al., 2004, 2005, 2006). Surprisingly, however, IN-hydrolyzing activity of all 10 IgGs was inhibited by iodoacetamide by 12-98 % (Baranova et al., 2009).

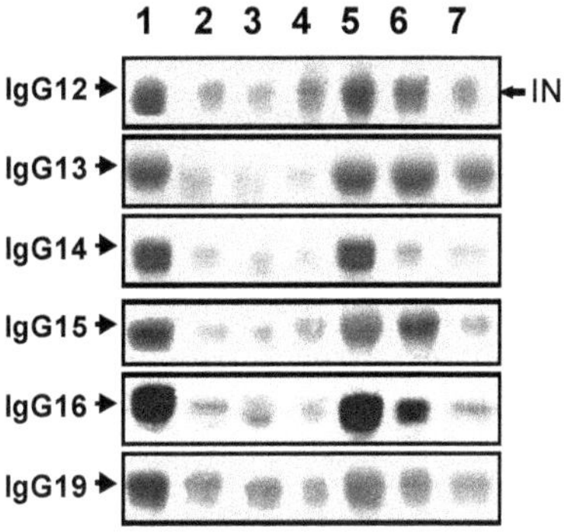

Fig. 6. SDS-PAGE analysis of a decrease in the intensity of protein band after its incubation with pIgGs from AIDS patients in different conditions. IN was incubated alone (1); in the presence of AIDS pIgGs from the sera of six different AIDS patients (IgG-12 - IgG19) and in the absence of other components (2) or in the presence of AEBSF (3), leupeptin (4), iodoacetamide (5), EDTA (6), and pepstatin A (lane 7). Arrows indicate the positions of molecular mass markers.

Similar surprising situation was observed for ten AIDS pIgMs with IN-hydrolyzing activity (Table 2) (Baranova et al., 2010). Leupeptin, significantly inhibited the proteolytic activity of only two of ten individual AIDS IgMs, and very weak inhibition was observed for one more preparation (Table 2). A specific inhibitor of acidic proteases, pepstatin A, significantly inhibited the IN-hydrolyzing activity of only three pIgMs and demonstrated weak inhibition of two preparations (Table 2). Surprisingly, a significant inhibition of serine protease-like activity by AEBSF was found only for two and weak suppression of the activity for another of ten AIDS IgMs. Proteolytic activity of five of ten AIDS IgMs was inhibited by 33–91% after incubating the IgMs with 0.01 M EDTA, while this chelating reagent at 0.1 M concentration decreased the relative activity of six preparations by 64–98% and inhibited three more preparations for ~8-10% (Table 2). As for AIDS IgGs, iodoacetamide inhibited the IN-hydrolyzing activity of all ten of ten Abs by 30–99% (Table 2). The inhibition of AIDS IgGs and IgMs with EDTA was comparable with that for IgGs from patients with MS (Polosukhina et al., 2004, 2005, 2006).

Iodoacetamide, a specific inhibitor of thiol proteases, usually does not significantly affect the activity of proteolytic Abzs (≤ 3–7% inhibition) (see above). Therefore, it was surprising that the IN-hydrolyzing activity of AIDS IgGs was suppressed by iodoacetamide in all 100% preparations by 12–98% (average value 65.7 ± 20.6%) in a stark contrast with other known proteolytic Abzs. A similar result was observed for AIDS IgMs; iodoacetamide suppressed the IN-hydrolyzing activity by 30–99% (average value 75.6 ± 21.2%) in all ten Ab preparations. Interestingly, there was no statistically significant difference in the inhibition of AIDS pIgGs and pIgMs by iodoacetamide ($p = 0.2$). Our findings support the idea that the pools of pIgGs and IgMs of AIDS patients can contain IN-hydrolyzing Abzs of four types

Number of prep.	Inhibition, %*					
	AEBSF	Leupeptin	Pepstatin A	Iodoacetamide	0.1 M EDTA	Sum of effects**
IgG9	42±5	74±8	51±5	85±9	0	252
IgG10	0	70±7	0	83±9	96±9	249
IgG11	0	0	0	66±7	0	66
IgG12	0	0	0	66±5	44±5	110
IgG13	0	0	59±6	98±8	98±8	255
IgG14	0	0	0	87±7	3±1	90
IgG15	0	11±3	0	33±4	45±4	89
IgG16	0	0	0	78±8	40±3	118
IgG17	49±5	0	0	12±1.5	0	61
IgG19	0	0	0	49±5	2±1	51
IgM4	0	0	48 ± 5	97 ± 8	98 ± 2	243
IgM5	0	47 ± 5	36 ± 5	36 ± 5	80 ± 7	199
IgM7	8 ± 1	68 ± 7	0	95 ± 9	94 ± 8	265
IgM8	0	0	7 ± 2	99 ± 8	8 ± 2	114
IgM9	0	0	0	76 ± 6	0	76
IgM10	0	0	0	83 ± 7	93 ± 8	176
IgM11	0	0	0	94 ± 7	8 ± 3	102
IgM12	0	7 ± 1	0	55 ± 5	98 ± 8	153
IgM13	46 ± 5	0	88 ± 9	91 ± 10	64 ± 4	289
IgM23	80 ± 8	0	5 ± 2	30± 5	10 ± 2	125

**The decrease in the intensity of initial IN band estimated from SDS-PAGE electrophoresis data in the absence of inhibitor was taken for 100 %, for each preparation, a mean of 3 repeats are used.
**Sum of the effects of different compounds on the proteolytic activity (leupeptin+Pepstatin+iodoacetamide + EDTA).

Table 2. Inhibition of proteolytic activity of individual IgGs and IgMs (from 10 AIDS patients) in the hydrolysis of HIV integrase by specific inhibitors of proteases of different types

resembling thiol, serine, acidic, and metal-dependent proteases, the ratio of which may be individual for every HIV-infected patient.

Interestingly, only IgM9 and three of IgGs (IgG11, IgG14, and IgG19) demonstrated significant inhibition by one inhibitor (iodoacetamide). At the same time other IgG and IgM preparations were sensitive to two or three inhibitors (Table 2). For example, IgM10 and IgM11 was strongly suppressed by iodoacetamide and EDTA; IgM23 was sensitive to AEBSF and iodoacetamide; IgM4 and IgM8 showed strong or at least some inhibition of the activity by three inhibitors (iodoacetamide, EDTA, and pepstatin A), while IgM12 was sensitive to leupeptin instead of pepstatin A (Table 2). Surprisingly, three of ten preparations (IgM5, IgM7, and IgM13) could be significantly inhibited by four different inhibitors. Of these, iodoacetamide and EDTA were common inhibitors for all three IgM preparations, while two other inhibitors were different: pepstatin A and leupeptin for IgM5, leupeptin and AEBSF for IgM7, and pepstatin A and AEBSF for IgM13 (Table 2). Very comparable situations were observed for AIDS IgGs and IgMs (Table 2).

In principle it is possible that the pools of IgGs and IgMs from AIDS patients may be "cocktails" of Abz molecules, with each molecule possessing only one of four alternative types of proteolytic activity: serine-, acidic-, thiol-, or metal-dependent. Yet the effects of two, three, and four inhibitors of different protease types did not always add to 100% inhibition. Only in three of ten IgM preparations (IgM8, IgM9, and IgM11) this sum was less or comparable with 100% (76–114%), while for other seven IgMs it varied from 125% to 289% (Table 2). Three IgG preparations (IgG9, IgG10, and IgG13) demonstrated this sum from 249 to 255 % (Table 2). Since IgM9 had only thiol protease-like activity, and IgM8 and IgM11 could be significantly suppressed (94-99%) only with iodoacetamide but lost their activity only marginally in the presence of EDTA or pepstatin A (by 7–8 %), it is most likely that in these patients most of the Abz molecules possess only the thiol protease type of proteolytic activity (Table 2). However, since the proteolytic activity in seven of ten IgMs and five of ten IgGs was summarily suppressed by specific inhibitors of serine, acidic, metal-dependent, and thiol proteases by more than 100% (110–289%, Table 2), it is possible that the immune system of HIV-infected patients produces anti-IN Abzs with a combined structure of the active center, carrying amino acid residues typical of different proteases. For example, we suggest that the pools of IgM4, IgM7, and IgM13 (209–289% of the summarized inhibition) contain IgM molecules with extremely complicated active centers containing structural elements of thiol and metal-dependent proteases, which may be additionally combined with structural elements of the active centers of acidic proteases (IgM4), serine proteases (IgM7), or both (IgM13). Similar suggestion is reason in the case of several AIDS IgGs (Table 2) (Baranova et al., 2009, 2010).

5.2 pH optima diversity of AIDS abzymes

Theoretically, a mammalian immune system can produce up to 10^6 variants of Abs against one antigen. An extreme diversity of RNase and DNase IgG and/or IgM Abzs from the sera of patients with MS and SLE and autoimmune prone MRL-lpr/lpr mice was observed (Baranovskii *et al.*, 1998, 2001; Andrievskaya *et al.*, 2000, 2002; Kuznetsova *et al.*, 2007; Nevinsky *et al.*, 2003, 2005, 2010[a], 2010[b]). It was shown that different patients (and animals) may have a relatively small or an extremely large pool of polyclonal nuclease Abzs containing different relative amounts of light chains of κ- and λ-types, demonstrating maximal activity at various optimal pHs, having a different net charge, activated or not by different metal ions, characterized by different substrate specificities. MS IgGs of all four subclasses (IgG1-IgG4) were catalytically active in the hydrolysis of hMBP (Legostaeva *et al.*, 2010) and DNA (Parkhomenko *et al.*, 2010).

We have analyzed the pH dependencies of the initial rates of DNA hydrolysis by AIDS catalytic IgGs (Odintsova et al., 2006[a]). Fig. 7A demonstrates three pH dependencies of different types which were revealed for catalytic pIgGs from the sera of 3 different patients. In contrast to all human DNases having one pronounced pH optimum in hydrolysis of DNA (Baranovskii et al., 2004), catalytic Abs usually show high DNase activity at a wide range of pH values between 5.5-9.0. Nevertheless, as one can see from Fig. 7A, one of the IgG preparations has a pronounced optimum at pH 8.0; second at pH 7.5, while third one demonstrates two marked pH optima at pH 7.5 and 8.5.

We have analyzed the pH dependencies of the initial rates of human casein hydrolysis by four individual AIDS IgGs. In contrast to all human proteases having one pronounced pH optimum (Horl et al., 1987; Rao et al., 1998), catalytic AIDS IgGs demonstrated high specific casein-hydrolyzing activity within a wide range of pH values (5.0–9.0) and the pH profile for each IgG was unique (Fig. 7B) (Odintsova et al., 2006).

It is well known that canonical mammalian, bacterial, and plant proteases, depending on their biological function, can have optimal pH values ranging from acidic (2.0) to neutral and alkaline (8-10) (Horl et al., 1987; Rao et al., 1998). We have measured the relative activity of AIDS IgGs and IgMs at pH from 3.0 to 10.5. In contrast to all human proteases, catalytic IgGs demonstrated high specific IN-hydrolyzing activity within a wide range of pH values (3.0–10).

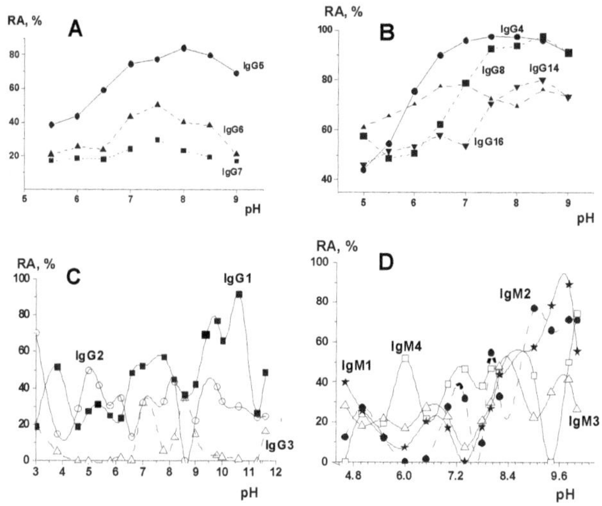

Fig. 7. pH dependences of the relative DNase (A), casein-hydrolyzing (B) activity of IgGs, and IN-hydrolyzing activity (RA) of individual pIgGs (C) and pIgMs (D) from the sera of several different AIDS patients (number of Ab correspond to number of patient). The average error in the initial rate determination at each pH from two experiments did not exceed 7-10 %.

The pH profile for each IgG and IgM was unique; each preparation demonstrated from three to seven brightly expressed optima at different pH from 3 to 11 (Fig. 7). Taking into account the effective hydrolysis of IN at pH 3.0, one cannot exclude that human immune system of AIDS patients could in principle produce IgGs and IgMs with a proteolytic activity similar to that of stomach acidic proteases. The above results clearly demonstrate that pIgGs and pIgMs from individual AIDS patients can consist of different sets of catalytic Ab subfractions demonstrating quite distinct enzymic properties in the hydrolysis of DNA, human casein, and integrase.

Overall, a pool of many auto-Abs may contain very different monoclonal Abzs with various pH optima. It should be mentioned that the RAs of Abzs from patients with different AI and viral diseases are usually compared at one fixed pH, in which all samples are more or less active. Changing the reaction pH, one can reveal not only the major fraction of Abzs in different individuals analyzed, but also other subfractions of Abs, the activity of which may be comparable with or less than that of the major subfraction. In addition, the number of K_m and V_{max} values, characterizing interaction of different monoclonal of polyclonal Abzs with their specific substrates, can significantly increase when they measured at several pH values (Nevinsky, 2010[b]).

5.3 Affinity and relative catalytic activity diversity of AIDS abzymes

It was shown previously, that nuclease and protease Abzs from the sera of AI patients and animals are very heterogeneous in their affinity for cognate substrate and can be separated into many fractions by chromatography on affinity resins bearing immobilized substrate (Baranovskii et al., 2001; Andrievskaya et al., 2002; Semenov et al., 2004; Kuznetsova et al., 2007; Nevinsky et al., 1998, 2005, 2010[a], 2010[b]). We have analyzed the affinity of AIDS pIgGs for human β-casein by chromatography on casein-Sepharose (Odintsova et al., 2006[b]). Interestingly, when IgGs were eluted from casein-Sepharose by a KCl gradient (0–3 M), the protein (and casein-hydrolyzing activity) was distributed all over the chromatography profile. A similar result was obtained at AIDS IgGs chromatography on RT- and HSA-Sepharoses (Odintsova et al., 2006[b]). The data indicate for extreme affinity heterogeneity of casein-, RT-, and HSA-hydrolyzing abzymes to cognate protein substrates (Odintsova et al., 2006).

We have subjected an equimolar mixture of pIgGs (and IgMs) from five AIDS patients to affinity chromatography on IN-Sepharose. Only 15±3 % of the total IgGs (Fig. 8A) and 17±3 % of the total IgMs (Fig. 8B) were bound to IN-Sepharose (Baranova et al., 2009, 2010).

As we have shown previously, the fraction of Abzs with different catalytic activities including in the serum of AI patients usually does not exceed 0.1-5 % of total Igs (Nevinsky et al., 2005, 2010[a], 2010[b]). Therefore, it was surprising that IN-Sepharose can bind up to 15-17 % of the total pIgGs and pIgMs. At the same time, IN is known as a very hydrophobic protein which can interact nonspecifically with different hydrophobic compounds including other proteins. Taking this into account we could suppose that immobilized IN binds anti-IN pIgGs and pIgMs in a specific manner, and interacts with some other IgGs and IgMs non-specifically.

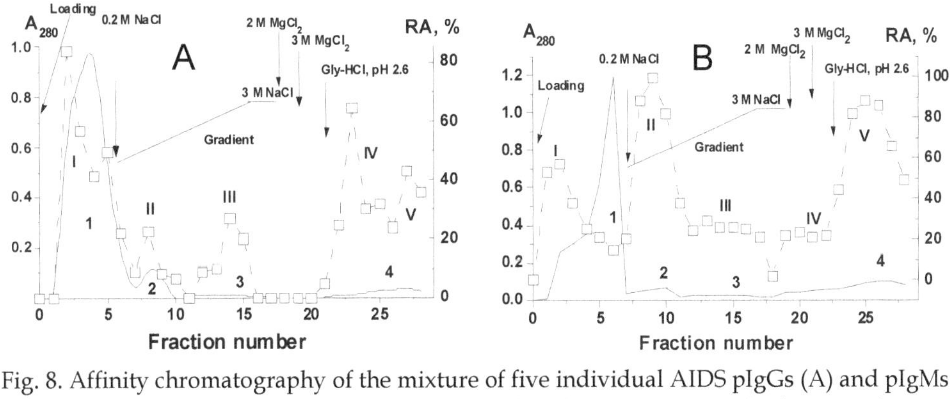

Fig. 8. Affinity chromatography of the mixture of five individual AIDS pIgGs (A) and pIgMs (B) on IN-Sepharose: (—), absorbance at 280 nm; the relative activity (RA) of IgGs and IgMs (5 μl of dialyzed eluate, total volume of the reaction mixture 10 μl) corresponding to complete hydrolysis of 0.3 mg/ml IN after 16 h of incubation was taken for 100%.

The pIgG and IgM fractions of the first peak (~83-85% of protein loaded on IN-Sepharose) with a very low affinity for IN possess high IN-hydrolyzing activity (peak 1, Fig. 8). As it was shown previously non-separated on affinity resins pIgGs and IgMs from AIDS patients contain small subfractions hydrolyzing specifically not only HIV IN (Baranova et al., 2009, 2010), but also HIV RT, HSA and human casein (Odintsova et al., 2006). However, the fractions of pIgGs and pIgMs having high affinity to IN-Sepharose and eluted from this sorbent with different concentrations of NaCl, $MgCl_2$ and acidic buffer (protein peaks 2-4, activity peaks II-V; Fig. 8) hydrolyzed only IN. Thus, IgGs and IgMs with IN-independent activities do not have affinity for IN-Sepharose, but some other Abs can be bound with IN non-specifically.

The total IN-hydrolyzing activities of pIgGs and pIgMs were distributed all over the chromatography profiles and in the case of both Abs five peaks of IN-hydrolyzing activity (I - V, Fig. 8) were brightly expressed. The data obtained are indicative of extreme heterogeneity of IN-hydrolyzing pIgGs and pIgMs in their affinity to IN.

When Abzs are highly heterogeneous, the dependence of V on the substrate concentration for non-fractionated Abs may appear inconsistent with simple Michaelis-Menten kinetics and may be described by a sum of several hyperbolic curves corresponding to different Ab subfractions. However, the contribution of some subfractions to the total curve may be small, or they may have comparable K_m and V_{max} (k_{cat}) values. As a rule, only when significant differences (≥ 5-fold) exist between the K_m and V_{max} values for different Ab subfractions it is possible to determine these parameters characterizing individual subfractions of polyclonal Abz from the aggregated initial rate curves.

First, we have measured the K_m and V_{max} values in the reaction of IN hydrolysis using two individual preparations of pIgGs and pIgMs not fractionated on IN-Sepharose. The initial rate data obtained for these Abs at the increasing IN concentration were inconsistent with the Michaelis-Menten kinetics and the dependences corresponded to at least three or four hyperbolic curves with several segments reflecting different K_m values, which were approximately in the ranges of 5-10, 15-20, 30-50, and higher than 70-100 μM (Fig. 9). Similar situation was observed for the mixtures of equal amounts of electrophoretically homogeneous IgGs ($pIgG_{mix}$) and IgMs ($pIgM_{mix}$) from the sera of five AIDs patients.

For more detailed analysis of K_m and k_{cat} values characterizing different Ab fractions within total pool of Abzs ($pIgG_{mix}$ and $pIgM_{mix}$) we have analyzed several individual $pIgG_{mix}$ and $pIgM_{mix}$ fractions eluted from IN-Sepharose (Fig. 8). First, we have measured the K_m and V_{max} values in the reaction catalyzed by IgG_{mix} (IgG_{load}) and IgM_{mix} (IgM_{load}) corresponding to the second fraction eluted under loading of Abs on IN-Sepharose (Fig. 8). The dependencies of V/[S] (hyperbolic curves; Fig. 10A) and 1/V *vs* 1/[S] (Fig. 10B) demonstrated virtually normal Michaelis-Menten character for second fractions of pIgGs and pIgMs. The K_m and k_{cat} for IgG_{load} (156± 40 μM; 0.3±0.1 min^{-1}) and IgM_{load} (130± 30 μM; 2.0±0.4 min^{-1}) were determined. The V/[S] and 1/V *vs* 1/[S] dependences for individual fractions of pIgGs and pIgMs eluted from IN-Sepharose in gradient of NaCl concentration (IgG_{salt} and IgM_{salt}) and by acidic buffer (IgG_{acid} and IgM_{acid}) had also typical Michaelis-Menten character.

The affinity of pIgGs for IN (in terms of K_m values) increased with the increase of their affinity to IN-Sepharose; for IgG_{salt} (K_m = 44±4.0 μM) corresponding to fraction 8 (eluted with the salt) and IgG_{acid} (K_m = 14±1.0 μM) corresponding to fraction 24 (eluted with an acidic buffer) the affinity was 3.5- and 11-fold respectively higher than that for IgG_{load} (156±40 μM). Similar situation was observed for the separated individual fractions of IgM_{mix} (Fig. 8B); $pIgM_{solid}$ (K_m =43±4.0 μM; fraction 10 eluted with NaCl) and $pIgM_{acid}$ (K_m = 12.8±1.0 μM;

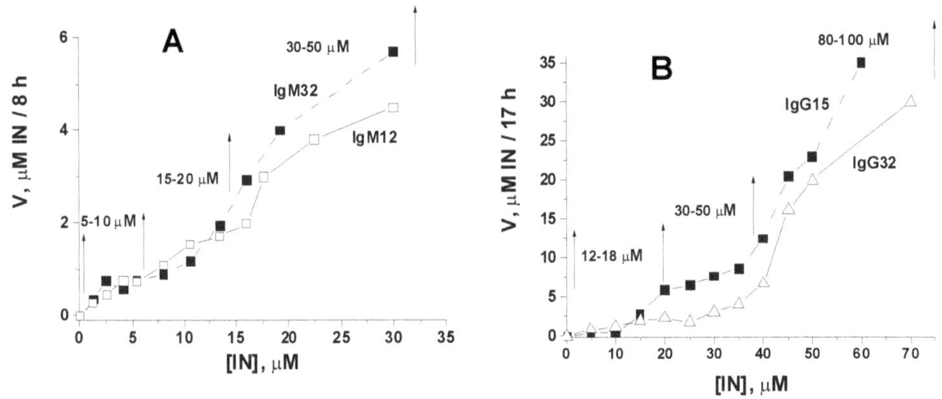

Fig. 9. The dependencies of the initial rates of IN hydrolysis upon the IN concentration in the reaction catalyzed by non-separated by affinity chromatography two individual pIgMs (A) and two pIgGs (B) from different patients in coordinates V *vs* [S]. IgM12, IgM32, IgG15, and IgG32 were used in different concentrations. Arrows show different hyperbolic fragments of complicated curves corresponding to the total dependencies.

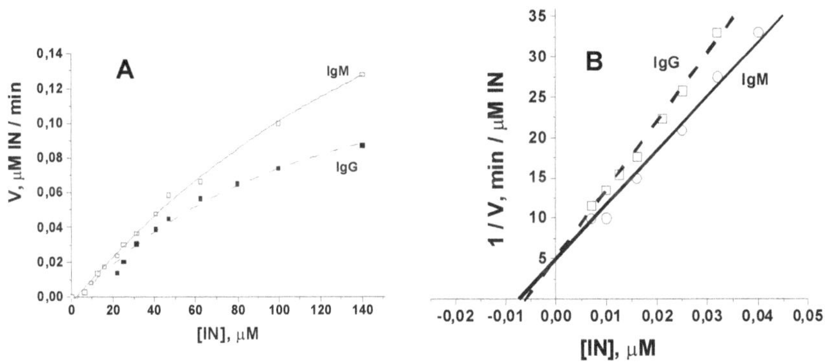

Fig. 10. The dependencies of the initial rates of IN hydrolysis upon the IN concentration in the reaction catalyzed by fractions of $pIgG_{mix}$ and $pIgM_{mix}$ purified on IN-Sepharose (Fig. 8; fractions number 2; IgG_{load} and IgM_{load}) in coordinates V vs [S] (A). Determination of the K_m for IN and V_{max} values using the Lineweaver-Burk plot in the case of the same IgG_{load} and IgM_{load} (B).

fraction 24 eluted with an acidic buffer) demonstrated 3- and 10-fold respectively higher affinity than that for $pIgM_{load}$ fraction (130⊥ 30 μM). The K_m and k_{cat} values corresponding to fractionated pIgGs and pIgMs agree with the relative contents and specific activities of the major Ab subfractions isolated by affinity chromatography (Fig. 8). On overall, the above data demonstrate extreme diversity of HIV IgGs and IgMs in their affinity to IN and in the relative k_{cat} values (Figs 8-10).

Affinity chromatography of DNase and RNase Abs from AI patients and animals (Baranovskii et al., 2001; Andrievskaya et al., 2002; Kuznetsova et al., 2007), healthy rabbits immunized with DNA, RNA, DNase I, DNase II, pancreatic RNase (Krasnorutskii et al.

2008[a], 2008[b], 2008[c], 2008[d], 2009) as well as AI Abs with proteolytic and other activities (Nevinsky et al, 1998; Semenov et al., 2004; Legostaeva et al., 2010) on resins bearing immobilized specific substrates using elution of Abs with different concentration of NaCl and an acidic buffer always leads to separation of Abs into many Abz subfractions with different affinity to immobilized substrate. In addition, the affinity of separated fractions for immobilized substrate increased gradually with the increase in eluting NaCl concentration, but the K_m (and V_{max}) values corresponding to each fraction eluted from affinity sorbent are individual for every patient analyzed. It means, that the apparent number of monoclonal Abzs with different catalytic properties within the polyclonal Abs pool may be significantly underestimated since it is impossible to separate Abzs with comparable affinities for a specific substrate or to distinguish monoclonal Abzs with similar kinetic parameters. Some minor monoclonal Abzs with a relatively high activity and even major Abzs with low activity may be hidden by major Abzs with high activity. As a consequence, the K_m (and V_{max}) values determined using Abzs not fractionated on affinity sorbents more often characterize the interaction of substrates with a major fraction of Abzs with the maximal content and highest relative enzymatic activity at condition used. At the same time, these characteristic are very useful for comparisons of Abs with different substrate specificities and from patients with different diseases. For example, it was shown that affinity of specific major fractions of AIDS IgGs non-fractionated on affinity resins to HSA (K_m = (1.8 ± 0.6)×10^{-8} M, k_{cat} = (3.6± 1.1)×10^{-5} min^{-1}) is 270-290-fold higher than to HIV RT (K_m = (4.9 ± 0.5)×10^{-6} M, k_{cat} = (2.2± 0.2)×10^{-3} min^{-1}) and to β-casein (K_m = (5.3 ± 0.5) ·10^{-6} M, k_{cat} = (2.0± 0.2)×10^{-2} min^{-1}) (Odintsova et al., 2006). At the same time, the relative rate of β-casein hydrolysis was 9- and 550-fold higher than that for HIV RT and HSA, respectively. The K_m for casein ((7.3±1.2)×10^{-6} M; k_{cat} = 0.75±0.05 min^{-1}) estimated in the reaction catalyzed by polyclonal sIgAs from human milk (Odintsova et al., 2005) is comparable with that for IgGs from AIDS patients, while the k_{cat} is ~38-fold higher. This difference is most likely due to a higher content of anti-casein proteolytic Abzs in human milk in comparison with blood of AIDS patients.

The affinity of AIDS pIgGs hydrolyzing HIV RT, human casein, and HSA (K_m = 0.018 – 5.3 μM; see above) as well as IN-Sepharose-purified AIDS pIgGs and pIgMs for IN (K_m = 12.8-156 μM) in terms of K_m values is comparable with typical affinities (K_m = 0.038–7.3 μM) (Paul et al., 1989; Kalaga et al., 1995; Legostaeva et al., 2010; Nevinsky et al., 2005, 2010[a], 2010[b]) of Abzs hydrolyzing different proteins.

The K_m (and k_{cat}) values for plasmid scDNA in the reaction catalyzed by two individual non-fractionated AIDS IgG preparations were determined (Odintsova et al., 2006[a]). In the case of one of two preparations analyzed, the initial rate of DNA hydrolysis increases with increase in DNA concentration according to the Michaelis–Menten kinetics and only one pair of K_m (53 ± 9 nM) and k_{cat} ((2.1 ± 0.1)×10^{-2} min^{-1}) was observed. For the second pIgG preparation two pairs of K_m (2.6 ± 0.1 and 4.4 ± 0.7 nM) and k_{cat} values ((6.7 ± 0.1)×10^{-2} and (29.6 ± 5.0)×10^{-2} min^{-1}) were revealed. Thus, the affinity the scDNA substrate for AIDS IgGs varied (in terms of K_m values) in the range 2.6–53 nM, which correspond to typical K_d values for Ab–antigen interactions and is about 3–4 orders of magnitude higher than affinity of scDNA for DNase I (K_M = 46–58 μM) (Gololobov et al., 1995). These K_m values for scDNA are comparable with the K_m for plasmid DNA (43 nM) reported previously for IgG from SLE patients (Gololobov et al., 1995).

The catalysis mediated by artificial Abzs against reaction transition states is usually characterized by relatively low reaction rates: k_{cat} values are 10^2–10^6-fold lower than for canonical enzymes (Keinan, 2005). The known k_{cat} values for natural Abzs from AI patients vary in the range of 0.001–40 min^{-1} (Gololobov et al., 1995; Kalaga et al., 1995; Nevinsky et al., 2005, 2010[a], 20010[b]). There are only several exceptions. For example, the specific activity of RNase IgGs from AI patients was about 1-20% of that for RNase A and of six known human sera RNases, while poly(A) was hydrolyzed by Abzs 2-10-fold faster than by RNase A, one of the most active RNases known (Buneva et al., 1994; Baranovskii et al., 1997, 1998; Vlasov et al., 1998). At the same time, the specific activity of homogeneous Abzs of several SLE and MS patients was about 40-400% of that for RNase A (Baranovskii et al., 1998). In addition, the specific nucleotide-hydrolyzing activities of mouse polyclonal IgGs is ~1–4 orders of magnitude higher that those of known natural Abzs (Andryushkova et al., 2009). The k_{cat} values for AIDS pIgGs hydrolyzing scDNA ($(2.1\text{-}29.6)\times10^{-2}$ min^{-1}), human casein (2.0×10^{-2} min^{-1}), HSA (3.6×10^{-5} min^{-1}), and HIV RT (2.2×10^{-3} min^{-1}), as well IgGs (0.3-2.9 min^{-1}) and IgMs (2.0-6.4 min^{-1}) purified on IN-Sepharose (Table 2) in the IN hydrolysis were comparable with those for known Abzs (Odintsova et al., 2006[a], 2006[b]; Baranova et al., 2009, 2010).

Currently there are no methods that can efficiently separate Abzs from catalytically inactive Abs against the same antigen. In addition, as it was shown above, IN-Sepharose interact not only with anti-IN IgMs and IgGs but bind non-specifically some other Abs. Even partial purification of IgGs and IgMs on IN-Sepharose (or other specific affinity resins) leads to significant increase in the k_{cat} value for IN and other substrates hydrolysis. Since the specific activities in all cases were calculated using the total concentration of purified pIgGs and pIgMs and affinity chromatography on IN-Sepharose (and other affinity sorbents) cannot separate catalytically active and inactive anti-IN Abs, the specific IN-hydrolyzing activities of the individual monoclonal subfractions in the pIgG and pIgM pools may be higher than those of non-fractionated or partially fractionated Abs. It should be mentioned that specific activities of some Abzs are often significantly lower than those for canonical enzymes with the same catalytic activities. However, it is impossible to dismiss the RAs of Abs from patients with AI and viral infection as biologically inessential since they are comparable with those for many canonical and very important enzymes, for example, restriction endonucleases and repair enzymes (Gololobov et al., 1995; Nevinsky et al., 2005, 2010, 2010). Thus, IN-hydrolyzing IgGs and IgMs from HIV-infected patients are very heterogeneous in their affinity to IN-Sepharose, demonstrate different K_m and V_{max} values and different subfractions of Abzs can hydrolyze various substrates at pH from 3 to 10. In addition, in contrast to other Abzs with proteolytic activity they can possess for different types of proteolytic activities: thiol-, metal-dependent, serine- and acidic-like.

6. Peculiarities of protein hydrolysis by AIDS abzymes and canonical proteases

6.1 Casein hydrolysis by AIDS abzymes

Casein hydrolyzing Abzs was found not only in the sera of HIV-infected patients (Odintsova et al., 2006[b]) but also in the milk of lactating women (Odintsova et al., 2005; 2011). At the first glance, no obvious immunizing factors could be found in clinically healthy pregnant and lactating women. However, pregnancy could "activate" or "trigger" autoimmune-like manifestations in clinically healthy women, and a sharp exacerbation of AI reactions can occur in some cases soon after childbirth (Amino *et al.*, 1982; Freeman *et al.*, 1986). Postnatal AI pathologies arise sometimes, including SLE, Hashimoto's thyroiditis, phospholipids syndrome, polymyositis, AI myocarditis, etc. (Amino *et al.*, 1982; Freeman *et al.*, 1986).

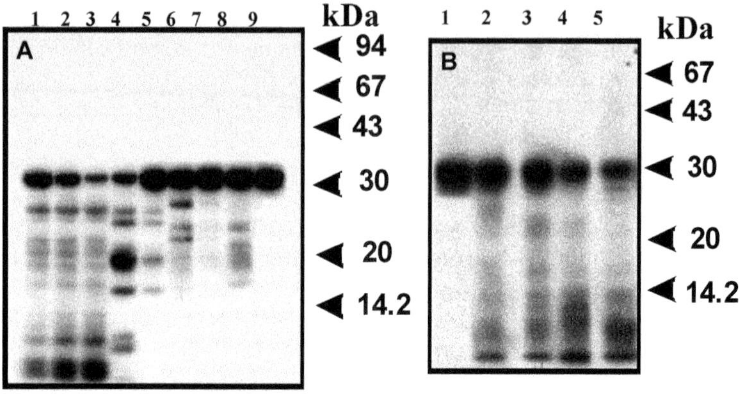

Fig. 11. SDS-PAGE analysis of products of [32P]casein hydrolysis by human milk sIgA and different proteases (A) or AIDS IgGs (B) (autoradiograph). A, Lanes 1, 2, and 3 correspond to [32P]β-casein incubated with sIgAs for 20, 40, and 60 min, respectively; lanes 4 and 5, incubation with trypsin for 10 and 15 min; lanes 6 and 7, incubation with proteinase K for 10 and 15 min; lane 8, incubation with chymotrypsin for 10 min; 9, casein incubated alone for 60 min. The reaction mixture (10 μl) for analysis of proteolytic activity of different proteases contained 6.2 μg/ml casein and sIgAs or enzymes at the following concentrations: 0.32 μg/ml trypsin, 0.064 μg/ml chymotrypsin, 0.1 μg/ml proteinase K, and 20 μg/ml sIgA. B, [32P]casein was incubated for 14 h in the absence of Abs (lane 1) and in the presence IgGs from the sera of different AIDS patients: lane 2, IgG-1 (14 h), lanes 3 and 4, IgG2 (7 and 14 h, respectively), lane 5, IgG-3 (14 h).

Parenteral or oral administration of various proteins to animals late in pregnancy leads to the production of the corresponding Abs at high levels (Fey *et al.*, 1973; Mestecky *et al.*, 1987). Thus, pregnant women may be effectively immunized by contacts with compounds of viruses and bacteria that are not immunogenic in other healthy humans. There may be also some degree of autoimmunization during pregnancy similar to that in AI patients (Nevinsky et al., 2005, 2010a, 2010b and refs therein).

It was shown that lactation is associated with the appearance of sIgA and IgG abzymes with DNase, RNase (Kanyshkova *et al.*, 1997; Nevinsky *et al.*, 2000a, 2000b), ATPase (Semenov *et al.*, 2004), amylolytic (Savel'ev *et al.*, 2001), protein- (Nevinsky *et al.*, 1998), lipid- (Gorbunov *et al.*, 2005) and polysaccharide (Karataeva *et al.*, 2006a, 2006b) kinase activities in human milk. The specific activities of milk Abzs are significantly higher than those of Abzs from the blood of healthy lactating women and patients with different AI pathologies (Nevinsky *et al.*, 2003, 2005, 2010a, 2010b and refs therein).

We have compared the hydrolysis of β-casein by canonical proteases, human milk sIgA (Fig. 11A) and three different individual AIDS IgGs (Fig. 11B) (Odintsova et al., 2006b; 2011). The patterns of β-casein hydrolysis by milk sIgA, AIDS IgG, trypsin, chymotrypsin, and proteinase K were quite different. In addition, there was observed remarkable difference in the hydrolysis of β-casein by three individual AIDS IgG-1, IgG-2, and IgG-3 (Fig 11B).

It should be mentioned that AIDS IgGs demonstrated only serine-like protease activity (Odintsova et al., 2006b), while milk IgAs additionally possess Me-dependent activity (Odintsova et al., 2011). Thus, possible ways of the production of Abzs with casein-hydrolyzing activity in healthy human mothers and in AIDS patients may be different.

6.2 Integrase hydrolysis by AIDS abzymes

6.2.1 Specific regularities of integrase interaction with DNA

HIV-1 integrase catalyzes insertion of a DNA copy of the viral genome into the host genome (Asante-Appiah & Skalka, 1999). Therefore IN, together with RT and protease, is the main important target of anti-HIV drugs.

Specific interactions between HIV IN and long terminal repeats are required for insertion of viral DNA into the host genome. The use of a method based on stepwise increase in ligand complexity allowed an estimation of the relative contributions of each nucleotide from oligonucleotides (ODNs) to the total affinity for IN (Bugreev et al., 2003). It was shown that IN interacts with ODNs through superposition of weak contacts with their bases and, more importantly, with the internucleotide phosphate groups. Formation of the IN complex with specific DNA cannot by itself account for the major contribution of enzyme specificity, which lies in the k_{cat} term; the rate of 3′-processin reaction is increased by more than 5 orders of magnitude upon transition from non-specific to specific oligonucleotides (Bugreev et al., 2003).

In solution, HIV-1 IN exists in a dynamic equilibrium of monomers, dimers, tetramers and high-order oligomers (Deprez et al., 2000). We have recently analyzed the activity of different purified oligomeric forms of recombinant IN obtained after stabilization by platinum crosslinking and shown that these forms do not share the same *in vitro* catalytic properties (Faure et al., 2005). While monomers were inactive for all specific IN activities, dimers were able to catalyze the 3′-processing and the insertion of only one LTR into a short target DNA. In contrast, a tetramer of IN catalyzed the full-site integration of the two viral LTR ends into a target DNA.

To characterize the influence of the determinants of DNA substrate specificity on the oligomerization status of IN, the small-angle X-ray scattering technique was used (Baranova et al., 2007). Under special conditions in the absence of ODNs IN existed only as monomers. IN preincubation with specific ODNs led mainly to formation of dimers, the relative amount of which correlated well with the increase in the enzyme activity. Under these conditions, tetramers were scarce. Nonspecific ODNs stimulated formation of catalytically inactive dimers and tetramers. Complexes of monomeric, dimeric and tetrameric forms of IN with specific and nonspecific ODNs had varying radii of gyration (R_g), suggesting that the specific sequence-dependent formation of IN tetramers occurs by dimerization of two dimers of different structure. From the data it was concluded that the DNA-induced oligomerization of HIV-1 IN is of extreme importance to provide substrate specificity and to increase the enzyme activity (Baranova et al., 2007).

6.2.2 Effect of DNA on the integrase hydrolysis by different proteases

It is known that a formation of multiple contacts between the same or various subunits of oligomeric enzymes is usually provided by multiple hydrophobic and electrostatic contacts and hydrogen bonds. A similar situation was observed for the dimeric forms of HIV-1 IN by X-ray crystallography (for review see Wlodawer 1999; Chiu & Davies, 2004). Analysis of effects of specific and nonspecific ODNs on the rate of IN proteolysis by chymotrypsin, trypsin, and proteinase K can provide useful information concerning a possible decrease in the accessibility of aromatic and positively charged amino acid residues after an enzyme binds its substrates, changes its conformation, or forms contacts between its subunits. It was interesting to compare the effect of different ODNs on the cleavage of IN by Abzs and canonical proteases. The specific single-stranded (ss) 5′-GTGTGGAAAATCTCTAGCA (19-CA), ss 5′-GTGTGGAAAATCTCTAGCAGT (21-GT), ss 5′-ACTGCTAGAGATTTTCCACAC (21-COM, complementary to 21-GT and to 19-CA), double-stranded (ds) 21-GT (21-GT•21-COM) and ds 19-CA (19-CA•21-COM) corresponding to terminal repeats of viral DNA were used.

While nonspecific $d(pT)_n$ markedly decreased the IgG-dependent hydrolysis of IN, $d(pA)_n$ and $d(pA)_n \bullet d(pT)_n$ demonstrated no detectable protective effect (Fig. 12) (Odintsova E., Baranova S., and Nevinsky G.A., personal communication).

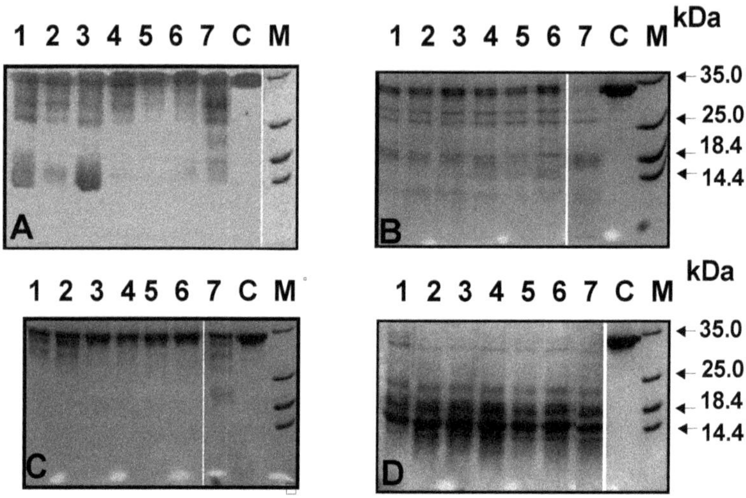

Fig. 12. SDS-PAGE analysis of HIV IN hydrolysis by IgGs and canonical proteases. Polyclonal IgGs from HIV-infected patients (A), chymotrypsin (B), trypsin (C), and proteinase K (D) were used for hydrolysis of IN after its preincubation in the absence and in the presence of various ODNs leading to the formation of different IN oligomeric forms. IN was pre-incubated for 1 h at 30°C in the absence (lane 7) or in the presence of saturating concentrations (0.2–1 mM) of ss $d(pA)_{24}$ (lane 1), ss $d(pT)_{24}$ (lane 2), ds $d(pA)_{24} \bullet d(pT)_{24}$ (lane 3), ss 21-COM (lane 4), ss 21-GT (lane 5), ds 21-GT•21-COM (lane 6). Then, pre-incubated mixture was diluted 3-fold and one of three canonical proteases or pIgGs from HIV-infected patients was added. After 5–10 min incubation in the presence of trypsin (19 μM), chymotrypsin (1.6 μM), proteinase K (19 μM) and 6 h in the presence of pIgGs (0.17 μM) the reaction was stopped and the efficiency of IN hydrolysis was analysed by SDS-PAGE.

The best protection from the hydrolysis by IgGs was observed for ss and especially ds specific ODNs (Fig. 12). Overall, the protective effects of all specific and nonspecific ss and ds ODNs from hydrolysis of IN by chymotrypsin were comparable. Therefore, one can suggest that the formation of IN complex with specific and nonspecific ODNs led to a similar decrease in the accessibility of aromatic amino acid residues as a result of their shielding by ODNs and/or involvement of these residues to the formation of multiple contacts at the interfaces of IN oligomer subunits. In contrast to chymotrypsin, nonspecific ODNs strongly protects IN from hydrolysis by trypsin, which cleaves peptide chains mainly at the carboxyl side of lysine and arginine residues (Fig. 12). Thus, these ODNs most probably stimulate formation of dimeric forms of IN with more Lys- and Arg-dependent electrostatic contacts between the monomers. A weak protective effect of specific and nonspecific ODNs was observed in the case of proteinase K, which is mostly sequence-independent. Thus, specific and nonspecific DNAs stimulate the formation of different IN oligomeric forms, in which aromatic and charged amino acid residues in different extent accessible for Abzs, chymotrypsin, and trypsin. The findings correlate with the results obtained by small-angle X-ray scattering, which show that all nonspecific and specific ODNs stimulate different changes in the structure of IN monomers and dimers free of DNA (Baranova et al., 2007).

MALDI-TOF analysis of the fragments formed after IN incubation with pIgG and pIgM purified on IN-Sepharose was carried out (Odintsova E., Baranova S., and Nevinsky G.A., personal communication). The cross-sections of longitudinal slices of the gel corresponding to the products with approximate mol. masses 29 ± 2 (P1), 22 ± 2 (P2), 16 ± 2 (P3), and 12 ± 2 (P4), as well as 30± 2 (P0) kDa were cut out as shown on Fig. 13 and the proteins were eluted from the gel. MALDI-TOF analysis has shown that P1–P4 fractions contain from four to eight major fragments with different molecular masses. The peptides found in the P1–P4 fractions were digested with trypsin under standard conditions for MALDI analysis, and the hydrolyzates were studied.

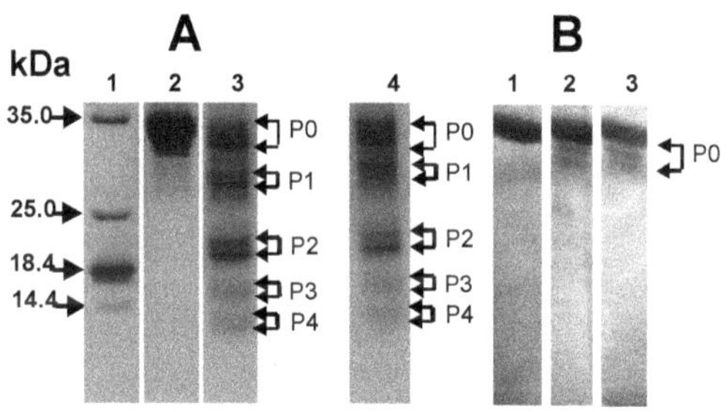

Fig. 13. SDS-PAGE analysis of IN hydrolysis by pIgG-1 (lane 3, A), IgG-6 (lane 2, B), pIgM-2 (lane 4, A) and pIgM-6 (lane 3, B) purified on IN-Sepharose after 9 h (A) and 2 h (B) of incubation in a nonreducing 12% gel followed by silver staining. Lanes 1 (B) and 2 (A), IN incubated in the absence of Abs. Lane 1 (A) protein molecular mass markers. Gel zones P1, P2, P3, and P4 (A) as well as P0 (B) were used for MALDI-TOF analysis (see the text).

Seven antigenic determinants (AGDs) have been reported for HIV IN corresponding to amino acid residues 5–22 (AGD1), 14–35 (AGD2) (Yi et al., 2000), 58–141 (AGD3), 141–172 (AGD4), 248–264 (AGD5) (Bizub-Bender et al., 1994), 208–228 (AGD6), and 251–271(AGD7) (Nilsen et al., 1996) (underlined in Fig. 14). Interestingly, 6–7 cleavage sites found by MALDI corresponded to the N-terminal stretch of residues 11–35, belonging to two overlapping antigenic determinants AGD1 and AGD2 (Fig. 14). Three clusters of cleavage sites were located within the long AGD3. A block of 12 closely spaced cleavage sites corresponded to the N-terminal part of AGD4. Only one cleavage site was located within AGD5 and four sites corresponded to AGD6 and AGD7. At the same time, some sites of IN cleavage, most notably a cluster of 16 sites between residues 175 and 202, did not corresponds to any IN AGD known at this moment.

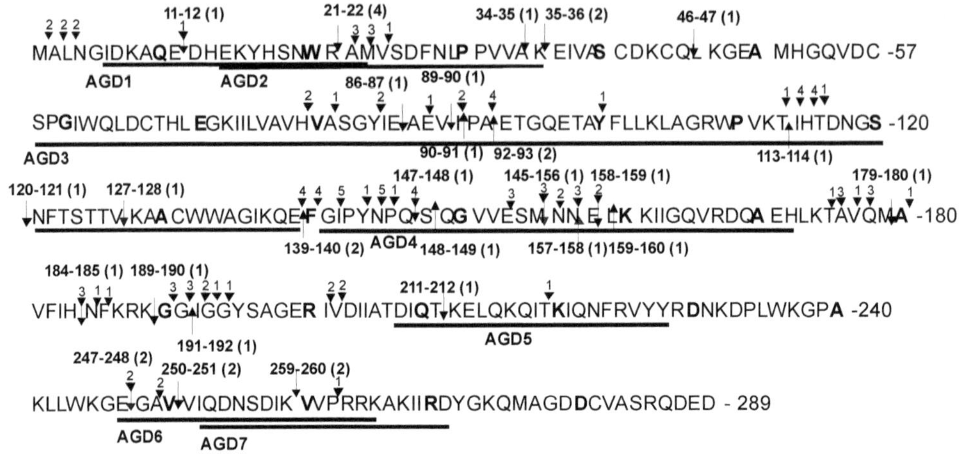

Fig. 14. All trypsin-independent points of IN cleavage determined from the MALDI-TOF analysis directly mol. masses of the P0–P4 fractions and after their cleavage by trypsin. Numbers next to the arrows show the position of the residue within the IN sequence; numbers under short arrows and in parentheses correspond to the frequency of these cleavage sites found using different approaches. Seven known antigenic determinants of IN are underlined in the figure.

Interestingly, a similar situation was observed for MS IgGs specifically hydrolyzing MBP; in addition to the sites of cleavage within four known AGDs of MBP, several sites were outside these determinants (Ponomarenko et al., 2006). Thus, the number of structurally different antigenic determinants in the case of IN may be great.

Interestingly, in contrast to the absence of hydrolysis of non-specific globular proteins by anti-IN Abs, they first cleave IN with the accumulation of long fragments corresponding mainly to known AGDs and then are capable of further degradation of these long intermediates, and the formation of very short products was observed after 72–100 h of IN incubation In with Abzs (Odintsova E., Baranova S., and Nevinsky G.A., personal communication). AIDS anti-IN pIgGs and IgMs hydrolyze specific 20-25-mer oligopeptides corresponding to the IN AGDs ~30–70-fold faster than nonspecific long 20-25-mer oligopeptides corresponding to AGDs of human myelin basic protein and HIV RT. In addition, AIDS anti-IN Abzs can hydrolyze very short 3-4-mer nonspecific oligopeptides 100–300-fold more slowly than specific ones. Therefore, the recognition and digestion of globular proteins and relatively short oligopeptides by the Abzs proceeds in different ways. Since catalytic centers of Abzs specifically hydrolyzing different proteins including IN are usually located on the light chains of Abs (Nevinsky et al., 2005, 2010[a], 2010[b], and refs therein), the observed hydrolysis of short oligopeptides can be a consequence of their interaction with light or heavy chains without significant contacts with alternative chains.

Interestingly, separated light chains of pIgGs, pIgMs, and pIgAs from the sera of patients with different AI and viral diseases usually significantly more active than intact Abs in the hydrolysis of DNA, RNA, oligosaccharides, and proteins (Nevinsky et al., 2005, 2010[a], 2010[b], and refs therein). This phenomenon may be a consequence of a higher affinity of intact Abs, as compared with separated light chains, for different substrates due to interaction of the substrates with both light and heavy chains of Abzs. The separation of the light chains can lead to a decrease in the lifetime of the existence of the complex and, as a consequence, to an increase in the turnover number and V_{max} (k_{cat}) of the reaction catalyzed by L-chains. Taken together, the absence or very weak interaction of short substrates with heavy chains of AIDS Abzs in contrast with globular molecules proteins (and higher rate of the reaction) may be a main reason of a decrease of specificity of Abzs action in the case of short oligopeptides; one cannot exclude that light (or heavy) chains of some Abzs can effectively hydrolyzed short oligopeptides of any sequences.

We have shown that *in vitro* IgGs and IgMs hydrolyzing IN significantly decrease the 3′-processing and integration reaction catalyzed by IN (for example, Fig. 15) (Odintsova E., Baranova S., and Nevinsky G.A., personal communication).

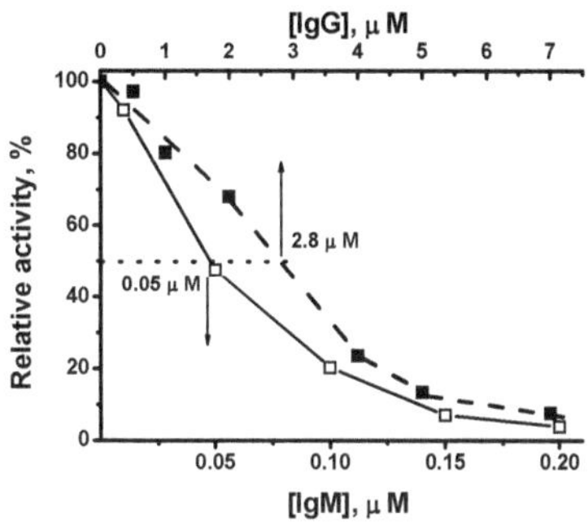

Fig. 15. Effect of IN-hydrolyzing IgGs and IgMs from AIDS patients on the rate of the 3′-processing reaction.

7. Conclusion

According to modern point of view, the immune response to the viral components is the most important factor providing slow transition of HIV infection to the stage of AIDS (Fauci et al., 2008). Since AIDS anti-IN anti-RT Abs can efficiently hydrolyze IN and RT (Odintsova et al., 2006[b]; Baranova et al., 2009, 2010), a positive role of abzymes in counteracting the infection cannot be excluded and these polyclonal and corresponding monoclonal Abzs with proteolytic activities are potentially interesting for designing new anti-HIV agents. In addition, detection of IN-hydrolyzing activity can be useful for diagnostic purposes and for assessment of the immune status in AIDS patients.

The field of monoclonal Abzs with immunotherapeutic potential has recently been reviewed (see "Introduction"). Abzs that cleave HIV envelope gp120 protein may find their use in the treatment of AIDS (Tellier, 2002; Stockwin & Holmes, 2003). pIgG degrading gp120 was also obtained taking advantage of the susceptibility of SJL mice to a peptide-induced AI disorder, experimental AI encephalomyelitis (Ponomarenko et al., 2006). Immunization of specific pathogen-free SJL mice with structural fragments of gp120 fused in-frame with the encephalitogenic MBP(85-101) peptide resulted in a pronounced disease-associated immune response against these antigens. This strategy can be generalized to create catalytic vaccines against viral pathogens (Ponomarenko et al., 2006). In addition, Abzs with different catalytic activities can be used for different purposes (see "Introduction").

In conclusion, a number of studies of Abzs show the extremely wide potential of the immune system in producing Abzs possessing very different enzymatic activities, which very often are not comparable with those of known enzymes, and natural Abs with specified and novel functions may have wide potential for biotechnology and medicine.

8. Acknowledgments

This research was made possible in part by grants from Analytical Departmental Special program "Development of Scientific Potential of High School (No. 2.1.1/5580)" from the Presidium of the Russian Academy of Sciences ("Molecular and Cellular Biology Program" No. 22.7, "Fundamental Sciences to Medicine" No. 21.16), Russian Foundation for Basic Research (08-04-00315, 09-04-00804), and funds from the Siberian Division of the Russian Academy of Sciences.

9. Abbreviations

Abs - antibodies
Abzs - abzymes - or catalytically active antibodies
AG - antigen
AI - autoimmune
AD - autoimmune disease
AIDS - human autoimmune deficit syndrome
BSA - bovine serum albumin
CC - correlation coefficient
HSCs - hematopoietic stem cells
sc - supercoiled
ss and ds - single- and double-stranded - respectively
CBA - (CBAxC57BL)F1 mice
HT - Hashimoto's thyroiditis
hMBP - human myelin basic protein
MFT - microsomal fraction of thyrocytes
MBP - myelin basic protein
MS - multiple sclerosis
nat-DNA and den-DNA - native and denatured DNA - respectively
MHO - maltoheptaose
pAbs and pIgGs - polyclonal Abs and IgGs - respectively
RF - rheumatoid factor
SLE- systemic lupus erythematosus - SDS-PAGE - SDS-polyacrylamide gel electrophoresis
TBE - tick-borne encephalitis
VIP - vasoactive intestinal peptide
RA - relative activity
CFU-GM - granulocytic-macrophagic colony-forming unit
BFU-E - erythroid burst-forming unit
CFU-GEMM - granulocytic-erythroid-megakaryocytic- macrophagic colony-forming unit

10. References

Amino, N.; Mori, H.; Iwatani, Y.; Tanizawa, O.; Kawashima, M.; Tsuge, I.; Ibaragi K. & Kumahara, Y.; Miyai, K. (1982). High prevalence of transient post-partum thyrotoxicosis and hypothyroidism. *N. Engl. J. Med.*, 306(14), 849-852, ISSN 0028-4793

Asante-Appiah, E. & Skalka, A. M. (1999). HIV-1 integrase: structural organization, conformational changes, and catalysis. *Adv. Virus Res.*, 52, 351-369, ISSN 0065-3527

Andrievskaya, O. A.; Buneva, V. N.; Naumov, V. A. & Nevinsky, G. A. (2000). Catalytic heterogeneity of polyclonal RNA-hydrolyzing IgM from sera of patients with lupus erythematosus. *Med. Sci. Monit.*, 6(3), 460 –470, ISSN 1234-1010

Andrievskaya, O. A.; Buneva, V. N.; Baranovskii, A. G.; Gal'vita, A. V.; Benzo, E. S.; Naumov, V. A. & Nevinsky, G. A. (2002). Catalytic diversity of polyclonal RNA-hydrolyzing IgG antibodies from the sera of patients with systemic lupus erythematosus. *Immunol. Lett.*, 81(3), 191-198, ISSN 0165-2478

Andryushkova, A. A.; Kuznetsova, I. A.; Orlovskaya, I. A.; Buneva, V. N. & Nevinsky, G. A. (2006). Antibodies with amylase activity from the sera of autoimmune-prone MRL/MpJ-lpr mice. *FEBS Lett.*, 580(21), 5089-5095, ISSN 0014-5793

Andryushkova, A. S.; Kuznetsova, I. A.; Buneva, V. N.; Toporkova, L. B.; Sakhno, L. V.; Tichonova, M. A.; Chernykh, E. R.; Orlovskaya, I. A. & Nevinsky, G. A. (2007) Formation of different abzymes in autoimmune-prone MRL-lpr/lpr mice is associated with changes in colony formation of haematopoetic progenitors. *J. Cell. Mol. Med.*, 11(3), 531-551, ISSN 1582-1838

Andryushkova, A. S.; Kuznetsova, I. A.; Orlovskaya, I. A.; Buneva, V. N. & Nevinsky, G. A. (2009) Nucleotide-hydrolyzing antibodies from the sera of autoimmune-prone MRL-lpr/lpr mice. *Int. immunol.*, 21(8), 935-945, ISSN 0953-8178

Baranova S.; Tuzikov F. V.; Zakharova O. D.; Tuzikova N. A.; Calmels C.; Litvak S.; Tarrago-Litvak L.; Parissi V. & Nevinsky G. A. (2007). Small-angle X-ray characterization of the nucleoprotein complexes resulting from DNA-induced oligomerization of HIV-1 integrase. *Nucleic Acids Res.*, 35(3), 975-987, ISSN 0305-1048

Baranova, S. V.; Buneva, V. N.; Kharitonova, M. A.; Sizyakina, L. P.; Calmels, C.; Andreola, M. L.; Parissi, V. & Nevinsky, G. A. (2009). HIV-1 integrase-hydrolyzing antibodies from sera of HIV-infected patients. *Biochimie*, 91(9), 1081-1086, ISSN 0300-9084

Baranova, S. V.; Buneva, V. N.; Kharitonova, M. A.; Sizyakina, L. P.; Calmels, C.; Andreola, M. L.; Parissi, V. & Nevinsky, G. A. (2010). HIV-1 integrase-hydrolyzing IgM antibodies from sera of HIV-infected patients. *Int. Immunol.*, 22(8), 671-680, ISSN 0953-8178

Baranovskii, A. G.; Matushin, V. G.; Vlassov, A. V.; Zabara, V. G.; Naumov, V. A.; Buneva, V. N. & Nevinskii, G. A. (1997). DNA- and RNA-hydrolyzing antibodies from the blood of patients with various forms of viral hepatitis. *Biochemistry (Moscow)*, 62(12), ISSN 0006-2979

Baranovskii, A. G.; Kanyshkova, T. G.; Mogelnitskii, A. S.; Naumov, V. A.; Buneva, V. N.; Gusev, E. I.; Boiko, A. N.; Zargarova, T. A.; Favorova, O. O. & Nevinsky, G. A. (1998). Polyclonal antibodies from blood and cerebrospinal fluid of patients with multiple sclerosis effectively hydrolyze DNA and RNA. *Biochemistry (Moscow)*, 63(11), 1239-1248, ISSN 0006-2979

Baranovskii, A. G.; Ershova, N. A.; Buneva, V. N.; Kanyshkova, T. G.; Mogelnitskii, A. S.; Doronin, B. M.; Boiko, A. N.; Gusev, E. I.; Favorova, O. O. & Nevinsky, G. A. (2001). Catalytic heterogeneity of polyclonal DNA-hydrolyzing antibodies from the sera of patients with multiple sclerosis. *Immunol. Lett.*, 76(3), 163-167, ISSN 0165-2478

Baranovskii, A. G.; Buneva, V. N. & Nevinsky, G. A. (2004) Human deoxyribonucleases. *Biochemistry (Mosc)*, 69(6), 587-601, ISSN 0006-2979

Barbas, C. F. 3rd; Heine, A.; Zhong, G.; Hoffmann, T.; Gramatikova, S.; Bjornestedt, R.; List, B.; Anderson, J.; Stura, E. A.; Wilson, I. A. & Lerner, R. A. (1997) *Science*, 278(5346), 2085-2092, ISSN 0036-8075

Barzilai, O.; Ram, M. & Shoenfeld, Y. (2007). Viral infection can induce the production of autoantibodies. *Curr. Opin. Rheumatol.*, 19(8), 636-643, ISSN 1040-8711

Bigazzi, P. E. (1983). In: *Mechanisms of Immunology*, Cohen, S.; Wozd, P. E. & McKlaskie, R. T. (Ed.), pp. 181-206, Moscow: Meditsina.

Bizub-Bender, D.; Kulkosky, J. & Skalka, A. M. (1994). Monoclonal antibodies against HIV type 1 integrase: clues to molecular structure. *AIDS Res. Hum. Retroviruses*, 10(9), 1105-1115, ISSN 0889-2229

Blanco, F.; Kalsi, J. & Isenberg, D. A. (1991) Analysis of antibodies to RNA in patients with systemic lupus erythematosus and other autoimmune rheumatic diseases. *Clin. Exp. Immunol.*, 86(1), 66-70, ISSN 0009-9104

Bugreev, D. V.; Baranova, S.; Zakharova,O. D.; Parissi, V.; Desjobert, C.; Sottofattori, E.; Balbi, A.; Litvak, S.; Tarrago-Litvak, L. & Nevinsky, G. A. (2003). Dynamic, thermodynamic, and kinetic basis for recognition and transformation of DNA by HIV-1 integrase. *Biochemistry*, 42(30), 9235-9247. ISSN 0006-2960

Buneva, V. N.; Andrievskaia, O. A.; Romannikova, I. V.; Gololobov, G. V.; Iadav, R. P.; Iamkovoi, V. I. & Nevinskii, G. A. (1994) Interaction of catalytically active antibodies with oligoribonucleotides. *Mol. Biol. (Moscow)*, 28(4), 738 - 743, ISSN 0026-8933

Chiu, T. K. & Davies D. R. (2004) Structure and function of HIV-1 integrase. *Curr. Top. Med. Chem.*, 4(9) 965-977, ISSN 1568-0266

Deprez, E.; Tauc, P.; Leh, H., Mouscadet, J. F.; Auclair, C. & Brochon, J. C. (2000). Oligomeric states of the HIV-1 integrase as measured by time-resolved fluorescence anisotropy. *Biochemistry*, 39(31), 9275-9284, ISSN 0006-2960

Dias, S.; Jovic, F.; Renard, P. Y.; Taran, F.; Créminon, C.; Mioskowski, C. & Grassi, J. (2002) Immunologically driven chemical engineering of antibodies for catalytic activity. *J. Immunol. Methods*, 269(1-2), 81-98, ISSN 0022-1759

Gabibov, A. G.; Ponomarenko, N. A.: Tretyak, E. B.: Paltsev, M. A. & Suchkov, S. V. (2006) Catalytic autoantibodies in clinical autoimmunity and modern medicine. *Autoimmun. Rev.*, 5(5), 324-330, ISSN 1568-9972

Dubrovskaya, V. V.; Andryushkova, A. S.; Kuznetsova, I. A.; Toporkova, L. B.; Buneva, V. N.; Orlovskaya, I. A. & Nevinsky, G. A. (2003). DNA-hydrolyzing antibodies from sera of autoimmune-prone MRL/MpJ-lpr mice, *Biochemistry (Mosc.)*, 68(10), 1081-1088, ISSN 0006-2979

Earnshaw, W. C. & Rothfield, N. (1985). Identification of a family of human centromere proteins using autoimmune sera from patients with scleroderma. *Chromosoma*, 91(3-4), 313-321, ISSN 0009-5915

Faure, A.; Calmels, C.; Desjobert, C.; Castroviejo, M.; Caumont-Sarcos, A.; Tarrago-Litvak, L.; Litvak, S. & Parissi, V. (2005) HIV-1 integrase crosslinked oligomers are active in vitro. *Nucleic Acids Res.*, 33(3), 977-986, ISSN 0305-1048

Founel, S. & Muller, S. (2002) Antinucleosome antibodies and T-cell response in systemic lupus erythematosus. *Ann. Med. Interne (Paris),* 153(8), 513-519.

Freeman, R.; Rosen, H. & Thysen, B. (1986). Incidence of thyroid dysfunction in an unselected postpartum population. *Arch. Intern. Med.,* 146(7), 1361-1364, ISSN 0003-9926

Galvita, A. V.; Baranovskii, A. G.; Kuznetsova, I. A.; Vinshu, N. V.; Galenok, V. A.; Buneva, V. N. & Nevinsky, G. A. (2007). A peculiarity of DNA hydrolysis by antibodies from patients with diabetes. *Russ. J. Immunol.,* 1, 116-131.

Gao, Q. S.; Sun, M.; Tyutyulkova, S.; Webster, D.; Rees, A.; Tramontano, A.; Massey, R. J. & Paul, S. (1994). Molecular cloning of a proteolytic antibody light chain. *J. Biol. Chem.,* 269(51), 32389-32393, ISSN 0021-9258

Garmashova, N. V.; Kazanskii, V. E.; Tyshkevich, O. B.; Doronin, B. M.; Buneva, V. N. & Nevinskii, G. A. (2004). Antibodies to DNA in the blood of patients with tick-borne encephalitis. *Mol. Biol. (Moscow),* 38(4), 723-730, ISSN 0026-8933

Goldfarb, M. F. (2001). Analysis of casein using two-dimensional electrophoresis, western blot, and computer imaging. *Adv. Exp. Med. Biol.,* 501, 535-539, ISSN 0065-2598

Golinelli-Pimpaneau, B.; Gigant, B.; Bizebard, T.; Nazava, J.; Saludjian, P.; Zemel, R.; Tawfik, D. S.; Eshhar, Z.; Green, B. S. & Knossow, M. (1994). Crystal structure of catalytic antibody Fab with esterase-like activity. *Current Biology, Structure,* 2(3), 175-183, ISSN 0960-9822

Gololobov, G. V.; Mikhalap, S. V.; Starov, A. V.; Kolesnikov, A. F. & Gabibov, A. G. (1994). DNA-protein complexes. Natural targets for DNA-hydrolyzing antibodies. *Appl. Biochem. Biotechnol.,* 47(2-3), 305-314, ISSN 0273-2289

Gololobov, G. V.; Chernova, E. A.; Schourov, D. V.; Smirnov, I. V.; Kudelina, I. A. & Gabibov, A. G. (1995) Cleavage of supercoiled plasmid DNA by autoantibody Fab fragment: application of the flow linear dichroism technique. *Proc. Natl. Acad. Sci USA,* 92(1), 254-257, ISSN 0027-8424

Gottlieb, A. A. & Shwartz, R. H. (1972) Antigen-RNA interactions. *Cell Immunol.,* 5(2), 341-362, ISSN 0008-8749

Grusby, M. J.; Mitchell, S. C.; Nabavi, N.; & Glimcher, L. H. (1990) Casein expression in cytotoxic T lymphocytes. *Proc. Natl. Acad. Sci. USA,* 87(17), 6897-6901, ISSN 0027-8424

Fauci, A. S., Braunwald, E., Kasper, D. L., Hauser, S. L., Longo, D. L., Jameson, J. L. & Loscalzo, J. (2008). *Harrison's Principles of Internal Medicine,* 17th Edition. McGraw-Hill Professional, ISBN 0071466339 / 9780071466332, USA

Fey, H.; Butler, R. & Marti, F. (1973). The production in the pregnant cow of anti-human immunoglobulin to be used for the antiglobulin test. *Vox. Sang.,* 25(3), 245-253, ISSN 0042-9007

Hanson, C. V.; Nishiyama, Y. & Paul, S. (2005). Catalytic antibodies and their applications. *Curr. Opin. Biotechnol.,* 16(6), 631-636, ISSN 0958-1669

Hentati, B.; Sato, M. N.; Payelle, B.; Avrameas, S. & Ternynck, T. (1994). Beneficial effect of polyclonal immunoglobulins from malaria-infected BALB/c mice on the lupus-like syndrome of (NZB x NZW)F1 mice. *Eur. J. Immunol.,* 24(1), 8-15, ISSN 0014-2980

Hhachn B. Ch. (1996). Systemic lipus erythematosus. In: *Internal diseases,* E.E. Braunvald, K.D., Isselbakher, R.G. Petersdorf, D. D. Wilson, D.B. Martin & A.S. Fauchi (Eds.), 407-419, Moscow: Medicine.

Horl, W.H.; Wanner, C. & Schollmer, P. (1987). Proteinases in catabolism and malnutrition. *JPEN J. Parenter. Enteral. Nutr.* 11(5 Suppl), 98S-103S, ISSN 0148-6071

Ikeda, R.; Takasaki, Y.; Hirokawa, K.; Takeuchi, K. & Hashimoto, H. (2003). Clinical significance of antibodies to TS1-RNA in patients with mixed connective tissue disease. *J. Rheumatol.*, 30(5), 998-1005, ISSN 0315-162X

Ikehara, S.; Kawamura, M. & Takao, F. (1990). Organ-specific and systemic autoimmune diseases originate from defects in hematopoietic stem cells. *Proc. Natl. Acad. Sci. USA,* 87(21), 8341-8344, ISSN 0027-8424

Ivanen, D. R.; Kulminskaya, A. A.; Eneyskaya, E. V.; Ershova N. A.; Shabalin, K. A.; Savel'ev, A. N.; Kanyshkova, T. G.; Buneva V. N.; Nevinsky G. A. & Neustroev, K. N. (2002) Human autoantibodies with amylolytic activity. *Biologia (Bratislava), 57*(suppl. 11), 253-260.

Ivanen, D. R.; Kulminskaya, A. A.; Shabalin, K. A.; Isaeva-Ivanova, L. V.; Ershova N. A.; Saveliev, A. N.; Nevinsky, G. A.; & Neustroev, K. N. (2004). Catalytic properties of IgMs with amylolytic activity isolated from patients with multiple sclerosis. *Med. Sci. Monit.*, 10(8), BR273-BR280, ISSN 1234-1010

Janda, K. D.; Lo, L. C.; Lo, C. H.; Sim, M. M.; Wang, R.; Wong, C. H. & Lerner, R. A. (1997). Chemical selection for catalysis in combinatorial antibody libraries. *Science,* 275(5302), 945-948, ISSN 0036-8075

Jerne, N. K. (1974) Towards a network theory of the immune system. *Ann. Immunol. (Paris),* 125C(1-2), 373-389.

Li, L.; Paul, S.; Tyutyulkova, S.; Kazatchkine, M. D. & Kaveri, S. (1995). Catalytic activity of anti-thyroglobulin antibodies. *J. Immunol.,* 154(7), 3328-3332, ISSN 0022-1767

Kalaga, R., Li, L., O'Dell, J. R., & Paul, S. (1995). Unexpected presence of polyreactive catalytic antibodies in IgG from unimmunized donors and decreased levels in rheumatoid arthritis. *J. Immunol.,* 155(5), 2695-2702, ISSN 0022-1767

Kanyshkova, T. G.; Semenov, D. V.; Khlimankov, D.; Buneva, V. N. & Nevinsky, G. A. (1997) DNA-hydrolyzing activity of the light chain of IgG antibodies from milk of healthy human mothers. *FEBS Lett..* 416(1), 23-26, ISSN 0014-5793

Karataeva, N. A.; Gorbunov, D.; Prokudin, I. V.; Buneva, V. N.; Kulminskaya, A. A.; Neustroev, K. N. & Nevinsky, G. A. (2006[a]). Human milk antibodies with polysaccharide kinase activity. *Immunol. Lett.,* 103(1), 58-67, ISSN 0165-2478

Karataeva, N. A.; Buneva, V. N. & Nevinsky, G. A. (2006[b]) Polysaccharide kinase activity of human milk IgG antibodies. *Biochemistry (Mosc.),* 71(11), 1207-1221, ISSN 0006-2979

Keinan E.E. (Ed.), (2005). *Catalytic antibodies,* Wiley VCH Verlag GmbH and Co. KgaA, ISBN 3-527-30688-9, Morlenbach, Germany

Kim, J. S.; Lee, S. Y.; Lee, W. R.; Sohn, J. N.; Chung, Y. C.; Shim, H. K.; Lee, S. C.; Kwon, M. H. & Kim, Y. S. (2006). Heavy and light chain variable single domains of an anti-DNA binding antibody hydrolyze both double- and single-stranded DNAs without sequence specificity. *J. Biol. Chem.,* 281(22), 15287-15295, ISSN 0021-9258

Kozyr, A. V.; Kolesnikov, A. V.; Aleksandrova, E. S.; Sashchenko, L. P.; Gnuchev, N. V.; Favorov, P. V.; Kotelnikov, M. A.; Iakhnina, E. I.; Astsaturov, I. A.; Prokaeva, T. B.; Alekberova, Z. S.; Suchkov, S. V. & Gabibov, A. G. (1998). Novel functional activities of anti-DNA autoantibodies from sera of patients with lymphoproliferative and autoimmune diseases. *Appl. Biochem. Biotechnol.*, 75(1), 45-61, ISSN 0273-2289

Krasnorutskii, M. A.; Buneva, V. N. & Nevinsky, G. A. (2008[a]). Antibodies against DNA hydrolyze DNA and RNA. *Biochemistry (Moscow)*, 73(11), 1547-1560, ISSN 0006-2979

Krasnorutskii, M. A.; Buneva, V. N. & Nevinsky, G. A. (2008[b]). Antibodies against RNA hydrolyze RNA and DNA. *J. Mol. Recognit.*, 21(5), 337–346, ISSN 0952-3499

Krasnorutskii, M. A.; Buneva, V. N. & Nevinsky, G. A. (2008[c]). Immunization of rabbits with DNase I produces polyclonal antibodies with DNase and RNase activities. *J. Mol. Recognit.*, 21(4), 233–242, ISSN 0952-3499

Krasnorutskii, M. A.; Buneva, V. N. & Nevinsky, G. A. (2008[d]) Anti-RNase Antibodies against pancreatic ribonuclease A

hydrolyze RNA and DNA. *Int. Immunol.*, 20(8), 1031-1040, ISSN 0953-8178

Krasnorutskii, M. A.; Buneva, V. N. & Nevinsky, G. A. (2009). Immunization of rabbits with DNase II leads to formation of polyclonal antibodies with DNase and RNase activities. *Int. Immunol.*, 21(4), 349-360, ISSN 0953-8178

Kuznetsova, I. A.; Orlovskaya, I. A.; Buneva, V. N. & Nevinsky, G. A. (2007). Activation of DNA-hydrolyzing antibodies from the sera of autoimmune-prone MRL-lpr/lpr mice by different metal ions. *Biochim. Biophys. Acta*, 1774(7), 884-896, ISSN 1570-9639

Lacroix-Desmazes, S.; Moreau, A.; Sooryanarayana; Bonnemain, C.; Stieltjes, N.; Pashov, A.; Sultan, Y.; Hoebeke, J.; Kazatchkine, M. D. & Kaveri, S. V. (1999). Catalytic activity of antibodies against factor VIII in patients with hemophilia A. *Nat. Med.*, 5(9), 1044-1047, ISSN 1078-8956

Lacroix-Desmazes, S.; Bayry, J.; Kaveri, S.V.; Hayon-Sonsino, D.; Thorenoor, N.; Charpentier, J.; Luyt, C.E.; Mira, J. P.; Nagaraja, V.; Kazatchkine, M. D.; Dhainaut, J. F. & Mallet, V. O. (2005). High levels of catalytic antibodies correlate with favorable outcome in sepsis. *Proc. Natl. Acad. Sci. USA*, 102(11) 4109-4113, ISSN 0027-8424

Legostaeva, G. A.; Polosukhina, D. I.; Bezuglova, A. M.; Doronin, B. M.; Buneva, V. N. & Nevinsky, G. A. (2010) Affinity and catalytic heterogeneity of polyclonal myelin basic protein-hydrolyzing IgGs from sera of patients with multiple sclerosis. *J. Cell Mol. Med.*, 14(3), 699–709, ISSN 1582-1838

Li, L.; Paul, S.; Tyutyulkova, S.; Kazatchkine, M. D. & Kaveri, S. (1995). Catalytic activity of anti-thyroglobulin antibodies. *J. Immunol.*, 154(7), 3328-3332, ISSN 0022-1767

Martin, A. B. & Schultz, P. G. (1999). Opportunities at the interface of chemistry and biology. *Trends Cell Biol.*, 9(12), 24-28, ISSN 0962-8924

Matsiota-Bernard, P.; Mahana, W.; Avrameas, S. & Nauciel, C. (1993). Specific and natural antibody production during *Salmonella typhimurium* infection in genetically susceptible and resistant mice. *Immunology*, 79(3), 375-380, ISSN 0019-2805

Matsiota-Bernard, P.; Hentati, B.; Pie, S.; Legakis, N.; Nauciel, C. & Avrameas, S. (1996) Beneficial effect of *Salmonella typhimurium* infection and of immunoglobulins from *S. typhimurium*-infected mice on the autoimmune disease of (NZB x NZW) F1 mice. *Clin. Exp. Immunol.*, 104(2), 228-235, ISSN 0009-9104

Mestecky, J. & McGhee, J. R. (1987) Immunoglobulin A (IgA): molecular and cellular interactions involved in IgA biosynthesis and immune response. *Adv. Immunol.*, 40, 153-245, ISSN 0065-2776

Mitsuhashi, S.; Saito, R.; Kurashige, S. & Yamashugi, N. (1978) Ribonucleic acid in the immune response. *Moll. Cell. Biochem.* 20(3), 131-147, ISSN 0300-8177

Nagata, S. & Suda, T. (1995). Fas and Fas ligand: *lpr* and *gld* mutations. *Immunol. Today,* 16(1), 39–43.

Nevinsky, G. A.; Kit, Y. Y.; Semenov, D. V.; Khlimankov, D. Y. & Buneva, V. N. (1998). Secretory immunoglobulin A from human milk catalyzes milk protein phosphorylation. *Appl. Biochem. Biotechnol.,* 75(1), 77-91, ISSN 0273-2289

Nevinsky, G. A.; Semenov, D. V. & Buneva, V. N. (2000[a]) Catalytic antibodies (abzymes) induced by stable transition-state analogs. *Biochemistry (Moscow), 65*(11), 1233-1244, ISSN 0006-2979

Nevinsky, G. A.; Kanyshkova, T. G. & Buneva, V. N. (2000[b]) Natural catalytic antibodies (abzymes) in normalcy and pathology. *Biochemistry (Mosc),* 65(11), 1245-1255, ISSN 0006-2979

Nevinsky, G. A.; Kanyshkova, T. G.; Semenov, D. V.; Vlassov, A. V.; Gal'vita, A. V. & Buneva, V. N. (2000[c]). Secretory immunoglobulin A from healthy human mothers' milk catalyzes nucleic acid hydrolysis. *Appl. Biochem. Biotechnol.,* 83(1-3), 115-129, ISSN 0273-2289

Nevinsky, G. A.; Breusov, A. A.; Baranovskii, A. G.; Prints, A. V.; Kanyshkova, T. G.; Galvita, A. V.; Naumov, V. A. & Buneva, V. N. (2001). Effect of different drugs on the level of DNA-hydrolyzing polyclonal IgG antibodies in sera of patients with Hashimoto's thyroiditis and nontoxic nodal goiter. *Med. Sci. Monit.,* 7(2), 201-211, ISSN 1234-1010

Nevinsky, G. A. & Buneva, V. N. (2002[a]). Human catalytic RNA- and DNA-hydrolyzing antibodies. *J. Immunol. Methods* 269(1-2), 235-249, ISSN 0022-1759

Nevinsky, G.A.; Favorova, O.O. & Buneva, V.N. (2002[b]). *Catalytic* antibodies: New characters in the protein repertoire. In:*Protein-protein interactions. A molecular cloning manual.* E. Golemis, (Ed.), 523-534, Cold Spring Harbor, NY

Nevinsky, G.A. & Buneva, V.N. (2003). Catalytic antibodies in healthy humans and patients with autoimmune and viral pathologies. *J. Cell. Mol. Med.,* 7(3), 265-276, ISSN 1582-1838

Nevinsky, G.A. & Buneva, V.N. (2005). Natural catalytic antibodies-abzymes. In: *Catalytic antibodies.* E. Keinan, (Ed.), 503-567, VCH-Wiley press, ISBN 3-527-30688-9, Morlenbach, Germany

Nevinsky, G. A. & Buneva, V. N. (2010[a]). Natural catalytic antibodies in norm, autoimmune, viral, and bacterial diseases. *ScientificWorldJournal,* 10, 1203-1233, ISSN 1537-744X

Nevinsky GA. (2010[b]). Natural catalytic antibodies in norm and in autoimmune diseases. In: *Autoimmune Diseases: Symptoms, Diagnosis and Treatment,* K. J. Brenner, (Ed), 1-107, Nova Science Publishers, Inc., ISBN 9781616680077, USA

Nilsen, B. M.; Haugan, I. R.; Berg K.; Olsen L.; Brown P. O. & Helland D. E. (1996). Monoclonal antibodies against human immunodeficiency virus type 1 integrase: epitope mapping and differential effects on integrase activities in vitro. *J. Virology,* 70(3), 1580-1587, ISSN 0022-538X

Nishi, Y. (2002). Evolution of catalytic antibody repertoire in autoimmune mice. *J. Immunol. Methods,* 269(1-2), 213-233, ISSN 0022-1759

Nishi, Y. (2003). Enzyme/abzyme prodrug activation systems: potential use in clinical oncology. *Curr. Pharm. Des.,* 9(26), 2113-2130, ISSN 1381-6128

Odintsova, E .S.; Buneva, V. N. & Nevinsky, G. A. (2005). Casein-hydrolyzing activity of sIgA antibodies from human milk. *J. Mol. Recognit.*, 18(5) 413-421, ISSN 0952-3499

Odintsova, E. S.; Kharitonova, M. A.; Baranovskii, A. G.; Siziakina, L. P.; Buneva, V. N. & Nevinskii, G. A. (2006[a]). DNA-hydrolyzing IgG antibodies from the blood of patients with acquired immune deficiency syndrome. *Mol. Biol. (Moscow)*, 40(5), 857-864, ISSN 0026-8933

Odintsova, E. S.; Kharitonova, M. A.; Baranovskii, A. G.; Siziakina, L. P.; Buneva, V. N. & Nevinskii, G. A. (2006[b]). Proteolytic activity of IgG antibodies from blood of acquired immunodeficiency syndrome patients. *Biochemistry (Mosc)*, 71(3), 251-261, ISSN 0006-2979

Odintsova, E. S.; Zaksas, N. P.; Buneva, V. N. & Nevinsky, G. A. (2011). Metal dependent hydrolysis of β-casein by sIgA antibodies from human milk. *J. Mol. Recognit.*, 24(1), 45-59, ISSN 0952-3499

Parkhomenko, T. A.; Odintsova, E. S.; Buneva, V. N.; Kunder, E. V.; Zhyltsov, I. V.; Senkovich, S. A.; Generalov, I. I. & Nevinsky, G. A. (2009). DNA-hydrolyzing activity of IgG antibodies from the sera of patients with diseases caused by different bacterial infections. *J. Cell. Mol. Med.*, 13(9A), 2875-2887, ISSN 1582-1838

Parkhomenko, T. A.; Buneva, V. N.; Tyshkevich, O. B.; Generalov, I. I.; Doronin, B. M. & Nevinsky, G. A. (2010). DNA-hydrolyzing activity of IgG antibodies from the sera of patients with tick-borne encephalitis. *Biochimie*, 92(5), 545-554, ISSN 0300-9084

Parkhomenko, T.A.; Legostaeva, G.A.; Doronin, B.M.; Buneva, V.N. & Nevinsky, G.A. (2010). IgGs containing light chains of the lambda and kappa type and of all subclasses (IgG1-IgG4) from sera of patients with multiple sclerosis hydrolyze DNA. *J. Mol. Recognit.*, 23(5), 486-494, ISSN 0952-3499

Paul, S.; Volle, D. J.; Beach, C. M.; Johnson, D. R.; Powell, M. J. & Massey, R. J. (1989). Catalytic hydrolysis of vasoactive intestinal peptide by human autoantibody. *Science*, 244(4909), 1158-1162, ISSN 0036-8075

Paul, S.; Li, L.; Kalaga, R.; Wilkins-Stevens, P.; Stevens, F. J. & Solomon, A. (1995). Natural catalytic antibodies: peptide-hydrolyzing activities of Bence Jones proteins and VL fragment. *J. Biol. Chem.*, 270(25), 15257-15261, ISSN 0021-9258

Paul, S.; Li, L.; Kalaga, R.; O'Dell, J.; Dannenbring, R. E. Jr.; Swindells, S.; Hinrichs, S.; Caturegli, P. & Rose, N. R. (1997). Chacterization of thyroglobulin-directed and polyreactive catalytic antibodies in autoimmune disease. *J. Immunol.*, 159(3), 1530-1536, ISSN 0022-1767

Paul, S.; Nishiyama, Y.; Planque, S. & Tagushi, H. (2006). Theory of proteolytic antibody occurrence. *Immunol Lett.*, 103(1), 8-16, ISSN 0165-2478

Pauling, L. (1946). Molecular basis of biological specificity. *Chem. Eng. News*, 24, 13751-13777.

Pollack, S. J.; Jacobs, J. W.; & Schultz, P. G. (1986). Selective chemical catalysis by an antibody. *Science*, 234(4783), 1570-1573, ISSN 0036-8075

Pisetsky, D. (2001). Immune response to DNA in systemic lupus erythematosus. *Isr. Med. Ass. J.*, 39, 850-853.

Planque, S.; Nishiyama, Y.; Taguchi, H.; Salas, M.; Hanson, C. & Paul, S. (2008). Catalytic antibodies to HIV: physiological role and potential clinical utility. *Autoimmun. Rev.*, 7(6), 473-479, ISSN 1568-9972

Polosukhina, D. I.; Kanyshkova, T. G.; Doronin, B. M.; Tyshkevich, O. B.; Buneva, V. N.; Boiko, A. N.; Gusev, E. I.; Favorova, O. O. & Nevinsky, G. A. (2004). Hydrolysis of myelin basic protein by polyclonal catalytic IgGs from the sera of patients with multiple sclerosis. *J. Cell Mol. Med.*, 8(3), 359-368, ISSN 1582-1838

Polosukhina, D. I.; Buneva, V. N.; Doronin, B. M.; Tyshkevich, O. B.; Boiko, A. N.; Gusev, E. I.; Favorova, O. O. & Nevinsky, G. A. (2005). Hydrolysis of myelin basic protein by IgM and IgA antibodies from the sera of patients with multiple sclerosis. *Med. Sci. Monit.*, 11(8), BR266- BR272, ISSN 1234-1010

Polosukhina, D. I.; Buneva, V. N.; Doronin, B. M.; Tyshkevich, O. B.; Boiko, A. N.; Gusev, E. I.; Favorova, O. O. & Nevinsky, G. A. (2006). Metal-dependent hydrolysis of myelin basic protein by IgGs from the sera of patients with multiple sclerosis. *Immunol. Lett.*, 103(1), 75-81, ISSN 0165-2478

Rao, M. B.; Tanksale, A. M.; Ghatge, M. S. & Deshhange, V. V. (1998). Molecular and biotechnological aspects of microbial proteases. *Microbiol. Mol. Biol Rev.*, 62(3), 597-635.

Raptis, L. & Menard, H. A. (1980). Quantitation and characterization of plasma DNA in normals and patients with systemic lupus erythematosus. *J. Clin. Invest.*, 66(6), 1391-1399.

Sun, M.; Li, L.; Gao, Q. S. & Paul, S. (1994). Antigen recognition by an antibody light chain. *J. Biol. Chem.*, 269(1), 734-738, ISSN 0021-9258

Sun, M.; Gao, Q. S.; Kirnarskiy, L.; Rees, A. & Paul, S. (1997). Cleavage specificity of a proteolytic antibody light chain and effects of the heavy chain variable domain. *J. Mol. Biol.*, 271(3), 374-385, ISSN 0022-2836

Sato, T.; Uvhiumi, T.; Arakawa, M. & Kominami, R. (1994) Serological association of lupus autoantibodies to a limited functional domain of 28S ribosomal RNA and to the ribosomal proteins bound to the domain. *Clin. Exp. Immunol.*, 98(1), 35-39, ISSN 0009-9104

Savel'ev, A. N.; Kanyshkova, T. G.; Kulminskaya, A. A.; Buneva, V. N.; Eneyskaya, E. V.; Filatov, M. V.; Nevinsky, G. A. & Neustroev, K. N. (2001). Amylolytic activity of IgG and sIgA immunoglobulins from human milk. *Clin. Chim. Acta,* 314(1-2), 141-152.

Savel'iev, A. N.; Ivanen, D. R.; Kulminskaya, A. A.; Ershova, N. A.; Kanyshkova, T. G.; Buneva, V. N.; Mogelnitskii, A. S.; Doronin, B. M.; Favorova, O. O.; Nevinsky, G. A. & Neustroev, K. (2003). Amylolytic activity of IgM and IgG antibodies from patients with multiple sclerosis. *Immunol. Lett.*, 86(3), 291-297, ISSN 0165-2478

Schochetman, G. & Massey, R. (1985). International Patent no. W085/02414.

Semenov, D. V.; Kanyshkova, T. G.; Karotaeva, N. A.; Krasnorutskii, M. A.; Kuznetsova, I. A.; Buneva, V. N. & Nevinsky, G. A. (2004). Catalytic nucleotide-hydrolyzing antibodies in milk and serum of clinically healthy human mothers. *Med. Sci. Monit.*, 10(2), BR23-BR33, ISSN 1234-1010

Shoenfeld, Y.; Ben-Yehuda, O.; Messinger, Y.; Bentwitch, Z.; Rauch, J.; Isenberg, D. I. & Gadoth, N. (1988) Autoimmune diseases other than lupus share common anti-DNA idiotypes. *Immunol. Lett.*, 17(3), 285-291, ISSN 0165-2478

Shoenfeld, Y.; Teplizki, H. A.; Mendlovic, S.; Blank, M.; Mozes, E. & Isenberg, D. A. (1989). The role of the human anti-DNA idiotype 16/6 in autoimmunity. *Clin. Immunol. Immunopathol.*, 51(3), 313-325.

Shuster, A. M.; Gololobov, G. V.; Kvashuk, O. A.; Bogomolova, A. E.; Smirnov, I. V. & Gabibov, A. G. (1992). DNA hydrolyzing autoantibodies. *Science,* 256(5057), 665-667, ISSN 0036-8075

Steinman, L. (2001). Multiple sclerosis: a two-stage disease. *Nat. Immunol.*, 2(9), 2762-2764, ISSN 1529-2908

Stockwin, L. H. & Holmes, S. (2003). Antibodies as therapeutic agents: vive la renaissance! *Expert. Opin. Biol. Ther.*, 3(7), 1133-1152, ISSN 1471-2598

Sugiama, Y. & Yamamota, T. (1996). Characterization of serum anti-phospholipid antibodies in patients with multiple sclerosis. *Tohoku J. Exp. Med.*, 178, 203-215, ISSN 10040-8727

Suzuki, H. (1994). Recent advances in abzyme studies. *J. Biochem. (Tokyo),* 115(4), 623-628.

Tanaka, A.; Lindor, K.; Ansari, A. & Gershwin, M. E. (2000). Fetal microchimerisms in the mother: immunologic implications. *Liver Transpl.*, 6(2) 138-143, ISSN 1527-6465

Tanaka, F. (2002). Catalytic antibodies as designer proteases and esterases. *Chem. Rev.*, 102(12), 4885-4906, ISSN 0009-2665

Tanaka, F. & Barbas, C. F., 3rd. (2002). Reactive immunization: a unique approach to catalytic antibodies. *J. Immunol. Methods,* 269(1-2), 67-79, ISSN 0022-1759

Tawfik, D. S.; Chap, R.; Green, B. S.; Sela, M. & Eshhar, Z. (2002). Unexpectedly high occurrence of catalytic antibodies in MRL/lpr and SJL mice immunized with a transition-state analog: is there a linkage to autoimmunity? *Proc. Natl. Acad. Sci. USA*, 92, 2145-2149, ISSN 0027-8424

Tellier, C. (2002). Exploiting antibodies as catalysts: potential therapeutic applications. *Transfus. Clin. Biol.*, 9(1), 1-8, ISSN 1246-7820

Ternynck, P., Falanga, B., Unterkircher, C., Gregoire. J., Da Silva, L. P. & Avrameas S. (1991). Induction of high levels of IgG autoantibodies in mice infected with *Plasmodium chabaudi*. *Int. Immunol.*, 3, 29-37, ISSN 0953-8178

Thayer, M. M.; Olender, E. H.; Arvai, A. S.; Koike, C. K.; Canestrelli, I. L.; Stewart, J. D.; Benkovic, S. J.; Getzoff, E. D. & Roberts, V. A. (1999). Structural basis for amide hydrolysis catalyzed by the 43C9 antibody. *J. Mol. Biol.,* 291(2), 329-345, ISSN 0022-2836

Thiagarajan, P.; Dannenbring, R.; Matsuura, K.; Tramontano, A.; Gololobov, G. & Paul, S. (2000). Monoclonal antibody light chain with prothrombinase activity. *Biochemistry,* 39(21), 6459-6465, ISSN 0006-2960

Tramontano, A.; Janda, K. D. & Lerner, R. A. (1986[a]). Catalytic antibodies. *Science,* 234(4783), 1566-1570, ISSN 0036-8075

Tramontano, A.; Janda, K. D. & Lerner, R. A. (1986[b]). Chemical reactivity at an antibody binding site elicited by mechanistic design of a synthetic antigen. *Proc. Natl. Acad. Sci. USA,* 83(18), 6736-6740, ISSN 0027-84Tyutyulkova, S.; Gao, Q. S.; Thompson, A.; Rennard, S. & Paul, S. (1996). Efficient vasoactive intestinal polypeptide hydrolyzing autoantibody light selected by phage display. *Biochim. Biophys. Acta,* 1316(3), 217-223, ISSN 1570-9639

Vlasov, A. V.; Baranovskii, A. G.; Kanyshkova, T. G.; Prints, A. V.; Zabara, V. G.; Naumov, V. A.; Breusov, A. A.; Giege R.; Buneva, V. N. & Nevinskii, G. A. (1998). Substrate specificity of serum DNA- and RNA-hydrolyzing antibodies of patients with polyarthritis and autoimmune thyroiditis. *Mol. Biol. (Mosk),* 32(3), 559-569, ISSN 0026-8933

Vlasov, A. V.; Helm, M.; Naumov, V. A.; Breusov, A. A.; Buneva, V. N.; Florentz, C.; Giege, R. & Nevinskii, G. A. (1999). Features of tRNA hydrolysis by autoantibodies from blood serum of patients with certain autoimmune and virus diseases. *Mol. Biol. (Moscow)*, 33(5), 866-872, ISSN 0026-8933

Vlassov, A.; Florentz, C.; Helm, M.; Naumov, V.; Buneva, V.; Nevinsky, G. & Giege, R. (1998). Characterization and selectivity of catalytic antibodies from human serum with RNAse activity, *Nucleic Acid Res.*, 26(3), 5243-5250, ISSN 0305-1048

Watanabe-Fukunaga, R.; Brannan, C. I. & Copeland, N. G. (1992). Lymphoproliferation disorder in mice explained by defects in Fas antigen that mediates apoptosis. *Nature*, 356(6367), 314-317, ISSN 0968-0004

Wentworth, P. Jr.; Liu, Y.; Wentworth, A. D.; Fan, P.; Foley, M. J. & Janda, K. D. (1998). A bait and switch hapten strategy generates catalytic antibodies for phosphodiester hydrolysis. *Proc. Natl. Acad. Sci. USA*, 95(11), 5971-5975, ISSN 0027-8424

Wlodawer, A. (1999). Crystal structures of catalytic core domains of retroviral integrases and role of divalent cations in enzymatic activity, *Adv.Virus. Res.*, 52, 335-350, ISSN 0065-3527

Wójcik, T. & Kieć-Kononowicz, K. (2008). Catalytic activity of certain antibodies as a potential tool for drug synthesis and for directed prodrug therapies. *Curr. Med. Chem.*, 15(16), 1606-1615, ISSN 0929-8673

Yi, J.; Arthur, J. W.; Dunbrack, R. L.; Jr. & Skalka A. M. (2000). An inhibitory monoclonal antibody binds at the turn of the helix-turn-helix motif in the N-terminal domain of HIV-1 integrase. *J. Biol. Chem.*, 275(49), 38739-38748, ISSN 0021-9258

Zandman-Goddard, G.; Shoenfeld, Y. (2002). HIV and autoimmunity. *Autoimmun. Rev.*, 1(6), 329-337, ISSN 1568-9972

Zhou, Y. X.; Karle, S.; Taguchi, H.; Planque, S.; Nishiyama, Y. & Paul, S. (2002). Prospects for immunotherapeutic proteolytic antibodies. *J. Immunol. Methods*, 269(1-2), 257-268, ISSN 0022-1759

Zouali, M. (2001). B cell tolerance to self in systemic autoimmunity. *Arch. Immunol. Ther. Exp. (Warsz)*, 49(5), 361-365, ISSN 0004-069X

11

Exponential Equilibria and Uniform Boundedness of HIV Infection Model

E. Castellanos-Velasco[1] and J. Santos-Ferreira[2]
[1]*Facultad de Ciencias, Electrónica, Universidad Autónoma de San Luis Potosí, San Luis Potosí, S.L.P.*
[2]*Centro Universitário do Leste de Minas Gerais, Campus Coronel Fabriciano-M.G., Programa de Mestrado em Engenharia Industrial, Minas Gerais*
[1]*Mexico*
[2]*Brasil*

1. Introduction

According to data and statistics in a global summary of the Acquired immune deficiency syndrome (AIDS) epidemic from The World Health Organization (WHO), by the end of 2007 an estimated 33 million people worldwide were living with human immunodeficiency virus, HIV. That same year, some 2 million died of AIDS, and the number of people receiving antiretroviral therapy (ART) was reported in 2.990.000, while an estimated of about 9.700.000 the people needing ART. In other words, globally, less than one person in five at risk of HIV has access to basic HIV prevention services. The same study indicates a total 31% as the ART coverage at that same period (WHO, 2007).

Highly Active Antiretroviral Therapy (HAART) has demonstrated to be effective at slowing the progression of (HIV) infection to Acquired immune deficiency syndrome (AIDS) and, subsequently, to improve quality of life for infected people. However, if on the one hand the cocktail of drugs has been making possible to extend patient's lives, on the other hand the many problems associated with it and its high cost, particularly to poor people are a clear indication that new approaches to address the situation are needed. Most efforts to control HIV replication has been focused on developing and optimizing antiretroviral therapies.

The immune system of human beings contains different types of cells that help protect the body from infections. One of these types of specialized cells are called Cluster of Differentiation Antigen 4 (CD4) or T-cells, by the fact that CD4 is a glycoprotein predominantly found on the surface of helper T cells. The Human Immunodeficiency Virus (HIV) is a retrovirus and therefore it needs cells from a host so that it can make copies of itself. The CD4 cells are receptors for HIV and they aid the virus to initiate its replication process by enabling it to enter into its host. HIV is essentially considered as an infection of the immune in the sense that this virus infects and damages CD4 during the virus replication process. The more virus is produced by infected cells, the higher is the viral load and consequently, lower will be the number of functioning CD4 cells. When this number of uninfected cells declines below a critical value, the immune system is seriously deteriorated by HIV.

In section 2, it is shown the theoretical reference used to analyze the asymptotic behavior of the solution to the nonlinear perturbed system. The analysis concerning the origin, x=0 as a stable equilibrium point. On the other hand, the functions that represent the perturbation have the nonlinear dynamic and the function that force the localization of equilibrium point. That function allows to characterize the behavior of the trajectory around origin, x=0. In section 3 are analyzed the properties of the equilibrium in the origin that corresponds to the infected state and the asymptotic behavior of the solution to the model of 3 EDO presented by (Barao & Lemos, 2007; Perelson & Nelson, 1999; Santos & Middleton, 2008). The model is used to characterize the dynamic infection of the disease. In the last section are made some conclusions about exponential equilibrium and uniform boundedness of the model solution.

2. Perturbed system

Consider the following perturbed system

$$\dot{x} = h(t, x), \tag{1}$$

where $h : [0, \infty) \times D \to R^n$ is continuous and t is locally Lipschitz in x on domain $D \subset R^n$, and D is an open connected set that contains the origin $x = 0$. Now, consider the right-hand side of (1), then by adding and subtracting $f(x)$ known as the nominal system around the origin, we can rewrite the right-hand side as

$$h(t, x) = f(x) + [h(t, x) - f(x)],$$

and define

$$g(x) + d(t) = h(t, x) - f(x),$$

Hence, the perturbed system (1) can be written as

$$\begin{aligned} \dot{x} &= h(t, x) = f(x) + g(x) + d(t) \\ \dot{x} &= e(x) + d(t), \end{aligned} \tag{2}$$

where $f : D \to R^n$ and $g : D \to R^n$ are locally Lipschitz in x on domain $D \subset R^n$, $d(t)$ is a uniformly bounded disturbance that satisfies $|d(t)| \leq \delta$ for all $t \geq 0$ and $e(x) = f(x) + g(x)$. The nominal system in $f(x)$ could have a stable or asymptotically stable equilibrium point at the origin. The approach of the Lyapunov method will allow us to draw conclusions about the system when the nominal system is perturbed, whether such perturbation is an autonomous or a non autonomous perturbation respectively.

2.1 Nonlinear autonomous perturbation

Consider the autonomous system

$$\dot{x} = h(x), \tag{3}$$

where $h : D \to R^n$ is locally Lipschitz map from a domain $D \subset R^n$.
Suppose $\tilde{x} \in D$ is an equilibrium point of (3), that is $h(\tilde{x}) = 0$. The aim is to characterize the stability for the case when the equilibrium point is at the origin, that is $\tilde{x} = 0$. For autonomous system, there is a convergence of the trajectory to a set, the same as the asymptotic stability of the origin. A major concern in analysing the stability of dynamical system is the robustness of various stability properties to uncertainties in the system's model. In the following, it is introduced the stability definition.

Definition 1. *The equilibrium point $x = 0$ of (3) is*

- *Stable, if for each $\varepsilon > 0$, there is $\delta = \delta(\varepsilon) \geq 0$ such that*

$$\|x(0)\| < \delta \Rightarrow \|x(t)\| < \varepsilon, \ \ \forall t \geq 0.$$

- *Unstable, if not stable.*
- *Asymptotically stable if it is stable and $\delta > 0$ can be chosen such that*

$$\|x(0)\| < \delta \Rightarrow \lim_{t\to\infty} x(t) = 0.$$

Let $V : D \to R$ be a differentiable function defined in a domain $D \subset R^n$ that contains the origin. The derivative of $V(x)$ along the trajectories of (3), denoted by $\dot{V}(x)$, is given by

$$\dot{V}(x) = \sum_{i=1}^{n} \frac{\partial V}{\partial x_i}\dot{x}_i = \sum_{i=1}^{n} \frac{\partial V}{\partial x_i}h_i(x). \tag{4}$$

The function $\dot{V}(x)$ is dependent on the system's equation. Hence, if $\dot{V}(x)$ is negative, $V(x)$ will decrease along the solution of (3). The following lemma (Khalil, 2002) states Lyapunov's stability sense.

Lemma 1. *Let $x = 0$ be an equilibrium point for (3). Let $V : D \to R$ be a continuously differentiable function on a neighbourhood D of $x = 0$, such that*

$$\begin{aligned} V(0) = 0 \ \ and \ \ V(x) > 0 \ \ in \ D - \{0\}, \\ \dot{V}(x) \leq 0 \ \ in \ D. \end{aligned} \tag{5}$$

Then, $x = 0$ is stable. Moreover, if

$$\dot{V}(x) < 0 \ \ in \ D - \{0\}. \tag{6}$$

Then $x = 0$ is asymptotically stable.

Proof. Given $\varepsilon > 0$, choose $r \in (0, \varepsilon]$ such that

$$B_r = \{x \in R^n | \|x\| \leq r\} \subset D.$$

Let $\alpha = min_{\|x\|=r} V(x)$. Then, $\alpha > 0$ by (5). Take $\beta \in (0, \alpha)$, and let

$$\Omega_\beta = \{x \in B_r | V(x) \leq \beta\}.$$

The set Ω_β has the property that any trajectory starting in Ω_β at $t = 0$, stays in Ω_β for all $t \geq 0$. This follows from (5) since

$$\dot{V}(x(t)) \leq 0 \Rightarrow V(x(t)) \leq V(x(0)) \leq \beta, \ \ \forall t \geq 0.$$

Since Ω_β is a compact set (is closed and bounded since it is contained in B_r), the system in (3) has a unique solution defined for all $t \geq 0$, whenever $x(0) \in \Omega_\beta$. Since $V(x)$ is continuous and $V(0) = 0$, there is $\delta > 0$ such that

$$\|x\| \leq \delta \Rightarrow V(x) < \beta.$$

Then

$$B_\delta \subset \Omega_\beta \subset B_r,$$

and

$$x(0) \in \beta_\delta \Rightarrow x(0) \in \Omega_\beta \Rightarrow x(t) \in \Omega_\beta \Rightarrow x(t) \in B_r.$$

Therefore,

$$\|x(0)\| < \delta \Rightarrow \|x(t)\| < r \leq \varepsilon, \ \ \forall t \geq 0.$$

which shows that the equilibrium point $x = 0$ is stable. Now, to show asymptotic stability it is necessary to show that $x(t) \to 0$ as $t \to \infty$, that is, for every $a > 0$, there is $T > 0$ such that $\|x(t)\| < a$, for all $t > T$. For every $a < 0$, we can choose $b > 0$ such that $\Omega_b \subset B_a$. Therefore, it is sufficient to show that $V(x(t)) \to 0$ as $t \to \infty$. Since $V(x)$ is monotonically decreasing and bounded from below by zero,

$$V(x(t)) \to c \geq 0 \ \ as \ \ t \to \infty.$$

To show that $c = 0$, suppose by contradiction $c > 0$. By continuity of $V(x)$, there is $d > 0$ such that $B_d \subset \Omega_c$. The limit $V(x(t)) \to c > 0$ implies that the trajectory $x(t)$ lies outside the ball $B_d \subset \Omega_c$ for all $t \geq 0$. When $\dot{V}(x)$ is integrated on t, it follows by (6) that

$$V(x(t)) = V(x(0)) + \int_0^t \dot{V}(x(\tau))d\tau \leq V(x(0)) + kt,$$

where $k = -max_{a \leq \|x\| \leq r} \dot{V}(x) < 0$. Since the right-hand side will eventually become negative, the inequality contradicts the assumption that $c > 0$. □

Remark 1. *The origin is stable if there is a continuously differentiable positive definite function $V(x)$ so that $\dot{V}(x)$ is negative semi-definite, and it is asymptotically stable if $\dot{V}(x)$ is negative definite.*

Remark 2. *The theorem's conditions are only sufficient. Failure of a Lyapunov function candidate to satisfy the conditions for stability or asymptotic stability does not mean that the equilibrium is not stable or asymptotically stable. It only means that such a stability property cannot be established by using this Lyapunov function candidate.*

For the case when the origin $x = 0$ is asymptotically stable, it is often interesting to determine how far from the origin can the trajectory be and still converges to the origin as $t \to \infty$. This gives rise to the definition of the region of attraction or basin.

Definition 2. *Let $x(t, x(0))$ be the solution of (3) that starts at initial state x_0 at time $t = 0$. Then, the region of attraction is defined as the set of all points x such that $\lim_{t\to\infty} x(t, x(0)) = 0$.*

To find the exact region of attraction analytically might be difficult or even impossible. However, Lyapunov functions can be used to estimate the region of attraction, that is, to find sets contained in the region of attraction. From the proof of Lemma 1, we say that if there is a Lyapunov function that satisfies the conditions of asymptotic stability over a domain D, and if

$$\Omega_c = \{x \in R^n | V(x) \leq c\}, \tag{7}$$

is bounded and contained in D, then every trajectory starting in Ω_c remains in Ω_c, and approaches the origin as $t \to \infty$. The set in (7) with $\dot{V}(x) \leq 0, \forall x \in \Omega_c$ is a positively invariant set, since, as we showed in the proof of Lemma 1, a solution starting in Ω_c remains in Ω_c for all $t \geq 0$. Now, it is introduced the following corollaries known as the LaSalle invariance principle and the Barbashin-Krasovskii theorem.

Corollary 1. *Let Ω_c be a compact (closed and bounded) set with the property that every solution of (3) which starts in Ω_c remains for all future time in Ω_c. Let $V : \Omega_c \to R$ be a continuously differentiable function such that $\dot{V}(x) \leq 0, \forall x \in \Omega_c$. Let E be the set of all points in Ω_c where $\dot{V}(x) = 0$. Let M be the largest invariant set in E. Then every solution starting in Ω_c approaches M as $t \to \infty$.*

Corollary 2. *Let $x = 0$ be an equilibrium point for (1). Let $V : \Omega_c \to R$ be a continuously differentiable positive definite function on a neighbourhood Ω_c of $x = 0$, such that $\dot{V}(x) \leq 0, \forall x \in \Omega_c$. Let $S = \{x \in \Omega_c | \dot{V}(x) = 0\}$, and suppose that no solution can stay forever in S, other than the trivial solution. Then, the origin $x = 0$ is asymptotically stable.*

Remark 3. *When $\dot{V}(x)$ is negative definite, $S = 0$. Then, corollary 2 coincide with lemma 1.*

With the previous stability criteria for equilibria point about the origin, it is necessary to introduce the specific analysis for autonomous perturbed system.

2.1.1 Mean value

Consider the autonomous case in (2), when $d(t) = 0$ for all $t \geq 0$. Suppose that the origin $x = 0$ is inside of D and is an equilibrium point for the nominal system $f(x)$, that is, $f(0) = 0$. By the mean value

$$f(x) = f(0) + \frac{\partial f(z)}{\partial x} x,$$

where z is a point on the line segment connecting x to the origin. The above equality is valid for any point $x \in D$ such that the line segment connecting x to the origin lies entirely in D. Since $f(0) = 0$, we can write $f(x)$ as

$$f(x) = \frac{\partial f(z)}{\partial x} x = \frac{\partial f(0)}{\partial x} x + \left[\frac{\partial f(z)}{\partial x} - \frac{\partial f(0)}{\partial x}\right] x,$$
$$f(x) = Ax + g(x),$$

where

$$A = \frac{\partial f(0)}{\partial x}, \quad and \quad g(x) = \left[\frac{\partial f(z)}{\partial x} - \frac{\partial f(0)}{\partial x}\right] x.$$

The function $g(x)$ satisfies

$$\|g(x)\|_2 \leq \left| \frac{\partial f(z)}{\partial x} - \frac{\partial f(0)}{\partial x} \right|_2 \|x\|_2 \leq k\|x\|_2,$$

for any $k > 0$, there exists $r > 0$, such that $\forall \|x\|_2 < r$. It is possible to approximate in a small neighbourhood of the origin the nonlinear system $f(x)$ by its linearization about the origin

$$\dot{(x)} = Ax, \quad where \quad A = \frac{\partial f(0)}{\partial x}. \tag{8}$$

The following corollary characterizes the stability properties of the origin.

Corollary 3. *The equilibrium point $x = 0$ of (8) is stable if and only if all eigenvalues of A satisfy $Re(\lambda_i) \leq 0$. The equilibrium point $x = 0$ is asymptotically stable if and only if all eigenvalues of A satisfy $Re(\lambda_i) < 0$. When all eigenvalues of A satisfy $Re(\lambda_i) < 0$, A is called a stability matrix or a Hurwitz matrix. The origin of (8) is asymptotically stable if and only if A is a stability matrix.*

Consider a quadratic Lyapunov function candidate

$$V(x) = x^T P x,$$

where P is a real symmetric positive definite matrix. The derivative of V along the trajectories of the linear system (8) is given by

$$\dot{V}(x) = \dot{x}^T P x + x^T P \dot{x} = x^T \left(PA + A^T P \right) x = -x^T Q x.$$

Asymptotic stability of the origin can be also investigated using Lyapunov's equation, as it is shown on corollary 4.

Corollary 4. *A matrix A is a stability matrix, that is, $Re(\lambda_i) < 0$ for all eigenvalues of A, if and only if for any given positive definite symmetric matrix Q there exists a positive definite symmetric matrix P that satisfies the Lyapunov equation*

$$PA + A^T P = -Q. \tag{9}$$

If Q is positive definite, then the origin is asymptotically stable, that is, $Re(\lambda_i) < 0$, for all eigenvalues of A. Here it follows the usual procedure of Lyapunov's method, where it choose $V(x)$ to be positive definite and then check negative definiteness of $\dot{V}(x)$.

Remark 4. *If matrix A is a stability matrix, then P is a unique solution of (9).*

The Lyapunov equation can be used to test whether or not a matrix A is a stability matrix, as an alternative to calculating the eigenvalues of A. The existence of a Lyapunov function will allow us to draw conslusions about the system when the linear term Ax is perturbed, whether such perturbation is a linear perturbation in the coefficients of A or a nonlinear autonomous perturbation. The following lemma is known as Lyapunov's indirect method or Lyapunov first method.

Lemma 2. *Let $x = 0$ be an equilibrium point for the nonlinear system*

$$\dot{x} = f(x), \tag{10}$$

where $f : D \to R^n$ is continuously differentiable and D is a neighbourhood of the origin. Let

$$A = \left. \frac{\delta f(x)}{\delta x} \right|_{x=0}.$$

Then, the origin is asymptotically stable if $Re(\lambda_i) < 0$ for all eigenvalues of A.

Proof. Let A be a stability matrix. Then, by corollary 4 it is known that for any positive definite symmetric matrix Q, the solution P of the Lyapunov equation (9) is positive definite. Consider

$$V(x) = x^T P x,$$

as a Lyapunov function candidate for the nonlinear system. The derivative of $V(x)$ along the trajectories of the system is given by

$$\dot{V}(x) = x^T P e(x) + e^T(x) P x = x^T P \left(Ax + g(x) \right) + \left(x^T A^T + g^T(x) \right) P x,$$
$$\dot{V}(x) = x^T \left(PA + A^T P \right) x + 2x^T P g(x) = -x^T Q x + 2x^T P g(x).$$

The first term on the right-hand side is negative definite, while the second term is indefinite. But the function $g(x)$ satisfies

$$\|g(x)\|_2 \leq k\|x\|_2, \quad \forall \|x\|_2 < r.$$

For any $k > 0$, there exists $r > 0$. Hence, after majorize the right-hand side

$$\dot{V}(x) \leq -x^T Qx + 2k\|P\|_2\|x\|_2^2,$$

but

$$x^T Qx \geq \lambda_{min}(Q)\|x\|_2^2,$$

where $\lambda_{min}(\cdot)$ denotes the minimum eigenvalue of a matrix. Note that $\lambda_{min}(Q)$ is real and positive since Q is symmetric and positive definite. Thus

$$\dot{V}(x) \leq -\left(\lambda_{min}(Q) - 2k\|P\|_2\|\right)\|x\|_2^2.$$

By choosing

$$k < \frac{1}{2}\frac{\lambda_{min}(Q)}{\|P\|_2},$$

ensures that $\dot{V}(x)$ is negative definite. By lemma 1, we conclude that the origin is asymptotically stable. □

2.2 Non linear non autonomous perturbation

Consider the system given in (2)

$$\dot{x} = h(t,x) = f(x) + g(x) + d(t),$$
$$\dot{x} = e(x) + d(t),$$

where $f : D \to R^n$ and $g : D \to R^n$ are locally Lipschitz in x on domain $D \subset R^n$, $d(t)$ is a uniformly bounded disturbance that satisfies $|d(t)| \leq \delta$ for all $t \geq 0$ and $e(x) = f(x) + g(x)$. The notions of stability and asymptotic stability of the equilibrium of a non autonomous system are basically the same as Definition 1 for autonomous system, see (Khalil, 2002). The difference here is that, while the solution of an autonomous system depends only on $(t - t_0)$, the solution of a non autonomous system may depend on both t and t_0. Here, in that case the function $d(t) \neq 0$ for all $t \geq 0$ about the origin.
Therefore, the stability behavior of the equilibrium point will be dependent on t_0.

Definition 3. *The equilibrium point $x = 0$ of (2) is*

- *Stable, if for each $\varepsilon > 0$, and any $t_0 \geq 0$ there is $\delta = \delta(\varepsilon, t_0) \geq 0$ such that*

$$\|x(t_0)\| < \delta \Rightarrow \|x(t)\| < \varepsilon, \quad \forall t \geq 0.$$

- *Unstable, if not stable.*
- *Asymptotically stable if it is stable and $\delta > 0$ can be chosen such that*

$$\|x(t_0)\| < \delta \Rightarrow \lim_{t\to\infty} x(t) = 0.$$

It is necessary to introduce special scalar functions that will help to characterize and study the behavior of a solution for the non autonomous system.

Definition 4. *A scalar function $w(r) \in R$ is said to be positive definite, if it is continuous and $w(r) > 0$ for $|r| > 0$ and $w(0) = 0$. The scalar function is radially unbounded if $w(r) \to \infty$ as $|r| \to \infty$.*

Definition 5. *A scalar function $u(r,s) \in R$ is said to be positive definite and decreasing, if for each fixed s, the function $u(r,s) > 0$ and $u(r,0) = 0$ is continuous with respect to r, and for each fixed r the function $u(r,s)$ is continuous and decreasing with respect to s and $u(r,s) \to 0$ as $|s| \to \infty$.*

The following corollary states some properties of positive definite functions.

Corollary 5. *Let $w_1(\cdot)$ and $w_2(\cdot)$ be positive definite functions on domain $D = \{x \in R^n, \|x\| < r\}$. Consider the following difference between scalar functions*

$$k_1 w_1(r) - k_2 w_2(\|x\|) \geq 0, \quad \text{where} \quad \|x\| < r.$$

If the leading term can be factorized, then the bound is given by

$$\|x\| \leq \gamma, \quad \text{where} \quad \gamma = w_2^{-1}[w_1(r)].$$

The following stability properties of the origin are given.

Definition 6. *The equilibrium point $x = 0$ of (2) is*

1. *Uniformly stable, if there exists a positive definite function $w(\cdot)$ and a positive constant r, independent of t_0 such that*

$$\|x(t)\| \leq w(\|x(t_0)\|), \forall t \geq t_0 > 0, \forall \|x(t_0)\| < r. \tag{11}$$

2. *Uniformly asymptotically stable, if there exist a positive definite and decreasing function $u(\cdot,\cdot)$ and a positive constant r, independent of t_0 such that*

$$\|x(t)\| \leq u(\|x(t_0)\|, t - t_0), \forall t \geq t_0 > 0, \forall \|x(t_0)\| < r. \tag{12}$$

3. *Globally uniformly asymptotically stable, if inequality (12) is satisfied for any initial state $x(t_0)$.*
4. *Exponentially stable if inequality (12) is satisfied with*

$$u(r,s) = kre^{-\alpha s}, \quad k > 0, \ \alpha > 0. \tag{13}$$

To establish uniform asymptotic stability of the origin, it is necessary to verify inequality (12) with the aid of an auxiliary scalar differential equation. The following corollary defines a scalar solution of a special equation.

Corollary 6. *Consider the scalar differential equation*

$$\dot{y} = -w(y), \quad y(t_0) = y_0.$$

where $w(\cdot)$ is a locally Lipschitz positive definite function. Then, this equation has a unique solution $y(t)$ defined for all $t \geq t_0$

$$y(t) = \sigma(y(t_0), t - t_0)$$

where $\sigma(r,s)$ is a positive definite and decreasing function, see Definition 5.

Lyapunov stability theorems give sufficient conditions for stability, asymptotic stability, and so on. They do not say whether the given conditions are also necessary. There are converse theorems which establish, that for many Lyapunov stability theorems the given conditions are indeed necessary (Hahn, 1967; Krasovskii, 1967). The converse theorems are proved by actually constructing auxiliary functions that satisfy the conditions of the respective theorems. Almost always this construction assumes the knowledge of the solution of the differential equation. The origin $x = 0$ of the perturbed non-autonomous system (2), may not be an equilibrium point. We can no longer study stability of the origin as an equilibrium point, nor should we expect the solution of the perturbed system to approach the origin as $t \to \infty$. If the perturbation terms $g(x)$ and $d(t)$ are small in some sense, then the solution $x(t)$ will be bounded by a small bound, that is $\|x(t)\|$ will be small for sufficiently large t.

Definition 7. *The solution of $\dot{x} = h(t,x)$ is said to be uniformly bounded if there exist constants a and b, and for every $\mu \in (0,b)$ there is a constant T such that*

$$\|x(t_0)\| < \mu \Rightarrow \|x(t)\| < a, \ \ \forall t > t_0 + T. \tag{14}$$

It is said globally uniformly bounded if (14) holds for arbitrarily large μ.

The following Lyapunov like theorem is useful to show uniform boundedness.

Theorem 1. *Let $D = \{x \in R^n \mid \|x\| < r\}$ and $h : [0,\infty) \times D \to R^n$ be continuous in t and locally Lipschitz in x. Let $V : [0,\infty) \times D \to R$ be a continuously differentiable function such that*

$$w_1(\|x\|) \le V(t,x) \le w_2(\|x\|), \tag{15}$$

$$\frac{\partial V}{\partial t} + \frac{\partial V}{\partial x} h(t,x) \le w_3(x), \tag{16}$$

for all $\|x\| \ge \mu > 0$, and for all $x \in D$, where $w_1(\cdot)$, $w_2(\cdot)$ and $w_3(\cdot)$ are positive definite functions and $\mu < w_2^{-1}(w_1(r))$. Then, there exists a positive definite and decreasing function $u(\cdot,\cdot)$ and a finite time t_1 (dependent on $x(t_0)$ and μ) such that

$$\|x(t)\| \le u(\|x(t_0)\|, t - t_0), \ \ \forall t_0 \le t < t_1, \tag{17}$$

$$\|x(t)\| \le w_1^{-1}(w_2(\mu)), \ \ \forall t \ge t_1, \tag{18}$$

for all $\|x(t_0)\| < w_2^{-1}(w_1(r))$. Furthermore, if $w_i(r) = k_i r^c$, for some positive constants k_i and c, then $u(r,s) = kre^{-\alpha s}$, with $k = (k_2/k_1)^{1/c}$, and $\alpha = (k_3/k_2 c)$.

Proof. By definition 6, it is necessary to prove that the origin is uniformly asymptotically stable in order to have an uniformly bounded solution. First, consider the derivative of $V(t,x)$ along the trajectories of (2)

$$\dot{V}(t,x) = \frac{\partial V}{\partial t} + \frac{\partial V}{\partial x} h(t,x) < -w_3(\|x\|).$$

Let $\rho < r$, and define a time-dependent set $\Omega_{t,\rho}$ by

$$\Omega_{t,\rho} = \{x \in D | V(t,x) \le w_1(\rho)\}.$$

The set $\Omega_{t,\rho}$ contains the ball $\left\{ \|x\| \le w_2^{-1}(w_1(\rho)) \right\}$ since

$$w_2(\|x\|) \le w_1(\rho) \ \ and \ \ V(t,x) \le w_1(\rho).$$

Also, the set $\Omega_{t,\rho}$ is a subset of the ball $\{\|x\| \leq \rho\}$ since $w_1(\|x\|) \leq w_1(\rho)$. Thus

$$\left\{x \in R^n | \|x\| \leq w_2^{-1}(w_1(\rho))\right\} \subset \Omega_{t,\rho},$$
$$\Omega_{t,\rho} \subset \{x \in R^n | \|x\| \leq \rho\} \subset D,$$

for all $t \geq 0$. For any $t_0 \geq 0$ and any $x(t_0) \in \Omega_{t,\rho}$, the solution starting at $(t_0, x(t_0))$ stays in $\Omega_{t,\rho}$ for all $t_0 \geq 0$. This follows from the fact that $\dot{V}(t,x)$ is negative on $D - \{0\}$; hence $V(t,x)$ is decreasing. Therefore, the solution starting at $(t_0, x(t_0))$ is defined for all $t \geq t_0$ and $x(t) \in D$. Now, it will assume that $\left\{\|x(t_0)\| \leq w_2^{-1}(w_1(\rho))\right\}$. Then

$$\dot{V}(t,x) \leq -w_3\left(\|x(t_0)\|\right) \leq -w_3\left(w_2^{-1}(w_1(\rho))\right).$$

Let $y(t)$ satisfy the auxiliary autonomous first order differential equation

$$\dot{y} = w(y), \;\; y(t_0) = V(t_0, x(t_0)) \geq 0.$$

It is clear that

$$V(t, x(t)) \leq y(t), \;\; \forall t \geq t_0.$$

By corollary 6, there exists a positive definite and decreasing function $\sigma(r,s)$ such that

$$V(t, x(t)) \leq \sigma(V(t_0, x(t_0)), t - t_0), \;\; \forall t \geq t_0.$$

Therefore, any solution starting in $\Omega_{t,\rho}$ satisfies the inequality

$$w_1(\|x(t)\|) \leq V(t, x(t)),$$
$$\|x(t)\| \leq w_1^{-1}(V(t, x(t))),$$
$$\|x(t)\| \leq w_1^{-1}(\sigma(V(t_0, x(t_0)), t - t_0)),$$
$$\|x(t)\| \leq w_1^{-1}(\sigma(w_2(\|x(t_0)\|), t - t_0)),$$
$$\|x(t)\| \leq u(\|x(t_0)\|, t - t_0).$$

Since $\mu < w_2^{-1}(w_1(r))$, we can choose $\rho < r$ such that $\mu < w_2^{-1}(w_1(\rho))$.
Furthermore, for any $\|x(t_0)\| < w_2^{-1}(w_1(r))$, we can choose ρ close enough to r such that $\|x(t_0)\| < w_2^{-1}(w_1(\rho))$. Let $\eta = w_1^{-1}(w_2(\mu))$. Then

$$B_\mu \subset \Omega_{t,\eta} \subset B_\eta \subset B_\rho \subset D,$$

and

$$\Omega_{t,\eta} \subset \Omega_{t,\rho} \subset B_\rho \subset D.$$

The sets $\Omega_{t,\rho}$ and $\Omega_{t,\eta}$ have the property that a solution starting inside either set cannot leave it because $\dot{V}(t,x)$ is negative on the boundary. Therefore, if $\|x(t_0)\| \leq w_2^{-1}(w_1(\rho))$, the solution $x(t)$ will belong to $\Omega_{t,\rho}$ for all $t \geq t_0$. For a solution starting inside $\Omega_{t,\eta}$, the inequality (18) is satisfied for all $t \geq t_0$. For a solution starting inside $\Omega_{t,\rho}$, but outside $\Omega_{t,\eta}$, let t_1 be the first time it enters $\Omega_{t,\eta}$. This time t_1 could be t_0 (if the solution starts inside $\Omega_{t,\eta}$) or infinite (if it never enters $\Omega_{t,\eta}$). Since $u(\|x(t_0)\|, t - t_0) \to 0$ as $t \to \infty$, there is a finite time after which $u(\|x(t_0)\|, t - t_0) < \mu$ for all t. Therefore, the time t_1 must be finite; that is, the solution must enter the set $\Omega_{t,\eta}$ in finite time. Once inside the set, the solution remains inside for all $t \geq t_1$. Therefore,

$$V(t, x(t)) \leq w_1(\eta), \quad \forall t \geq t_1,$$

and

$$\|x(t)\| \leq \eta, \quad \forall t \geq t_1.$$

Hence, any initial state $x(t_0)$ can be included in the set $\{\|x\| \leq w_2^{-1}(w_1(\rho))\}$. Thus, inequality (12) is satisfied for all $\{\|x(t_0)\| \leq w_2^{-1}(w_1(\rho))\}$, which implies that the origin $x = 0$ is uniformly asymptotically stable. The exponentially decaying for $w_1(\cdot)$, $w_2(\cdot)$ and $w_3(\cdot)$ is given by

$$w_i(r) = k_i r^c, \quad k_i > 0, \quad c > 0, \quad i = 1, 2, 3.$$

Further, for scalar function

$$w(r) = k_3 \left[\left(\frac{r}{k_2} \right)^{1/c} \right]^c = \frac{k_3}{k_2} r.$$

Hence, the positive definite and decreasing function $\sigma(\cdot, \cdot)$ is given by

$$\sigma(r, s) = re^{-(k_3/k_2)s}.$$

Subsequently, the function $u(\cdot, \cdot)$ is given by

$$u(r, s) = \left[\frac{k_2 r^c e^{-(k_3/k_2)s}}{k_1} \right]^{1/c}.$$

Hence, the origin is exponentially stable. The property completes the proof. □

Inequalities (17) and (18) show that the solution $x(t)$ is uniformly bounded for all $t \geq t_0$.

Remark 5. *Let $w_1^{-1}(w_2(\mu))$ be a positive definite function called the bound of μ. As $\mu \to 0$, the bound approaches zero. Sometimes, it is possible to combine inequalities (17) and (18) in one inequality*

$$\|x(t)\| \leq u(\|x(t_0)\|, t - t_0) + w_1^{-1}(w_2(\mu)), \quad \forall t \geq t_0. \tag{19}$$

Now, let us illustrate how Theorem 1 is used in the analysis of the perturbed system (2), when the origin of the nominal system is exponentially stable and the system has a uniform bounded solution.

Lemma 3. *Let $x = 0$ be an exponentially stable equilibrium point of the nominal system (8). Let $V : [0, \infty) \times D \to R$ be a Lyapunov function of the nominal system that satisfies inequalities (15) and (16), where $D = \{x \in R^n, \|x\| < r\}$. Suppose the perturbation term $g(x) + d(t)$ satisfies*

$$\|g(x)\| \leq c_4 \|x\|, \quad \|d(t)\| \leq \delta < \frac{\zeta}{c_5} r\theta \sqrt{\frac{c_1}{c_2}},$$

for all $t \geq 0$, $x(t) \in D$, and some positive constants $0 < \theta < 1$, $0 < \zeta < 1$, $c_2 > 0$, $c_4 > 0$, $c_5 > 0$ respectively. Then, for all $\|x(t_0)\| < r\sqrt{c_1/c_2}$, the solution of the perturbed system $x(t)$ satisfies

$$\|x(t)\| \leq k \|x(t_0)\| exp(-\alpha(t - t_0)), \quad \forall t_0 \leq t < t_1,$$

and

$$\|x(t)\| \leq b, \quad \forall t \geq t_1,$$

for some finite time t_1, where

$$k = \sqrt{\frac{c_2}{c_1}}, \quad \alpha = \frac{(1-\theta)\zeta}{2c_2}, \quad b = \frac{c_5}{\zeta}\frac{\delta}{\theta}k,$$
$$c_1 = \lambda_{min}(P), \; c_2 = \lambda_{max}(P),$$
$$c_3 = \lambda_{min}(Q), \; c_4 \leq c_3 - \zeta.$$

Proof. Consider $V(t,x)$ as a Lyapunov function candidate. The derivative of $V(t,x)$ along the trajectories of (2) satisfies

$$\dot{V}(t,x) \leq -c_3\|x\|_2^2 + \left\|\frac{\partial V}{\partial x}\right\|_2 \|g(x)\|_2 + \left\|\frac{\partial V}{\partial x}\right\|_2 \|d(t)\|_2,$$
$$\dot{V}(t,x) \leq -c_3\|x\|_2^2 + c_4\|x\|_2^2 + c_5\delta\|x\|_2,$$
$$\dot{V}(t,x) \leq -(c_3 - c_4 - \zeta)\|x\|_2^2 - \zeta\|x\|_2^2 + c_5\delta\|x\|_2,$$
$$\dot{V}(t,x) \leq -\zeta\|x\|_2^2 + c_5\delta\|x\|_2, \; 0 < \zeta < 1,$$
$$\dot{V}(t,x) \leq -(1-\theta)\zeta\|x\|_2^2 - \theta\zeta\|x\|_2^2 + c_5\delta\|x\|_2,$$
$$\dot{V}(t,x) \leq -(1-\theta)\zeta\|x\|_2^2, \; 0 < \theta < 1, \; \forall\|x\|_2 \geq \delta c_5/\theta\zeta.$$

By following application of theorem 1 completes the proof. □

The bound b is proportional to the upper bound on the perturbation δ. Once again, this result can be viewed as a robustness property of nominal system having exponentially uniform equilibria at the origin, because it shows that arbitrarily small (uniformly bounded) perturbations, will not result in large steady-state derivations from the origin.

3. HIV infection model approximation: Third order ODE

Consider the following model for HIV infection that involves a 3rd order ODE (Barao & Lemos, 2007), (Perelson & Nelson, 1999), and (Santos & Middleton, 2008)

$$\begin{aligned} \frac{dT}{dt} &= s - d_\tau T - \beta T V, \\ \frac{d\tilde{T}}{dt} &= \beta T V - \delta \tilde{T}, \\ \frac{dV}{dt} &= p\tilde{T} - cV, \end{aligned} \tag{20}$$

where T denotes the concentration of uninfected target cells (specially, CD4+helper T cells), $\tilde{T}$ is the concentration of infected target cells and V denotes the concentration of virions. There are two equilibrium points for the system given in (20). One of these is termed the uninfected state and is given by

$$T = \frac{s}{d_T}, \quad \tilde{T} = 0, \quad V = 0. \tag{21}$$

The other equilibrium is termed the infected state and is given by

$$T = \frac{\delta c}{\beta p}, \quad \tilde{T} = \frac{s}{\delta} - \frac{c d_\tau}{\beta p}, \quad V = \frac{ps}{\delta c} - \frac{d_\tau}{\beta}. \tag{22}$$

Parameter	Description	Value/units
s	Source term for uninfected cells	10mm^{-3} per day
d_T	Death rate of uninfected cells	0.02 per day
β	Infection rate of free virus particles	2.4×10^{-5} mm^{-3} per day
δ	Death rate of infected cell	0.24 per day
p	Rate of virions produced per infected cells	100 per day
c	Death rate of free particle virions	2.4 per day
t	Time	days

Table 1. Parameters for HIV model

3.1 Linearisation on infected and uninfected equilibrium point

On reference (Santos & Middleton, 2008), both equilibrium points (21) and (22) were studied. The uninfected state (21), see parameter values on Table 1, is an unstable equilibrium, where even a small perturbation (e.g introduction of HIV virus to system's dynamic) leads to divergence. For infected state in (22), it is concluded that the infected equilibrium is locally stable for the parameter values given on Table 1. The qualitative behavior of a non linear system near an equilibrium point can be determined via linearisation (Khalil, 2002). The system can be linearised by computing the Jacobian which for (20) is given by

$$A = \left.\frac{\partial f}{\partial x}\right|_{x=[T,\tilde{T},V]} = \begin{bmatrix} -(d_T+\beta V) & 0 & -\beta T \\ \beta V & -\delta & \beta T \\ 0 & p & -c \end{bmatrix}, \tag{23}$$

where A is a stability matrix for the evaluation of infected state given in (22) that leads to the characteristic polynomial

$$|\lambda I - A| = \lambda^3 + a_1\lambda^2 + a_2\lambda + a_3 \tag{24}$$

where $a_1 = \left(c+\delta+\frac{\beta sp}{\delta c}\right)$, $a_2 = \frac{\beta sp}{\delta c}(c+\delta)$, and $a_3 = (\beta sp - \delta c d_T)$.

From (24), the Hurwitz stability conditions are $a_k > 0$, for $k = 1,2,3$ and $a_1a_2 - a_3 > 0$. This stability domain is very conservative, because of the local behavior about the equilibrium point in (22). In next subsection, for equilibrium point in (22), we need to probe the exponentially uniform stable property and describe boundedness of the region of attraction. We propose to work with the converse Lyapunov stability analysis in order to obtain a uniformly bounded estimation for the equilibria point behavior at perturbation.

3.2 Non autonomous perturbation analysis

Now, it is necessary to study the dynamics for the perturbation and to determine the extent of stability region to know how large a perturbation from the equilibrium can be allowed and it can still be sure that the solution remains toward the equilibrium (Hahn, 1967), (Khalil, 2002). Consider the following change of variables in (20)

$$x = [T, \tilde{T}, V]^T = [x_1, x_2, x_3]^T.$$

The HIV model equations (20) can be rewritten as a perturbed model

$$\begin{aligned} \dot{x}_1 &= s - d_T x_1 - \beta x_1 x_3 = -d_T x_1 + (s - \beta x_1 x_3), \\ \dot{x}_2 &= \beta x_1 x_3 - \delta x_2 = -\delta x_2 + (\beta x_1 x_3), \\ \dot{x}_3 &= p x_2 - c x_3. \end{aligned} \tag{25}$$

The compact form of (25) is

$$\dot{x} = f(x) + g(x) + d(t), \tag{26}$$

where $\beta \geq 0$ is unknown, d is bounded disturbance that satisfies $|d(t)| \leq \delta$, for $t \geq 0$, and

$$f(x) = Ax = \left.\frac{\partial f}{\partial x}\right|_{x=0} x = \begin{bmatrix} -d_T & 0 & 0 \\ 0 & -\delta & 0 \\ 0 & p & -c \end{bmatrix} \begin{bmatrix} x_1 \\ x_2 \\ x_3 \end{bmatrix},$$

$$g(x) = \begin{bmatrix} -\beta x_1 x_3 \\ \beta x_1 x_3 \\ 0 \end{bmatrix}, \quad d(t) = \begin{bmatrix} s \\ 0 \\ 0 \end{bmatrix}. \tag{27}$$

Suppose the perturbation $g(x)$ satisfies the uniform bound

$$\|g(x)\|_2 \leq \beta \begin{bmatrix} |x_1||x_3| \\ |x_1||x_3| \\ 0 \end{bmatrix} \leq \frac{\beta}{2} \begin{bmatrix} \|x\|_2 \\ \|x\|_2 \\ 0 \end{bmatrix}. \tag{28}$$

The linearisation about the origin $x = 0$ for the perturbed system in (20) is described by matrix A in (27). The stability analysis of matrix A is given by the eigenvalues

$$|\lambda I - A| = \begin{vmatrix} \lambda + d_T & 0 & 0 \\ 0 & \lambda + \delta & 0 \\ 0 & -p & \lambda + c \end{vmatrix},$$

$$|\lambda I - A| = (\lambda + d_T)(\lambda + \delta)(\lambda + c).$$

Matrix A is Hurwitz when $d_T > 0, \delta > 0, c > 0$.

The converse theorem of Lyapunov is based on linearisation about the origin, $x = 0$. The theorem supposes that matrix A is Hurwitz, in other words the nominal system. Then, there exists a candidate Lyapunov function $V(x) = x^T P x$, which permit to analyse the stability by evaluating its derivative along the trajectories of the nominal system (27) such that

$$\begin{aligned} \dot{V}(x) &= \dot{x}^T P x + x^T P \dot{x}, \\ \dot{V}(x) &= x^T A^T P x + x^T P A x, \\ \dot{V}(x) &= x^T [A^T P + PA] x. \end{aligned}$$

By solving the Lyapunov equation

$$A^T P + PA = -Q, \;\; Q = Q^T > 0. \tag{29}$$

It is possible to find the unique solution with matrix $P = P^T > 0$ be positive definite. By taking the parameter values in Table 1 the matrix P is

$$P = \begin{bmatrix} 25 & 0 & 0 \\ 0 & 3.2902 \times 10^3 & 7.8914 \\ 0 & 7.8914 & 0.2083 \end{bmatrix}. \tag{30}$$

The candidate Lyapunov function $V(x) = x^T Px$ needs to satisfy the following four conditions, for being a positive definite scalar function

1. $\lambda_{min}(P)\|x\|_2^2 \leq V(x) \leq \lambda_{max}(P)\|x\|_2^2$,
   $\lambda_{min}(P) = 0.1894, \ \ \lambda_{max}(P) = 3.2902 \times 10^3$.

2. $\frac{\partial V}{\partial x} f(x) = \frac{\partial V}{\partial x} Ax = -x^T Qx$,
   $\|\frac{\partial V}{\partial x}\|_2 \|Ax\|_2 \leq -\lambda_{min}(Q)\|x\|_2^2$,
   $\lambda_{min}(Q) = 1, \ \ Q = I = Q^T > 0$.

3. $\|\frac{\partial V}{\partial x}\|_2 = \|2x^T P\|_2 \leq 2\|P\|_2\|x\|_2 \leq 2\lambda_{max}(P)\|x\|_2$,
   $2\lambda_{max}(P) = 6.5804 \times 10^3$.

4. $\|\frac{\partial V}{\partial x}\|_2 |d(t)| = |2x^T P||d(t)|$,
   $\|\frac{\partial V}{\partial x}\|_2 |d(t)| \leq 2|P||x||d(t)|$,
   $\leq 2\sum_{i=1}^{3} \lambda_i(P)|x_i||d_i(t)| = 0.5|x_1|$.

Remark 6. *A candidate Lyapunov function $V(x)$ is used to investigate for the nominal system and its stable or asymptotically stable equilibrium point at the origin, and determine if perturbed system (26) can obtain a uniform bounded value.*

By evaluation the derivative of $V(x)$ along the trajectories of perturbed system (26)

$$\dot{V}(x) = \frac{\partial V}{\partial x}\dot{x} = \frac{\partial V}{\partial x} f(x) + \frac{\partial V}{\partial x} g(x) + \frac{\partial V}{\partial x} d(t), \tag{31}$$

where $f(x)$ is a function which describes the nominal system in (26), $g(x)$ is a function which describes the perturbation about the origin in (26) and satisfy the growing bound given in (28) and $d(t)$ is a function for a bounded perturbation in (26). Hence, by using the bound (28) given for $g(x)$, their corresponding results for the function $V(x)$ are given by

$$\dot{V}(x) \leq -\|x\|_2^2 + \left\|\frac{\partial V}{\partial x}\right\|_2 \|g(x)\|_2 + \left\|\frac{\partial V}{\partial x}\right\|_2 \|d(t)\|_2,$$
$$\dot{V}(x) \leq \ \ \|x\|_2^2 + \frac{6.5804 \times 10^3}{2}\beta\|x\|_2^3 + 50s\|x\|_2,$$
$$\dot{V}(x) \leq -\zeta\|x\|_2^2 + 50s\|x\|_2^2; \ \ 0 < \zeta < 1, \ \ M > 0,$$
$$\dot{V}(x) \leq (1-\theta)\zeta\|x\|_2^2; \ \ 0 < \theta < 1.$$

Then, the function $\dot{V}(x)$ will be negative definite if the following conditions are satisfied

$$\forall\|x\|_2 \geq \min\left\{\frac{50s}{\theta\zeta}, M\right\}, \tag{32}$$

where

$$M = \frac{\beta 6.5804 \times 10^3}{2(1-\zeta)} > 0, \;\; 0 < \theta < 1, \;\; 0 < \zeta < 1.$$

Therefore, the function $\dot{V}(x)$ is negative definite inside the ball $\|x\| < r\sqrt{c_1/c_2}$. The ball defines the region of attraction for the solution, when condition (32) is satisfied. It is concluded that the origin $x = 0$ is exponentially uniform stable and the solution for system (20) is uniformly bounded in the large for disturbances that satisfy $|d(t)| \leq \delta$, for all $t \geq 0$.

3.3 Simulation of trajectories and the region of attraction

For the bound given in (32), the following simulations are shown, with initial condition $T(0) = 520$, $\tilde{T}(0) = 0$ and $V(0) = 1$. The phase space for system (20) is depicted in Figure 1 for parameter values $s = 10$, and $\beta = 2.4 \times 10^{-5}$.

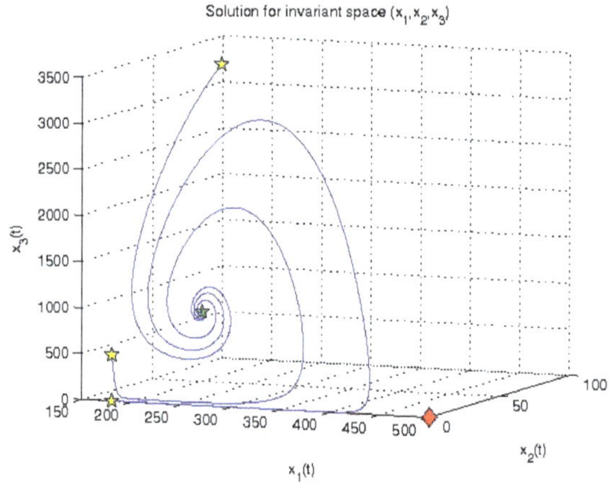

Fig. 1. Phase space for: $s = 10$, $\beta = 2.4 \times 10^{-5}$ with three initial conditions (order from above to bottom): a) $T(0) = 180.2$, $\tilde{T}(0) = 77.6$, $V(0) = 3305$; b) $T(0) = 180.2$, $\tilde{T}(0) = 0$, $V(0) = 500$; c) $T(0) = 180.2$, $\tilde{T}(0) = 0$, $V(0) = 1$.

The result describing the region of attraction is useful for the clinical personal studying HIV behavior, since it allows to predict the infection development and then choose treatment options. This model does not describe the infection behavior when AIDS has already developed. The region of attraction describes the zone for which, given any initial state condition within it, its future dynamics will be particularly slow, i.e. exponentially uniform. In the positive sector ($x_i > 0, i = 1,2,3$) of the trajectory space, the solutions will be exponentially uniform, but two different types of conditions are analysed: those starting outside and those starting inside of the domain. The latter are from an invariant set. In Fig. 2, the trajectory corresponds to initial condition given in the paper (Barao & Lemos, 2007). That trajectory belongs to solution with fast dynamics that becomes slow as soon as it traverses the invariant set.

One point which is closer to conditions found in reality is the point $(180.2, 0, 1)$, which is depicted in Fig. 1, c). Here, the viral load is small, but the number of uninfected cells is zero. This makes us think of an HIV-infected patient who is not having a large viral load. This information may be useful to configure control law that locate the starting condition at a point such that no large viral load is generated. It is important to keep in mind that the attraction

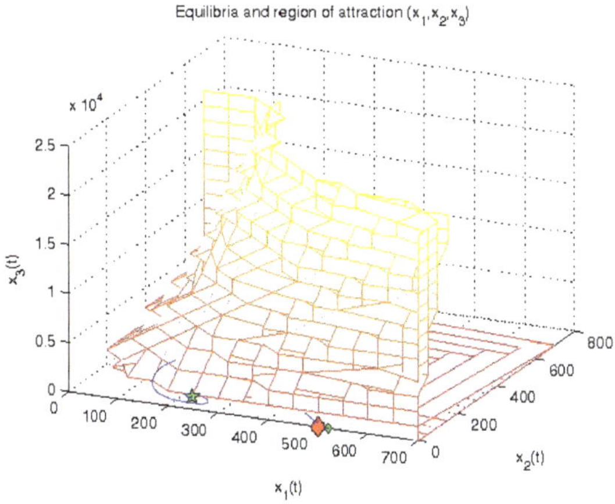

Fig. 2. Region of attraction for: $T(0) = 520$, $\tilde{T}(0) = 0$, $V(0) = 1$.

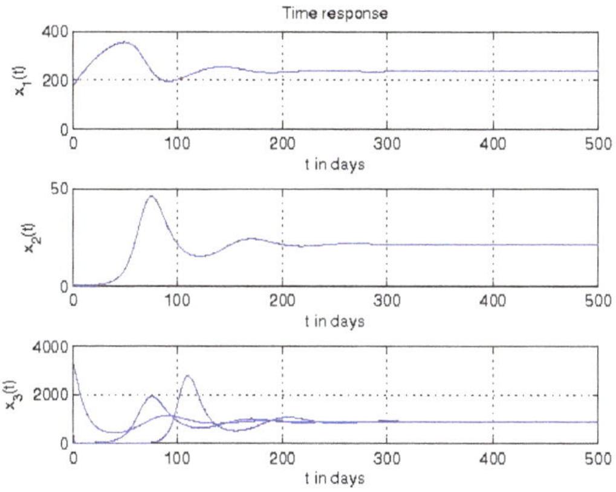

Fig. 3. Time response for three initial conditions: a) $T(0) = 180.2$, $\tilde{T}(0) = 77.6$, $V(0) = 3305$; b) $T(0) = 180.2$, $\tilde{T}(0) = 0$, $V(0) = 500$; c) $T(0) = 180.2$, $\tilde{T}(0) = 0$, $V(0) = 1$.

point is the same, regardless of the the given initial condition. The proposed change in the values causes a shift in the response for the viral load for variable V, without modifying the time response for T and $\tilde{T}$, see Fig. 3. Also, the possibility of the initial condition $(180.2, 0, 500)$ is worth considering in Fig. 1,b) and Fig. 3. That represents the beginning of an infection with a high viral load. This generates a more benign transient concerning the viral load dynamics. The aim of plotting the trajectories generated from different initial conditions is to depict the dynamics generated by the three state HIV model. Remember that the perturbation term $d(t)$ is constant.

4. Conclusions

In the paper of (Barao & Lemos, 2007), the study is made for 3rd order ODE, which focus on the analysis of eigenvalues resulting from linearisation around the equilibrium points (Santos

& Middleton, 2008). The disadvantage of linearizing about the equilibrium point when it is not the origin, is that the non linearities of the system are not taken into account.

Lyapunov converse analysis allows to obtain bounds on the phase space so that the exponential stability of the equilibrium point at the origin is guaranteed.

This means that the system trajectory describes an exponentially uniform trajectory as it approaches to stable equilibrium point. It can be seen that, there are initial conditions which are not within the given sets but their respective trajectories eventually reach the stable equilibrium point.

This dynamic characteristic is studied for the kind of nonlinear system which is studied in this chapter. It must be emphasized that the region of attraction will always determined by the initial conditions and the parameter values. It is also interesting in the future, to study the repulsion region, that means, the region which corresponds to the unstable equilibrium region. Both regions, attraction and repulsion are located in a manifold. The closer the initial condition is to the manifold in which the equilibrium point is located, the less stressful will the patient suffer from the dynamics. That is the main reason to justify the search for manifolds where the uniformly exponentially stable trajectories are found.

5. References

Barao, M. & Lemos, J.M. (2007). Nonlinear control of HIV-1 infection with a singular perturbation model. *Biomedical signal precessing and control,* Vol. 2, September 2007, 248–257, ISSN 1746-8094.

Perelson, A.S. & Nelson, P.W. (1999). Mathematical analysis of HIV-1 dynamics in vivo. *SIAM Review,* Vol.41, No.1, 3-44, ISSN 0036-1445.

Santos-Ferreira, J. & Middleton, R. (2008). A preliminary analysis of HIV infection dynamics, *Proceedings of ISSC-2008*, pp. 1-6, Galway, Rep. of Ireland, (June 2008).

Hahn, W. (1967). *Stability of motion*, Springer-Verlag, ISBN 67-23956, New York, USA.

Khalil, H.K. (2002). *Nonlinear systems*, Prentice-Hall, ISBN 013-0673-89-7, New Jersey, USA.

Krasovskii, N.N. (1967). *Stability of motion*, Stanford University Press, ISBN engrus, Stanford, USA.

Part 4

Treatment, Care and Support of HIV/AIDS Patients

12

Drug-Drug Interactions as a Challenge in the Treatment of HIV/AIDS

Norah L. Katende-Kyenda
Walter Sisulu University, Department of Pharmacology, P Bag X 1, Mthatha, South Africa

1. Introduction

Human immunodeficiency virus (HIV) is a major challenge in the medical fraternity worldwide. According to the UNAIDS report on the global AIDS epidemic, in 2004 it had affected more than 42 million people, and of these 25 million resided in the sub-Sahara Africa (UNAIDS, 2004 & Bhigjee, 2005).

This virus has no cure; the lives of the infected patients can only be prolonged using lifelong highly active antiretroviral (ARV) therapy (HAART). HAART has been proven to suppress HIV-1 viral replication continuously thus reducing mortality and morbidity in treated patients. It has further been proven that HAART is only highly effective if prescribed in combination of more than 2 drugs. However these drug combinations can be presented with potential drug-drug interactions (DDIs) an important cause of adverse drug reactions (ADRs) (Highleyman, 2007).

DDIs are well-recognised causes of adverse drug effects (ADEs) (Bates *et al.*, 1995). According to Juurlink *et al.* (2003), DDIs do cause particularly important type of adverse drug event because they are often predictable based on previous reports, clinical studies, and an understanding of pharmacological principles.

According to Johnson *et al.* (1999), DDIs are classified as an important category of ADEs. Drug interactions result in undesirable modification of the action of one or more concurrently administered agents. The interaction may cause treatment failure, an increased pharmacologic effect, or a toxic effect, which may be fatal. Because DDIs usually have a specific time course (i.e., onset and duration), they are more predictable (and preventable) then ADRs (adverse drug reactions). Bates *et al.* (1999) state that Preventable DDIs account for about one third of ADEs but incur about one half of the total ADE costs.

In HIV-infected patients, the introduction of HAART has led to reduced morbidity and mortality in treated patients (Egger *et al.*, 2002). However, in a substantial proportion of patients, the effectiveness of HAART has not been sufficient due to occurrence of virological failure and immunological decay (Bartlett *et al.*, 2001). All this has been due to failure to determine drug interactions and prevention of toxic effects. (Boffito *et al.*, 2005).

The possible causes of DDIs include drug combinations, lack of communication between the prescribers and medical history, increase in the number of newly marketed drugs and polypharmacy. Specific patients who are risk for DDIs include the elderly, people living with HIV/AIDS. Patients with HIV are more at risk for the virus because they are treated

using HAART which consist of at least three agents with the risk rising from 13% in patients taking two drugs to 82% in those taking seven drugs or more (Sanderson, 2005).
The main focus in this abstract will be on the pharmacological aspects of DDIs between ARVs. The topics to be covered in this chapter will include:

1. The concept of DDIs.
2. The different types of DDIs.
3. Drug-drug interactions rating systems and their significance levels.
4. The possible causes of DDIs.
5. Patients that are at risk for DDIs.
6. The pharmacological aspects of DDIs between ARVs.
7. The role of pharmacists in preventing DDIs in clinical practice and;
8. Recommendations on the clinical management of DDIs.
9. Conclusion.

2. Concept of DDIs

The term drug-drug interactions can be defined as *"the pharmacological or clinical response to the administration of a drug combination different from that anticipated from the known effects of the two agents when given alone"* (Tatro, 2009). As described by Tatro (2009), the effect of a DDI may be one of the following:

- Antagonism, such as a loss of blood pressure control by clonidine when tricyclic antidepressants are added to a regimen.
- Synergism, as an example of which is the increased anticoagulant effect resulting from administering salicylates and warfarin.
- Idiosyncratic, such as the possible though rare severe effects that have been associated with patients concurrently receiving pethidine and monoamine oxidase inhibitor (Jankel & Fitterman, 1993).

3. Different types of DDIs

According to Seden *et al.* (2009), DDIs may arise due to the pharmacokinetics or pharmacodynamics of administered compounds. DDIs can be classified as pharmacokinetic or pharmacodynamics (Young, 2005; Cohen *et al.*, 2002) or pharmaceutical (Hall, 1986).

3.1 Pharmaceutical interactions

Pharmaceutical interactions occur when two drugs are given together, e.g., in an infusion, or when a drug reacts with the infusion solution. While it is necessary to be aware of this type of interaction, it is relatively uncommon (Hall, 1986).

3.2 Pharmacokinetic interactions

Pharmacokinetic interactions may be defined as those interactions in which the disposition of the first drug is altered by the second drug or precipitant drug. As a result, the effect of the first drug is either diminished or increased. Pharmacokinetic interactions are divided into those that affect (Swart & Harris, 2005; Young, 2005; Cohen *et al.*, 2002):

- **Drug absorption**: An example of this interaction is when didanosine containing an aluminium-magnesium antacid buffer, is administered with ciprofloxacin, the metallic ions in the buffer may chelate with ciprofloxacin, resulting in subtherapeutic blood levels of ciprofloxacin (Sahai *et al.*, 1993).

- **Drug binding**: This was illustrated by in vivo work which showed that methadone concentrations were decreased when administered with ritonavir, due to displacement of methadone from plasma binding sites (Piscitelli & Gallicano, 2001).
- **Drug metabolism:** An example of this kind of interaction is between PIs and NNRTIS that act as inhibitors or inducers of cytochrome P450 (CYP450). Ritonavir is the most potent CYP450 and therefore the most likely to interact with other drugs such as amiodarone, cisapride or pethidine. Likewise efavirenz induces the metabolism of indinavir and saquinavir by reducing their plasma concentrations (Piscitelli & Gallicano, 2001).
- **Excretion:** In this case, the NRTIs may have additive or synergistic adverse effects, so if for example stavudine is administered with zalcitabine or didanosine, because these drugs are eliminated primarily by the kidney peripheral neuropathy caused by stavudine (Lee & Henderson, 2001).
- **Transport system:** One case report demonstrated a 48% decrease in valproic acid concentration after a patient had been started on lopinavir/ritonavir-based regimen. This interaction was likely to be due to the ability of ritonavir to induce valproic acid metabolism via glucuronidation (Sheehan *et al.*, 2006).

The result of pharmacokinetic DDIs may be an increase or decrease in the concentration of the drug at the site of action. The mechanism most common is drug metabolism.

3.2.1 Drug metabolism interactions

Drugs are metabolised by two types of reactions: phase 1 reactions that involve oxidation, reduction or hydrolysis in which drugs are turned into more polar compounds and phase 11 reactions that involve coupling drugs with some other substance (e.g. glucuronic acid) to make (usually) inactive compounds (Cohen *et al.*, 2002). These reactions make drugs more easily excretable. Drug metabolism interactions can increase or decrease the amount of drug available by inhibition or induction of metabolism (Cohen *et al.*, 2002).

3.2.1.1 Enzyme induction

Enzyme induction frequently affects phase 1 oxidation, which requires the presence of the reduced form of nicotinamide adenine dinucleotide phosphate (NADPH) and the haem-containing protein cytochrome P450. Enzyme inducers like carbamazepine, phenytoin, phenobarbital, PIs and NNRTIs, increase the activity of the microsomal enzymes (cytochrome P450 isoenzyme), increasing the rate of metabolism and excretion. One study reported that there was a decreased metabolism and subsequent toxicity of carbamazepine when concomitantly administered with ritonavir (Bates & Herman, 2006; Young, 2005). A case study reported of a patient who was prescribed ritonavir with midazolam concomitantly, and developed extreme sedation and possibly respiratory depression due to the inhibition of midazolam metabolism.

3.2.1.2 Enzyme inhibition

Enzyme inhibitors inhibit the microsomal enzymes (cytochrome P450 isoenzymes), decreasing the rate of metabolism and excretion of other drugs that are metabolised by these same enzymes (Cohen *et al.*, 2002). Examples of these drugs are PIs and delavirdine presenting drug interactions with statins because they are metabolised by the same enzyme (Geletko & ZuWallack, 2001). These drugs begin to accumulate in the body and toxicity may develop within 2 to 3 days. The clinical significance of the enzyme inhibition interaction depends on the extent to which serum levels rise. Some drugs may have additive or synergistic adverse effects. For example, zidovudine may cause anaemia and neutropnenia, so drugs causing bone marrow suppression should be prescribed with caution if used concomitantly (Matheny *et al.*, 2001). Another example of this metabolism was the administration of simvastatin with saquinavir/ritonavir, the interaction leading to increased levels of simvastatin by more than 3000% (Fichenbaum *et al.*, 2002b). This could put the patient at risk for adverse effects like myalgias, rhabdomyolysis, elevated creatinine phosphokinase and hepatic dysfunction (Dube *et al.*, 2003).

3.2.2 Cytochrome P450 isoenzymes

Cytochrome P450 is a large family of related isoenzymes of which about 30 have been identified. The most frequently involved in drug interactions are CYP3A4 and CYP2D6. There are many drugs that are metabolised by these cytochrome P450 isoenzymes including ARVs (Clarke *et al.*, 2008). Drugs may be metabolised by more than one cytochrome isoenzyme. For example, the majority of PIs and NNRTIs and antidepressants are substrates for, and can inhibit or induce the CYP450 system and have the potential to cause clinical drug interactions including serotonin syndrome, a potential fatal complication. According to Swart and Harris (2005) it is of value to know which particular isoenzymes are responsible for the metabolism of a specific drug as this makes it possible to predict with which other drugs it may possibly interact.

3.3 Pharmacodynamic interactions

Pharmacodynamic interactions are those where the effects of one drug are changed by the presence of another drug at its site of action, without alterations in the concentrations of either drug (Young, 2005; Cohen *et al.*, 2002). Sometimes one drug competes directly with another for particular receptors, but often the reaction is more indirect and involves the interference with physiological mechanisms, making pharmacodynamic interactions more difficult to classify than pharmacokinetic interactions (DeVane as quoted by Delafuente, 2003). There are four basic subdivisions as quoted by Swart and Harris (2005):

- Additive or synergistic interactions and combined toxicity
- Antagonistic or opposing interactions
- Interactions due to changes in drug transport mechanisms
- Interactions due to disturbances in fluid and electrolyte

3.3.1 Mechanisms of drug-drug interactions

Drugs interact with one another through various mechanisms which include altered absorption, altered distribution, altered metabolism and altered elimination.

3.3.1.1 Altered absorption

Drug interactions can occur where one drug changes the absorption characteristics of another drug. The binding of one drug to another causes changes in gastric pH, and changes in gastrointestinal motility and can cause these drug interactions (Cohen *et al.*, 2002). One example is that of didanosine which contains an aluminium-magnesium antacid buffer. When administering didanosine with ciprofloxacin, the metallic ions in the buffer may chelate concomitantly with ciprofloxacin resulting in subtherapeutic levels of the antibiotic

(Sahai *et al.*, 1993). It is therefore recommended that the two drugs be administered at different times. Absorption of many drugs, such as delavirdine, atazanavir, aspirin, ciprofloxacin, and digoxin, can be significantly impaired by concurrent administration of antacids by a variety of mechanisms (Fulco *et al*, 2006).

3.3.1.2 Gastrointestinal motility

A mechanism of DDIs that may go unrecognised is where one drug changes the gastrointestinal transit time. In doing so, the pharmacokinetics of not altering the transit time can be changed, leading to changes in the drug's pharmacological actions. Drugs with anticholinergic properties and opioids will slow gastrointestinal motility, while drugs, such as metoclopramide and laxatives will increase gastric emptying and gastric transit and generally increase the rate of absorption (Benet *et al.*, 1990).

3.3.1.3 Altered gastric pH

Drugs that change the normal pH of the stomach can affect absorption characteristics of other drugs. This is an essentially important point, considering the widespread use of proton pump inhibitors, although only a few clinically relevant interactions have been identified (e.g. ketoconazole) (Delafuente, 2003). The results of data in a study done by O'Connor-Semmes *et al.* (2001) suggested that the elderly may be more sensitive to the increase in gastric pH compared to younger adults.

According to Piscitell and Gallicano (2001), when didanosine is administered with indinavir, changes in pH may significantly alter drug absorption of indinivarir because of an increase in pH due to the didanosine buffer. It is therefore recommended that didanosine and indinavir be administered at least one hour apart.

It has been reported by Fulco *et al.* (2006) and Tran *et al.* (2001) that acid-suppressive therapy with histamine-2 (H_2) blockers, proton pump inhibitors or antacids can cause a decrease in the absorption of some PIs. This is due to changes in the pH of the gastrointestinal tract. PIs like atazanavir, fosamprenavir, tipranavir have been found to have significant interactions with acid-suppressive therapy that require intervention due to the potential for virological failure from inadequate ARV concentration (Fulco *et al.*, 2006).

3.3.1.4 Altered distribution

The most common DDI affecting drug distribution is alteration in protein binding. This type of interaction occurs when there is competitive inhibition for protein binding sites. This allows for the unbound fraction of the drugs to be increased, and it is the free fraction that is responsible for pharmacological activity (Young, 2005). Most of the clinically significant interactions involve drugs that are highly protein bound and have a narrow therapeutic index. An example of this is when the cytidine analogue lamivudine inhibits phosphorylation of another cytidine analog, zalcitabine, resulting in high incidence of toxicities. Therefore such combinations should be avoided (Young, 2005).

An example of this DDI is when zidovudine and stavudine are co-administered, the two NRTIs do compete for cellular thymidine kinase, the enzyme that is responsible for the monophosphorylation of both drugs to nucleotides. The inhibitory effect impairs the efficacy of stavudine when combined with zidovudine (Havril *et al.*, 2000).

3.3.1.5 Altered metabolism

3.3.1.5.1 Cytochrome P450 isoenzyme

Most of the clinically important types of pharmacokinetic DDIs are those altering a drug's metabolism. Many elderly patients, but not all, have underlying impaired CYP450

metabolising capability. According to Flockhart and Tanus-Santos (2002), six CYP450 isoenzymes that have been identified to be involved in oxidative metabolism of most commonly used drugs are: CYP1A2, CYP2C9, CYP2C19, CYP2D6, CYP2E1, and CYP3A4.
Interactions involving the CYP450 enzymes are often due to either inhibition of an isoenzyme, leading to increased blood or tissue concentrations of the substrate, or induction of an isoenzyme, causing enhanced metabolism and lower substrate concentrations (Delafuente, 2003:137). According to Johnson *et al.* (1999) enzyme inhibition is the mechanism most often responsible for life-threatening interactions.[32] Such interactions have been observed when zalcitabine is combined with stavudine or didanosine producing severe peripheral neuropathy, pancreatitis, and lactic acidosis (Simpson & Tagliati, 1995).
Induction of certain CYP450 isoenzymes, for example CYP2C9/19 by lopinavir/ritonavir and nelfinavir was reported by Honda *et al.* (1999) that it could lead to an increase in the matabolism of antiepileptic drugs like phenytoin, a norrow therapeutic index drug. The reduction in the anticonvulsant serum concentration could lead to seizures.

3.3.1.5.2 Cytochrome P450 inhibition

Competitive binding at the enzyme's binding site between two drugs is often responsible for inhibition of a drug's metabolism. The onset of CYP450 inhibition depends on the inhibiting drug's half-life. For drugs with short half-lives, enzyme inhibition occurs quickly and clinically significant interactions can be apparent within 1 or 2 days (Cheng *et al.*, 2009). Inhibition of CYP450 is also dose-dependent. Higher doses of an inhibitory drug will cause greater amounts of competitive inhibition than lower doses. Although sufficient data are not available to help in clinical situations as stated by Delafuente (2003), knowing the CYP450 enzymes involved in a drug's metabolism can be used to predict and avoid clinical problems resulting from drug interactions.
All currently marketed PIs - atazanavir, amprenavir, fosamprenavir, indinavir, lopinavir, nelfinavir, ritonavir and saquinavir (Young, 2005) - and the NNRTI delavirdine inhibit CYP3A4 (Piscitelli & Gallicano, 2001) decrease the hepatic clearance of CYP3A4 substrates and increase their plasma levels.

3.3.1.5.3 Cytochrome P450 induction

The onset of enzyme induction is usually longer than that of enzyme inhibition (Chapron, 2001). Enzyme induction is dependent on the half-life of the synthesis of new CYP450 isoenzymes and is dependent on the half-life of the inducing drug. Like inhibition of CYP450 enzymes, shorter half-life drugs will have a shorter onset of induction. A drug with half life, such as phenobarbital, may take one week before enzyme induction is seen.
Drugs often involved in induction of CYP450 isoenzymes are carbamazepine, phenytoin, phenobarbital, primidone, and rifampicin (Clarke *et al.*, 2008). Aging may impair enzyme induction, but this is not a universal finding as stated by Chapron (2001).
Of the ARVs, the NNRTIs nevirapine and efavirenz induce CYP3A4, thus increasing the hepatic clearance of CYP3A4 substrates and decreasing their plasma levels (Piscitelli & Gallicano, 2001). Other ARVs like PIs induce CYP450 isoenzymes, and it has been reported that drugs like phenytoin, rifampin, carbamazepine, phenobarbital, and dexamethasone can increase the hepatic clearance and therefore decrease plasma concentrations of the PIs (Lesho & Gey, 2003).

3.3.1.5.4 Altered renal elimination

Many drugs and drug metabolites are excreted in the urine via renal tubular secretion. Two drugs can compete for the same active secretion sites in the tubule allowing for decreased elimination and potentially toxic serum concentrations (Lesho & Gey, 2003). Alteration in urine pH can also affect drug elimination. Alkalinisation of the urine will decrease elimination of drugs that are weak bases and decreases in urine pH will increase their elimination. Acidification of the urine will decrease renal elimination of drugs that are weak acids (Hasten, 1995).

This mechanism happens in interactions that alter drug bioavailability by decreasing it and these are commonly found in PIs. The reason is that PIs induce CYP450 isoenzymes, so drugs like phenytoin, rifampin, carbamazepine, phenobarbitone, and dexamethasone can increase the hepatic clearance, thereby decreasing plasma concentrations of the PIs (Lesho & Gey, 2003). All this result in increase in toxicity of the drugs (Lesho & Gey, 2003). In the elderly as stated by Delafuente (2003), more common and potentially more significant are DDIs that affect renal function. Glomerular filtration rates decline with advanced aging. To compensate for this physiologic change, a compensatory production of vasodilatory renal prostaglandins occurs (Delafuente, 2001). However, according to Swedko *et al.* (2003) in frail elderly patients, serum creatinine concentrations may be very misleading, often in the normal range despite poor renal function.

4. DDIs rating system: significance levels

Most rating systems as employed by Tatro (2009) and De Maat *et al.* (2004) indicate:

- major significance,
- moderate significance; and
- minor significance.

4.1 Major significance: level 1

Significance level 1 indicates a major contradiction or a drug interaction that requires very careful monitoring. According to Strain *et al.* (2002b) the effects are potentially life-threatening or capable of causing permanent damage. The clinician needs to document why he or she is prescribing this combination, and the medical necessity to use both drugs concomitantly only if there is no alternative or the potential benefit outweighs the risk. Drug combinations producing an interaction with a significance level 1 are combinations that result in serious and potentially life-threatening adverse effects such as arrhythmia, respiratory depression and/or death (Winston & Boffito, 2005).

Obviously, if this combination is to be used the drug(s) in question must be prescribed with an explanation as to the need for their concomitant use and must be preceded by very cautious monitoring. Documentation of the clinician's awareness of the potential serious - level 1 - interaction should be accomplished at the time of prescribing this potentially dangerous combination. In addition, it is obligatory to alert the other health care providers' of the potential interactions and adverse outcomes which they could expect. Obviously, the optimum choice, if possible, is to use an alternative medication to avoid significance level 1 interactions (Strain *et al.*, 2002a).

4.2 Moderate significance: level 2

With significance level 2, the effects may cause deterioration in a patient's status. Additional treatment, hospitalisation or extension of hospital stay may be necessary (Strain *et al.*,

2002b). The potential interaction must also be documented and the clinical outcome(s) must be monitored carefully so that unacceptable, pernicious reactions are halted as soon as possible. According to Strain *et al.* (2002b) it is essential that the clinician document that the potential drug interactions were considered when using this combination. It is also essential to alert the patient's health care providers to the potential interactions so that they are observed early in their course.

4.3 Minor significance: level 3

As stated by Strain *et al.* (2002b) the effects are usually mild. Consequences may be bothersome or unnoticeable, but should not significantly affect the therapeutic outcome. Additional treatment is usually not required (Tatro, 2005 & Sewester, 2001). According to Strain *et al.* (2002a) significance level 3 does not preclude the use of a specific drug, but clinical decision making requires acknowledging if the adverse reactions (e.g. nausea and rash) might be precluded by choosing an alternative drug. The potential interaction and its mechanism(s) needs documentation in the patient's medical chart and the patient's health care providers need to be informed.

Another rating system is employed by *Drug Interaction Facts* which utilises 5 point significance classification scheme (Tatro, 2009) and *Facts and Comparisons* (McEvoy, 2000) and they recommended the following:

- Avoid combination: risk always outweighs benefit.
- Usually avoid combination: use combination only under special circumstances.
- Minimise risk: take action as necessary to reduce risk.
- No action needed: risk of adverse outcomes appears small.
- No interaction: evidence suggests no interaction.

5. Possible causes of DDIs

5.1 Drug combinations

Drug combinations of interacting drugs are among the major causes leading to DDIs (Seden *et al.*, 2009). Drug combinations are more common in an elderly population using many drugs (Bjőrkman *et al*,. 2002). A large proportion of these combinations are likely to be part of a normal drug regimen. In a study done by Bjőrkman *et al.* (2002), in DDIs most of the drug combinations increased the risk of ADRs and lowered therapeutic effects as stated by Seymour and Routledge (1998). In all potential DDIs, 50% of the combinations could result in an adverse drug reaction and 50% in a suboptimal therapeutic effect. However, combination ARV treatment is a potent and effective therapy for HIV infection (Pontali, 2008). This is also a disadvantage because ARV drugs frequently interact amongst themselves and other drugs as was identified by KatendeKyenda et al (2007). Since some of these drug combinations have negative effects, more attention must be focused on detecting and monitoring patients using such combinations and could also be addressed by dose adjustment.

5.2 Lack of communication and medication history

Communication between emergency departments and primary care physicians often does not occur (Beers *et al.*, 1990), and primary care physicians do not take down medication histories optimally and therefore, the physicians responsible for follow-up may be unaware of the changes made in therapy.

Emergency department physicians do not routinely screen for potential drug interactions due to unavailability of a medication history. In a study by Beers *et al.* (1990) it was stated that groups of patients at higher risk of drug complications, the elderly and those taking multiple medications, did not appear to receive more cautious care. Neither the physician's record nor the instructions given to the patient indicated that prescribing physicians recognised the potential adverse reactions that were introduced. There is need for physians to screen for interactions. A patient's advanced age or a long list of medications should cause the physicians to be more reticent in prescribing. Fewer medications should be given to the elderly and to high medication users.

5.3 Increase in number of newly marketed drugs

There is a considerable number of newly marketed drugs with a growing number of possible combinations. Complex disease states often require the concurrent use of these drug combination therapies so as to be highly effective (Bergk *et al.*, 2004). Nevertheless, as supported by Merlo *et al.* (2001) multiple drug use is also associated with the occurrence of DDIs. Therefore the majority of these interactions can be compensated by dose adjustment or prevented by a well-considered sequence of administration (Bergk *et al.*, 2004). The considerable number of newly marketed drugs with a number of possible combinations raises the need to support general practitioners with the pertinent information for careful approach to patients.

5.4 Polypharmacy

Polypharmacy, the use of two or more medications by one patient, has become prevalent especially in elderly patients (Gaeta *et al.*, 2002). Beers *et al.* (1990) in their study showed that those 65 years of age and older used an average of two to six prescribed medications and one to four non-prescribed medications per day. The frequency of polypharmacy in the elderly increases the incidence of adverse drug reactions and interactions, and it is the most significant contributing factor for DDIs. Patient's past medical history and medication has to be evaluated by the physicians. According to Seden *et al.* (2009), polypharmacy is largely unavoidable for patients receiving ARVs in both the developed and developing world and resource-poor setting, with life-long treatment and change of drug combinations along the way.

6. Patients at risk for DDIs

Patients that are at risk for DDIs are discussed in this section with specific reference to the elderly and the HIV/AIDS patients.

6.1 The elderly

The incidence of adverse drug reactions and interactions in the elderly has been reported to be two to three times the incidence in younger patients (Nolan & O'Malley, 1998). According to Sloan (1992), this increased risk for the elderly may be related to impaired organ reserve capacity, multiorgan dysfunction, and altered pharmacokinetics and pharmacodynamics.

6.2 People living with HIV/AIDS

The HIV infection is treated by using HAART, which involves a regimen of at least three agents to be effective (Seden *et al.*, 2009). In a study on DDIs in general medical patients,

Sanderson (2005) found that the risk of DDIs rose from 13% in patients taking two drugs to 82% in patients taking seven drugs or more.

7. Pharmacological aspects of DDIs between ARVs

DDIs are a serious complication of taking multiple medications and account for 3% to 5% of all hospital medication errors (Leape *et al.,* 1995). According to Clarke *et al.* (2008), the consequences of drug interactions vary ranging from drug toxicities to therapeutic failures, or loss of effectiveness and can significantly affect a patient's clinical outcome. Of particular concern are drug interactions in patients infected with HIV who are receiving HAART because it involves a regimen of a least three agents (Seden *et al.*, 2009).

HAART has revolutionised the management of HIV-1 infection and the ARV therapy has improved steadily in terms of efficacy, tolerability, and dosing convenience since the advent of HAART in 1995 (Chandwani & Shuter, 2008). HAART consists of four classes that are available for ARV therapy: (Nucleoside/nucleotide reverse transcriptase inhibitors (N(t)RTIs; non-nucleoside reverse transcriptase inhibitors (NNRTIs); protease inhibitors (PIs); and a fusion inhibitor). The strongly recommended regimen based on the existing efficacy data, is either NNRTI-based or PI-based HAART (Yeni *at al.*, 2004).

7.1 Clinically significant drug interactions associated with Highly Active Antiretroviral Therapy

One of the most challenging issues faced by health care providers treating patients with HIV-1 infection is the complex problem of DDIs associated with HAART (Seden *et al.*, 2009; Clarke *et al.*, 2008; Pontali, 2007; Cohen *et al.*, 2002). The guidelines for the initial treatment of HIV infection recommend the use of at least three ARVs (Bartlett *et al.*, 2006a), each of which is associated with significant drug interactions (DHHS, 2003). Drug interactions associated with HIV medications can be classified into those that alter the pharmacokinetics and those that alter pharmacodynamics (Seden *et al.*, 2009).

Pharmacokinetic drug interactions result in a change in pharmacokinetic parameters, such as the area under the curve (AUC), which measures drug exposure, peak concentration (Cmax), through concentration or half-life (Young, 2005; Cohen, 2002). Pharmacodynamic interactions result in alterations in the pharmacologic activity of the medication; not causing a change in the pharmacokinetic (Young, 2005; Cohen, 2002). The most common drug interactions in HIV medicine are pharmacokinetic interactions as a result of a change in the absorption, distribution and metabolism and the result of the concurrently administered medication (Piscitelli & Gallicano, 2001).

7.2 Influence of cytochrome P450 (CYP450) on DDIs in HIV

The cytochrome P450 enzyme system is responsible for the biotransformation of drugs from active to inactive metabolites that are readily excreted by the body. DDIs are more common in PIs and NNRTIs (Seden *et al.*, 2009; Winston & Boffito, 2005; Young, 2005; Cohen *et al.*, 2002). Of the numerous isoenzymes of CYP450 that have been identified, the ones responsible for elimination of drugs used in HAART are CYP3A, CYP1A2, and CYP2D2 (Clarke *et al.*, 2008).

7.3 Nucleoside/Nucleotide Reverse Transcriptase Inhibitors (NRTIs & NtRTIs)

The NRTIs are valuable ARV agents in the treatment of HIV infection because they constitute the "backbone" of highly active ARV therapy regimens (Waters & Boffito, 2007).

Drug interactions associated with NRTIs and NtRTIs are few because these drugs are not metabolised by the CYP450 system (Clarke *et al.*, 2008). However, drug interactions may still occur within these drugs as was demonstrated by Katende-Kyenda et al. (2008a). One of the few pharmacodynamic interactions encountered in HIV medicine occurs, for example with co-administered zidovudine and stavudine, since both drugs are thymidine analogues and they can compete for the same phosphorylation site in the growing chain of HIV DNA, resulting in an antagonistic, pharmacodynamic interaction (Piscitelli & Gallicano, 2001). It is therefore recommended that these two drugs never to be combined.

The use of didanosine (ddl) is complicated by drug interactions (Cohen *et al*, 2002). It is a buffered tablet form containing magnesium and calcium to improve systemic absorption. It, however, interacts with certain antibiotics like ciprofloxacin, tetracycline and therefore, to minimise the interaction, didanosine should be administered at least two hours after or six hours before the fluoroquinolone (Knupp & Barbhaiya, 1999). Concurrent use of didanosine-buffered tablets may also impair the absorption of the PI atazanavir, since atazanavir requires an acidic environment for absorption (Product Information Videx EC, 2003). To minimise the interaction, patients should take a didanosine-buffered tablet two hours after or one hour before taking atazanavir.

The most significant didanosine drug interaction reported occurs when didanosine is used concurrently with the NrRTI tenofovir. The didanosine AUC increases by 60% and therefore it is recommended that in patients receiving these two drugs concurrently and weighing > 60 kg, the didanosine dosage should be reduced from 400 mg to 250 mg once daily or from 250 mg to 200 mg in patients who weigh less than 60 kg (Young, 2005). For severely underweight patients, the dose should be further reduced to 125mg once daily (Faragon & Piliero, 2004). All patients receiving concurrent tenofovir and didanosine should be closely monitored for didanosine -related toxicities such as pancreatitis, hyperlactatemia, and lactic acidosis, regardless of didanosine dosage adjustments.

7.4 Non-Nucleoside Reverse Transciptase Inhibitors (NNRTIs)

Drugs in this group are prone to drug interactions because they are extensively metabolised via CYP3A4 and can act as either inducers or inhibitors of CYP3A4. Nevirapine and efavirenz are inducers of CYP3A4, while delavirdine is an inhibitor of CYP3A4 (Pfister *et al.*, 2003). Therefore, when one of these drugs is combined with a drug that is also metabolised by CYP3A4, a drug interaction may occur (Clarke *et al.*, 2008).

Nevirapine presents with numerous drug interactions, being a CYP3A4 inducer, and drug interactions associated with it lead to an increase in metabolism and reduced concentration of the co-administered drug. For example, when nevirapine is concurrently given with methadone, withdrawal symptoms may occur as a result of reduced methadone levels (Pinzanni *et al.*, 2000). Efavirenz is a potent inducer of CYP3A4 in vivo. Like the PIs, EFV is extensively metabolised primarily by the CYP3A4 (Pfister *et al.*, 2003).

The induction properties of efavirenz can result in reduced concentrations of concurrently administered drugs that are metabolised by CYP3A4 and it is therefore contraindicated with midazolam, triazolam and ergotamine derivative since there is a potential for increased drug concentrations of these medications and associated toxicity (Product Infomation Sustiva, 2003). Efavirenz, as a potent inducer of CYP3A4 is suggested to have a potential interaction with lopinavir and ritonavir, both of which inhibit CYP3A4. This interaction was assessed in a parallel group study in which PI-experienced, NNRTI-naive, HIV-infected patients received different doses of these agents (Young, 2005).

7.5 Non-Nucleoside Reverse Transcriptase and Protease Inhibitors Interactions

When predicting potential drug interactions, it is important to know which P450 isoenzyme is responsible for the metabolism of a drug. Drug interactions between NNRTIs and PIs are common as was observed in a study by Katende-Kyenda (2008b), as all currently available agents in these two classes are metabolised mainly by the 3A4 isoenzyme of the CYP450 system (Fichtenbaum & Gerber, 2002). NNRTIs and PIs also inhibit or induce CYP3A4, decreasing or increasing hepatic clearance and, thereby, increasing or decreasing plasma levels, respectively, of drugs metabolised by CYP3A4. Therefore, depending primarily on the potency of each NNRTI or PI as an inhibitor or inducer of CYP3A4 and on the substrate affected, each one has a different drug interaction profile.

All currently marketed PIs - atazanavir, amprenavir, fosamprenavir, indinavir, lopinavir, nelfinavir, ritonavir, and saquinavir - and the NNRTI delavirdine inhibit CYP3A4 (Piscitelli & Gallicano, 2001). According to Von Moltke *et al.* (1998), ritonavir is the most potent CYP3A4 inhibitor and, consequently, has the most drug interactions, while amprenavir, indinavir, lopinavir, and nelfinavir appear to inhibit CYP3A4 equally, and saquinavir with the lowest inhibitory effect.

7.6 Effect of Protease Inhibitors on Nucleoside Analogues

The nucleoside analogue reverse transcriptase inhibitor, tenofovir, does not appear to inhibit CYP3A4 isoenzyme significantly and, like most inhibitors, is excreted by the kidneys. Tenofovir, unlike other NRTIs, is associated with several drug interactions, particularly a bidirectional effect (i.e. agent can alter plasma levels of the other) with atazanavir, while atazanavir raises plasma levels of tenofovir (Holder, 2003).

Indinavir does not alter the pharmacokinetics of zidovudine, stavudine or lamivudine (Perry & Belfour, 1996:928). This is because the optimal absorption of indinavir requires a normal (acidic) gastric pH whereas an acid medium rapidly degrades didanosine, which is formulated with buffering agents to increase the pH. Therefore the administration of indinavir and didanosine should be separated by at least 1 hour to avoid an interaction mediated by altered drug absorption (Perry & Balfour, 1996).

7.7 Effect of Non-Nucleoside Reverse Transciptase Inhibitors on Nucleoside Analogues

Nevirapine is a potent and selective non-competitive inhibitor of reverse transcriptase (De Maat *et al.*, 2003). It does not compete with template or nucleoside triphosphates, and therefore a significant interaction would not be expected. Nevirapine may reduce plasma zidovudine concentrations by 25% but does not influence plasma concentrations of didanosine or zalcitabine (Murphy & Montaner, 1996).

NRTIs, unlike NNRTIs and PIs, are not metabolised by the hepatic CYP3A4 ezyme system and – the exception of zidovudine and abacavir - undergo renal rather than biliary excretion. Zidovudine undergoes hepatic glucuronidation and abacavir is metabolised in the liver by alcohol dehydrogenase (Barry *et al.*,1999). Therefore, there is little potential for interaction between NRTIs and NNRTIs or between NRTIs and PIs. In addition, the NRTI class as a whole has fewer drug interactions than the NNRTI and PI classes have.

7.8 Protease inhibitor interactions

The PIs are extensively metabolised by the cytochrome P450 (CYP) enzymes present in the liver and small intestine (Winston & Boffito, 2005). Therefore drug interactions involving PIs will occur largely as a result of enzyme induction or enzyme inhibition (Barry *et al.*, 1999). Some PIs can alter metabolism and thus the plasma concentration of other PIs, creating complex drug interactions when a second PI is added to HAART. According to Van Heeswijk *et al.* (2001), additionally, favourably positive DDIs can increase the exposure to PIs, allowing the use of lower doses at reduced dosing frequencies with fewer dietary restrictions.

Protease inhibitors have differing affinities for the CYP3A4 isoenzyme. The most potent inhibitor of CYP3A4 is ritonavir (Cooper *et al.*, 2003), whereas the least potent is saquinavir. CYP3A4 inhibition associated with indinavir, nelfinavir, and amprenavir, and atazanavir tends to be intermediate. Ritonavir is often the most likely medication in the PI class to cause drug interactions because in addition to its CYP3A4 inhibition, it also inhibits CYP2D6 and induces CYP1A2 and CYP2C9 (Clarke *et al.*, 2009). However, ritonavir is often used to enhance the pharmacokinetic parameters of co-administered PIs like indinavir (Kappelhoff *et al.*, 2005), due to its potent inhibition of their metabolism by CYP3A4 (Zeldin & Petruschke, 2004).

The use of boosted double PI regimen is presented with complex unexpected pharmacokinetic interactions (Winston & Boffito, 2005). Therefore combinations like tipranavir/ritonavir with others must be avoided because such combinations have shown to significantly reduce plasma concentrations of saquinavir, amprenavir and lopinavir (Boffito *et al.*, 2005). Another interesting interaction that was observed by Boffito *et al.* (2005) was with the boosted double combinations of atazanavir/saquinavir/ritonavir. Saquinavir levels are enhanced in this regimen further than when dosed with ritonavir alone, thus suggesting a role for this as a once daily regimen.

8. Role of pharmacists in preventing DDIs in clinical practice

Although the number of clinically relevant DDIs is probably low, DDIs may be responsible for a substantial number of hospital admissions. Therefore the pharmacist is responsible for preventing the use of unsafe or non-effective drug regimens. Specifically, pharmacists should avoid the dispensing of combinations of drugs that may cause serious DDIs (Becker *et al.*, 2005).

Many drug interactions can be avoided or managed safely if adequate time and precautions are taken by a patient's pharmacist. Having the pharmacist provide patient counselling on the use of prescription and non-prescription medication, disease state(s), and the safety of concurrent use of herbal products plays a major role in avoiding drug interactions (Brown, 2004).

According to Lien and Lien (1994), many patients visit more than one doctor for their different diseases and receive more than one drug at a time, and often doctors are unaware of all the medications their patients are taking and the risks to which their patients are exposed when treated with multiple drugs. Since pharmacists in the community setting or hospital, are the most accessible health care providers, they are able to intervene when faced with potential drug interactions that may occur during patients' multiple drug therapy.

Adverse DDIs are the major cause of morbidity and mortality. Cancer patients, for example, are particularly at high risk of such interactions because they commonly receive multiple medications, including cytotoxic chemotherapy, hormonal agents and supportive care drugs (Blower *et al.,* 2005). Increased awareness by pharmacists of the potential for drug interactions will allow health care providers to minimise the risk by selecting appropriate drugs and also by monitoring for signs of interaction.

According to Pezella (2005), in 2000, the number of patient deaths attributable to ADRs in the United States of America, was estimated to be 218 000 annually. More than 51% of approved drugs in the market in 2009 may have serious side-effects not detected before marketing approval. Therefore health plans and pharmacy benefit managers must work together to take effective steps to increase ADR monitoring and reporting and to proactively avoid ADRs through pharmacy management tools.

9. Recommendations regarding management of level 2 ARV DDIs in clinical practice

The overall review revealed that most DDIs are identified between ARVs interacting at level 2 as identified by Tatro guidelines. Therefore the following recommendations can be formulated to manage these DDIs, based on the standard treatment guidelines for ARVs.

- Patients must be told the importance of consulting their doctors before using over- the counter drugs that might interact with their prescribed ARVs;
- The prescriber should always check for potential DDIs then prescribing any concomitant drug for a patient who is on ARV therapy;
- Drug level monitoring of concurrent patients' medications should be done;
- While DDIs involving HIV drugs are essentially unavoidable, many can be managed through dosage adjustments as recommended by McNicholl & Coffey, (2007 & 2009) and McNicholl, (2009).

10. Conclusion

This chapter dealt with drug-drug interactions as a challenge presented to healthcare providers in the management of HIV/AIDS. This worldwide epidemic can be managed using HAART which according to the recommended treatment guidelines, three or more drugs have to be prescribed. However some these combinations present with DDIs, the major cause of adverse drug events. DDIs can nevertheless be managed accordingly either by switching the drug combinations or by dosage adjustments. It is therefore the role both prescribers and specifically the pharmacists to identify the DDIs and working in collaboration manage them.

11. References

Barry, M.; Mulcahy, F.; Merry, C. et al. (1999). Pharmacokinetics and potential interactions amongst ARV agents used to treat patients with HIV infection. *Clinical Pharmacokinetics,* vol.36, No.4 pp. 289-304.

Bartlett, J.A.; Faith, M.J.; DeMasi, R. et al. (2006a). An updated systematic overview of triple combination therapy in ARV-naive HIV-infected adults. *AIDS,* Vol.20, No.16, pp:2051-2064.

Bates, DW.; Collen, DJ.; Laird, N. et al. (1995). Incidence of adverse drug events and potential adverse drug events: implications for prevention: ADE prevention study group. *Journal of the American Medical Association*, Vol.274 No.1, pp.29-34.

Becker, E.E.; Ceerecker, M.L.; Kallewwrd, M.; et al. (2005). Potential determinants of DDI associated with dispensing in community pharmacies. *Drug safety*, Vol.28, No.5, pp.371-378.

Beers, M.H.; Storrie, M. & Lee, G. (1990). Potential adverse drug interactions in the emergency room. *Annals of internal medicine*, Vol.112, No.1, pp.61-64.

Benet, L.Z.; Mitchell, J.R. & SHEINER, L.B. (1990). Pharmacokinetics: the dynamics of drug absorption, distribution, and elimination. (*In*: Goodman, G.A. Rall, T.W. Nies, A. & Taylor. P.. *Goodman & Gilman's: the pharmacological basis of therapeutics*. 1990: XVI-1811p Pergamons Press, Ney York NY).

Bergk, V.; Gasse, C.; Schnell, R. & Haefeli, W.E. (2004). Requirements for a successful implementation of drug interaction information systems in general practice: results of a questionnaire survey in Germany. *European journal of clinical pharmacology*, Vol. 60, No.8, pp: 595-602.

Bhigjee AL. (2005). Seizure in HIV/AIDS: a southern African perspective. Acta Neurology Scandinavia Vol.112. Suppl.131, pp:4-7.

Blower, P.; De Wit, R.; Goodin, S. & Apro, M. (2005). DDIs in oncology: why are they important and can they be minimised? *Critical Reviews in Oncology/Hematology*, Vol.55, No.2, pp:117-142.

Boffito, M,; Acosta, E,; Burger, D. et al. (2005). Current status and future prospects of therapeutic drug
monitoring and applied clinical pharmacology in ART. *AIDS*, Vol.10, No.3, pp:375-92.

Bjorkman, I.; Fastbom, J.; Schmidt, I.K. & Bernsten, C.B. (2002). DDIs interactions in the elderly. *The Annals of pharmacotherapy*, Vol.36, No.11, pp: 1675-1681.

Brown, CH. (2004). Overview of drug interactions: role of pharmacist in managing drug-drug interactions.
http://www.uspharmacist.com. Date of access: 3 August 2005.

Chandwan, A. & Shuter, J. (2008). Lopinavir/ritonavir in the treatment of HIV-1 infection: a review. *Therapeutics and Clinical Risk Management*, Vol.4, No.5, pp: 1023-1033.

Chapron, D.J. (2001). Drug disposition and response. (*In*: Delafuente, J.C., Stewart, R.B, editors, *Therapeutics in the elderly*. 3rd ed. Cincinnati: Harvey Whitney Books Co.; 2001. Pp: 257-88).

Cheng, J. W. M.; Frishman, W. H.; Aronow, W. S. (2009). Updates on Cytochrome P450-Mediated Cardiovascular Drug Interactions. *American Journal of Therapeutics*, Vol.16, No. 2. pp:155-163.

Clarke S,; Stein, C. & Townsed ML. (2008). Drug-drug interactions with HIV antiretroviral therapy. *US pharmacist*, Vol. 33, No.4, pp:HS-3-HS-21.

Cohen, B.H. & Lea, R.B. (2004). Essentials of statistics for the social and behavioral sciences. Hooken: Wiley, 2004.

Cohen, J. (1988). Statistical power analysis for the behavioural sciences. Hillsdale: Erlbaum, 1988.

Cohen, K.; Andrews, S. & Maartens, G. (2002). Drug interactions with antiretroviral therapy. *The South African Journal of HIV medicine, pp*: 42-37.

Cooper, C.L.; Van Heeswijik, R.P.G.; Gallicano, K. & Cameron, D.W. (2003). A. Review of low-dose ritonavir in protease inhibitor combination therapy. *Clinical Infectious Diseases,* Vol.36, No.12, pp:1585-92.

De Maat, M,; Ekhart,G,; Huitema, A. et al. (2003). Drug interactions between ARV drugs and comedicated agents. *Clinical pharmacokinetics,* Vol.42, No.3, pp: 223-282.

Delafuente, J.C. (2003). Understanding and preventing drug interactions in elderly patients. *Clinical reviews in oncology/haematology,* Vol.48, No.2, pp: 133-143.

Devane, C.L. & Nemeroff, C.B. (2000). Guide to psychotropic drug interactions. New York: MedWorks Media Inc.

DHHS (Department of Health and Human Services). 2004. Department of Health and Human Services and Henry J. Kaiser Family Foundation. 2003. Guidelines for the use of antiretroviral agents in HIV-infected adults and adolescents. November 10, 2003. [Web:] http://www.aidsinfo.nih.gov/contentsfiles/AdultandAdolescentsGL.pdf. Date of access: 6 June 2009.

Dube, M.P.; Stein, J.H.; Aberg, J.A. et al. (2003). Guidelines for the evaluation of and management of dyslipidemia in HIV-infected adults receiving antiretroviral therapy: recommendations of the HIV Medical Association of the IDSA and the adult AIDS Clinical Trials Group. *Clinical Infectious Diseases,* Vol.37, No.5, pp:613-627.

Egger, M. May, M. Chêne, G. et al. (2002). Prognosis of HIV-1 infected patients starting highly active antiretroviral therapy: a collaborative analysis of prospective studies. *Lancet,* 360(9327):119-29.

F aragon , J.J. & Piliero, P.J. (2003). Drug interactions associated with HAART: focus on treatments for addiction and recreational drugs. *AIDS read,* Vol.13, No.9, pp:433-4, 437-41, 446-50.

Fargon, J.J. & Piliero, P.J. (2004). Clinically significant drug interactions associated with highly active antiretroviral therapy. Infectious Diseases in Corrections. HEPP Report. January 2004. http://www.thebody.com/contents/art/3000.html. Date accessed: 21 Nov. 2007.

Fichtenbaum , C.J. & Gerber. J.G. (2002). Interactions between Antiretroviral drugs and drugs used for therapy of the metabolic complications encountered during HIV infection. *Clinical Pharmacotherapy,*Vol.41, No.14, pp:1196-1211.

Flockhart, D.A. & Tanus-Santos, J.E. (2002). Implications of cytochrome P450 interactions when prescribing medication for hypertension. *Archives of internal medicine,* Vol.162, No.4, pp:405-12.

Fulco, P.P.; Vora, U.B. & Bearman, G.M. (2006). Acid suppressive therapy and the effects on protease inhibitors. *Annals of Pharmacotherapy,* Vol.40, No.11, pp:1974-1983.

Gaeta, T. J.; Fiorini, M. & Ender, (2002). Potential drug-drug interactions in elderly patients presenting with syncope. *The Journal of emergency medicine,* 22(2): 159-162.

Geletko, S.M. & Zuwallack, A.R. (2001). Treatment of hyperlipidemia in HIV-infected patients. *American Society of Health- System Pharmacists,* Vol.58, No.7, pp:607-614.

Hall, M.R.P. (1986). Drug interactions in geriatric patients. *Drugs and Aging* ed. By D.Platt. Springer - Verlag Berlin Heidelberg. 1986.

Hasten, P.D. (2002). Appendix 11: important drug interactions. (*In*: Katzung BG, editor. Basic and clinical harmacology. 6th ed. Norwalk Connecticut: Appleton & Lange; 1995. p. 986-95.

Havril, D.V.; Tierney, C. Fiedland, G.H. et al. (2000). In vivo antagonism with zidovudine plus stavudine combination therapy. *Journal of infectious diseases,* Vol.182, No.1, pp:321-325.

Highleyman L. (2007). Drug interactions and anti-HIV therapy. The body: the complete HIV/AIDS resource. Available at: http://www.thebody.com/content/treat/art2579. (Accessed on 2 August 2007).

Holder, S. (2003). Important new pharmacokinetic data for Reyataz™ (atazanavir sulphate) in combination with Vired® (tenofovir disoproxil fumarate) [Letter to health care providers]. Bristol-Meyers Squibb Company. August 8.

Honda, M.; Yasuoka, A.; Aokil, M. & Oka. S. (1999). A generalized seizure following initiation of nelfinavir in a patient with HIV type 1, suspected due to interaction between nelfinavir and phenytoin. *Internal Medicine,* Vol.38, No.3, pp:302-303.

Jankel, C.A. & Fitterman L.K. (1993). Epidemiology of drug-drug interactions as a cause of hospital admissions. *Drug safety,* Vol.9, No.1, pp:51-59.

Johnson, M.D.; Newkirk, G. & White, J.R. (1999). Clinically significant drug interactions. What you need to know before writing prescriptions. *Drug interactions,* Vol.105, No.2. pp:193-219.

Juurlink DN, Mamdani M, Kopp A et al. (2003). DDIs among eldely patients hospitalized for drug toxicity. *Journal of the American Medical Association,* Vol.289, No.13, pp: 1652-1658.

Kappelhoff, B.S.; Huutelma, D.R. & Sankatsing, N. (2005). Population pharmacokinetics of indinavir alone and in combination with ritonavir in HIV-1-infected patients. *British journal of clinical pharmacology,* Vol.60, No.3, pp:276-286.

Katende-Kyenda N L, Lubbe MS. Serfontein JHP, Truter I. (2008a). Prevalence of drug-drug interactions of antiretroviral agents in the private health care sector in South Africa. *South African Medical Journal*, Vol.98, No.2, pp: 109-113.

Katende-Kyenda NL, Lubbe MS, Serfontein JHP and Truter I. (2008b). Prevalence of drug-drug interactions between antiretroviral agents in different age groups in a section of the private health care sector setting in South Africa.*Journal of Clinical Pharmacy and Therapeutics,* Vol. 33, pp: 393-400.

Katende-Kyenda NL, Lubbe MS, Serfontein JHP, Truter I. (2007). Effect of prescribed minimum benefits on the prevalence of possible drug-drug interactions of antiretroviral agents in a section of the private health care sector in South Africa: a 2 year comparative study. *International Journal of Pharmacy Practice* Vol.16, pp: 403-408.

Knupp, C.A & Barbhaiya, F.H. (1999). A multiple-dose pharmacokinetic interaction study between didanosine (Videx) and ciprofloxacin in male subjects seropositive for HIV but asymptomatic. *Biopharmaceutical drug disposition,* Vol.18, No.1, pp:65-77.

Leape, L.L. Bates, D. W. Cullen, D.J. (1995). Systems analysis of adverse drug events. ADE Prevention Study Group. *Journal of American medical association,* Vol.274, No.1, pp:35-43.

Lee, D. & Bergman, U. (1994). Studies of drug utilization. (*In* STROM, B.L., ed. *Pharmacoepidemiology.* 2nd ed. Chichester: John Wiley & Sons. p. 380).

Lee, L.M. & Henderson, D.K. (2001). Torelability of postexposure ARV prophylaxis for occupational exposures to HIV. *Drug Safety,* Vol.24, No.8, pp:587-597.

Lesho, E.P. & Gey, D.C. (2003). Managing issues related to ARV therapy. *American family physician,* Vol.68, No.44, pp:675-686.

Lien, L.L. & Lien, E.J. (1994). Preventing potential drug interactions in community pharmacy. *Journal of clinical pharmacology and therapeutics,* Vol.19, No.6, pp: 371-9.

Lim, M.L. Min, S.S. Eron, J.J. et al. (2004). Coadministration of lopinavir/ritonavir and phenytoin results in two -way drug interaction through cytochrome P-450 induction. *Journal of acquired immune deficiency syndrome,* Vol.36, No.5, pp:1034-1040.

Matheny, C.J.; Lamb, M.W.; Brower, K.L.R. & Pollack, G.M. 2001. Pharmacokinetic and pharmacodynamic implications of P-glycoprotein modulation. *Pharmacotherapy,* Vol.21, No.7, pp:778-798.

McEvoy, G.K. 2000. (ed). American hospital formulary service drug information. *American society of health system pharmacists.* Bethesda, MD. 2000.

McNicholl, I.A. & Coffey, S. (2007). Dosage adjustments for ARV-ARV drug interactions (Adult Dosing).

The AIDS Education & Training Centers (AETC) National Resource Center and UCSF Center for

HIV Information, October 2007.
http://www.aidsetc.org/aidsetc?page=et-03-00-04. Date of access: 26 Jun 2008.

McNicoll, I.R. & Coffey, S. (2009). Dosage Adjustments for ARV-ARV Drug Interactions. AETC National Resource Center and UCSF Center for HIV Information. July 2009. http://www.aidsetc.org/aidsetc?page=et-03-00-04. Date of access: 6 Oct 2009.

McNicholl, I.R. (2009). Dosage adjustments for ARV-ARV Drug Interactions (Adult Dosing). AETC (The AIDS Education &Training Centers) National Resource Center and ACSF Center for HIV Information.
http://www.aids-etc.org/aidsetc?page=etres-display&resource=etres-320. Date of access: 25 June 2008.

Merlo, J.; Liedholm, H.; Lindbland, U. et al. (2001). Prescriptions with potential drug interactions dispensed at Swedish pharmacies in January 1999: cross sectional study. *British medical journal,* Vol.323, No.3710, pp: 427-428.

Nolan, L. & O'Malley, K. (1998). Prescribing for the elderly: Part 1 – sensitivity of the elderly to adverse drug reactions. *Journal of American geriatric society,* Vol.36, No.2, pp: 142-149.

O'Connor-Semmes, R.L.; Kersey, K.; Williams, D.H. (2001). Effect of ranitidine on the pharmacokinetics of triazolam and a-hydroxytriazolam in both young (19-60 years) and older (61-78 years) people *Clinical pharmacology and therapeutics,* Vol.70, No.2, pp: 126-31.

Perry , CM. & Balfour, JA. (1996). Fomiviresn. *Drugs,* Vol.52, No.6, pp:928-62.

Pezella, E. (2005). Preventing adverse drug reactions in the general population. *Managed care interface,* Vol.18, No.1, pp: 49-52.

Pfister M,; Labbe. L.. & Hammer S.C. (2003). Population pharmacokinetics and pharmacodynamics of efavirenz, nelfinavir and indinavir: adult AIDS clinical trial group study. *Antimicrobial agents and chemotherapy,*Vol.47, No.1, pp: 130-137.

Pinzanni,V.; Faucherre, V.; Peyiere, H. & Blayac, J.P. (2000). Methadone withdrawal symptoms with nevirapine and efavirenz. *Annals of Pharmacotherapy,* Vol.34, No.3, pp:405-407.

Piscitelli, S.C. & Gallicano, K.D. (2001). Interactions among drugs for HIV and opportunistic infections. *The New England journal of medicine,* Vol.344, No.13, pp:984-996.

Pontali, E. (2007). Interactions of antiretroviral drugs with anti-infectives and other antiretrovirals. *Chemotherapy,* Vol.53, No.1, pp:26-29.

Sahail, J. Gallicano, K. Oliveras, L. (1993). Cations in the didanosine tablet reduce ciprofloxacin bioavailability. *Clinical pharmacology and therapeutics,*Vol.53, No.3, pp:292-297.

Saanderson. N. (2005). DDIs: the silent epidemic. *Psychiatric service* , Vol.56, No.1, pp: 22-24.

Seden, K.; Back D & Khoo S. (2009). ARV drug interactions:often recognised, frequently unavoidable, sometimes unmanageable. *Journal of Antimicrobial therapy.* Vol.64, No.1, pp: 5-8.

Sewester, C.S.; Olin, B. & Hebel, S.K. (editors). (2001). Drug facts and comparisons. Facts and comparisons. St. Louis, MO 2000. *Monthly update July.*

Seymor, R.M. & Routledga, P.A. (1998). Important drug-drug interactions in the elderly. *Drugs Aging,* Vol.12, No.6, pp: 485-94.

Sheehah, N.L.; Brouillette, M.J. Delisle, M.S. & Allan, J. 2006. Possible interaction between lopinavir/ritonavir and valproic acid exacerbates bipolar disorder. *The annals of pharmacotherapy,* Vol.40, No.1, pp:147-150.

Simpon, D.M. & Tagliati, M. (1995). Nucleoside analogue-associated peripheral neuropathy in human immunodeficiency virus infection. *Journal of Acquired Immune Deficiency Syndrome & Human Retrovirology,*Vol.9, No.2, pp:153-161.

Sloan, R. (1992). Principles of drug therapy in geriatric patients. *American family physician,* Vol.45, No.6, pp:2709-18.

Stannic, A,; Granarana, JC. (2009). Review of antiretroviral agents for the treatment of HIV infection *Formulary,* Vol. 44, No.1, pp: 47-54.

Strain, J.J.; Karim, A.& Caliendo, G. (2002b). Cardiac drug-psychotropic drug update. *General hospital psychiatry,* Vol.24, No.5, pp: 283-289.

Strain J.J. Karim, A. Caliendo, G. Brodsky, M. et al. (2002a). Neurologic drug-psychotropic drug update. *General hospital psychiatry,* Vol.24, No.5, pp: 290-310.

Swart, A. & Harris V. (2005). Drug interactions with TB therapy. *Community Medical Education,* Vol.23, No.2, pp: 56-60.

Swedko, P.J. Clark, H.D. Paramsothy, K. & Akbari, A. (2003). Serum creatinine an inadequate screening test for renal failure in elderly patients. *Archives of internal medicine,* Vol.163, No.3, pp:356-60.

Tatro DS., ed. (2009). Drug interaction facts, and comparisons: drug interaction facts.TM St. Louis, MO: WolterKluwer Health.

Tran, J.Q.; Gerber, J.G. & Kerr, B.M. (2001). Delavirdine: clinical pharmacokinetics and drug interactions. *Clinical Pharmacokinetics,* Vol.40, No.3, pp:207-226.

UNAIDS Report on the global AIDS epidemic. Bangkok: XV International AIDS Conference, 2004. http://www.unaids.org/bangkok2004/report.html (accessed March 25, 2007).

Van Heeswijk, R.P. Veldkamp, A. Mulder, J. W. et al. (2001). Combinations of protease inhibitors for the treatment of HIV-1-infected patients. A review of pharmacokinetics and clinical experience. *Antiviral therapy,* Vol.6, No.4, pp:201-229.

Von Moltke, L.L. Greenblatt, D.J. Grassi, J.M. et al. (1998). Protease inhibitors as inhibitors of human cytochromes P450: High risk associated with ritonavir. *The journal of clinical pharmacotherapy,* Vol.38, No.2, pp:106-111.

Waters, L & Boffito, M. (2007). Pharmacology of current and investigational human immunodeficiency virus (HIV) nucleoside/nucleotide reverse transcriptase inhibitors in adults. *Anti-Infective Agents in Medicinal Chemistry,* Vol. 6, No.3, pp:213-221.

Winston, A. & Boffito, M. 2005. The management of HIV-1 protease inhibitor pharmacokinetic interactions. *Journal of antimicrobial chemotherapy,* Vol.56, No.1, pp:1-5.

Yeni, P.G.; Hammer, S.M.; Carpenter, C.C. et al. (2002). Antiretroviral treatment for adult HIV infection in 2002: updated recommendations of the International AIDS Society-USA Panel. *Journal of American Association,* Vol.288, No.2, pp:222-235.

Young, B. 2005. Mixing New Cocktails: Drug Interactions in ARV Regimens. *Aids patient care and STDs* Vol.19, No.5, pp:286-297.

Zeldin, R.K. & Peetruschke, R.A. (2004). Pharmacological and therapeutic properties of ritonavir-boosted protease inhibitor therapy in HIV-infected patients. *The Journal of antimicrobial chemotherapy* Vol.53, No.1, pp:4-9.

13

Glycosphingolipids in HIV/AIDS: The Potential Therapeutic Application

Clifford A. Lingwood[2,3,6] and Donald R. Branch[1,2,4,5]

[1]Department of Medicine, University of Toronto,
[2]Department of Laboratory Medicine and Pathobiology, University of Toronto,
[3]Department of Biochemistry, University of Toronto,
[4]Division of Cell and Molecular Biology, Toronto General Research Institute,
[5]Research and Development, Canadian Blood Services, Toronto, Ontario,
[6]Research Institute, Hospital for Sick Children, Toronto, Ontario
Canada

1. Introduction

It has been 30 years since the original description of acquired immunodeficiency syndrome (AIDS) was first reported (Gottlieb et al., 1981). Since this initial discovery, human immunodeficiency virus (HIV) and HIV pathogenesis ranks near the top as one of the most studied human diseases in the history of medical science. Unfortunately, we are no closer now than we were back in the early 1980s at finding a cure. Although there has been significant progress in treatment, there continues to be an increase in the numbers of infected people and those dying from AIDS throughout the world.

Current dogma says that HIV type 1 (HIV-1) is the most common HIV virus and that it infects immune cells called helper T-cells. HIV can also infect other cells involved in the immune response such as monocytes, macrophages and dendritic cells. The virus has an envelope that mediates its tropism for immune cells. The viral envelope protein gp120 first recognizes and binds to the CD4 molecule located on the cell-surface of $CD4^+$ helper T-cells (Dalgleish et al., 1984). Although researchers insisted for over a decade that CD4 was the only cellular receptor required for HIV to infect cells, some in the research community were sceptical and aware from clinical and laboratory findings that something else must be required for HIV infection. Indeed, in 1996 it was discovered that CD4 does not act alone. Another family of cell-surface receptors, the chemokine receptors, were shown to be required, in conjunction with CD4, for successful infection with HIV-1 (Feng et al., 1996, Alkhatib et al., 1996). These receptors are important for the tropism of the virus. Thus, the CXCR4 chemokine receptor, directs infection of T cells by T cell-tropic HIV-1, whereas the CCR5 and CCR3 chemokine receptors are responsible for infection of monocytes with monocyte-tropic HIV-1 virions. However, as more studies were undertaken, it became clear that many other chemokine receptors could support HIV-1 infection and that the tropism was directed more to the chemokine co-receptor than to the cell type. Thus, HIV viruses that require CXCR4 are now known as X4 HIV-1 while virus that recognizes CCR5, or other members of this family of chemokine receptor, are now known as R5 HIV-1. (Dragic et al.,

1996, Littman, 1998).Thus, the current paradigm for HIV infection is that X4 or R5 HIV-1 first binds via its envelope gp120 to CD4 on T-cells expressing either CXCR4 or CCR5. The binding to CD4 results in a conformational change in the structure of a part of the virus envelope gp120 known as the variable V3 loop. This change in conformation of the gp120 exposes a binding site for either chemokine co-receptor. Following binding of the virus to the chemokine co-receptor, another conformational change occurs in the gp120 that exposes another viral membrane protein called gp41. It is the gp41 that then is able to cause the fusion of the virus envelope to the host cell membrane so that the virus can release its contents into the host target cell and begin the infectious process.

Perhaps not that surprising given the history of HIV/AIDS, the HIV-1 paradigm for productive infection continues to change as more studies are undertaken. A role for a family of cell-surface-expressed neuropeptide receptors has been proposed to be important for productive HIV infection (Branch et al., 2002) and cell-surface-expressed glycosphingolipids (GSLs) have been proposed to act as HIV-1 fusion receptors (Fantini et al., 1997; Nehete et al., 2002). Thus, despite 30 years of intense research, we continue to find new and surprising aspects of HIV pathogenesis that have eluded us over the years. One of these more recent findings is the possible therapeutic potential of GSLs in HIV/AIDS.

2. Glycosphingolipids

2.1 Biochemistry, biosynthesis and degradation

GSLs are carbohydrate-lipid conjugates almost exclusively restricted to the outer leaflet of the plasma membrane bilayer of mammalian cells. The hydrophobic backbone, ceramide, consists of a fatty acid chain linked to a sphingosine base, and is common to all GSLs. The alkyl chains of the lipid moiety (ceramide) are embedded in the bilayer and vary in chain length, saturation and hydroxylation (Huwiler et al., 2000; Hakomori, 1993) (Figure 1).

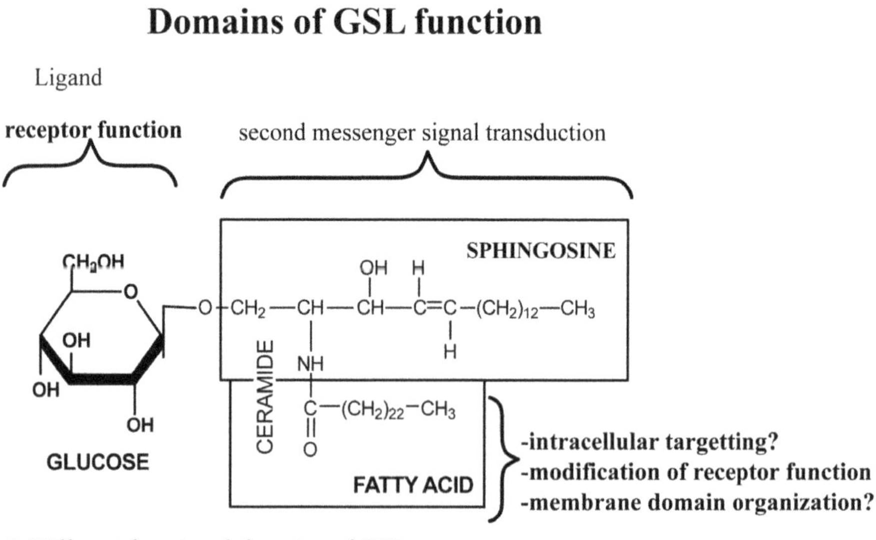

Fig. 1. Different functional domains of GSLs.

The hydrophilic core sugar sequence defines the carbohydrate moieties, and these protrude into the extracellular space (Stults et al., 1989). The different moieties comprising GSLs have different roles in these multifunctional membrane lipids. GSLs are classified as neutral, acidic (anionic) and basic (cationic) glycolipids (Hakomori, 1986). Acidic GSLs usually contain either a sialic acid, which largely encompass the gangliosides, or a sulphate group. Basic glycolipids are very rare, but include plasmalopsychosine or glyceroplasmalopsychosine (Hikita et al., 2002). For the most part, GSLs are comprised of four groups, characterised by their basic core structure: globo- (defined by Galα1-4 Gal), lacto- (Galβ1-3GlcNAc), neolacto- (Galβ1-4GlcNAc) and ganglio- (Galβ1-3GalNAc) series.

The ceramide backbone of GSLs is synthesized on the cytosolic leaflet of the rough ER, through condensation of L-serine and fatty-acyl co-enzymeA and subsequent enzymatic modification (Huwiler et al., 1998). Ceramide may be converted in the lumen of the ER into gala-series glycolipids by addition of galactose, via β-glycosidic linkage, producing the first in the series, galactosylceramide (GalCer) (Sprong et al., 1998). The addition of a sulphate group to the 3-position of the sugar residue on GalCer will give rise to sulphatide (SGC). Ceramide may alternatively be transported to the Golgi apparatus where the first sugar added is glucose, via β-glycosidic link, producing glucosylceramide (GlcCer). The precursor for most GSL structures is GlcCer, which is synthesised by glucosyltransferase located in the cytosol (Futerman & Pagano, 1991). GlcCer can be then translocated by the flippase function of the drug resistance pump, P-glycoprotein (P-gp), to the Golgi lumen (De Rosa et al., 2004, Lala et al., 2000). Here subsequent synthesis of all other GSLs takes place through highly specific glycosyltransferases (Lannert et al., 1998). The first product that is formed from GlcCer is lactosyl ceramide (Galβ1-4Glc cer, LC), which can then be sialylated, to give monosialoganglioside (sialic acid α2-3 Galβ1-4Glc cer, GM3). Alternatively, LC is galactosylated to form globotriaosyl ceramide (Galα1-4 Galβ1-4Glc cer, Gb_3), which can be further converted to globotetraosyl ceramide (GalNAcβ1-3 Galα1-4 Galβ1-4Glc cer, Gb_4) (Figure 2). The major GSLs contain ~5 sugars or less although GSLs containing over 60 sugar residues have been described (Miller-Podraza et al., 1993), and more than 400 GSL species have been reported (Hakomori, 2008). Newly synthesised GSLs follow anterograde vesicular traffic through the Golgi compartments and are directed to the plasma membrane, where they are integrated into the outer leaflet. GSLs follow a process of recycling between intracellular compartments and the plasma membrane, before final endocytosis and transportation through endosomal compartments to the lysosomes (Huwiler et al., 1998). Here, highly specific glycosylhydrolases remove the terminal sugar sequentially from the GSLs, to release the ceramide backbone, which is subsequently catabolised or recycled. It is important to note here, that deficiencies in specific glycosylhydrolases manifest specifically as lysosomal storage diseases, where there is an accumulation of GSL in the lysosome (Kolter & Sandhoff, 1998). These include: Tay-Sachs disease, which accumulates GM2; Gaucher's disease, which accumulates glucocerebroside; and Fabry's disease, which accumulates Gb_3 (Kanfer & Hakomori, 1983).

2.2 Cellular functions

The biological functions of GSLs are many and varied, and may particularly relate to the distribution pattern within the membrane. One such functional role is attributed to the maintenance of membrane structural rigidity, and the ordering of the membrane structure in lipid rafts (discussed below).

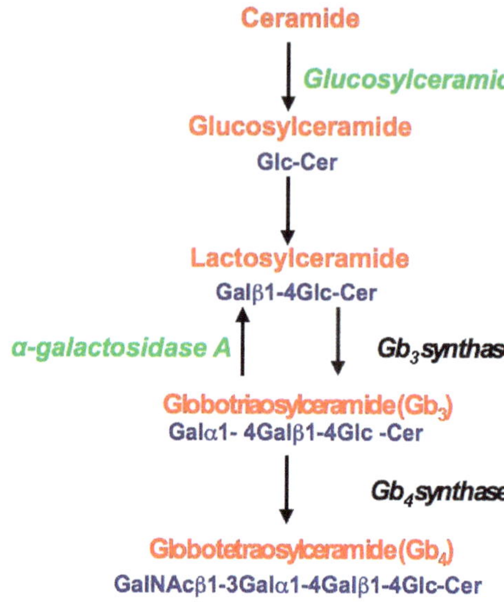

Fig. 2. Biosynthesis of Globotriaosylceramide (Gb_3).

Several GSLs act as cellular antigens or cell-type specific markers, although the functional significance of this is not well understood. Perhaps the most well-known cell-type specific antigens are the GSLs that comprise the histo-blood group antigens, which include members of the Lewis (Le), ABH, I/i and $P/P_1/P^k$ blood groups. Differential expression of GSLs is also particularly depicted during development. The GSLs Le^x (stage-specific embryonic antigen 1, SSEA-1), which is also a Lewis blood-group antigen, Gb_5 (SSEA-3) and monosialyl-Gb_5 (SSEA-4) are variably expressed at specific stages of embryonic development (Kannagi et al., 1983a, Kannagi et al., 1982, Kannagi et al., 1983b, Solter & Knowles, 1978). This differential expression profile has been shown to be important for cell adhesion and cell-cell contact, and such (carbohydrate-carbohydrate) interactions may be essential in developmental processes (Eggens et al., 1989). Indeed, SSEA-4 is a human multipotent stem cell marker.

Interestingly, cell-specific expression of GSLs is also common during differentiation and this is well demonstrated in the haematopoietic cell system. Myeloid cells are characterised by Le^x, Neutrophils specifically express the GSL marker LC (CDW17) and the major T-cell (and monocyte) GSL is ganglioside GM3 (Schwartz-Albeiz et al., 1991, Sorice et al., 2004). Furthermore Gb_3, which has been defined as CD77, is a marker of germinal centre B cells in humans, and thus a marker of differentiation (Mangeney et al., 1991, Wiels et al., 1991).

Given the role of GSLs in development and differentiation, it is not surprising that GSL expression may be aberrant in tumour development, and several have been identified as tumour-associated antigens (Hakomori, 1985). Developmentally regulated GSLs may be re-expressed, or the GSL profile modified, to specifically aid in tumour progression through adhesion functions or tumour growth modulation (Hakomori, 1996, Hakomori, 2002).

It is interesting to note that certain GSLs have been documented to act as cell adhesion molecules, and even as functional receptors, on the cell surface. The GSL sialyl 6-sulfo Le^x acts as an adhesion ligand for selectins on leukocytes and activated endothelial cells, facilitating the process termed "rolling", a critical step in migration of cells from the blood stream during an immune response (Sperandio, 2006) Furthermore, cell-cell interactions can take place between GSLs, and these interactions have been documented between GM3-Gg3, GM3-LacCer, and SGC-GalCer (Kojima & Hakomori, 1991, Koshy et al., 1999) and more recently, between Gb3-GalCer and Gb3-GlcCer (Mahfoud et al., 2010) and between Gg4-GM1, Gg4-Gg3 and Gg4-LacCer(Emam et al., 2010). GSLs acting as functional receptors include sulphated galactolipids (SGC, SGG), which are receptors for hsp70's (Boulanger et al., 1995, Mamelak et al., 2001b); GM1, a co-receptor for FGF2 (Rusnati et al., 2002); and nerve cell gangliosides GD1a and GT1b that bind myelin-associated glycoprotein (MAG), and inhibit nerve regeneration (Vyas et al., 2002).

GSLs, particularly gangliosides, may also have an impact on cell growth and motility (Hakomori & Igarashi, 1993). In terms of cell growth, several GSLs have been shown to interact with growth factor receptors, such as FGFR and EGFR, and modulate growth (Bremer, 1994, Weis & Davis, 1990). GM3 interaction with the insulin receptor is important in type 2 diabetes (Tagami et al., 2002, van Eijk et al., 2009). While the mechanisms of inhibitory or stimulatory effects are not well understood, in many cases receptor-associated tyrosine kinases are inhibited. Cell motility is controlled by integrin function, and is specifically affected by gangliosides. The GSL, GM3 is able to inhibit motility by interaction within a complex of N-glycosylated alpha3 integrin and tetraspanin CD9 (Ono et al., 2001).

2.3 Lipid rafts

Biological membrane lipids are not homogeneously distributed but can be organized into heterogeneous microdomains or lipid rafts of increased membrane order. Lipid rafts within the plasma membrane of eukaryotic cells present different physical assemblies of proteins and lipids. Specifically, rafts are comprised of increased concentrations of GSLs, certain phospholipids, and cholesterol, as well as scaffold and/or functional membrane proteins (Hooper, 1999, Simons & Ehehalt, 2002, Simons & Ikonen, 1997). Several membrane proteins preferentially associate with lipid rafts, and these include glycosylphosphatidylinositol (GPI)-anchored cell surface proteins within the outer leaflet, and cytosolic palmitoylated and myristoylated proteins, and cholesterol- or phospholipid-binding proteins (Rajendran & Simons, 2005). The proteins and lipids cooperate to form dynamic membrane assemblies to facilitate transmembrane information flow (Lingwood & Simons, 2010) One morphologically identifiable raft structure is caveolae, which are flask-shaped invaginations of the membrane associated with caveolin scaffolding protein (Kurzchalia & Parton, 1999).

Lipid rafts are small, highly dynamic and detergent-insoluble, and while these assemblies are fluid, they represent a more ordered region within the membrane. This "liquid-ordered" domain is more tightly packed than the surrounding bilayer, and this is largely due to the saturated hydrocarbon chains of raft-associated GSL and phospholipids (Simons & Vaz, 2004). Thus, the degree of saturation and hydroxylation of GSLs may greatly affect the "liquid-ordered" state of the membrane, as well as the degree of clustering or association with membrane proteins (Brown & London, 1997, Hakomori et al., 1998b). Because raft formation is dependant on lipid structure, lipids of the appropriate structure are capable of forming microdomains in model membranes (Dietrich et al., 2001, Radhakrishnan et al., 2000). However such model membrane systems do not fully reflect plasma membrane microdomains (Kaiser et al., 2009).

Two fundamental properties of lipid rafts associated with their physical attributes, are their capacity to selectively incorporate proteins, and their ability to coalesce to form larger domains. It is not surprising therefore, that lipid rafts play a role in protein sorting, membrane trafficking and signal transduction (Brown & London, 2000, Lajoie & Nabi, 2010). Because of the thermodynamic formation of lipid rafts, the cell utilizes them as centres or "hot spots" for transmembrane signal transduction for a variety of membrane receptors (Hakomori & Igarashi, 1995, Simons & Toomre, 2000). Ligand-induced receptor dimerization and successive cytosolic phosphorylation cascades occur in microdomains, and as such membrane receptors often partition into such domains upon ligation, and may subsequently be internalised and traffic through said domains (Dykstra et al., 2001). This can result in direct ligand interaction with GSLs (Hakomori et al., 1998a, Iwabuchi et al., 2000) without necessarily, the involvement of a transmembrane protein (Katagiri et al., 1999, Mori et al., 2000). This implies a mechanism of communication between the cell surface and the cytosolic lipid bilayer leaflets. Cytosolic signal transduction proteins, such as *src*-family tyrosine kinases and small G-proteins, are often associated with the cytosolic surface of such domains in a transient and surface ligand-regulated manner (Dykstra et al., 2001, Hakomori, 2000, Katagiri et al., 1999).

Lipid rafts are also involved in internalisation and intracellular trafficking of proteins and lipids(Lajoie & Nabi, 2010, Mukherjee & Maxfield, 2000) and likely, their attendant signalling. An endocytic role has been established for cavolae and lipid rafts, which may translocate and endocytose GPI-anchored proteins in particular (Parton & Richards, 2003). Other raft-mediated routes of internalisation have been identified where the GPI-anchor acts as a targeting signal in the traffic to an endosomal organelle called the GPI-anchored protein enriched early endosomal compartment (Sabharanjak et al., 2002). It is clear therefore that several distinct raft-mediated trafficking pathways exist. It is important to note however, that lipid rafts are not distributed randomly in the endosomal pathway, but are excluded from the degradative compartments, although this is not well understood (Nichols et al., 2001, Simons & Gruenberg, 2000).

2.3.1 Defining a new assay for lipid raft formation

Lipid rafts are isolated from cells from the Triton insoluble fraction separated on a discontinuous sucrose ultracentrifuge gradient. Due to their atypical density, the rafts separate as a band above the 30% sucrose layer. The majority of proteins sediment to the bottom, while components found in this fraction are deemed lipid raft associated. This has not been studied for purified (glyco)lipids. We have developed this procedure as a new method for examining the 'raft' forming capability of glycolipids. Soluble adamantylGb_3 (adaGb_3), natural Gb_3 or Gb_3+cholesterol were mixed with Triton and placed at the bottom of the sucrose gradient, below the 30% layer, the lower half of which now contains FITC-labeled VT1 B subunit. The gradients are centrifuged at 66K rpm for 3 days. Any rafts structures formed will float up through the FITC-VT1 B layer and the raft band should thus be fluorescently labeled. When this was performed with Gb_3 alone, no fluorescent band was formed. In contrast, a distinct fluorescent band was formed for Gb_3+cholesterol. However adaGb_3 formed the strongest labeled 'raft' band (Mahfoud et al., 2002b). While the characteristics of the structures formed by adaGb_3 in this band remain to be fully characterized, this supports the "raft-like" character of adaGb_3. Moreover, this is an excellent method for determining the properties and components required for optimal raft formation (Nutikka & Lingwood, 2004). We have shown that cholesterol is one requirement. A fifty fold molar excess of the SPC3 peptide from the glycolipid binding V3 loop of gp120 of HIV, which strongly binds adaGb_3 (Mahfoud et al., 2002b) is able to eliminate FITC-VT1 B labeling of the adaGb_3 'raft" band. The raft band is still formed –seen under visible light- in the presence of SPC3. Thus both the SPC3 peptide (and presumably, gp120 and the intact HIV virus) and VT1 B selectively bind the same Gb_3 containing raft structures. This would correlate with the raft requirement for HIV infectivity and VT cytotoxicity (Falguieres et al., 2001).

2.4 Pathogens and GSL receptors

GSLs have been shown to play a role in many pathogen interactions with host cells. As previously described, several GSLs represent histo-blood group molecules, and there is a longstanding association between pathogens and these particular blood groups, which are not necessarily limited to expression on erythrocytes. Such interactions have been defined both in protective qualities conferred by a specific blood type, and in pathogen interactions with blood group antigens (Moulds & Moulds, 2000, Rios & Bianco, 2000)

Several GSLs, including those categorised as blood group antigens, have been identified as adherence receptors for bacteria, or bacterial toxins (Lingwood, 1998). The globo-series of GSLs expressed on urogenital epithelia, particularly monosialyl-Gb5, are infection sites for *Escherichia coli* (Stapleton et al., 1992). The Le^b antigen is required for surface adherence of *Helicobacter pylori*, known to cause gastritis and peptic ulcers, to gastric mucosa, and Group O Le (b+) secretors are thus likely most susceptible to this pathogen (Borén et al., 1993). The minimal structure of sialyl-lactosylceramide (GM3) is crucial for colonization and adherence to epithelium via fimbria-dependant binding of *Haemophilus influenzae*, which causes a variety of diseases from meningitis to upper respiratory infection (van Alphen et al., 1991).Ganglioseries GSLs such as asialoGM1(Gg4), are binding targets for the pili of certain *Pseudomonas aeruginosa* strains, which are opportunistic pathogens that target and colonize epithelial cells of the lung (Comolli et al., 1999). These GSLs are not receptors for these organisms (Emam et al., 2006) but can assist host cell invasion (Emam et al., 2010). Finally, bacterial toxins, which are soluble proteins, often bind to GSLs to elicit their effects. Glycolipid receptors include ganglioside GM1, bound by cholera toxin (De Haan & Hirst, 2004) from *Vibrio cholerae*, and Gb_3, which is utilized by *Escherichia coli* elicited verotoxins (VT) (Petruzziello et al., 2009), susceptibility to cholera toxin (and *E. Coli* LT) is blood group O related.

The involvement of GSLs in the host cell attachment of viruses, and also fusion in terms of enveloped viruses, has long been recognised (Haywood, 1994). The initial step of viral attachment to the susceptible cell is crucial in the process of establishing an infection. The sialic acid motif, which is widely presented on acidic GSLs, is perhaps the most broadly recognised adhesion component utilised by viruses, from small non-enveloped DNA polyomaviruses to larger enveloped RNA influenza viruses (Gilbert & Benjamin, 2004, Miller-Podraza et al., 2000, Tsai et al., 2003). The GSL neolactotetraosylceramide (nLc_4Cer) is a key receptor for the enveloped Dengue virus, an infectious agent transmitted by mosquitoes (Aoki et al., 2006). The ganglioside GD1a has been identified as a critical component for viral binding of Sendai virus, and fusion of this enveloped virus with its target is abolished if GD1a is not present for initial contact (Epand et al., 1995).

2.5 Pathogens and lipid rafts

GSLs and lipid rafts themselves are important for many microbial pathogens and often form preferential sites for pathogen interactions (Lafont et al., 2002, Samuel et al., 2001, van der Goot & Harder, 2001, Vieira et al., 2010). Pathogenic interactions may be vast and varied. For example, lipid rafts serve as key platforms for entry of parasitic agents, such as *Plasmodium falciparum,* which causes malaria. Following attachment of the *P. falciparum* merozoite to erythrocytes, the membrane invaginates taking up the parasite within a parasitophorous vacuolar membrane (PVM) (Haldar et al., 2002). Lipid rafts are critical for the formation of the PVM, as are the raft-associated proteins internalized with the vacuole (Lauer et al., 2000). Indeed, even 'non-classic' infectious agents require lipid rafts, as demonstrated by the requirement for the prion proteins which partition into rafts during the conversion of PrP^{c} to infectious PrP^{sc} (Simons & Ehehalt, 2002).

Bacteria often favour lipid rafts during host-cell interactions (Heung et al., 2006),. Raft association may provide a platform for colonisation, through signalling, cytoskeleton rearrangements and membrane ruffling (Manes & Martinez, 2004). Intracellular bacteria rely on lipid rafts to enter host-cells, which provides protection from degradation and immune detection. This is demonstrated by *Mycobacterium* spp., which exploits rafts to generate phagosomes in which to survive within the cell, allowing the bacterium to evade antigen processing (Gatfield & Pieters, 2000). Toxins produced by non-intracellular bacteria, are particularly dependant on rafts for host-cell interaction, which mediates oligomerization, internalization and intracellular trafficking (Fivaz et al., 1999). Cholera toxin binding ganglioside GM1 is the current "gold standard' for identification of such rafts (Lencer, 2001) Lipid rafts are integral in the retrograde transport of cholera toxin to the Golgi (Lencer & Saslowsky, 2005).VT is also dependant on the organization of its receptor, Gb_3, into rafts for intracellular routing (Falguieres et al., 2001) and cytopathology (Khan et al., 2009).

Lipid rafts are also fundamental in viral infection, predominantly in the process of viral entry, both for enveloped and non-enveloped viruses (Manes et al., 2003). In the case of non-enveloped viruses, lipid rafts are important in the process of viral attachment and subsequent internalization and trafficking to the appropriate sub-cellular niche. Caveolae lipid rafts are required for non-enveloped simian virus 40 (SV40) interactions with MHC-I and viral entry, a process that can be inhibited with cholesterol chelators (Norkin, 1999). Lipid rafts facilitate the traffic of SV40 to the ER through the Golgi (Parton, 1994). Interestingly, rafts appear to be involved in a sorting process in viral trafficking, as other viruses, such as the echovirus, enter by caveolae but do not traffic to the ER(Marjomaki et al., 2002). Enveloped viruses are particularly dependant on lipid raft domains for the process of viral/cell membrane fusion. Cholesterol and sphingolipids, which define these domains, have been identified as critical in the process of fusion for alphaviruses, such as the Semliki-forest virus (Ahn et al., 2002). Interestingly, disrupting raft formation by replacing cholesterol with androstenol did not hinder envelope glycoprotein insertion, but replacing sphingolipids with dipalmitoylphosphatidylcholine was inhibitory, emphasizing the importance of GSLs in the process of fusion (Waarts et al., 2002). Finally, lipid rafts are critical in the process of enveloped virus assembly and budding for many viruses, including influenza, measles, filoviruses and HIV (Bavari et al., 2002 , Luo et al., 2008, Manie et al., 2000, Scheiffele et al., 1999). Membrane rafts are an efficient system of concentrating viral proteins in a specific region, may provide a specific lipid composition for the virus, and also exclude/include host-proteins from the viral envelope (Manes et al., 2003).

3. Globotriaosylceramide

3.1 Characteristics and expression

The neutral glycolipid, globotriaosylceramide (Gb_3), is defined by the trisaccharide core unit (Galα1-4Galβ1-4Glc) linked to a ceramide backbone, and as such belongs to the globo-series of GSLs. Gb_3 shares the amphipathic characteristics of all GSLs, and their fatty acid chain length, saturation and hydroxylation, may vary yielding various Gb_3 isoforms. Gb_3 may also partition into lipid-rafts and interact with raft-associated proteins. Gb_3 is widely expressed in a variety of tissues, but is a major GSL of human renal cortex(Boyd & Lingwood, 1989), heart, spleen and placenta; (Kojima et al., 2000). Moreover, it has been described in a number of epithelial and endothelial cell lines. Gb_3, or CD77, is expressed as a differentiation antigen on a subset of tonsillar B lymphocytes in the germinal center, where expression is very specific, and only occurs at a restricted stage (Mangeney et al., 1991, Wiels et al., 1991). It is interesting to note that human Burkitt lymphoma cells, which are characteristically derived from B cells, also express Gb_3 (Wiels et al., 1981; Kim et al., 2011). Finally, human erythrocytes are characterized by two major globo-series GSLs, Gb_3 or P^k, being one, the other being Gb_4, or P. Gb_3 is also upregulated in many human tumours (Devenica et al., 2010)

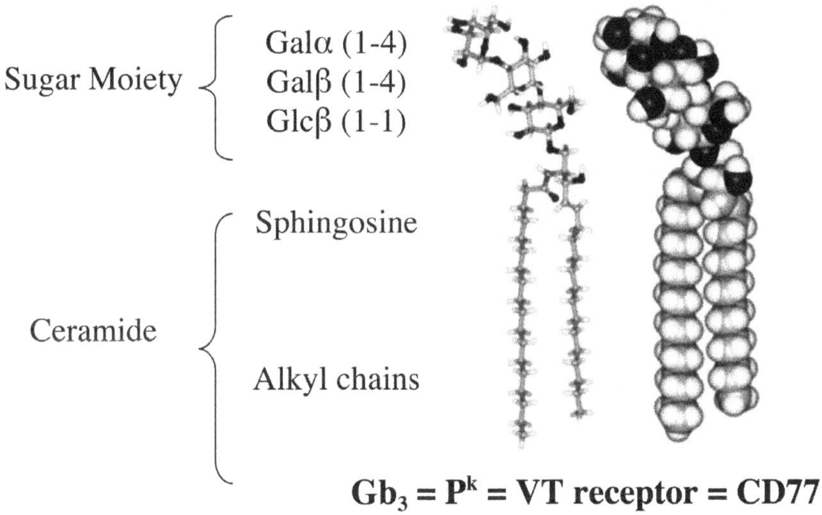

Fig. 3. Chemical structure of globotriaosylceramide.

3.2 Function

Gb_3 expressed on B-lymphocytes, has specifically been implicated in signal transduction resulting from CD19 engagement (Maloney & Lingwood, 1994). Indeed, the extracellular domain of CD19 presents a Gb_3 binding site, (with sequence similarity to the Gb_3-binding VT1B subunit of *Escherichia coli*). Gb_3 is crucial for CD19 induced homotypic adhesion of B cells and this suggests a potential role for Gb_3 in adhesion during B cell development (Maloney & Lingwood, 1994). Gb_3 has further been shown to mediate CD19 directed apoptosis of B cells, which may be important during B cell selection (Khine et al., 1998). This occurs following CD19 ligation, where Gb_3 mediates targeting and intracellular traffic of CD19 to the ER and nuclear envelope (Khine et al., 1998).

Gb_3 expression has also been shown to affect the binding capacity of IFN-α for its receptor, α2 interferon receptor IFNAR1, on B lymphoid cells (Ghislain et al., 1992). The amino terminus of IFNAR1 is able to bind to Gb_3, sharing sequence similarity with the VT1B subunit (Lingwood & Yiu, 1992) and binding to Gb_3 likely affects the subsequent signaling. Gb_3 has thus been shown to be critical for IFNAR1-dependant α2IFN induced growth inhibition, mediated by short chain fatty acid Gb_3 isoforms (Khine & Lingwood, 2000). Furthermore, Gb_3 is important in α2IFN IFNAR1 signaling to induce antiviral activity, which is mediated by long fatty acid isoforms of Gb_3 (Khine & Lingwood, 2000). Gb_3 has been implicated in angiogenesis and is found in tumour neovasculature (Heath-Engel & Lingwood, 2003), and can promote tumour metastases (Kovbasnjuk et al., 2005)

3.3 Blood group antigens

Gb_3 belongs to the P1PK and GLOB blood group system, that have red cell phenotypes termed $P/P_1/P^k$ (Table 1) and whose expression profile is not limited to erythrocytes. The structure galabiose (Galα1-4Gal) is the terminal structure of P^k, also known as Gb_3, and P_1 blood group antigens, whilst it is the precursor for P antigen, also known as globoside or Gb_4, which terminates with β1-3GalNAc(Spitalnik & Spitalnik, 1995). P_1 and P_2 are the two common $P/P_1/P^k$-related blood group phenotypes. P_1 individuals (~80% of Caucasians but only ~20% of Asians)(Daniels, 2002) express P and P_1 but only expose low amounts of P^k antigens on their cell surfaces. P_2 individuals (~20% of Caucasians and ~80% of Asians)(Daniels, 2002) express only P and low amounts of P^k antigens. There are also rare phenotypes defined by a deficiency in one or more of the $P/P_1/P^k$ blood group antigens. Individuals deficient in P antigen have mutations in the *B3GALNT1* gene causing lack of functional Gb_4 synthase (β3GalNAc transferase) (Hellberg et al., 2002, Hellberg et al., 2004), and consequently express high amounts of unmodified precursor, P^k. These individuals may express P_1 antigen (P_1^k phenotype) or not (P_2^k). Although uncertain for many years (Hellberg et al., 2005; Iwamura et al., 2003), the molecular basis for P_1/P_2 has recently been elucidated (Thuresson et al., 2011). Individuals who do not express any $P/P_1/P^k$ antigens have mutations in the *A4GALT* gene, causing lack of functional Gb_3 synthase (α4Gal transferase), and have the rare p blood group phenotype (Furukawa et al., 2000, Hellberg et al., 2002, Hellberg et al., 2003, Steffensen et al., 2000). Similar to the ABO blood group system, naturally occurring antibodies are formed against the $P/P_1/P^k$ antigens when missing (Spitalnik & Spitalnik, 1995). Recent studies show anti-P^k is present in all normal sera (Pochechueva et al., 2010)

Phenotype	Frequency	Red Blood Cell Antigens	Serum Antibodies
P_1	75%	P_1, P, P^k	None
P_2	25%	P, P^k	Anti-P_1
P_1^k	Rare	P_1, P^k	Anti-P
P_2^k	Rare	P^k	Anti-P_1, anti-P
P	Rare	None	Anti-P_1, anti-P, anti-P^k

Table 1. Red Blood Cell Phenotypes in the P1Pk and GLOB Blood Group System (Spitalnik & Spitalnik, 1995; Branch, 2010)

4. Relationship to disease

The P1PK and GLOB blood group system antigens are of particular interest, with many defined pathogen interactions. Both P^k (or Gb_3) and P (or Gb_4) are receptors for P pili of uropathogenic *E. coli* (Leffler & Svanborg-Eden, 1981). P^k has been shown to act as a receptor for the porcine bacteria *Streptococcus suis* (Haataja et al., 1994). Indeed, P^k is also known to act as a receptor for bacterial toxins, Shigella or Verotoxins specifically, produced by *Shigella dysenteriae* and Enterohemorrhagic *E. coli* (Bitzan et al., 1994, Pellizzari et al., 1992) but no association with P blood group status has been found (Jelacic et al., 2002). Viruses have also been shown to have interactions with blood group antigens. In terms of the P blood group system, Parvovirus B19 utilizes the P antigen as its receptor to infect cells, and individuals with the p phenotype lacking P are resistant to the virus (Brown et al., 1994). More recently, the P1PK and GLOB blood group system antigens, specifically, P^k, has been implicated as having a role in HIV infection (Branch, 2010)(see below).

4.1 Verotoxin-induced disease

Enterohemorrhagic *Escherichia coli* induce disease, characteristically haemolytic uremic syndrome (HUS), by the production of verotoxins (VT). VTs are capable of binding to Gb_3, thus Gb_3 contributes to the pathology of VT-induced disease (Lingwood, 2000, Lingwood et al., 1987) VT is comprised of a single toxic 'A' subunit and non-covalently associated pentameric 'B' subunits responsible for receptor (Gb_3) binding. Only cells with Gb_3 surface expression are sensitive to VT toxicity (Okuda et al., 2006, Waddell et al., 1990). VT interaction with the sugar moiety of Gb_3 is dependant on the lipid moiety in its membrane environment (Arab & Lingwood, 1996, Kiarash et al., 1994, Pellizzari et al., 1992), which is crucial in internalization and subcellular targeting of VT (Arab & Lingwood, 1998 , Smith et al., 2006). The intracellular routing of VT thus is also dependant on the organization of Gb_3 into lipid rafts (Falguieres et al., 2001). Indeed, VT binding to cell surface Gb_3 within lipid microdomains has been shown to activate cytosolic raft-associated src kinase ((Katagiri et al., 1999, Mori et al., 2000)) indicating Gb_3 can mediate transmembrane signals. Furthermore, Gb_3 containing cells where Gb_3 is not present in rafts are insensitive to VT cytotoxicity (Falguieres et al., 2001, Ramegowda & Tesh, 1996). In cells sensitive to VT cytotoxicity, the toxin is internalized via both clathrin independant/dependant pathways(Lauvrak et al., 2004) and undergoes retrograde transport via the reverse of the secretory system to the Golgi and ER/nucleus (Arab & Lingwood, 1998, Khine & Lingwood, 1994, Sandvig et al., 1994) Highly VT sensitive cells contain higher levels of short fatty acid containing Gb_3 isoforms and retrograde transport the VT/Gb_3 complex to the ER/nucleus. Less VT sensitive cells have longer fatty acid containing Gb_3 isoforms and retrograde transport VT to the Golgi only (Arab & Lingwood, 1998). Interestingly, Gb_3 is maintained in lipid rafts during retrograde transport (Smith et al., 2006).

4.2 Fabry disease

Fabry disease is an X-linked lysosomal storage disorder, as a result of a genetic defect in the lysosomal enzyme α-galactosidase A, which results in reduced enzyme activity (Brady, 1967). This enzyme is normally responsible for the removal of the terminal Gb_3 galactose residue, through hydrolysis of the α1-4 glycosidic linkage. Thus, Gb_3, and potentially other α-galactose terminal lipids accumulate in the lysosomes to abrogate their normal function and the function of these organelles. Clinical manifestations of the disorder are related to the cell-type-specific expression of Gb_3 (Huwiler et al., 2000). Thus patients with Fabry disease typically experience renal dysfunction, myocardial and skin lesions, and joint pain, which relate to the major tissue distribution of Gb_3 (Hakomori, 1986).

5. HIV and GSLs

5.1 GSL receptors

Initial contact of HIV with the host cell surface must occur before the virus can initiate infection. HIV envelope glycoprotein gp120 targets CD4 and CCR5 or CXCR4 chemokine co-receptors on monocytes and T-cells respectively, as the major HIV-host cell interaction (Alkhatib et al., 1996, Dalgleish et al., 1984, Feng et al., 1996). GSLs have been implicated in HIV infection since the original description of the binding of GalCer and sulfatide (3′ sulfogalactosyl ceramide, SGC) by the HIV adhesin gp120 (Bhat et al., 1993, Bhat et al., 1991) and indeed gp120 binding to these species is considered the primary mechanism by which non-CD4 expressing cells are 'infected' by HIV(Dorosko & Connor, 2010, Harouse et al., 1995, Magerus-Chatinet et al., 2007, Ullrich et al., 1998). GSLs bound by gp120 include GalCer, SGC, Gb_3 and the ganglioside GM3 (Delezay et al., 1996, Hammache et al., 1998a). It has been suggested that GM3 is bound only by gp120 from R5 strains whereas Gb3 is bound by both X4 and R5 strains (Hammache et al., 1999). GSL analogues have been shown to inhibit HIV infection(Fantini et al., 1997, Faroux-Corlay et al., 2001, Garg et al., 2008, Lund et al., 2006, Weber et al., 2000)and the efficacy of such analogues depends on the nature of both the carbohydrate and lipid moieties. In addition, GalCer binds to gp120 associated gp41 (Alfsen & Bomsel, 2002), the fusion heptad repeat C-terminal peptide of which, mediates viral/host membrane fusion (Shnaper et al., 2004). Nevertheless, the exact role of the GSLs in HIV infection remains unclear. Early suggestions were that GSL binding within lipid rafts facilitated a simultaneous recognition of CD4 and chemokine receptor by gp120(Fantini, 2003). However, the fact that the GSL-binding site (Delezay et al., 1996), defined as 2 alpha helixes with a central aromatic amino acid sequence(Mahfoud et al., 2002a), responsible for gp120-GSL binding, is contained within the same V3 loop as amino acids crucial for chemokine receptor binding (Xiao et al., 1998), suggest that the binding of GSLs within the V3 loop would more likely provide an inhibitory, rather than stimulatory effect on chemokine receptor binding. To address this potential dichotomy the unusual membrane properties of GSLs must be considered.

5.1.1 GSL conformation and lipid heterogeneity

A single glycosphingolipid (i.e. a single carbohydrate species with a heterogeneous ceramide moiety) can differentially recognize two or more ligands, specific for the carbohydrate sequence. This can be based on differential recognition of the hydroxyl groups within the sugar sequence as has been shown for Verotoxin variants and monoclonal anti-Gb_3 (Chark et al., 2004). Differential binding of anti-GM1 and cholera toxin to GM1 lipid isoforms has also been reported (Iglesias-Bartolome et al., 2009). This is consistent with differential ligand recognition of GSL lipid isoforms by ligands which bind the same carbohydrate sequence. The oligosaccharide moiety of glycolipids shows considerable flexibility in conformation and nine potential energy minima have been defined by molecular modeling (Nyholm & Pascher, 1993). This potential for differential carbohydrate conformation which can be regulated by the relative plane of the plasma membrane may therefore reflect the lipid composition and its membrane microenvironment. Indeed, cholesterol can induce a fatty acid-dependent GSL conformational change (Lingwood et al., 2011). The identification of a family of fatty acyl co-A selective ceramide synthases (Stiban et al., 2010, Teufel et al., 2009) provides the metabolic means to regulate the differential synthesis of such GSL fatty acid isoforms.

As indicated, cell membrane GSLs can be organized into cholesterol enriched microdomains. Such microdomains are typically correlated with resistance to detergent extraction *in vitro* (Lingwood & Simons, 2007). While this procedure can induce domain pooling and the relationship between detergent resistance and natural cell membrane GSL domains has yet to be established (Westerlund & Slotte, 2009), detergent resistance indicates stronger lateral membrane interactions. Detergent resistant, cholesterol enriched plasma membrane domains have been shown to be important for HIV infection by most studies (Del Real et al., 2002 , Gummuluru et al., 2003, Liao et al., 2001 , Manes et al., 2000, Nguyen & Hildreth, 2000 , Popik et al., 2002 , Raulin, 2002) but not all (Percherancier et al., 2003).

5.1.2 GSLs and HIV infection

The role of GSLs in HIV infection must be considered both in terms of GSL species generally distributed in the membrane or restricted to lipid microdomains. Several studies have shown that the binding of the gp120 HIV adhesin to GSL is dependent not only on the carbohydrate, but also the lipid moiety of the GSL (Mahfoud et al., 2009, Mahfoud et al., 2002b, Villard et al., 2002).

The interaction of GSLs with cholesterol is modulated by the fatty acid chain length and the binding of HIV gp120 to Gb_3/cholesterol vesicles has been shown to be a function of the fatty acid composition in that C16 fatty acid Gb_3 was bound but C17, C18 and C20 Gb_3 were not. C22 and C24 fatty acid containing Gb_3s were bound(Mahfoud et al., 2009). The Gb_3 fatty acid isoforms not recognized by gp120 in this context, have fatty acid chain lengths which are of the order of the dimensions of the cholesterol molecule, suggesting that these fatty acid isoforms have the minimum 'hydrophobic mismatch' (Niemela et al., 2009) and therefore interact more effectively with cholesterol. The interaction of GSLs with cholesterol has been shown in modeling studies to induce a conformation change in the headgroup to become parallel to the plane of the cholesterol containing membrane rather than perpendicular, as seen in the absence of cholesterol (Hall et al., 2010, Lingwood et al., 2011, Yahi et al., 2010). In such a membrane parallel carbohydrate format, the accessibility of the carbohydrate to carbohydrate binding ligands, such as gp120, will be restricted (but lateral interaction with the membrane may be enhanced). In GSL/cholesterol model detergent resistant membranes separated by sucrose gradient centrifugation, the major GSL fraction was not recognized by gp120 (GSLs -sulfatide, galactosyl ceramide and Gb_3) (Mahfoud et al., 2010). Only a minor fraction of smaller vesicles were bound. Such smaller vesicles may display the GSL in a more disperse format, even in the presence of cholesterol, and thereby defray the effect of this potential cholesterol-induced conformational change. Moreover, the fatty acid isoforms of Gb_3 negative for gp120 binding were dominant negative in mixtures of saturated Gb_3 fatty acid isoforms, whereas addition of the unsaturated C24:1 Gb_3 was dominant positive, suggesting that membrane fluidity in these vesicles could be a key factor in determining availability of the GSL carbohydrate for gp120 binding(Mahfoud et al., 2009). Thus the interaction of gp120 with membrane GSLs is extremely complex depending also, on the membrane bilayer organization and perhaps curvature and fluidity. In addition, host cell GSLs taken up into the viral membrane at the time of plasma membrane budding may also play a direct role in HIV dendritic cell targeting (Hatch et al., 2009) and T cell infection.

This differential availability of cell membrane Gb_3 for example, is dramatically highlighted by the differential binding of various monoclonal antibodies to Gb_3 and verotoxin B subunit to lymphoid cells which synthesize Gb_3 (Kim et al., 2011), despite the fact that these antibodies show similar efficacy to detect the Gb_3 once extracted from the cells and separated by TLC. Gb3 positive cells which do not bind any Gb_3 ligands have been reported(Sekino et al., 2004).

The masking of membrane GSL is also dependent on the relative cholesterol concentration. In model GSL membranes, the thickness of the carbohydrate layer was an inverse function of the cholesterol concentration, suggesting that the sugar can adopt intermediate conformations between the membrane perpendicular (thickest) and parallel (thinnest) conformation according to membrane cholesterol content (Lingwood et al., 2011), extending the potential for conformational regulation of GSL receptor function.

The differential expression of membrane GSLs within and without cholesterol enriched lipid rafts may provide the explanation for the differential function ascribed to GSLs in HIV infection; first as promotors of fusion/infection (Puri et al., 1998, Puri et al., 2004) and then as inhibitors of these functions (Lund et al., 2009, Ramkumar et al., 2009). It is conceivable that different GSL carbohydrate conformers can play different roles at different (or the same) times in infection.

Amino acids within the gp120 V3 loop defined by mutational analysis as crucial for chemokine receptor binding(Xiao et al., 1998) coincide with 3 amino acids of the concensus GSL binding site at the V3 loop apex (Delezay et al., 1996), together with 2 distinct amino acids, one in the base of each alpha helix comprising the V3 loop(Xiao et al., 1998). The GSL hexapeptide binding domain has been synthesized as a separate peptide and shown to bind the same GSLs *in vitro* as observed for the intact gp120 (Delezay et al., 1996). The V3 loop must open following CD4 -gp120 binding to allow the chemokine receptor to bind (Wang et al., 1999) whereas gp120 -GSL binding is observed in the absence of CD4 (Mahfoud et al., 2009). Thus GSL binding to the apex of the V3 loop could well alter the alpha helix conformation at the base of the V3 loop to modulate chemokine receptor binding. It is possible that binding of different GSLs, or different lipid isoforms of the same GSL, could differentially alter the conformation of the V3 loop to enhance or inhibit CCR5 binding.

This concept is consistent with NMR studies which indicate that the N terminus of CCR5 binds within the base of the V3 loop (Huang et al., 2007). In combination, soluble CD4 and CCR5 reduced proteolytic susceptibility of the V3 loop of gp120, consistent with binding. A model was proposed (Huang et al., 2007) by which the CCR5 N terminus bound to the base of the V3 loop (via tyrosine sulfate) and then the second extracellular loop of CCR5 associated with the V3 loop apex. Alternatively, the extracellular CCR5 loop associated with the V3 loop apex first, followed by CCR5 N terminus binding to the V3 loop base. The binding of the CCR5 N terminus to the V3 loop base was found to cause a conformational change to rigidify the V3 loop. Such a conformation change might be impeded or promoted by GSL binding within the GSL binding site at the V3 loop apex (Figure 4).

If the first GSL sugar is primarily responsible for binding, it is possible that the effect on V3 conformation could be dependent on the number and character of additional sugar residues. In the absence of the gp120 conformational change induced by CD4 binding, V3 loop binding to GSLs via this apical binding site could mediate a less effective mechanism for HIV internalization. Cell membrane GSLs undergo a natural process of internalization and recycling and GSLs function in receptor mediated endocytosis of appropriate GSL binding ligands. This could thereby provide a basis for the observed association of galactosyl

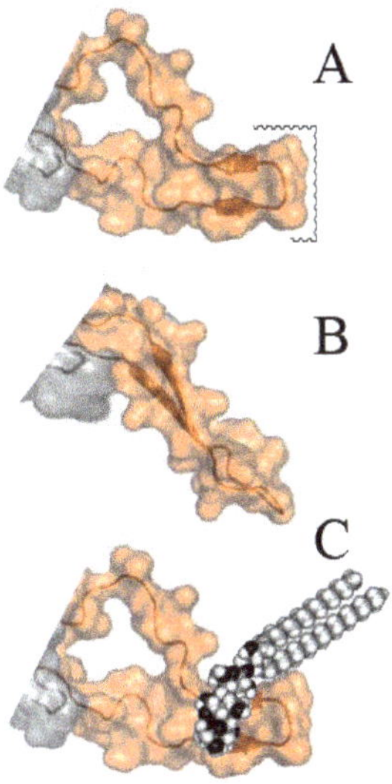

Fig. 4. **Conformational change in gp120 induced by CCR5 binding and relation to GSL binding.** The NMR structure of the V3 loop alone (A) or with bound CCR5 N terminus (B) is shown according to Huang et al., 2007. The amino acids of the GSL binding site at the loop apex are boxed in (A). The V3 loop initially disorganized, becomes more rigid on binding of the CCR5 N terminus to the V3 loop base. Gb_3 has been arbitrarily placed and oriented with its glucose moiety stacked over the phenylalanine of the CCR5 unbound loop (C) to illustrate the potential of GSL binding to affect this V3 loop conformational change.

ceramide in gastroepithelial/neuronal/renal cells targeted by HIV (Harouse et al., 1995). Infectious HIV utilizes GSLs and lipid rafts to traverse the host mucosa and access underlying susceptible target cells during transmission. This process is called transcytosis, whereby "receptors" mediate the transcellular traffic of the virus across the tight epithelial cell barrier, rather than productive infection (Bomsel and Alfsen 2003). Thus uptake of the virus occurs at one pole of the cells and infectious virus is released at the opposite pole, gaining access to the submucosa. GalCer has been shown to bind to both HIV-gp120 and gp41 (Alfsen and Bomsel 2001). However, HIV binding to GalCer in epithelial cells does not result in HIV/host cell fusion necessary for productive infection but rather mediates HIV transcytosis (Bomsel, 1997), Bomsel and David 2002). This has been demonstrated in epithelial cell lines, where HIV 'hijacks' the vesicular pathway in order to cross the cell. The process of transcytosis via GalCer has also been shown to occur in primary intestinal epithelial cells, specifically for R5 HIV-1 strains, and is particularly dependant on lipid rafts, as disruption of rafts substantially reduces uptake (Meng Wei 2002). It has further been suggested that transcytosis may occur across specialized M cells, which provide an epithelial barrier, to lymphoid Peyer's patches in the gastrointestinal tract (Fotopoulos 2002). Mucosal dendritic cells express GalCer which can mediate HIV uptake and transfer to T cells (Magerus-Chatinet et al., 2007). To date, the vast majority of evidence suggests transcytosis is a process that facilitates HIV transmission across the gastrointestinal mucosa, and limited data has been shown for vaginal mucosal transmission

5.2 Membrane fusion

For productive infection, HIV enters cells directly via plasma membrane penetration, which requires fusion of the viral envelope with the host cell membrane (Marsh & Helenius, 1989). Membrane fusion is particularly dependant on lipid rafts, which have a central role in HIV infection. Depletion of cholesterol, a key component of lipid rafts, renders cells resistant to infection and membrane fusion, a phenotype rescued upon re-introduction of cholesterol (Manes, del Real 2000, Liao, Cimakasky et al 2001). GSLs, important components of lipid rafts, have also been shown to play a role in membrane fusion. Complete lack of GSLs protects CD4 positive cells from HIV infection (Hug et al., 2000, Puri et al., 2004, Rawat et al., 2003).Interestingly, reconstitution of GSL deficient cells with Gb_3, and to a lesser extent GM3, was able to restore membrane fusion in these model systems (Hug et al., 2000, Puri et al., 1998, Puri et al., 1999). However, no other GSLs were able to rescue this phenotype. This impediment could also be overcome by the over-expression of CD4 and CXCR4, suggesting the role for GSLs is facilitative (Hammache et al., 1999, Puri et al., 1998, Puri et al., 1999, Rawat et al., 2003). These findings have been supported by reports that both Gb_3 and GM3, when introduced into the cell membrane of $CD4^+$ T lymphocytes, have the potential to enhance HIV-1 fusion and entry of a broad range of isolates (Hug et al., 2000). It has also been shown that non-human cells expressing CD4, ordinarily not permissive to HIV-1 infection, become permissive to membrane fusion upon introduction of Gb_3 (Puri et al., 1998). Our studies using a different glucosyl ceramide synthase inhibitor are conssitent with an inhibitory role for GSLs(Gb3)(Ramkumar et al., 2009) and HIV resistance is also conferred by high GM3 levels (Rawat et al., 2004).

For membrane fusion to proceed, HIV-gp120 binding to CD4 and chemokine co-receptor, must initiate conformational change in gp120 and the associated transmembrane gp41 (Freed et al., 1992, Jones et al., 1998). At physiological levels, CD4 and the co-receptors are not physically associated in the membrane in the absence of HIV-1 (Jones, korte et al 1998). However, CD4 and CCR5 are both present in lipid rafts, albeit separate rafts, and their associations with rafts have been shown to be required for infection. Indeed, both CD4 and CCR5 may interact with lipid rafts containing GM3 and Gb_3 (Hammache et al., 1999, Hammache et al., 1998b, Manes et al., 2001, Millan et al., 1999, Sorice et al., 1997). Interestingly, CXCR4 is not normally associated with rafts, and is separated from CD4, which is ordinarily associated with GM3 rafts. Upon HIV-gp120 interactions with CD4 however, CXCR4 is physically recruited into these rafts for membrane fusion (Sorice et al., 2000, Sorice et al., 2001).

CD4 has been shown to insert into Gb_3 or GM3 monolayers, as has HIV-gp120 (Hammache et al., 1999). Since both CD4 and chemokine receptors are found in, or are recruited to, lipid rafts for HIV infection, it was proposed that CD4 binds GSLs in rafts to promote gp120/GSL interactions (Fantini et al., 2000). GSL within rafts may then function to promote the migration of the CD4-gp120 complex to an appropriate, initially distal, coreceptor (Hammache et al., 1999). This would in turn promote clustering and thus co-operative interactions between the CD4-GSL-chemokine coreceptors (Rawat et al., 2006). HIV-gp120 binding interactions within the GSL-containing domain could then induce the conformational changes necessary to effect membrane fusion. Indeed, the fusion complex has specifically been shown to assemble in lipid rafts (Manes, et al., 2000).

5.3 Infectivity and viral egress

It is interesting to note that there appears to be an overall role for GSL containing lipid rafts in HIV infection (Manes et al., 2000, Popik et al., 2002). More specifically, HIV not only requires lipid rafts in the process of entry, but in immune evasion, suppressing host-cell signalling during replication, and egress of the virus from the host (Manes et al., 2000, Nguyen & Hildreth, 2000, Peterlin & Trono, 2003)

HIV Nef is a myristoylated protein that is associated with rafts, and this association is necessary for its function. Nef is involved in down-regulation of CD4 and MHC-I molecules, crucial for viral infectivity and immune evasion. These functions are dependant on the Nef targeting and trafficking function, through clathrin coated pits and early endosome associations, and are thus dependant on lipid raft (Bresnahan et al., 1998 , Piguet & Trono, 1999). Interestingly, Nef has been shown to inhibit Gb_3 retrograde transport (Johannes et al., 2003).

GSL-enriched lipid rafts are required for viral egress in addition to entry. Assembly and incorporation of envelope glycoproteins in the virion envelope is regulated by an interaction between the gp41 cytoplasmic tail and the MA domain of the Gag precursor peptide (Hourioux, Brand 2000). During post-transctiptional modification, the MA domain of Gag is myristoylated, and the envelope precursor gp160 is palmitoylated. These modifications target these proteins to lipid rafts, which promote the assembly of budding virions (Ono & Freed, 2001) . Furthermore, because HIV selectively buds from lipid rafts, the viral envelope is enriched in lipid raft components, including cholesterol and GlcCer (Brugger et al., 2006, Nguyen & Hildreth, 2000). The viral membrane GSL content can affect infectious potential (Hatch et al., 2009)

5.4 Clinical links to GSL

Increased Gb_3 and GM3 synthesis can be detected at an early stage in HIV-1 infected individuals. In addition, antibodies to these GSLs have been detected in HIV patients (Fantini et al., 1998b). These GSLs have important functions within the immune system, with regards to cell growth, signalling and motility. They are of particular importance as markers in lymphocyte differentiation, where Gb_3 is a marker of B cell development (Wiels et al., 1991)and GM3 of monocytes and T-cells. In addition, GM3 containing microdomains are functional in T cell motility (Gomez-Mouton et al., 2001) and signalling (Sorice et al., 2000). Thus, perturbations in GSL expression, and antibodies produced to GSL in HIV-1 infection may be immunosuppressive.

It is of interest to note that HIV infected patients are more prone to haemolytic uremic syndrome (HUS) (Turner et al., 1997). HUS is characterised by thrombotic microangiopathy of the renal glomeruli mediated by verotoxin/Gb_3 binding(Muthing et al., 2009). It is thus interesting that transgenic mice, in which the HIV genome has been incorporated into the germ line, show renal Gb_3 synthesis is selectively upregulated to induce renal disease (Liu et al., 1999)

5.5 Inhibiting HIV at the membrane level

In the quest for new drug targets, such as the entry inhibitors, and subsequent potential microbicide candidates, attention has been turned to HIV interactions with lipid rafts and GSLs. Several studies have investigated cholesterol-depletion as a means of disrupting lipid rafts to prevent HIV-1 fusion and entry (Liao et al., 2001; Liao et al., 2003) It has also been proposed that increasing ceramide levels in $CD4^+$ lymphocytes and monocyte-derived macrophages may block HIV infection, perhaps inhibiting HIV fusion by disrupting normal lipid raft organization and function (Finnegan & Blumenthal, 2006).These studies have used several mechanisms to increase ceramide, including pharmacological agents, such as *N*-(4-

hydroxyphenyl) retinamide and fenretinide, treatment with sphingomyelinase or addition of long-chain ceramide. Lipid-raft altering compounds may have dual efficacy in treatment of HIV/AIDS. Microorganisms causing opportunistic infections in AIDS patients often rely on lipid-raft mediated mechanisms to elicit their effect, thus HIV treatments altering lipid-rafts may be protective.

As GSLs are critical in the process of HIV infection and pathogenesis, targeting of these molecules may give rise to the development of novel therapeutics. Not only are GSLs key components of lipid rafts, but they also play several roles during HIV binding and host cell fusion. The efficacy of inhibiting HIV infection by targeting GSLs has already been demonstrated *in vitro*. Peptide analogues of the V3 loop of gp120, including those that define the GSL binding site, are effective as inhibitors of HIV-membrane fusion (Delezay et al., 1996, Savarino et al., 2003). Furthermore, analogues of galactosyl ceramide have been found to be protective against T cell infection *in vitro*, where the hydrophobic aglycone moiety of GalCer played an important role (Fantini, 2000, Fantini et al., 1997, Faroux-Corlay et al., 2001)

6. Generation of GSL mimics

Given the importance of GSLs in HIV infection, and the demonstrated anti-HIV potential of GalCer analogues, it is particularly advantageous to develop soluble GSL analogues. GSL binding and receptor function is significantly regulated by lipid modulation (Lingwood, 1996). Despite the fact that the carbohydrate moiety of the GSL defines the specificity of binding interactions, the lipid-free sugar shows minimal binding activity (Boyd et al., 1994, Mamelak et al., 2001a). Thus, gp120 binding to the GSL receptors is abrogated if the lipid moiety, that is the anchor to the cell membrane, is removed (Faroux-Corlay et al., 2001, Mylvaganam & Lingwood, 1999b, Villard et al., 2002).In the membrane bilayer, GSLs comprise three domains - the external aqueous sugar domain, the internal liquid crystalline domain and the "interface" between them. The "interface" region modulates the receptor function of the carbohydrate in response to the liquid crystalline domain, and likely plays a role in lipid raft organization.

In order to generate GSL analogues and maintain the interface character, an adamantane frame was used to replace the fatty acid (Mylvaganam & Lingwood, 2003). This rigid, globular, cage-like hydrophobic structure close to the interface region perturbs the lateral packing of the glycolipid, and thus bilayer structure formation, thereby promoting solubility. The Gb_3 analogue, adamantylGb_3 (adaGb_3), was shown to preferentially partition into water in an organic/aqueous solvent system (Mylvaganum & Lingwood, 1999a). This compound, unlike the lipid-free Gb_3 sugar, maintained its receptor function and was able to inhibit VT/ Gb_3 binding, protecting cells against this toxin (Mylvaganam & Lingwood, 1999a).

We utilized the same strategy to develop a soluble analogue of SGC and GalCer. We substituted the fatty acid of SGC with an adamantane or with a norbornane (smaller) frame and, as with the Gb_3 case, the conjugates partitioned into water (although adamantylGalCer was significantly less soluble), rather than the organic phase (Whetstone & Lingwood, 2003). AdamantylSGC retained its receptor activity (Mamelak et al., 2001a, Whetstone & Lingwood, 2003)

6.1 AdaGb_3 as a mimic of lipid rafts: a 'superligand' for HIV gp120

We have found that adaGb_3 has a variety of additional unusual physical properties which indicate that adamantyl-glycolipids may have unusual biological effects, particularly in modulating host/microbial interactions. In collaboration with Fantini's group , we showed that gp120 can insert into a Gb_3 monolayer at the water/air interphase in a Langmuir trough (Mahfoud et al., 2002b). However, there was a 2 hour lag-phase prior to binding/insertion which then proceeded at a sigmoidal rate. AdaGb_3, although water-soluble, also can form a monolayer at a water/air surface interface. Binding and insertion of gp120 into such a monolayer was exponential and immediate. Thus adaGb_3 is by far (>1000x), a superior ligand for gp120 than the native Gb_3. These results were duplicated using the SPC3 peptide from the V3 loop of gp120 which contains the GSL binding domain (Delezay et al., 1996). In the studies with the peptide, the lag-phase prior to Gb_3 binding/insertion was even more exaggerated, being three hours as compared to immediate insertion into adaGb_3. The lag phase observed for gp120 insertion into Gb_3 monolayers was removed if the monolayer is formed with 20% cholesterol. This suggests that the gp120 may be interacting with Gb_3 containing lipid rafts or microdomains (of which cholesterol is a key component). The lag phase seen in the absence of cholesterol, may be a function of the ability of Gb_3 to organize into suitable microdomains for gp120 binding and the sigmoidal curve suggests a cooperative effect, once a few domains have been formed. The immediate binding and insertion into adaGb_3 monolayers suggests that this organization required for gp120 insertion is already present in the adaGb_3 monolayer. Interestingly, although gp120 binds SGC, we found no evidence for gp120 insertion into SGC monolayers, even in the presence of cholesterol. Similarly, no gp120 insertion into adamantylSGC monolayers was seen(Mahfoud et al., 2002b). Our recent work showing that 50% cholesterol can mask membrane Gb_3 from gp120(Mahfoud et al., 2010) indicates a bimodal concentration dependent cholesterol effect.

SGC was shown to inhibit HIV infection of CD4 negative HT29 cells (Fantini et al., 1998a) without inhibition of HIV cell binding. In these studies, SGC was incorporated into the host cell membrane thereby increasing HIV binding, since gp120 binds SGC(Bhat et al., 1993), but fusion with the host cell membrane was inhibited(Fantini et al., 1998a). Although these studies also implicated GalCer in these cells as mediating HIV infection, HT29 cells are Gb_3 positive. Thus, this is consistent with a role for Gb_3 rather than SGC, in HIV-cell fusion. It is possible that in addition to forming microdomains poorly itself, SGC could interfere with rafts containing other GSLs. AdamantylSGC (Whetstone & Lingwood, 2003) is a soluble inhibitor of gp120-SGC binding and may prove more effective than the poorly soluble SGC.

6.2 AdaGb_3 inhibits HIV infection

Comparison of the "compressibility" of Gb_3 and adaGb_3 monolayers shows that the adaGb_3 structure is more rigid and able to withstand greater increases in surface pressure without collapsing (Mahfoud et al., 2002b). This is consistent with a microdomain format for the adaGb_3 monolayer. If adaGb_3 is a "superligand" for gp120 as our studies indicate, adaGb_3 might be able to interfere with the process of HIV infection even for (T) cells which do not express Gb_3 (Akashi et al., 1988). We therefore tested whether adaGb_3 was able to modify HIV infectivity *in vitro*. 200μM adaGb_3 was able to reduce HIV infectivity in Jurkat T cells using a multiplicity of infectivity ratio of 0.6 (60x higher than standard practice) by ~70% over a 4 day infection period (figure 9) as monitored by ELISA of host cell production of viral nucleoprotein $p24^{gag}$. Amino adamantane itself showed no inhibition. *Thus, this approach does represent a novel basis for the control of HIV infectivity*. Moreover, in our studies to use adaGb_3 to protect mice against VT, we have shown that adaGb_3 itself (4mg/kg) shows no side effects *in vivo*.

In collaboration with Blumenthal's group at NIH we have found that adaGb$_3$ is also able to inhibit gp120/CD4/chemokine coreceptor dependent host cell fusion irrespective of gp120 type (R5 or X4 tropic, HIV-1 or HIV-2) as monitored in an indicator system in which gp120 is transfected into one indicator cell and the chemokine receptor into another (Lund et al., 2006).

6.3 FSL-Gb$_3$

Recently, additional GSL analogues have been shown to act to inhibit HIV-1 infection *in vitro*. A completely synthetic water soluble analogue of Gb$_3$ termed **F**unctional head **S**pacer **L**ipid tail-Gb$_3$ (FSL-Gb$_3$) was shown to inhibit X4 and R5 HIV-1 infection with a similar 50% inhibitory activity (IC$_{50}$) as adaGb$_3$ (Harrison et al., 2010). This Gb$_3$ analogue was unique in that the lipid tails were replaced with phosphatidylethanolamine and a spacer region containing multiple ionic residues allowed for complete solubility in aqueous media. A novel synthetic process maintains the carbohydrate moiety of Gb$_3$ coupled to phosphatidylethanolamine through a phosphate linker. This molecule gains its solubility through the insertion of charged nitrogen and phosphate containing groups that are located between the glycone and aglycone moietites. The molecule is completely synthetic, completely soluble in aqueous solutions, and available in large quantities for testing. In addition. animal studies have shown no toxicity at millimolar quantities systemically. The unusual tail also allows for this analogue to insert itself into cell membranes and convert an HIV-permissive Gb$_3$-negative T-cell into a Gb$_3$-positive T-cell that resists HIV infection (Harrison et al., 2010).
Harrison et al. (2010) have used the FSL-Gb$_3$ to show that it can inhibit HIV infection by two different mechanisms. First, as with adaGb$_3$, mixing the FSL-Gb$_3$ with either X4 or R5 HIV-1 results in inhibition of HIV infection with approximately the same IC$_{50}$ as with adaGb$_3$ (Harrison et al., 2010). This was shown both for laboratory strains of HIV-1 as well as for clinical isolates of R5 HIV-1 viruses. In addition, FSL-Gb$_3$, apparently due to its particular hydrophobic tail structure, was shown to insert itself into cell membranes, retaining proper cell-surface conformation of the carbohydrate moieties. Cellular insertion of FSL-Gb$_3$ was able to result in conversion of a human CD4$^+$ T-cell that completely lacked Gb$_3$ expression into a T-cell that highly expresses Gb$_3$. This property of FSL-Gb$_3$ to convert a permissive HIV target cell into a less permissive cell for HIV infection is a major finding; thus, providing acquired resistance to HIV-1 infection as a possible therapeutic approach. The following: "In addition, preliminary work has shown potential for soluble Gb3 analogues, including FSL-Gb$_3$, to act as microbicides to inhibit mucosal HIV transmission (Harrison et al., 2011). FSL-Gb$_3$ shows great promise as a possible therapeutic, *in vivo*, as it would be potentially capable of inhibiting HIV infection both systemically to reduce viremia but also by its insertion into CD4$^+$ T cells resulting in inhibition of HIV infection by blocking viral entry into its normal primary host targets.

6.4 Multimeric GSLs

The finding that a soluble GSL analogue was capable of inhibiting HIV infection soon led to other studies where the investigators used a series of C-glycoside synthetic analogues of GalCer (Garg et al., 2008). These investigators showed that two of six analogues were able to bind gp120 and inhibit X4 and R5 strains and dual-tropic HIV-mediated fusion and entry in the absence of any significant cytotoxicity. In addition to HIV, these investigators also showed that soluble GSLs may inhibit additional enveloped viruses such as vesicular stomatitis virus (VSV) (Garg et al., 2008).

Rosa Borges et al. (2010) found that if the synthesized analogues utilized multimeric Gb_3 sites, increased efficacy for inhibition of HIV-1 could be achieved. These investigators covalently attached multiple head groups of either Gb_3 or GM3 to a dendrimer core to produce multivalent dendrimeric compounds that were water soluble and showed a much lower IC_{50} for inhibition of HIV-1 infection, compared to either FSL-Gb_3 or adaGb_3 (Rosa Borges et al., 2010). Thus, soluble Gb_3 analogues have important therapeutic potential to block HIV from interacting with $CD4^+$ target cells (Figure 5D).

7. Pharmacologic modulation of Gb_3 expression

1-Deoxygalactonojirimycin (DGJ) is an alkylated imino sugar with a galactose head and a one-carbon side chain. It was found to be highly tolerable *in vivo* and established as a potent competitive inhibitor of *a-galactosidase A* (α-Gal A)(Hamanaka et al., 2008). DGJ has been proposed as a specific chemical chaperone for treatment of diseases including Fabry (Fan et al., 1999). Studies have indicated that oral administration of DGJ to transgenic mice expressing a human mutant α-Gal A substantially elevated enzyme activity in major organs (Fan et al., 1999). Because Gb_3 has now been suggested by the studies of Lund et al. (Lund et al., 2006). as an important component for prevention of the HIV entry mechanism, the use of DGJ to pharmacologically increase Gb_3 expression may be useful for HIV prevention strategies.

Recent studies (Ramkumar et al., 2009) used DGJ to increase the cell-surface expression of Gb_3 on the monocyte cell line, THP-1, which is infectable with X4 HIV-1. DGJ used at 100 μM was able to increase the cell-surface expression of Gb_3 of THP-1 cells by approximately 20-fold. Subsequent X4 HIV-1 infection was decreased significantly.

To inhibit Gb_3 expression in these cells, these investigators used the compound, D-threo-1-phenyl-2-palmitoylamino-3-pyrrolidino-1-propanol (P4) which inhibits GlcCer synthase, the enzyme responsible for producing GlcCer (Inokuchi & Radin, 1987). This is a key enzyme in the biosynthesis of GSLs because most are glucosylceramide-based. P4 is the most potent inhibitor of this glycosyltransferase (Lee et al., 1999). Using 2 μM P4, Ramkumar et al (Ramkumar et al., 2009) were able to completely inhibit Gb_3 expression with subsequent X4 HIV-1 infection increased up to 20-fold. DGJ had little effect on the infection of a Gb_3-negative subclone of THP-1 cells and FACS analysis indicated that after DGJ treatment, CD4 and HIV co-receptor levels were similar in the Gb_3 expressing and non-expressing THP-1 cell lines by these two compounds. Also, as DGJ was found to be non-toxic in the THP-1 cells up to concentrations of 300 μM, the inhibitory effect was not a result of cytotoxicity of DGJ treatment. The authors concluded that their results indicated that the difference in HIV infection was due solely to the modulation of the expression of the levels of Gb_3.

To examine the effects of DGJ and P4 treatment on subsequent infection with R5 HIV-1 virus, the glioblastoma cell line, U87, that had been transfected to express CD4 and the chemokine co-receptor, CCR5, was used. Ramkumar et al. (Ramkumar et al., 2009) again found that treatment of these cells with DGJ resulted in a significant inhibition of R5 HIV-1 infection while treatment with P4 caused a doubling in the infection. They concluded that pharmacologically increasing Gb_3 expression using DGJ treatment or inhibition of Gb_3 expression using P4 demonstrates a linear relationship between Gb_3 expression and infection with either X4 or R5 HIV-1. In addition, their studies suggest that pharmacologically increasing Gb_3 is an effective and novel means to prevent HIV-1 infection *in vitro* and that this approach should be explored for *in vivo* treatment of HIV infection.

8. HIV infection of CD4 negative cells

The current paradigm indicates that infection with HIV-1 depends entirely on the recognition of its primary and co-receptors for viral fusion and entry into a target cell. Unfortunately, this paradigm is insufficient to completely explain the pathogenesis of HIV-1. This is because there are many instances of HIV-1 infection where either the primary and/or co-receptors are missing from the infected cell. Indeed, HIV-1-infected CD4 negative- cells have been identified *in vivo*, including various brain cells (Pumarola-Sune et al., 1987, Ward et al., 1987, Wiley et al., 1986)epithelial cells (Nelson et al., 1988), cardiomyocytes (Barbaro et al., 1998), CD4 negative- lymphocytes (Livingstone et al., 1996, Saha et al., 2001a), renal tubular epithelial cells(Marras et al., 2002, Wyatt & Klotman, 2007), hepatocytes (Fromentin et al., 2011) and thymocytes (Kitchen et al., 1997). HIV-1 has also been shown to infect CD4-negative neural and epithelial cells *in vitro*, although not productively (Clapham et al., 1989, Tateno et al., 1989). However, it has been shown that HIV-1 can productively infect $CD4^{-}CD8^{+}$ T lymphocytes *in vitro* (Saha et al., 2001b).

Our own work supports the idea of HIV infection of CD4-negative cells. Using kidney-derived cell lines such as ACHN and 293 as well as a colon-derived cancer cell line called Caco-2, we have been able to show transient infection with an X4 virus (Figure 5). We have also shown that soluble Gb_3 can inhibit the infection of CD4-negative Caco-2 epithelial cell lines (Figure 6) as well as human CD4-negative cell lines derived from the cervix or endometrium (Harrison et al., 2011). Although, the infection of these cell lines is not robust

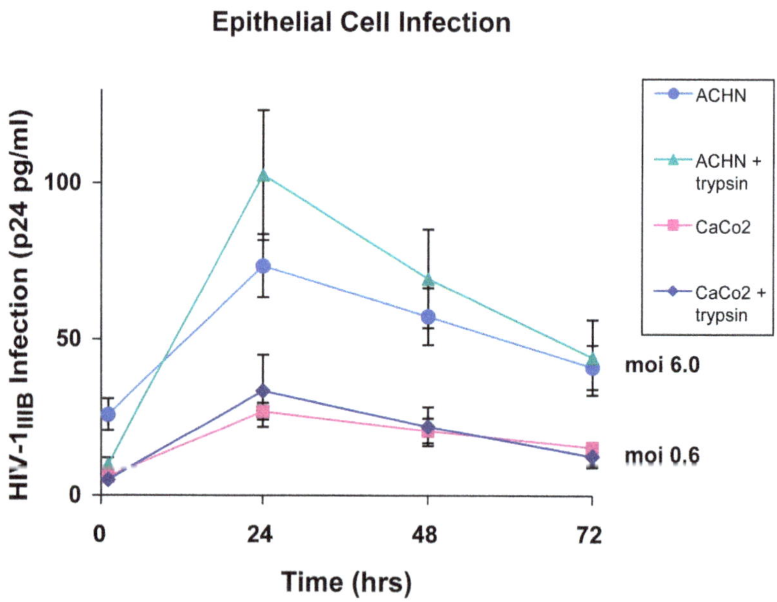

Fig. 5. **HIV can infect CD4-negative epithelial cells.** HIV infection of ACHN kidney-derived cell line and Caco-2 colon cancer derived epithelial cell line. Trypsin is used to insure that the p24 antigen being used as a measure of productive HIV infection is not derived from external virions sticking to the cell membranes but from budding virions indicating a round of replication of the virus.

and appears transient, these infected cells could serve as reservoirs of latent HIV provirus and may become activated under certain conditions to produce a round of progeny virions which would have the potential to infect other cells such as CD4+ T-cells and maintain or re-establish an active infection.

Several hypotheses have arisen to explain the infection of CD4-negative cells within the current paradigm of only CD4 and chemokine co-receptors playing a role. A popular theory is that the availability of CXCR4 in CD4-negative cells is sufficient for viral fusion and entry. However, the evidence addressing this idea is contradictory. In support, human $CD4^-CCR5^-CXCR4^+$ pre-T cell lines can be infected with HIV-1 (Borsetti et al., 2000). Furthermore, $CD4^+CXCR4^-$ human megakaryocytic cells are fully resistant to HIV-1 infection until they are transfected to over-express CXCR4 (Baiocchi et al., 1997). In contradiction, the CD4-negative human B-cell line Raji is not permissive to HIV-1 infection, even though it expresses functional CXCR4 (Speck et al., 1999). Therefore, the absolute dependence of HIV-1 on CXCR4, even in the absence of CD4, does not completely account for the ability of HIV-1 to infect $CD4^-$ cells.

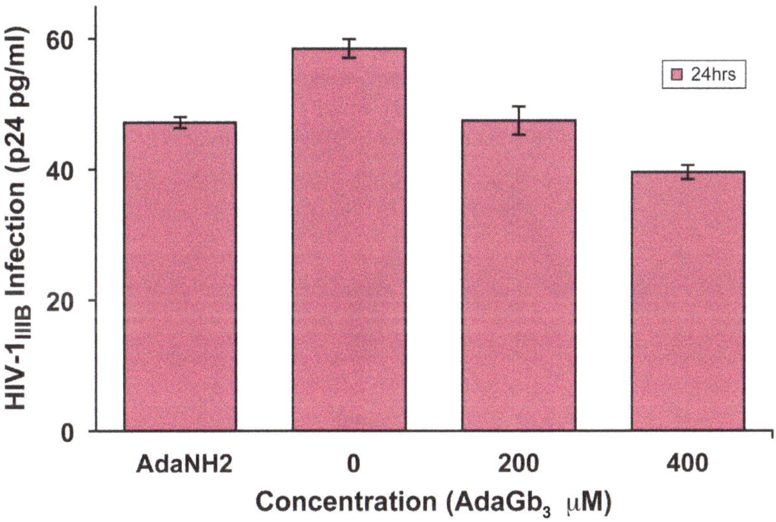

Fig. 6. **Inhibition of HIV infection of epithelial cells by soluble Gb_3.** Caco-2 CD4-negative epithelial cells are infected by HIV but the infection can be inhibited using soluble $adaGb_3$. adaNH2 is a control soluble GSL for $adaGb_3$

Taken together, the current paradigm that requires the availability of both a primary CD4 receptor plus a co-receptor, either CXCR4 or CCR5, in order for HIV to infect a target cell is not sufficient to explain other cell infections were either the primary receptor and/or the co-receptor are not present, or where there is a lack of infection when both receptors are present. Indeed, there is ample evidence that these receptors are not always sufficient for viral infection. Further examples include human CD4-negative astrocytes that express functional CCR5 and CXCR4 and are resistant to infection by HIV-1 strains (Boutet et al., 2001) and $CD4^+CXCR4^+$ cells, also resistant to infection with HIV-1 (Moriuchi et al., 1997). This was shown by infecting U937 monocyte-derived cell lines that were shown to be either permissive or nonpermissive for infection by HIV-1. All but one of these cell lines expressed both functional CXCR4 and CD4. One of these cell lines that was nonpermissive lacked CXCR4, but when this receptor was transfected back into this cell line, it remained nonpermissive to infection 1 (Moriuchi et al., 1997).

9. Summary

Studies have indicated that human PBMCs with an intracellular or cell-surface accumulation of Gb_3 were less susceptible to HIV infection (Lund et al., 2005, Lund et al., 2009).These PBMCs were derived from patients with Fabry disease and from healthy P_1^k blood group phenotype individuals having a pathologic or natural, respectively, elevation of Gb_3. AdaGb_3, FSL-Gb_3, and multivalent dendrimeric-Gb_3, all soluble Gb_3 analogues, have been shown to be effective inhibitors of HIV regardless of strain or tropism, and also to inhibit drug resistant HIV strains and prevent HIV infection of CD4-negative epithelial cells. Therefore, Gb_3 may be a natural host resistance factor and increasing its expression *in vitro* using soluble analogues, such as FSL-Gb_3, that can insert into T-cells that do not naturally express Gb_3, and/or the use of a pharmacologic agent, such as DGJ, to increase Gb_3 expression, may decrease HIV-1 susceptibility. Importantly, the further development of soluble Gb_3 analogues, especially multivalent analogues expressing multiple Gb_3 sugar moieties having increased affinity and avidity for the V3 loop of HIV gp120, may provide for novel and highly effective HIV therapeutics to prevent or treat HIV/AIDS (Figure 7).

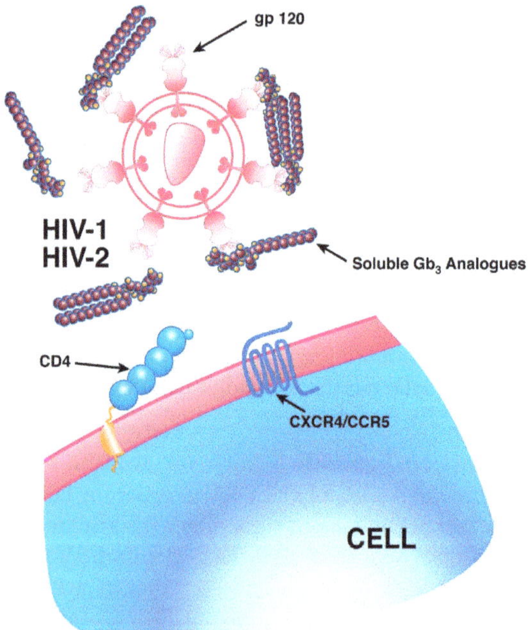

Fig. 7. **Potential novel HIV therapeutic.** Soluble Gb_3 analogues may be able to bind to HIV gp120 protruding from the HIV envelop and prevent HIV from interacting with the primary and/or co-receptors for HIV; thus, preventing HIV infection.

10. References

Ahn, A., D. L. Gibbons & M. Kielian (2002) The fusion peptide of Semliki Forest virus associates with sterol-rich membrane domains. *Journal of Virology*. 76, (pp. 3267-75).

Akashi, M., F. Takaku, H. Nojiri, Y. Miura, Y. Nagai & M. Saito (1988) Neutral and sialosyl glycosphingolipid composition and metabolism of human T-lymphoblastic cell line MOLT-3 cells: distinctive changes as markers specific for their differentiation. *Blood*. 72, (pp. 469-79).

Alfsen, A. & M. Bomsel (2002) HIV-1 gp41 envelope residues 650-685 exposed on native virus act as a lectin to bind epithelial cell galactosyl ceramide. *J Biol Chem*. 277, (pp. 25649-59.).

Alkhatib, G., C. Combadiere, C. C. Broder, Y. Feng, P. E. Kennedy, P. M. Murphy & E. A. Berger (1996) CC CKR5: a RANTES, MIP-1alpha, MIP-1beta receptor as a fusion cofactor for macrophage-tropic HIV-1. *Science*. 272, (pp. 1955-8).

Aoki, C., K. I. Hidari, S. Itonori, A. Yamada, N. Takahashi, T. Kasama, F. Hasebe, M. A. Islam, K. Hatano, K. Matsuoka, T. Taki, C. T. Guo, T. Takahashi, Y. Sakano, T. Suzuki, D. Miyamoto, M. Sugita, D. Terunuma, K. Morita & Y. Suzuki (2006) Identification and characterization of carbohydrate molecules in mammalian cells recognized by dengue virus type 2. *Journal of Biochemistry*. 139, (pp. 607-14).

Arab, S. & C. Lingwood (1998) Intracellular targeting of the endoplasmic reticulum/nuclear envelope by retrograde transport may determine cell hypersensitivity to Verotoxin: sodium butyrate or selection of drug resistance may induce nuclear toxin targeting via globotriaosyl ceramide fatty acid isoform traffic. *J Cell Physiol*. 177, (pp. 646-660).

Arab, S. & C. A. Lingwood (1996) Influence of phospholipid chain length on verotoxin/globotriaosyl ceramide binding in model membranes: comparison of a surface bilayer film and liposomes. *Glycoconj. J*. 13, (pp. 159-166).

Baiocchi, M., E. Olivetta, C. Chelucci, A. C. Santarcangelo, R. Bona, P. d'Aloja, U. Testa, N. Komatsu, P. Verani & M. Federico (1997) Human immunodeficiency virus (HIV)-resistant CD4+ UT-7 megakaryocytic human cell line becomes highly HIV-1 and HIV-2 susceptible upon CXCR4 transfection: induction of cell differentiation by HIV-1 infection. *Blood*. 89, (pp. 2670-8).

Barbaro, G., G. Di Lorenzo, B. Grisorio & G. Barbarini (1998) Cardiac involvement in the acquired immunodeficiency syndrome: a multicenter clinical-pathological study. Gruppo Italiano per lo Studio Cardiologico dei pazienti affetti da AIDS Investigators. *AIDS Res Hum Retroviruses*. 14, (pp. 1071-7).

Bavari, S., C. M. Bosio, E. Wiegand, G. Ruthel, A. B. Will, T. W. Geisbert, M. Hevey, C. Schmaljohn, A. Schmaljohn & M. J. Aman (2002) Lipid raft microdomains: a gateway for compartmentalized trafficking of Ebola and Marburg viruses. *The Journal of Experimental Medicine*. 195, (pp. 593-602).

Bhat, S., R. V. Mettus, E. P. Reddy, K. E. Ugen, V. Srikanthan, W. V. Williams & D. B. Weiner (1993) The galactosyl ceramide/sulfatide receptor binding region of HIV-1 gp120 maps to amino acids 206-275. *AIDS Res Hum Retroviruses*. 9, (pp. 175-81).

Bhat, S., S. L. Spitalinik, F. Gonzalez-Scarano & D. H. Silberberg (1991) Galactosyl ceramide or a derivative is an essential component of the neural receptor for human immunodeficiency virus type 1 envolope glycoprotein gp 120. *Proc. Natl. Acad. Sci*. 88, (pp. 7131-7134).

Bitzan, M., S. Richardson, C. Huang, B. Boyd, M. Petric & M. Karmali (1994) Evidence that Verotoxins (Shiga-like toxins) from *Escherichia coli* bind to P blood group antigens of human erythrocytes *in vitro*. *Infect Immun*. 62, (pp. 3337-3347).

Bomsel, M. (1997) Transcytosis of infectious human immunodeficiency virus across a tight human epithelial cell line barrier. *Nat Med*. 3, (pp. 42-7.).

Borén, T., P. Falk, K. A. Roth, G. Larson & S. Normark (1993) Attachment of *Helicobacter pylori* to human gastric epithelium mediated by blood group antigens. *Science*. 262, (pp. 1892-1895).

Borsetti, A., C. Parolin, B. Ridolfi, L. Sernicola, A. Geraci, B. Ensoli & F. Titti (2000) CD4-independent infection of two CD4(-)/CCR5(-)/CXCR4(+) pre-T-cell lines by human and simian immunodeficiency viruses. *J Virol*. 74, (pp. 6689-94).

Boulanger, J., D. Faulds, E. M. Eddy & C. A. Lingwood (1995) Members of the 70kDa heat shock protein family specifically recognize sulfoglycolipids: role in gamete recognition and mycoplasma related infertility. *J. Cell. Physiol*. 165, (pp. 7-17).

Boutet, A., H. Salim, Y. Taoufik, P. M. Lledo, J. D. Vincent, J. F. Delfraissy & M. Tardieu (2001) Isolated human astrocytes are not susceptible to infection by M- and T-tropic HIV-1 strains despite functional expression of the chemokine receptors CCR5 and CXCR4. *Glia*. 34, (pp. 165-77).

Boyd, B. & C. A. Lingwood (1989) Verotoxin receptor glycolipid in human renal tissue. *Nephron*. 51, (pp. 207-210).

Boyd, B., Z. Zhiuyan, G. Magnusson & C. A. Lingwood (1994) Lipid modulation of glycolipid receptor function: Presentation of galactose a1-4 galactose disaccharide for Verotoxin binding in natural and synthetic glycolipids. *Eur. J. Biochem*. 223, (pp. 873-878).

Brady, R. O. (1967) Enzymatic abnormalities in diseases of sphingolipid metabolism. *Clin Chem*. 13, (pp. 565-77).

Branch, D. R. (2010) Blood groups and susceptibility to virus infection: new developments. *Curr Opin Hematol*. 17, (pp. 558-64).

Branch, D. R., L. J. Valenta, S. Yousefi, D. Sakac, R. Singla, M. Bali, B. M. Sahai & X. Z. Ma (2002) VPAC1 is a cellular neuroendocrine receptor expressed on T cells that actively facilitates productive HIV-1 infection. *AIDS*. 16, (pp. 309-19).

Bremer, E. G. (1994). Glycosphingolipids as Effectors of Growth and Differentiation

Bresnahan, P. A., W. Yonemoto, S. Ferrell, D. Williams-Herman, R. Geleziunas & W. C. Greene (1998) A dileucine motif in HIV-1 Nef acts as an internalization signal for CD4 downregulation and binds the AP-1 clathrin adaptor. *Curr Biol*. 8, (pp. 1235-8).

Brown, D. & E. London (2000) Structure and function of sphingolipid- and cholesterol-rich membrane rafts. *J. Biol. Chem*. 275, (pp. 17221-17224).

Brown, D. A. & E. London (1997) Structure of detergent-resistant membrane domains: does phase separation occur in biological membranes? *Biochem Biophys Res Commun*. 240, (pp. 1-7).

Brown, K. E., J. R. Hibbs, G. Gallinella, S. M. Anderson, E. D. Lehman, P. McCarthy & N. S. Young (1994) Resistance to parvovirus B19 infection due to lack of virus receptor (erythrocyte P antigen). *The New England Journal of Medicine*. 330, (pp. 1192-6).

Brugger, B., B. Glass, P. Haberkant, I. Leibrecht, F. T. Wieland & H. G. Krausslich (2006) The HIV lipidome: a raft with an unusual composition. *Proc Natl Acad Sci U S A*. 103, (pp. 2641-6).

Chark, D., A. Nutikka, N. Trusevych, J. Kuzmina & C. Lingwood (2004) Differential carbohydrate epitope recognition of globotriaosyl ceramide by verotoxins and monoclonal antibody: Role in human renal glomerular binding. *Eur. J. Biochem.* 271, (pp. 1-13).

Clapham, P. R., J. N. Weber, D. Whitby, K. McIntosh, A. G. Dalgleish, P. J. Maddon, K. C. Deen, R. W. Sweet & R. A. Weiss (1989) Soluble CD4 blocks the infectivity of diverse strains of HIV and SIV for T cells and monocytes but not for brain and muscle cells. *Nature.* 337, (pp. 368-70.).

Comolli, J. C., A. R. Hauser, L. Waite, C. B. Whitchurch, J. S. Mattick & J. N. Engel (1999) Pseudomonas aeruginosa gene products PilT and PilU are required for cytotoxicity *in vitro* and virulence in a mouse model of acute pneumonia. *Infect Immun.* 67, (pp. 3625-30).

Dalgleish, A. G., P. C. Beverley, P. R. Clapham, D. H. Crawford, M. F. Greaves & R. A. Weiss (1984) The CD4 (T4) antigen is an essential component of the receptor for the AIDS retrovirus. *Nature.* 312, (pp. 763-7).

Daniels, G. (2002). Blackwell Science, Malden, MA

De Haan, L. & T. R. Hirst (2004) Cholera toxin: a paradigm for multi-functional engagement of cellular mechanisms (Review). *Mol Membr Biol.* 21, (pp. 77-92).

De Rosa, M. F., D. Sillence, C. Ackerley & C. Lingwood (2004) Role of Multiple Drug Resistance Protein 1 in neutral but not acidic glycosphingolipid biosynthesis. *J. Biol. Chem.* 279, (pp. 7867-7876).

Del Real, G., S. Jimenez-Baranda, R. A. Lacalle, E. Mira, P. Lucas, C. Gomez-Mouton, A. C. Carrera, A. C. Martinez & S. Manes (2002) Blocking of HIV-1 infection by targeting CD4 to nonraft membrane domains. *J Exp Med.* 196, (pp. 293-301.).

Delezay, O., D. Hammache, J. Fantini & N. Yahi (1996) SPC3, a V3 loop-derived synthetic peptide inhibitor of HIV-1 infection, binds to cell surface glycosphingolipids. *Biochemistry.* 35, (pp. 15663-71).

Devenica, D., V. Cikes Culic, A. Vuica & A. Markotic (2010) Biochemical, pathological and oncological relevance of Gb3Cer receptor. *Med Oncol.* (pp.

Dietrich, C., L. A. Bagatolli, Z. N. Volovyk, N. L. Thompson, M. Levi, K. Jacobson & E. Gratton (2001) Lipid rafts reconstituted in model membranes. *Biophys J.* 80, (pp. 1417-1428).

Dorosko, S. M. & R. I. Connor (2010) Primary human mammary epithelial cells endocytose HIV-1 and facilitate viral infection of CD4+ T lymphocytes. *J Virol.* 84, (pp. 10533-42).Dragic, T., V. Litwin, G. P. Allaway, S. R. Martin, Y. Huang, K. A. Nagashima, C. Cayanan, P. J. Maddon, R. A. Koup, J. P. Moore & W. A. Paxton (1996) HIV-1 entry into CD4+ cells is mediated by the chemokine receptor CC-CKR-5. *Nature.* 381, (pp. 667-73).

Dykstra, M. L., A. Cherukuri & S. K. Pierce (2001) Floating the raft hypothesis for immune receptors: access to rafts controls receptor signaling and trafficking. *Traffic.* 2, (pp. 160-6.).

Eggens, I., B. Fenderson, T. Toyokuni, B. Dean, M. Stroud & S.-I. Hamomori (1989) Specific interaction between Le^x and Le^x determinants. *J Biol Chem.* 264, (pp. 9476-9484).

Emam, A., W. G. Carter & L. C.A (2010) Glycolipid-dependent, protease sensitive internalization of *Pseudomonas aeruginosa* into cultured human respiratory epithelial cells *Open Microbiol J.* 4, (pp. 106-15).

Emam, A., A. Yu, H.-J. Park, R. Mahfoud, J. Kus, L. Burrows & C. Lingwood (2006) Laboratory and clinical *Pseudomonas aeruginosa* strains do not bind glycosphingolipids *in vitro* or during type IV pili-mediated initial host cell attachment. *Microbiol.* 152, (pp. 2789-2799).

Epand, R. M., S. Nir, M. Parolin & T. D. Flanagan (1995) The role of the ganglioside GD1a as a receptor for Sendai virus. *Biochemistry.* 34, (pp. 1084-9).

Falguieres, T., F. Mallard, C. Baron, D. Hanau, C. Lingwood, B. Goud, J. Salamero & L. Johannes (2001) Targeting of Shiga toxin b-subunit to retrograde transport route in association with detergent-resistant membranes. *Mol. Biol. Cell.* 12, (pp. 2453-68.).

Fan, J. Q., S. Ishii, N. Asano & Y. Suzuki (1999) Accelerated transport and maturation of lysosomal alpha-galactosidase A in Fabry lymphoblasts by an enzyme inhibitor. *Nat Med.* 5, (pp. 112-5).

Fantini, J. (2000) Synthetic soluble analogs of glycolipids for studies of virus-glycolipid interactions. *Methods in Enzymology.* 311, (pp. 626-638).

Fantini, J. (2003) How sphingolipids bind and shape proteins: molecular basis of lipid-protein interactions in lipid shells, rafts and related biomembrane domains. *Cell Mol Life Sci.* 60, (pp. 1027-32).

Fantini, J., D. Hammache, O. Delezay, G. Pieroni, C. Tamalet & N. Yahi (1998a) Sulfatide inhibits HIV-1 entry into $CD4^-/CXCR4^+$ cells. *Virology.* 246, (pp. 211-220).

Fantini, J., D. Hammache, O. Delezay, N. Yahi, C. Andre-Barres, I. Rico-Lattes & A. Lattes (1997) Synthetic soluble analogs of galactosylceramide (GalCer) bind to the V3 domain of HIV-1 gp 120 and Inhibit HIV-1-induced fusion and entry. *J. Biol. Chem.* 272, (pp. 7245-7252).

Fantini, J., D. Hammache, G. Pieroni & N. Yahi (2000) Role of glycosphingolipid microdomains in CD4-dependent HIV-1 fusion. *Glycoconj J.* 17, (pp. 199-204).

Fantini, J., C. Tamalet, D. Hammache, C. Tourrés, N. Duclos & N. Yahi (1998b) HIV-1-induced perturbations of glycosphingolipid metabolism are cell-specific and can be detected at early stages of HIV-1 infection. *Journal of Acquired Immune Deficiency Syndromes and Human Retrovirology.* 19, (pp. 221-229).

Faroux-Corlay, B., J. Greiner, R. Terreux, D. Cabrol-Bass, A. M. Aubertin, P. Vierling & J. Fantini (2001) Amphiphilic anionic analogues of galactosylceramide: synthesis, anti- HIV-1 activity, and gp120 binding. *J Med Chem.* 44, (pp. 2188-203.).

Feng, Y., C. C. Broder, P. E. Kennedy & E. A. Berger (1996) HIV-1 entry cofactor: functional cDNA cloning of a seven-transmembrane, G protein-coupled receptor. *Science.* 272, (pp. 872-7).

Finnegan, C. & R. Blumenthal (2006) Dissecting HIV fusion: identifying novel targets for entry inhibitors. *Infect Disord Drug Targets.* 6, (pp. 355-67).

Fivaz, M., L. Abrami & F. G. van der Goot (1999) Landing on lipid rafts. *Trends in Cell Biology.* 9, (pp. 212-3).

Freed, E. O., E. L. Delwart, G. L. Buchschacher, Jr. & A. T. Panganiban (1992) A mutation in the human immunodeficiency virus type 1 transmembrane glycoprotein gp41 dominantly interferes with fusion and infectivity. *Proc Natl Acad Sci U S A.* 89, (pp. 70-4).

Fromentin, R., M. R. Tardif & M. J. Tremblay (2011) Inefficient fusion due to a lack of attachment receptor/co-receptor restricts productive human immunodeficiency virus type 1 infection in human hepatoma Huh7.5 cells. *J Gen Virol.* 92, (pp. 587-97).

Furukawa, K., K. Iwamura, M. Uchikawa, B. N. Sojka, J. Wiels, T. Okajima & T. Urano (2000) Molecular basis for the p phenotype. Identification of distinct and multiple mutations in the alpha 1,4-galactosyltransferase gene in Swedish and Japanese individuals. *J Biol Chem.* 275, (pp. 37752-6).

Futerman, A. H. & R. E. Pagano (1991) Determination of the intracellular sites and topology of glucosylceramide synthesis in rat liver. *Biochem J.* 280 (Pt 2), (pp. 295-302).

Garg, H., N. Francella, K. A. Tony, L. A. Augustine, J. J. Barchi, Jr., J. Fantini, A. Puri, D. R. Mootoo & R. Blumenthal (2008) Glycoside analogs of beta-galactosylceramide, a novel class of small molecule antiviral agents that inhibit HIV-1 entry. *Antiviral Res.* 80, (pp. 54-61).

Gatfield, J. & J. Pieters (2000) Essential role for cholesterol in entry of mycobacteria into macrophages. *Science.* 288, (pp. 1647-50).

Ghislain, J., C. Lingwood, M. Maloney, L. Penn & E. Fish (1992) Association between the ifn alpha receptor and the membrane glycolipid globotriaosyl ceramide. *J Interfer Res.* 12, (pp. s114).

Gilbert, J. & T. Benjamin (2004) Uptake pathway of polyomavirus via ganglioside GD1a. *Journal of Virology.* 78, (pp. 12259-67).

Gomez-Mouton, C., J. L. Abad, E. Mira, R. A. Lacalle, E. Gallardo, S. Jimenez-Baranda, I. Illa, A. Bernad, S. Manes & A. C. Martinez (2001) Segregation of leading-edge and uropod components into specific lipid rafts during T cell polarization. *Proc Natl Acad Sci U S A.* 98, (pp. 9642-7.).

Gottlieb, M. S., R. Schroff, H. M. Schanker, J. D. Weisman, P. T. Fan, R. A. Wolf & A. Saxon (1981) Pneumocystis carinii pneumonia and mucosal candidiasis in previously healthy homosexual men: evidence of a new acquired cellular immunodeficiency. *N Engl J Med.* 305, (pp. 1425-31).

Gummuluru, S., M. Rogel, L. Stamatatos & M. Emerman (2003) Binding of Human Immunodeficiency Virus Type 1 to Immature Dendritic Cells Can Occur Independently of DC-SIGN and Mannose Binding C-Type Lectin Receptors via a Cholesterol-Dependent Pathway. *J Virol.* 77, (pp. 12865-74).

Haataja, S., K. Tikkanen, U. Nilsson, G. Magnusson, K. Karlsson & J. Finne (1994) Oligosaccharide-receptor interaction of the Gal alpha 1-4Gal binding adhesin of *Streptococcus suis*. Combining site architecture and characterization of two variant adhesin specificities. *J Biol Chem.* 269, (pp. 27466-27472).

Hakomori, S. (1985) Aberrant glycosylation in cancer cell membranes as focused on glycolipids: overview and perspectives. *Cancer Res.* 45, (pp. 2405-14).

Hakomori, S. (1986) Glycosphingolipids. *Scientific American.* 254, (pp. 40-53).

Hakomori, S. (1993) Structure and function of sphingoglycolipids in transmembrane signalling and cell-cell interactions. *Biochem Soc Trans.* 21 (Pt 3), (pp. 583-95).

Hakomori, S. (1996) Tumor malignancy defined by aberrant glycosylation and sphingo(glyco)lipid metabolism. *Cancer Res.* 56, (pp. 5309-5318).

Hakomori, S. (2002) Glycosylation defining cancer malignancy: new wine in an old bottle. *Proc Natl Acad Sci U S A.* 99, (pp. 10231-3).

Hakomori, S. & Y. Igarashi (1993) Gangliosides and glycosphingolipids as modulators of cell growth, adhesion, and transmembrane signaling. *Adv Lipid Res.* 25, (pp. 147-62).

Hakomori, S. & Y. Igarashi (1995) Functional role of glycosphingolipids in cell recognition and signaling. *J Biochem (Tokyo).* 118, (pp. 1091-1103).

Hakomori, S., S. Yamamura & A. K. Handa (1998a) Signal transduction through glyco(sphingo)lipids. Introduction and recent studies on glyco(sphingo)lipid-enriched microdomains. *Ann N Y Acad Sci.* 845, (pp. 1-10).

Hakomori, S.-I. (2000) Cell adhesion/recognition and signal transduction through glycosphingolipid microdomain. *Glycoconjugate J.* 17, (pp. 143-151).

Hakomori, S.-I., K. Handa, K. Iwabuchi, S. Yamamura & A. Prinetti (1998b) New insights in glycosphingolipid function: "glycosignaling domain," a cell surface assembly of glycosphingolipids with signal transducer molecules, involved in cell adhesion coupled with signaling. *Glycobiol.* 8, (pp. xi-xix).

Hakomori, S. I. (2008) Structure and function of glycosphingolipids and sphingolipids: recollections and future trends. *Biochim Biophys Acta.* 1780, (pp. 325-46).

Haldar, K., N. Mohandas, B. U. Samuel, T. Harrison, N. L. Hiller, T. Akompong & P. Cheresh (2002) Protein and lipid trafficking induced in erythrocytes infected by malaria parasites. *Cellular Microbiology.* 4, (pp. 383-95).

Hall, A., T. Rog, M. Karttunen & I. Vattulainen (2010) Role of glycolipids in lipid rafts: a view through atomistic molecular dynamics simulations with galactosylceramide. *J Phys Chem B.* 114, (pp. 7797-807).

Hamanaka, R., T. Shinohara, S. Yano, M. Nakamura, A. Yasuda, S. Yokoyama, J. Q. Fan, K. Kawasaki, M. Watanabe & S. Ishii (2008) Rescue of mutant alpha-galactosidase A in the endoplasmic reticulum by 1-deoxygalactonojirimycin leads to trafficking to lysosomes. *Biochim Biophys Acta.* 1782, (pp. 408-13).

Hammache, D., G. Piéroni, N. Yahi, O. Delézay, N. Koch, H. Lafont, C. Tamalet & J. Fantini (1998a) Specific interaction of HIV-1 and HIV-2 surface envelope glycoproteins with monolayers of galactosylceramide and ganglioside GM3. *J Biol Chem.* 273, (pp. 7967-7971).

Hammache, D., N. Yahi, M. Maresca, G. Pieroni & J. Fantini (1999) Human erythrocyte glycosphingolipids as alternative cofactors for human immunodeficiency virus type 1 (HIV-1) entry: Evidence for CD4-induced interactions between HIV-1 gp120 and reconstituted membrane microdomains of glycosphingolipids (Gb3 and GM3). *J Virol.* 73, (pp. 5244-5248).

Hammache, D., N. Yahi, G. Pieroni, F. Ariasi, C. Tamalet & J. Fantini (1998b) Sequential interaction of CD4 and HIV-1 gp120 with a reconstituted membrane patch of ganglioside GM3: Implications for the role of glycolipids as potential HIV-1 fusion cofactors. *Biochem. Biophys. Res. Commun.* 246, (pp. 117-122).

Harouse, J. M., R. G. Collman & F. Gonzalez-Scarano (1995) Human immunodeficiency virus type 1 infection of SK-N-MC cells: domains of gp120 involved in entry into a CD4-negative, galactosyl ceramide/3' sulfo-galactosyl ceramide-positive cell line. *J Virol.* 69, (pp. 7383-90).

Harrison, A., M.L. Olsson, R.B. Jones, S. Ramkumar, D. Sakac, B. Binnington, S. Henry, C.A. Lingwood & D.R. Branch (2010) A synthetic globotriaosylceramide analogue inhibits HIV-1 infection *in vitro* by two mechanisms. *Glycoconj. J.* 27, (pp. 515-524).

Harrison, A., S. Henry, R. Mahfoud, A. Manis, A. Albertini, Y. Gaudin, C. A. Lingwood & D.R. Branch (2011) A novel VSV/HIV pseudotype approach for the study of HIV microbicides without requirement for level 3 biocontainment. *Future Virol. In press*

Hatch, S. C., J. Archer & S. Gummuluru (2009) Glycosphingolipid composition of human immunodeficiency virus type 1 (HIV-1) particles is a crucial determinant for dendritic cell-mediated HIV-1 trans-infection. *J Virol.* 83, (pp. 3496-506).

Haywood, A. M. (1994) Virus receptors: binding, adhesion strengthening, and changes in viral structure. *Journal of virology.* 68, (pp. 1-5).

Heath-Engel, H. M. & C. A. Lingwood (2003) Verotoxin sensitivity of ECV304 cells *in vitro* and *in vivo* in a xenograft tumour model: VT1 as a tumour neovascular marker. *Angiogenesis.* 6, (pp. 129-41.).

Hellberg, A., M. A. Chester & M. L. Olsson (2005) Two previously proposed P1/P2-differentiating and nine novel polymorphisms at the A4GALT (Pk) locus do not correlate with the presence of the P1 blood group antigen. *BMC Genetics.* 6, (pp. 49).

Hellberg, A., J. Poole & M. L. Olsson (2002) Molecular basis of the globoside-deficient P(k) blood group phenotype. Identification of four inactivating mutations in the UDP-N-acetylgalactosamine: globotriaosylceramide 3-beta-N-acetylgalactosaminyltransferase gene. *The Journal of Biological Chemistry.* 277, (pp. 29455-9).

Hellberg, A., A. Ringressi, V. Yahalom, J. Safwenberg, M. E. Reid & M. L. Olsson (2004) Genetic heterogeneity at the glycosyltransferase loci underlying the GLOB blood group system and collection. *British Journal of Haematology.* 125, (pp. 528-36).

Hellberg, A., R. Steffensen, V. Yahalom, B. N. Sojka, H. E. Heier, C. Levene, J. Poole & M. L. Olsson (2003) Additional molecular bases of the clinically important p blood group phenotype. *Transfusion.* 43, (pp. 899-907).

Heung, L. J., C. Luberto & M. Del Poeta (2006) Role of sphingolipids in microbial pathogenesis. *Infect Immun.* 74, (pp. 28-39).

Hikita, T., K. Tadano-Aritomi, N. Iida-Tanaka, S. B. Levery, I. Ishizuka & S. Hakomori (2002) Cationic glycosphingolipids in neuronal tissues and their possible biological significance. *Neurochem Res.* 27, (pp. 575-81).

Hooper, N. (1999) Detergent-insoluble glycosphingolipid/cholesterol-rich membrane domains, lipid rafts and caveolae. *Molr Membr Biol.* 16, (pp. 145-156).

Huang, C. C., S. N. Lam, P. Acharya, M. Tang, S. H. Xiang, S. S. Hussan, R. L. Stanfield, J. Robinson, J. Sodroski, I. A. Wilson, R. Wyatt, C. A. Bewley & P. D. Kwong (2007) Structures of the CCR5 N terminus and of a tyrosine-sulfated antibody with HIV-1 gp120 and CD4. *Science.* 317, (pp. 1930-4).

Hug, P., H. Lin, T. Korte, X. Xiao, D. Dimitrov, J. Wang, A. Puri & B. R. (2000) Glycosphingolipids promote entry of a broad range of human immunodeficiency virus type 1 isolates into cell lines expressing CD4, CXCR4,and/or CCR5. *J Virol.* 74, (pp. 6377-6385).

Huwiler, A., D. Fabbro & J. Pfeilschifter (1998) Selective ceramide binding to protein kinase C-alpha and -delta isoenzymes in renal mesangial cells. *Biochem.* 37, (pp. 14556-14562).

Huwiler, A., T. Kolter, J. Pfeilschifter & K. Sandhoff (2000) Physiology and pathophysiology of sphingolipid metabolism and signaling. *Biochim Biophys Acta.* 1485, (pp. 63-99).

Iglesias-Bartolome, R., A. Trenchi, R. Comin, A. L. Moyano, G. A. Nores & J. L. Daniotti (2009) Differential endocytic trafficking of neuropathy-associated antibodies to GM1 ganglioside and cholera toxin in epithelial and neural cells. *Biochim Biophys Acta.* 1788, (pp. 2526-40).

Inokuchi, J.-I. & N. S. Radin (1987) Preparation of the active isomer of 1-phenyl-2-decanoylamino-3-morpholino-1-propanol, inhibitor of murine glucocerebroside synthetase. *J. Lipid Res.* 28, (pp. 565-571).

Iwabuchi, K., K. Handa & S. Hakomori (2000) Separation of glycosphingolipid-enriched microdomains from caveolar membrane characterized by presence of caveolin. *Methods Enzymol.* 312, (pp. 488-94).

Iwamura, K., K. Furukawa, M. Uchikawa, B. N. Sojka, Y. Kojima, J. Wiels, H. Shiku & T. Urano (2003) The blood group P1 synthase gene is identical to the Gb3/CD77 synthase gene. A clue to the solution of the P1/P2/p puzzle. *J Biol Chem.* 278, (pp. 44429-38).

Jelacic, S., C. L. Wobbe, D. R. Boster, M. A. Ciol, S. L. Watkins, P. I. Tarr & A. E. Stapleton (2002) ABO and P1 blood group antigen expression and stx genotype and outcome of childhood Escherichia coli O157:H7 infections. *J. Infect. Dis.* 185, (pp. 214-9).

Johannes, L., V. Pezo, F. Mallard, D. Tenza, A. Wiltz, A. Saint-Pol, J. Helft, C. Antony & P. Benaroch (2003) Effects of HIV-1 Nef on Retrograde Transport from the Plasma Membrane to the Endoplasmic Reticulum. *Traffic.* 4, (pp. 323-32).

Jones, P. L., T. Korte & R. Blumenthal (1998) Conformational changes in cell surface HIV-1 envelope glycoproteins are triggered by cooperation between cell surface CD4 and co-receptors. *J Biol Chem.* 273, (pp. 404-9).

Kaiser, H. J., D. Lingwood, I. Levental, J. L. Sampalo, L. Kalvodova, L. Rajendran & K. Simons (2009) Order of lipid phases in model and plasma membranes. *Proc Natl Acad Sci USA.* 106, (pp. 16645-50).

Kanfer, J. & S. Hakomori (1983). *Sphingolipid Biochemistry* Plenum Press, New York

Kannagi, R., S. B. Levery & S. Hakomori (1983a) Sequential change of carbohydrate antigen associated with differentiation of murine leukemia cells: i-I antigenic conversion and shifting of glycolipid synthesis. *Proc Natl Acad Sci U S A.* 80, (pp. 2844-8).

Kannagi, R., E. Nudelman, S. B. Levery & S. Hakomori (1982) A series of human erythrocyte glycosphingolipids reacting to the monoclonal antibody directed to a developmentally regulated antigen SSEA-1. *J Biol Chem.* 257, (pp. 14865-74).

Kannagi, R., R. Stroup, N. A. Cochran, D. L. Urdal, W. W. Young Jr. & S.-I. Hakomori, . (1983b) Factors affecting expression of glycolipid tumor antigens: Influence of ceramide composition and coexisting glycolipid on the antigenicity of gangliotriaosylceramide in murine lymphoma cells. *Cancer Res.* 43, (pp. 4997-5005,).

Katagiri, Y., T. Mori, H. Nakajima, C. Katagiri, T. Taguchi, T. Takeda, N. Kiyokawa & J. Fujimoto (1999) Activation of Src family kinase induced by Shiga toxin binding to globotriaosyl ceramide (Gb3/CD77) in low density, detergent-insoluble microdomains. *J. Biol. Chem.* 274, (pp. 35278-35282).

Khan, F., F. Proulx & C. A. Lingwood (2009) Detergent-resistant globotriaosyl ceramide may define verotoxin/glomeruli-restricted hemolytic uremic syndrome pathology. *Kidney Int.* 75, (pp. 1209-16).

Khine, A. A., M. Firtel & C. A. Lingwood (1998) CD77-dependent retrograde transport of CD19 to the nuclear membrane: Functional Relationship between CD77 and CD19 during germinal center B-cell apoptosis. *J. Cell. Physiol.* 176, (pp. 281-292).

Khine, A. A. & C. A. Lingwood (1994) Capping and receptor mediated endocytosis of cell bound verotoxin(Shiga-like toxin) 1; Chemical identification of an amino acid in the B subunit necessary for efficient receptor glycolipid binding and cellular internalization. *J. Cell. Physiol.* 161, (pp. 319-332).

Khine, A. A. & C. A. Lingwood (2000) Functional significance of globotriaosylceramide in a_2 interferon/ type I interferon receptor mediated anti viral activity'. *J. Cell. Physiol.* 182, (pp. 97-108).

Kiarash, A., B. Boyd & C. A. Lingwood (1994) Glycosphingolipid receptor function is modified by fatty acid content: Verotoxin 1 and Verotoxin 2c preferentially recognize different globotriaosyl ceramide fatty acid homologues. *J. Biol. Chem.* 269, (pp. 11138-11146).

Kim, M., D. Sakac, B. Binnington, K. Fernandes, S. Shi, LingwoodC. & D. Branch (2011) Comparison of detection methods for cell surface globotriaosylceramide. *J. Immunol. Methods* 371, (pp. 48-60).

Kitchen, S. G., C. H. Uittenbogaart & J. A. Zack (1997) Mechanism of human immunodeficiency virus type 1 localization in CD4-negative thymocytes: differentiation from a CD4-positive precursor allows productive infection. *J Virol.* 71, (pp. 5713-22).

Kojima, N. & S. Hakomori (1991) Cell adhesion, spreading, and motility of GM_3-expressing cells based on glycolipid -glycolipid interaction. *J. Biol. Chem.* 266, (pp. 17552-17558).

Kojima, Y., S. Fukumoto, K. Furukawa, T. Okajima, J. Wiels, K. Yokoyama, Y. Suzuki, T. Urano & M. Ohta (2000) Molecular cloning of globotriaosylceramide/CD77 synthase, a glycosyltransferase that initiates the synthesis of globo series glycosphingolipids. *J Biol Chem.* 275, (pp. 15152-6).

Kolter, T. & K. Sandhoff (1998) Glycosphingolipid degradation and animal models of GM2-gangliosidoses. *J Inherit Metab Dis.* 21, (pp. 548-63).

Koshy, K. M., J. Wang & J. M. Boggs (1999) Divalent cation-mediated interaction between cerebroside sulfate and cerebrosides: an investigation of the effect of structural variations of lipids by electrospray ionization mass spectrometry. *Biophys J.* 77, (pp. 306-18.).

Kovbasnjuk, O., R. Mourtazina, B. Baibakov, T. Wang, C. Elowsky, M. A. Choti, A. Kane & M. Donowitz (2005) The glycosphingolipid globotriaosylceramide in the metastatic transformation of colon cancer. *Proc Natl Acad Sci U S A.* 102, (pp. 19087-92).

Kurzchalia, T. & R. Parton (1999) Membrane microdomains and caveolae. *Curt Opin Cell Biol.* 11, (pp. 424-431).

Lafont, F., G. Tran Van Nhieu, K. Hanada, P. Sansonetti & F. G. van der Goot (2002) Initial steps of Shigella infection depend on the cholesterol/sphingolipid raft-mediated CD44-IpaB interaction. *Embo J.* 21, (pp. 4449-57.).

Lajoie, P. & I. R. Nabi (2010) Lipid rafts, caveolae, and their endocytosis. *Int Rev Cell Mol Biol.* 282, (pp. 135-63).

Lala, P., S. Ito & C. A. Lingwood (2000) Transfection of MDCK cells with the MDR1 gene results in a major increase in globotriaosyl ceramide and cell sensitivity to verocytotoxin: role of P-gp in glycolipid biosynthesis. *J Biol Chem.* 275, (pp. 6246-6251).

Lannert, H., K. Gorgas, I. Meißner, F. T. Wieland & D. Jeckel (1998) Functional organization of the Golgi apparatus in glycosphingolipid biosynthesis. Lactosylceramide and subsequent glycosphingolipids are formed in the lumen of the late Golgi. *J Biol Chem.* 273, (pp. 2939-2946).

Lauer, S., J. VanWye, T. Harrison, H. McManus, B. U. Samuel, N. L. Hiller, N. Mohandas & K. Haldar (2000) Vacuolar uptake of host components, and a role for cholesterol and sphingomyelin in malarial infection. *The EMBO Journal.* 19, (pp. 3556-64).

Lauvrak, S. U., M. L. Torgersen & K. Sandvig (2004) Efficient endosome-to-Golgi transport of Shiga toxin is dependent on dynamin and clathrin. *J Cell Sci.* 117, (pp. 2321-31).

Lee, L., A. Abe & J. A. Shayman (1999) Improved inhibitors of glucosylceramide synthase. *J Biol Chem.* 274, (pp. 14662-14669).

Leffler, H. & C. Svanborg-Eden (1981) Glycolipid receptors for uropathogenic Escherichia coli on human erythrocytes and uroepithelial cells. *Infection and Immunity.* 34, (pp. 920-9).

Lencer, W. (2001) Microbes and microbial toxins: paradigms for microbial-mucosal toxins. V. Cholera: invasion of the intestinal epithelial barrier by a stably folded protein toxin. *Am J Physiol - Gastro Liver Physiol.* 280, (pp. G781-786).

Lencer, W. I. & D. Saslowsky (2005) Raft trafficking of AB5 subunit bacterial toxins. *Biochim Biophys Acta.* 1746, (pp. 314-21).

Liao, Z., L. M. Cimakasky, R. Hampton, D. H. Nguyen & J. E. Hildreth (2001) Lipid rafts and HIV pathogenesis: host membrane cholesterol is required for infection by HIV type 1. *AIDS Res Hum Retroviruses.* 17, (pp. 1009-19.).

Lingwood, C. A. (1996) Aglycone Modulation of Glycolipid Receptor Function. *Glycoconj J.* 13, (pp. 495-503).

Lingwood, C. A. (1998) Oligosaccharide receptors for bacteria: a view to a kill. *Current Biology.* 2, (pp. 695-700).

Lingwood, C. A. (2000) Verotoxin/globotriaosyl ceramide recognition: angiopathy, angiogenesis and antineoplasia. *Bioscience Reports.* 19, (pp. 345-354).

Lingwood, C. A., H. Law, S. Richardson, M. Petric, J. L. Brunton, S. DeGrandis & M. Karmali (1987) Glycolipid binding of purified and recombinant *Escherichia coli*-produced verotoxin *in vitro*. *J. Biol. Chem.* 262, (pp. 8834-8839).

Lingwood, C. A. & S. C. K. Yiu (1992) Glycolipid modification of a2-interferon binding: Sequence similarity between a2-interferon receptor and the verotoxin (Shiga-like toxin) B-subunit. *Biochem. J.* 283, (pp. 25-26).

Lingwood, D., B. Binnington, T. Róg, I. Vattulainen, M. Grzybek, U. Coskun, C. Lingwood & K. Simons (2011) Cholesterol modulates glycolipid conformation and receptor activity. *Nature Chem. Biol.* 7, (pp. 260-2).

Lingwood, D. & K. Simons (2007) Detergent resistance as a tool in membrane research. *Nat Protoc.* 2, (pp. 2159-65).

Lingwood, D. & K. Simons (2010) Lipid rafts as a membrane-organizing principle. *Science.* 327, (pp. 46-50).

Littman, D. R. (1998) Chemokine receptors: keys to AIDS pathogenesis? *Cell.* 93, (pp. 677-80).

Liao, Z., D.R. Graham & J.E. Hildreth (2003) Lipid rafts and HIV pathogenesis: virion-associated cholesterol is required for fusion and infection of susceptible cells. *AIDS Res Hum Retroviruses.* 19, (pp. 675-87).

Liu, X.-H., C. A. Lingwood & P. Ray (1999) Recruitment of renal tubular epithelial cells expressing Verotoxin-1 (Stx1) receptors in HIV-1 transgenic mice with renal disease. *Kidney Int.* 55, (pp. 554-561).

Livingstone, W. J., M. Moore, D. Innes, J. E. Bell & P. Simmonds (1996) Frequent infection of peripheral blood CD8-positive T-lymphocytes with HIV-1. Edinburgh Heterosexual Transmission Study Group. *Lancet.* 348, (pp. 649-54).

Lund, N., D. Branch, M. Mylvaganam, D. Chark, X. Ma, D. Sakac, B. Binnington, J. Fantini, A. Puri, R. Blumenthal & C. Lingwood (2006) A novel soluble mimic of the glycolipid globotriaosylceramide inhibits HIV infection. *AIDS.* 20, (pp. 333-343).

Lund, N., D. R. Branch, D. Sakac, C. Lingwood, C. Siatskas, C. Robinson, R. Brady & J. Medin (2005) Lack of Susceptibility of Cells from Patients with Fabry Disease to Infection with R5 Human Immunodeficiency Virus. *AIDS.* 19, (pp. 1543-1546).

Lund, N., S. Ramkumar, M. L. Olsson, D. Sakac, Y. Yahalom, C. Levene, A. Hellberg, X. Ma, D. Jung, B. Binnington, C. A. Lingwood & D. R. Branch (2009) The human Pk histo-blood group antigen provides protection against HIVinfection. *Blood.* 113, (pp. 4980-91).

Luo, C., K. Wang, Q. Liu de, Y. Li & Q. S. Zhao (2008) The functional roles of lipid rafts in T cell activation, immune diseases and HIV infection and prevention. *Cell Mol Immunol.* 5, (pp. 1-7).

Magerus-Chatinet, A., H. Yu, S. Garcia, E. Ducloux, B. Terris & M. Bomsel (2007) Galactosyl ceramide expressed on dendritic cells can mediate HIV-1 transfer from monocyte derived dendritic cells to autologous T cells. *Virology.* 362, (pp. 67-74).

Mahfoud, R., N. Garmy, M. Maresca, N. Yahi, A. Puigserver & J. Fantini (2002a) Identification of a common sphingolipid-binding domain in Alzheimer, prion and HIV-1 proteins. *J Biol Chem.* 277, (pp. 11292-6).

Mahfoud, R., A. Manis, B. Binnington, C. Ackerley & C. A. Lingwood (2010) A major fraction of glycosphingolipids in model and cellular cholesterol containing membranes are undetectable by their binding proteins. *J Biol Chem.* 285, (pp. 36049-59).

Mahfoud, R., A. Manis & C. Lingwood (2009) Fatty acid-dependent globotriaosyl ceramide receptor function in detergent resistant model membranes *J Lip Res.* 50, (pp. 1744-55).

Mahfoud, R., M. Mylvaganam, C. A. Lingwood & J. Fantini (2002b) A novel soluble analog of the HIV-1 fusion cofactor, globotriaosylceramide(Gb_3), eliminates the cholesterol requirement for high affinity gp120/Gb_3 interaction. *J. Lipid Res.* 43, (pp. 1670-1679).

Maloney, M. D. & C. A. Lingwood (1994) CD19 has a potential CD77 (globotriaosyl ceramide)-binding site with sequence similarity to verotoxin B-subunits: Implications of molecular mimicry for B cell adhesion and enterohemorrhagic *Escherichia coli* pathogenesis. *J. Exp. Med.* 180, (pp. 191-201).

Mamelak, D., M. Mylvaganam, E. Tanahashi, H. Ito, H. Ishida, M. Kiso & C. Lingwood (2001a) The aglycone of sulfogalactolipids can alter the sulfate ester substitution position required for hsc70 recognition. *Carbohydr Res.* 335, (pp. 91-100.).

Mamelak, D., M. Mylvaganam, H. Whetstone, E. Hartmann, W. Lennarz, P. Wyrick, J. Raulston, H. Han, P. Hoffman & C. Lingwood (2001b) Hsp70s contain a specific sulfogalactolipid binding site. Differential aglycone influence on sulfogalactosyl ceramide binding by prokaryotic and eukaryotic hsp70 family members. *Biochemistry.* 40, (pp. 3572-3582).

Manes, S., G. del Real, R. A. Lacalle, P. Lucas, Gomez-Mouton, C., , S. Sanchez-Palomino, R. Delgado, J. Alcami, E. Mira & C. Martinez-A (2000) Membrane raft microdomains

mediate lateral assemblies required for HIV-1 infection. *EMBO Reports*. 1, (pp. 190-196).
Manes, S., G. del Real & A. C. Martinez (2003) Pathogens: raft hijackers. *Nature reviews. Immunology*. 3, (pp. 557-68).
Manes, S., R. Lacalle, C. Gomez-Mouton, G. del Real, E. Mira & A. C. Martinez (2001) Membrane raft microdomains in chemokine receptor function. *Sem Immunol*. 13, (pp. 147-157).
Manes, S. & A. C. Martinez (2004) Cholesterol domains regulate the actin cytoskeleton at the leading edge of moving cells. *Trends Cell Biol*. 14, (pp. 275-8).
Mangeney, M., Y. Richard, D. Coulaud, T. Tursz & J. Wiels (1991) CD77: an antigen of germinal center B cells entering apoptosis. *Eur. J. Immunol*. 21, (pp. 1131-1140).
Manie, S. N., S. de Breyne, S. Vincent & D. Gerlier (2000) Measles virus structural components are enriched into lipid raft microdomains: a potential cellular location for virus assembly. *Journal of virology*. 74, (pp. 305-11).
Marjomaki, V., V. Pietiainen, H. Matilainen, P. Upla, J. Ivaska, L. Nissinen, H. Reunanen, P. Huttunen, T. Hyypia & J. Heino (2002) Internalization of echovirus 1 in caveolae. *Journal of Virology*. 76, (pp. 1856-65).
Marras, D., L. Bruggeman, F. Gao, N. Tanji, M. Mansukhani, A. Cara, M. Ross, G. Gusella, G. Benson, V. D'Agati, B. Hahn, M. Klotman & P. Klotman (2002) Replication and compartmentalization of HIV-1 in kidney epithelium of patients with HIV-associated nephropathy. *Nature Medicine*. 8, (pp. 522-6).
Marsh, M. & A. Helenius (1989) Virus entry into animal cells. *Adv Virus res*. 36, (pp. 107-151).
Millan, J., J. Cerny, V. Horejsi & M. Alonso (1999) CD4 segregates into specific detergent-resistant T-cell membrane microdomains. *Tissue Antigens*. 53, (pp. 33-40).
Miller-Podraza, H., C. Andersson & K. A. Karlsson (1993) New method for the isolation of polyglycosylceramides from human erythrocyte membranes. *Biochim Biophys Acta*. 1168, (pp. 330-9).
Miller-Podraza, H., L. Johansson, P. Johansson, T. Larsson, M. Matrosovich & K. A. Karlsson (2000) A strain of human influenza A virus binds to extended but not short gangliosides as assayed by thin-layer chromatography overlay. *Glycobiology*. 10, (pp. 975-82).
Mori, T., N. Kiyokawa, Y. U. Katagiri, T. Taguchi, T. Suzuki, T. Sekino, N. Sato, K. Ohmi, H. Nakajima, T. Takeda & J. Fukimoto (2000) Globotriaosyl ceramide (CD77/Gb3) in the glycolipid-enriched membrane domain participates in B-cell receptor-mediated apoptosis by regulating Lyn kinase activity in human B cells. *Exp. Hemat*. 28, (pp. 1260-1268).
Moriuchi, H., M. Moriuchi, J. Arthos, J. Hoxie & A. S. Fauci (1997) Promonocytic U937 subclones expressing CD4 and CXCR4 are resistant to infection with and cell-to-cell fusion by T-cell-tropic human immunodeficiency virus type 1. *J Virol*. 71, (pp. 9664-71).
Moulds, J. M. & J. J. Moulds (2000) Blood group associations with parasites, bacteria, and viruses. *Transfusion Medicine Reviews*. 14, (pp. 302-11).
Mukherjee, S. & F. Maxfield (2000) Role of membrane organization and membrane domains in endocytic lipid trafficking. *Traffic*. 1, (pp. 203-211).

Muthing, J., C. H. Schweppe, H. Karch & A. W. Friedrich (2009) Shiga toxins, glycosphingolipid diversity, and endothelial cell injury. *Thromb Haemost.* 101, (pp. 252-64).

Mylvaganam, M. & C. Lingwood (1999a) Adamantyl globotriaosyl ceramide- a monovalent soluble glycolipid mimic which inhibits verotoxin binding to its glycolipid receptor. *Biochem. Biophys. Res. Commun.* 257, (pp. 391-394).

Mylvaganam, M. & C. A. Lingwood (1999b) A convenient oxidation of natural glycosphingolipids to their "ceramide acids"for neoglycoconjugation: Bovine serum albumin-glycoceramide acid conjugates as investigative probes for HIV coat protein gp120-glycosphingolipid interactions. *J Biol Chem.* 274, (pp. 20725-20732).

Mylvaganam, M. & C. A. Lingwood (2003). A preamble to aglycone reconstruction for membrane-presented glycolipids Wiley-VCH Press, Weinheim, Germany

Nehete, P.N., E.M. Vela, M.M. Hossain, A.K. Sarkar, N. Hahi, J. Fantini & K.J. Sastry (2002) A post-CD4-binding step involving interaction of the V3 region of viral gp120 with host cell surface glycosphingolipids is common to entry and infection by diverse HIV-1 strains. *Antiviral Res.* 56, (pp. 233-51).

Nelson, J. A., C. A. Wiley, C. Reynolds-Kohler, C. E. Reese, W. Margaretten & J. A. Levy (1988) Human immunodeficiency virus detected in bowel epithelium from patients with gastrointestinal symptoms. *Lancet.* 1, (pp. 259-62.).

Nguyen, D. H. & J. E. Hildreth (2000) Evidence for budding of human immunodeficiency virus type 1 selectively from glycolipid-enriched membrane lipid rafts. *J Virol.* 74, (pp. 3264-72).

Nichols, B., A. Kenworthy, R. Polishchuk, R. Lodge, T. Roberts, K. Hirschberg, R. Phair & L.-S. J. (2001) Rapid cycling of lipid raft markers between the cell surface and Golgi complex. *J Cell Biol.* 153, (pp. 529-41).

Niemela, P. S., M. T. Hyvonen & I. Vattulainen (2009) Atom-scale molecular interactions in lipid raft mixtures. *Biochim Biophys Acta.* 1788, (pp. 122-35).

Norkin, L. C. (1999) Simian virus 40 infection via MHC class I molecules and caveolae. *Immunological Reviews.* 168, (pp. 13-22).

Nutikka, A. & C. Lingwood (2004) Generation of receptor active, globotriaosyl ceramide/cholesterol lipid 'rafts' *in vitro*: a new assay to define factors affecting glycosphingolipid receptor activity. *Glycoconj. J.* 20, (pp. 33-38).

Nyholm, P.G. & I. Pascher (1993) Orientation of the saccharide chains of glycolipids at the membrane surface: conformational analysis of the glucose-ceramide and the glucose-glyceride linkages using molecular mechanics (MM3). *Biochem.* 32, (pp. 1225-34).

Okuda, T., N. Tokuda, S. Numata, M. Ito, M. Ohta, K. Kawamura, J. Wiels, T. Urano, O. Tajima & K. Furukawa (2006) Targeted disruption of Gb3/CD77 synthase gene resulted in the complete deletion of globo-series glycosphingolipids and loss of sensitivity to verotoxins. *J Biol Chem.* 281, (pp. 10230-5).

Ono, A. & E. O. Freed (2001) Plasma membrane rafts play a critical role in HIV-1 assembly and release. *Proc Natl Acad Sci U S A.* 98, (pp. 13925-30.).

Ono, M., K. Handa, S. Sonnino, D. A. Withers, H. Nagai & S. Hakomori (2001) GM3 ganglioside inhibits CD9-facilitated haptotactic cell motility: coexpression of GM3 and CD9 is essential in the downregulation of tumor cell motility and malignancy. *Biochemistry.* 40, (pp. 6414-21).

Parton, R. G. (1994) Ultrastructural localization of gangliosides; GM_1 is concentrated in caveolae. *J Histochem Cytochem.* 42, (pp. 155-166).
Parton, R. G. & A. A. Richards (2003) Lipid rafts and caveolae as portals for endocytosis: new insights and common mechanisms. *Traffic.* 4, (pp. 724-38).
Pellizzari, A., H. Pang & C. A. Lingwood (1992) Binding of verocytotoxin 1 to its receptor is influenced by differences in receptor fatty acid content. *Biochemistry.* 31, (pp. 1363-70).
Percherancier, Y., B. Lagane, T. Planchenault, I. Staropoli, R. Altmeyer, J. Virelizier, F. Arenzana-Seisdedos, D. Hoessli & F. Bachelerie (2003) HIV-1 Entry into T-cells Is Not Dependent on CD4 and CCR5 Localization to Sphingolipid-enriched, Detergent-resistant, Raft Membrane Domains. *J Biol Chem.* 278, (pp. 3153-61).
Peterlin, B. M. & D. Trono (2003) Hide, shield and strike back: how HIV-infected cells avoid immune eradication. *Nat Rev Immunol.* 3, (pp. 97-107).
Petruzziello, T. N., I. A. Mawji, M. Khan & P. A. Marsden (2009) Verotoxin biology: molecular events in vascular endothelial injury. *Kidney Int Suppl.* (pp. S17-9).
Piguet, V. & D. Trono (1999) The Nef protein of primate lentiviruses. *Rev Med Virol.* 9, (pp. 111-20).
Pochechueva, T., A. Chinarev, M. Spengler, E. Korchagina, V. Heinzelmann-Schwarz, N. Bovin & R. Rieben (2011) Multiplex suspension array for human anti-carbohydrate antibody profiling. *Analyst.* 136, (pp. 560-9).
Popik, W., T. M. Alce & W. C. Au (2002) Human immunodeficiency virus type 1 uses lipid raft-colocalized CD4 and chemokine receptors for productive entry into CD4(+) T cells. *J Virol.* 76, (pp. 4709-22.).
Pumarola-Sune, T., B. A. Navia, C. Cordon-Cardo, E. S. Cho & R. W. Price (1987) HIV antigen in the brains of patients with the AIDS dementia complex. *Ann Neurol.* 21, (pp. 490-6).
Puri, A., P. Hug, K. Jernigan, J. Barchi, H.-Y. Kim, J. Hamilton, J. Wiels, G. J. Murray, R. O. Brady & R. Blumenthal (1998) The neutral glycosphingolipid globotriaosylceramide promotes fusion mediated by a CD4-dependent CXCR4-utilizing HIV type 1 envelope glycoprotein. *Proc. Natl. Acad. Sci.* 95, (pp. 14435-14440).
Puri, A., P. Hug, K. Jernigan, P. Rose & R. Blumenthal (1999) Role of glycosphingolipids in HIV-1 entry: requirement of globotriosylceramide (Gb3) in CD4/CXCR4-dependent fusion. *Biosci Rep.* 19, (pp. 317-325).
Puri, A., S. S. Rawat, H. M. Lin, C. M. Finnegan, J. Mikovits, F. W. Ruscetti & R. Blumenthal (2004) An inhibitor of glycosphingolipid metabolism blocks HIV-1 infection of primary T-cells. *Aids.* 18, (pp. 849-58).
Radhakrishnan, A., T. G. Anderson & H. M. McConnell (2000) Condensed complexes, rafts, and the chemical activity of cholesterol in membranes. *Proc Natl Acad Sci.* 97, (pp. 12422-12427).
Rajendran, L. & K. Simons (2005) Lipid rafts and membrane dynamics. *J Cell Sci.* 118, (pp. 1099-102).
Ramegowda, B. & V. L. Tesh (1996) Differentiation-associated toxin receptor modulation, cytokine production, and sensitivity to Shiga-like toxins in human monocytes and moncytic cell lines. *Infect. Immun.* 64, (pp. 1173-1180).

Ramkumar, S., D. Sakac, B. Binnington, D. R. Branch & C. A. Lingwood (2009) Induction of HIV resistance: Cell susceptibility to infection is an inverse function of globotriaosyl ceramide levels. *Glycobiology*. 19, (pp. 76-82).

Raulin, J. (2002) Human immunodeficiency virus and host cell lipids. Interesting pathways in research for a new HIV therapy. *Prog Lipid Res*. 41, (pp. 27-65).

Rawat, S. S., S. A. Gallo, J. Eaton, T. D. Martin, S. Ablan, V. N. KewalRamani, J. M. Wang, R. Blumenthal & A. Puri (2004) Elevated expression of GM3 in receptor-bearing targets confers resistance to human immunodeficiency virus type 1 fusion. *J Virol*. 78, (pp. 7360-8).

Rawat, S. S., M. Viard, S. A. Gallo, R. Blumenthal & A. Puri (2006) Sphingolipids, cholesterol, and HIV-1: A paradigm in viral fusion. *Glycoconj J*. 23, (pp. 189-97).

Rawat, S. S., M. Viard, S. A. Gallo, A. Rein, R. Blumenthal & A. Puri (2003) Modulation of entry of enveloped viruses by cholesterol and sphingolipids (Review). *Mol Membr Biol*. 20, (pp. 243-54).

Rios, M. & C. Bianco (2000) The role of blood group antigens in infectious diseases. *Seminars in Hematology*. 37, (pp. 177-85).

Rosa Borges, A., L. Wieczorek, B. Johnson, A. J. Benesi, B. K. Brown, R. D. Kensinger, F. C. Krebs, B. Wigdahl, R. Blumenthal, A. Puri, F. E. McCutchan, D. L. Birx, V. R. Polonis & C. L. Schengrund (2010) Multivalent dendrimeric compounds containing carbohydrates expressed on immune cells inhibit infection by primary isolates of HIV-1. *Virology*. 408, (pp. 80-8).

Rusnati, M., C. Urbinati, E. Tanghetti, P. Dell'Era, H. Lortat-Jacob & M. Presta (2002) Cell membrane GM1 ganglioside is a functional coreceptor for fibroblast growth factor 2. *Proc Natl Acad Sci U S A*. 99, (pp. 4367-72).

Sabharanjak, S., P. Sharma, R. G. Parton & S. Mayor (2002) GPI-anchored proteins are delivered to recycling endosomes via a distinct cdc42-regulated, clathrin-independent pinocytic pathway. *Dev Cell*. 2, (pp. 411-23).

Saha, K., J. Zhang, A. Gupta, R. Dave, M. Yimen & B. Zerhouni (2001a) Isolation of primary HIV-1 that target CD8+ T lymphocytes using CD8 as a receptor. *Nat Med*. 7, (pp. 65-72).

Saha, K., J. Zhang & B. Zerhouni (2001b) Evidence of productively infected CD8+ T cells in patients with AIDS: implications for HIV-1 pathogenesis. *J Acquir Immune Defic Syndr*. 26, (pp. 199-207).

Samuel, B. U., N. Mohandas, T. Harrison, H. McManus, W. Rosse, M. Reid & K. Haldar (2001) The role of cholesterol and glycosylphosphatidylinositol-anchored proteins of erythrocyte rafts in regulating raft protein content and malarial infection. *J Biol Chem*. 276, (pp. 29319-29.).

Sandvig, K., M. Ryd, Ø. Garred, E. Schweda & P. K. Holm (1994) Retrograde transport from the Golgi complex to the ER of both Shiga toxin and the nontoxic Shiga B-fragment is regulated by butyric acid and cAMP. *J. Cell. Biol*. 126, (pp. 53-64).

Savarino, A., T. Bensi, A. Chiocchetti, F. Bottarel, R. Mesturini, E. Ferrero, L. Calosso, S. Deaglio, E. Ortolan, S. Butto, A. Cafaro, T. Katada, B. Ensoli, F. Malavasi & U. Dianzani (2003) Human CD38 interferes with HIV-1 fusion through a sequence homologous to the V3 loop of the viral envelope glycoprotein gp120. *FASEB J*. 17, (pp. 461-3).

Scheiffele, P., A. Rietveld, T. Wilk & K. Simons (1999) Influenza viruses select ordered lipid domains during budding from the plasma membrane. *The Journal of Biological Chemistry*. 274, (pp. 2038-44).

Schwartz-Albeiz, R., B. Dorken, P. Moller, N. T. Brodin, D. A. Monner & B. Kniep (1991) Neutral glycosphingolipids of the globo-series characterize activation stages corresponding to germinal center B cells. *Int Immunol.* 2, (pp. 929-936).

Sekino, T., N. Kiyokawa, T. Taguchi, H. Takenouchi, J. Matsui, W. R. Tang, T. Suzuki, H. Nakajima, M. Saito, K. Ohmi, Y. U. Katagiri, H. Okita, H. Nakao, T. Takeda & J. Fujimoto (2004) Characterization of a shiga-toxin 1-resistant stock of vero cells. *Microbiol Immunol.* 48, (pp. 377-87).

Shnaper, S., K. Sackett, S. A. Gallo, R. Blumenthal & Y. Shai (2004) The C- and the N-terminal regions of gp41 ectodomain fuse membranes enriched and not enriched with cholesterol, respectively. *J Biol Chem.* (pp.

Simons, K. & R. Ehehalt (2002) Cholesterol, lipid rafts, and disease. *J Clin Invest.* 110, (pp. 597-603).

Simons, K. & J. Gruenberg (2000) Jamming the endosomal system: lipid rafts and lysosomal storage diseases. *Trends Cell Biol.* 10, (pp. 459-62).

Simons, K. & E. Ikonen (1997) Functional rafts in cell membranes. *Nature.* 387, (pp. 569-572).

Simons, K. & D. Toomre (2000) Lipid rafts and signal transduction. *Nature Rev.* 1, (pp. 31-39).

Simons, K. & W. L. Vaz (2004) Model systems, lipid rafts, and cell membranes. *Annu Rev Biophys Biomol Struct.* 33, (pp. 269-95).

Smith, D. C., D. J. Sillence, T. Falguieres, R. M. Jarvis, L. Johannes, J. M. Lord, F. M. Platt & L. M. Roberts (2006) The Association of Shiga-like Toxin with Detergent-resistant Membranes Is Modulated by Glucosylceramide and Is an Essential Requirement in the Endoplasmic Reticulum for a Cytotoxic Effect. *Mol Biol Cell.* 17, (pp. 1375-87).

Solter, D. & B. B. Knowles (1978) Monoclonal antibody defining a stage-specific mouse embryonic antigen (SSEA-1). *Proc Natl Acad Sci U S A.* 75, (pp. 5565-9).

Sorice, M., T. Garofalo, L. Misasi R, A, , J. Mikulak, V. Dolo, G. Pontieri & P. A. (2000) Association between GM3 and CD4-Ick complex in human peripheral blood lymphocytes. *Glycoconj J.* 17, (pp. 247-252).

Sorice, M., T. Garofalo, R. Misasi, A. Longo, V. Mattei, P. Sale, V. Dolo, R. Gradini & A. Pavan (2001) Evidence for cell surface association between CXCR4 and ganglioside GM3 after gp120 binding in SupT1 lymphoblastoid cells. *FEBS Lett.* 506, (pp. 55-60.).

Sorice, M., A. Longo, T. Garofalo, V. Mattei, R. Misasi & A. Pavan (2004) Role of GM3-enriched microdomains in signal transduction regulation in T lymphocytes. *Glycoconj J.* 20, (pp. 63-70).

Sorice, M., I. Parolini, T. Sansolini, T. Garofalo, V. Dolo, M. Sargiacomo, T. Tai, C. Peschle, M. R. Torrisi & A. Pavan (1997) Evidence for the existence of ganglioside-enriched plasma membrane domains in human peripheral lymphocytes. *J Lipid Res.* 38, (pp. 969-80).

Speck, R. F., U. Esser, M. L. Penn, D. A. Eckstein, L. Pulliam, S. Y. Chan & M. A. Goldsmith (1999) A trans-receptor mechanism for infection of CD4-negative cells by human immunodeficiency virus type 1. *Curr Biol.* 9, (pp. 547-50.).

Sperandio, M. (2006) Selectins and glycosyltransferases in leukocyte rolling *in vivo*. *FEBS J.* 273, (pp. 4377-89).

Spitalnik, P. & S. Spitalnik (1995) The P blood group system: Biochemical, serological and clinical aspects. *Transfus Med Rev.* 9, (pp. 110-122).

Sprong, H., B. Kruithof, R. Leijendekker, J. W. Slot, G. van Meer & P. van der Sluijs (1998) UDP-galactose:ceramide galactosyltransferase is a class I integral membrane protein of the endoplasmic reticulum. *J Biol Chem.* 273, (pp. 25880-25888).

Stapleton, A., E. Nudelman, H. Clausen, S. Hakomori & W. E. Stamm (1992) Binding of uropathogenic Escherichia coli R45 to glycolipids extracted from vaginal epithelial cells is dependent on histo-blood group secretor status. *The Journal of Clinical Investigation.* 90, (pp. 965-72).

Steffensen, R., K. Carlier, J. Wiels, S. B. Levery, M. Stroud, B. Cederen, S. B. Nilsson, E. P. Bennett, C. Jersild & H. Clausen (2000) Cloning and expression of the histo-blood group Pk UDP-galactose: Galbeta 1-4Glcbeta 1-Cer alpha 1, 4-galactosyltransferase. Molecular genetic basis of the p phenotype. *J Biol Chem.* 275, (pp. 16723-16729).

Stiban, J., R. Tidhar & A. H. Futerman (2010) Ceramide synthases: roles in cell physiology and signaling. *Adv Exp Med Biol.* 688, (pp. 60-71).

Stults, C. L. M., C. H. Sweeley & B. A. Macher (1989) Glycosphingolipids; structure biological source and properties. *Methods Enzymol.* 179, (pp. 167-214).

Tagami, S., J. Inokuchi Ji, K. Kabayama, H. Yoshimura, F. Kitamura, S. Uemura, C. Ogawa, A. Ishii, M. Saito, Y. Ohtsuka, S. Sakaue & Y. Igarashi (2002) Ganglioside GM3 participates in the pathological conditions of insulin resistance. *J Biol Chem.* 277, (pp. 3085-92).

Tateno, M., F. Gonzalez-Scarano & J. A. Levy (1989) Human immunodeficiency virus can infect CD4-negative human fibroblastoid cells. *Proc Natl Acad Sci U S A.* 86, (pp. 4287-90.).

Teufel, A., T. Maass, P. R. Galle & N. Malik (2009) The longevity assurance homologue of yeast lag1 (Lass) gene family (review). *Int J Mol Med.* 23, (pp. 135-40).

Thuresson, B., J.S. Westman & M.L. Olsson (2011) Identification of a novel A4GALT exon reveals the genetic basis of the P1/P2 histo-blood groups. *Blood.* 117, (pp. 678-87).

Tsai, B., J. M. Gilbert, T. Stehle, W. Lencer, T. L. Benjamin & T. A. Rapoport (2003) Gangliosides are receptors for murine polyoma virus and SV40. *The EMBO Journal.* 22, (pp. 4346-55).

Turner, M., K. Kher, T. Rakussan, L. D'Angelo, S. Kapur, D. Selby & P. Ray (1997) Atypical hemolytic uremic syndrome in human immunodeficiency virus-1 infected children. *Ped Nephrol.* 11, (pp. 161-163).

Ullrich, R., W. Schmidt, T. Zippel, T. Schneider, M. Zeitz & E. O. Riecken (1998) Mucosal HIV infection. *Pathobiol.* 66, (pp. 145-150).

van Alphen, L., L. Gellen-van den Broek, L. Blaas, M. van Ham & J. Dankert (1991) Blocking of fimbria-mediated adherence of *Haemophilus influenzae* by sialyl gangliosides. *Infect Immun.* 59, (pp. 4473-4477).

van der Goot, F. G. & T. Harder (2001) Raft membrane domains: from a liquid-ordered membrane phase to a site of pathogen attack. *Semin Immunol.* 13, (pp. 89-97).

van Eijk, M., J. Aten, N. Bijl, R. Ottenhoff, C. P. van Roomen, P. F. Dubbelhuis, I. Seeman, K. Ghauharali-van der Vlugt, H. S. Overkleeft, C. Arbeeny, A. K. Groen & J. M. Aerts (2009) Reducing glycosphingolipid content in adipose tissue of obese mice restores insulin sensitivity, adipogenesis and reduces inflammation. *PLoS One.* 4, (pp. e4723).

Vieira, F. S., G. Correa, M. Einicker-Lamas & R. Coutinho-Silva (2010) Host-cell lipid rafts: a safe door for micro-organisms? *Biol Cell.* 102, (pp. 391-407).

Villard, R., D. Hammache, G. Delapierre, F. Fotiadu, G. Buono & J. Fantini (2002) Asymmetric synthesis of water-soluble analogues of galactosylceramide, an HIV-1 receptor: new tools to study virus-glycolipid interactions. *Chembiochem.* 3, (pp. 517-25.).

Vyas, A., H. Patel, S. Fromholt, M. Heffer-Lauc, K. Vyas, J. Dang, M. Schachner & R. Schnaar (2002) Gangliosides are functional nerve cell ligands for myelin-associated glycoprotein (MAG), an inhibitor of nerve regeneration. *Proc Natl Acad Sci.* 99, (pp. 8412-7).

Waarts, B. L., R. Bittman & J. Wilschut (2002) Sphingolipid and cholesterol dependence of alphavirus membrane fusion. Lack of correlation with lipid raft formation in target liposomes. *The Journal of Biological Chemistry.* 277, (pp. 38141-7).

Waddell, T., A. Cohen & C. A. Lingwood (1990) Induction of verotoxin sensitivity in receptor deficient cell lines using the receptor glycolipid globotriosyl ceramide. *Proc. Natl. Acad. Sci. USA.* 87, (pp. 7898-7901).

Wang, W. K., T. Dudek, M. Essex & T. H. Lee (1999) Hypervariable region 3 residues of HIV type 1 gp120 involved in CCR5 coreceptor utilization: therapeutic and prophylactic implications. *Proc Natl Acad Sci U S A.* 96, (pp. 4558-62).

Ward, J. M., T. J. O'Leary, G. B. Baskin, R. Benveniste, C. A. Harris, P. L. Nara & R. H. Rhodes (1987) Immunohistochemical localization of human and simian immunodeficiency viral antigens in fixed tissue sections. *Am J Pathol.* 127, (pp. 199-205).

Weber, K. T., D. Hammache, J. Fantini & B. Ganem (2000) Synthesis of glycolipid analogues that disrupt binding of HIV-1 gp120 to galactosylceramide. *Bioorg Med Chem Lett.* 10, (pp. 1011-4).

Weis, F. M. B. & R. J. Davis (1990) Regulation of epidermal growth factor receptor signal transduction. *J Biol Chem.* 265, (pp. 12059-12066).

Westerlund, B. & J. P. Slotte (2009) How the molecular features of glycosphingolipids affect domain formation in fluid membranes. *Biochim Biophys Acta.* 1788, (pp. 194-201).

Whetstone, D. & C. Lingwood (2003) 3′Sulfogalactolipid binding specifically inhibits Hsp70 ATPase activity *in vitro*. *Biochem.* 42, (pp. 1611-1617).

Wiels, J., M. Fellous & T. Tursz (1981) Monoclonal antibody against a Burkitt-lymphoma-associated antigen. *Proc Nat Acad Sci (Wash.).* 78, (pp. 6485-6488).

Wiels, J., M. Mangeney, C. Tetaud & T. Tursz (1991) Sequential shifts in the three major glycosphingolipid series are associated with B cell differentiation. *Int Immunol.* 3, (pp. 1289-300).

Wiley, C. A., R. D. Schrier, J. A. Nelson, P. W. Lampert & M. B. Oldstone (1986) Cellular localization of human immunodeficiency virus infection within the brains of acquired immune deficiency syndrome patients. *Proc Natl Acad Sci U S A.* 83, (pp. 7089-93).

Wyatt, C. M. & P. E. Klotman (2007) HIV-associated nephropathy in the era of antiretroviral therapy. *Am J Med.* 120, (pp. 488-92).

Xiao, L., S. M. Owen, I. Goldman, A. A. Lal, J. J. deJong, J. Goudsmit & R. B. Lal (1998) CCR5 coreceptor usage of non-syncytium-inducing primary HIV-1 is independent of phylogenetically distinct global HIV-1 isolates: delineation of consensus motif in the V3 domain that predicts CCR-5 usage. *Virology.* 240, (pp. 83-92).

Yahi, N., A. Aulas & J. Fantini (2010) How cholesterol constrains glycolipid conformation for optimal recognition of Alzheimer's beta amyloid peptide (Abeta1-40). *PLoS One.* 5, (pp. e9079).

14

Clinical Relevance of Drug Interactions in HIV-Infected Patients Receiving Antiretroviral Therapy

Pedro Amariles[1], Newar Giraldo Alzate[1] and Maria Jose Faus[2]
[1]*University of Antioquia, Medellin,*
[2]*University of Granada, Granada,*
[1]*Colombia*
[2]*Spain*

1. Introduction

The identification, prevention, and clinical solution of drug interactions (DIs) are a critical aspect to achieve desired pharmacotherapy goals in patients infected with human immunodeficiency virus and/or affected by acquired immunodeficiency syndrome (HIV/AIDS) receiving antiretroviral (ARV) therapy, mainly because DIs may lead that ARV therapy will be unsafe and/or ineffective and thus, DIs may be clinical relevant. Additionally, in this group of patients the DIs are more frequent among other aspects by:

- The use of Highly Active Antiretroviral Therapy (HAART) or combined Antiretroviral Therapy (cART) includes three or more ARV drugs; (DHHS, 2011) therefore it is associated with a greater likelihood of DIs.
- The pharmacokinetic properties of ARV drugs, for instance several of them are metabolized through complimentary cytochrome P450 isoenzymes, thus their therapeutic use could be accompanied by frequent DIs. (Miller et al., 2007)
- ARV drugs are concurrently used with other class of medications for other common conditions, mainly infections and cardiovascular disease; and many of these medications used to treat these conditions are metabolized through complimentary cytochrome P450 isoenzymes, so several pharmacokinetic DIs may occur.

Accordingly, some studies illustrate that the 96% of patients receiving HAART or cART has at least a clinical condition or use a concomitant drug that could cause that ARV therapy may be unsafe (adverse drug reactions) or ineffectiveness (therapeutic failure). (Grimes et al., 30 2002) Therefore, identifying, preventing, and solving clinically relevant DIs is recognized both as a topic of great importance in achieving therapeutic goals for drug therapy (Kashuba, 2005) as a constant challenge to health care providers to HIV-infected patients receiving HAAR or cART. In addition, the clinical significance of a DI depends on the disposition and toxicity profile of the drug being administered. Thus, in HIV-infected patients assessing the clinical relevance of a DI is complex due to the large interpatient variability in pharmacokinetics exhibited by most ARV drugs, and then the evaluation and prediction of clinical effect of a DI is critical in the pharmacotherapy of patients with HIV/AIDS.

Since most of ARV drug DIs are clinically relevant, it is considered appropriate both to outline **the concept, types, mechanisms, and effects of ARV DIs on drug therapy, and to present a comprehensive summary of those drugs that are affected and the clinical relevance of ARV DIs.** In this way, the aim of this chapter is provide evidence and systematize information about DIs in HIV-infected receiving ART therapy, which allow define, evaluate, and predict the clinical relevance of the DIs, highlight those associated to pharmacokinetic mechanism. In this way, a proposal to identify, evaluate, and predict DIs considered as clinically relevant is presented, in which clinical relevance of a DI is defined according to the probability of their occurrence and to the severity of clinical effect in patient health (adverse event or therapeutic failure). (Amariles et al., 2007a)

Previous review about DIs with ARV, (Amariles et al., 2007b; Giraldo et al., 2010) achieved as a result of searched in Pubmed/Medline database, have showed that, in the case of clinically relevant pharmacokinetic interactions, nearly 80% are related to changes in systemic clearance, mainly associated to the systemic inhibition or induction of the metabolic activity of the cytochrome P-450 (CYP-450), mostly CYP3A4 isoform, whereas approximately 15% are related to changes in bioavailability (changes in gastrointestinal pH, presystemic clearance [mediated by CYP3A4 hepatic or intestinal]) or in P-glycoprotein activity). (Amariles et al., 2007b; Giraldo et al., 2010)

For this chapter, the earlier published information (Amariles et al., 2007a, 2007b; Giraldo et al., 2010; Amariles, 2002.) have been complement with information achieved from both a structured and systematic review of publications on Pubmed/Medline and references cited in relevant articles, and in other electronic databases (SIETES, MEDSCAPE, and TRIPDATABASE), and supplemented by other primary and secondary information sources to identify DIs in HIV-infected patients. Thus, searched MeSH terms were drug interactions, antiretroviral agents (or drugs), drug food interactions, drug nutrient interactions, drug laboratory test interference, drug in special situations (age, diseases), drug herbal plant interactions, computerized drug interactions, decision clinical computer based, and clinical relevance, clinically relevant or significantly relevant.

Finally, according with clinical relevance of the DIs, pairs of the identified DIs have been classified in four levels, according to rate probability and severity, (Amariles et al., 2007a, 2007 b; Giraldo et al., 2010) and then, the different drug pairs have been structured in a software designed to facilitate the identification, evaluation, and prediction of clinical relevant DIs. Current, 1,082 drug pairs of potential DIs have been identified, near to 80% of them due to pharmacokinetic mechanism (changes in plasma concentration), mainly associated to systemic enzyme inhibition. The scaling of these 1,082 drug pairs of recognized DIs, according to different dosage forms and strengths of identified drugs, generates a total of 6,087 pairs of DIs, in which, according their clinical relevance, 4,158 (68.3%) are clinical relevant (Levels 1 and 2) in HIV-infected patients receiving ARV therapy. Thus, the designed software meets the requirements defined for this type of program (Gaikwad et al., 2007; Rodríguez et al., 2009) and most important it facilitates the assessment, prediction, and decision on clinical relevance of 4,158 ARV DIs, which are considered of clinical interest in patients with HIV/AIDS (levels 1 and 2).

2. Drug interactions in HIV-infected patients receiving antiretroviral therapy

2.1 Concept, type, and mechanism of drug interactions

Concept of DI. In patients with HIV/AIDS a DI could be assumed as **non-therapeutic and quantitative modification in the magnitude or duration of the drug effect** (decrease the efficacy or increase the toxicity) **that may lead to therapeutic failure or adverse drug reactions associated to a previous or a concomitant use** of another drug (**drug-drug interactions**), including herbal drug products (**herbal-drug interactions**), certain type of food (**drug-food interactions**) or due to a patient´s physio-pathological condition (**drug-disease interaction**). (Amariles et al., 2007a) Additionally, changes on the results of certain laboratory tests that may produce some drugs (**drug - laboratory tests interactions**) (Maddox et al., 1980) or on the bioavailability of several nutrients (**drug - nutrient interactions**) (Chan, 2002; Santos & Boullata, 2005) may be considered as a DI. (Amariles, 2002)

Elsewhere, the increasing use of herbal products worldwide and the growth of the herbal product industry have led to rising the identification and characterization of clinically relevant DIs among several drugs with some of these products, for instance St. John's Wort (Hypericum Perforatum L.), which has been the characterization of another type of DI: **herbal–drug drug interactions**. (Markowitz & DeVane, 2001)

Although from a pharmacological perspective, some DIs may lead to a required therapeutic effect, for instance "pharmacokinetic enhancement or ritonavir boosting, strategy in which low doses of ritonavir -100 to 200 mg- (a cytochrome P4503A inhibitor) are used in combination with other protease inhibitors to increase antiretroviral drug exposure (Rathbun & Rossi, 2002), from a risk perspective, the efforts should focus on evaluating, predicting, and solving DIs with high probability to produce effects that are undesirable and to arise **toxicities or therapeutic failures**, which are termed as **clinically relevant drug interactions.** (Amariles, 2002; Amariles et al., 2007a)

Pharmacological mechanism of drug interactions. The **previous or concomitant** use of a drug, herbal drug product, or food (like a patient´s physio-pathological condition) may cause a **non-therapeutic and quantitative modification in the magnitude or duration of the drug effect** because such substance or situation causes an alteration that involve one or more of the three pharmacologic processes namely biopharmaceutics, pharmacokinetics, or pharmacodynamics.

The biopharmaceutics is relating both to factors that influence the drug release from a drug product and the drug dissolution rate in the absorption site. Whereas, **the pharmacokinetics** is relating to drug absorption, distribution, metabolism, and excretion (ADME) (**what the body does to the drug**). As most drugs proceed through first order kinetics, and the process of ADME usually follows first order kinetics as well, the relationship between dose/time and drug plasma concentration for most drugs is linear. Thus, the **biopharmaceutics and pharmacokinetics phases determine the drug plasma concentration**. Similarly, since the relationship between plasma concentration and drug available on the site of action or biophase is linear, and the concentration on biophase is directly related to the intensity and duration of therapeutic response for most drugs as well, the relationship between drug plasma concentration and the magnitude of drug effect for most drugs is linear (figure 1).

Pharmacodynamics phase (what the drug does to the body): the pharmacodynamics studies the **mechanism of action** (specific molecular drug-target interaction, usually as a result of binding to a receptor or an enzyme, through which a drug causes its **pharmacological response or effect** (pharmacological surrogate or clinical effect as result of drug- target interaction).

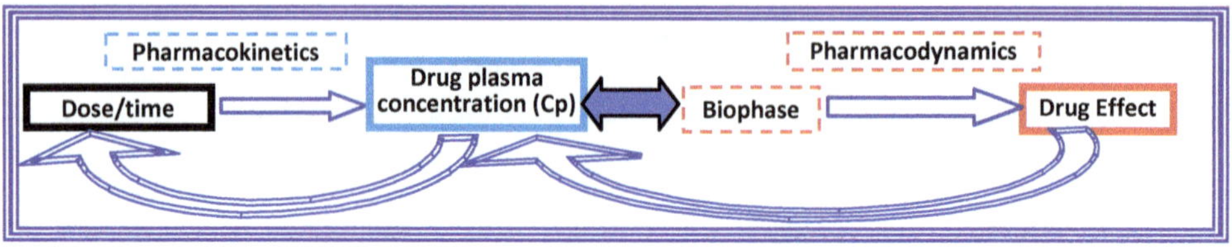

Fig. 1. Pharmacokinetics, plasmatic concentration (Cp), and pharmacologic effect.

Based on the pharmacological mechanism that explains the **non-therapeutic and quantitative modification in the magnitude or duration of the drug effect**, the DI may be classified as:

- Pharmacokinetic DI: The **non-therapeutic and quantitative modification in the magnitude or duration of the drug effect is explained mainly by a change in the drug plasma concentration** associate with substance or situation that causes the DI. The change in the drug plasma concentration may be attributed to a biopharmaceutic (drug release and dissolution) and/or pharmacokinetic (ADME) alteration. Thus, biopharmaceutic DIs are included in pharmacokinetic DIs (**both biopharmaceutic and pharmacokinetic DIs are attributed to a change in the drug plasma concentration**).
- Pharmacodynamic DI: The **non-therapeutic and quantitative modification in the magnitude or duration of the drug effect** occurs without **change in the drug plasma concentration.** This type of DIs are mainly due to drugs or substances that have either similar (synergism) pharmacological effect or opposing (antagonistic) pharmacological effect or physio-pathological condition (drug-disease interactions) that contributes or facilities (synergism) the therapeutic or toxic effect of the drug, or that diminish or counteract its therapeutic effect (antagonism). In general, in one patient, the use of drugs those have a similar unsafe profile increases the likelihood and severity of adverse drug effects, for instance the use of drug-induced hepatic or renal toxicity.

2.2 Proposal to evaluate and predict the clinical relevance of pharmacokinetic drug interactions in HIV-infected patients receiving antiretroviral therapy (Amariles et al., 2007b)

HAART or cART has improved survival of HIV-infected patients, but they currently have chronic co-morbidities which require pharmacologic interventions with several medications, increasing the risk of DIs. In clinical practice, it is known that DIs may lead important pharmacotherapy problems especially for illnesses which require using various medications. Therefore, clinically relevant DIs are frequent among HIV-infected patients who are receiving ARV therapy. (Miller et al., 2007) In this context, ARV drugs may lower the efficacy or enhance side effects or toxicity of several of these drugs, and similarly some of these drugs may cause therapeutic failure or increase the toxicity of ARV drugs. (Fletcher et al., 2000)

DIs are especially important for drugs with narrow therapeutic indices and may either be pharmacodynamic or pharmacokinetic in nature. However, pharmacokinetic DIs may be more frequent complex to evaluate and to predict the effect among HIV-infected patients receiving ARV therapy. For instance, protease inhibitors (PIs), non-nucleoside reverse transcriptase inhibitors (NNRTIs), and the CCR5 antagonist maraviroc are metabolized through the CYP450 system, mostly by CYP3A4. (DHHS, 2011) In addition, each of the NNRTIs and PIs induce and/or inhibit specific CYP450 enzymes and consequently are prone to cause pharmacokinetic DIs, (Pau & Boyd, 2010) mainly when they are concomitant used in patients with HIV and with others important co-morbidities, such as dyslipidaemia, hypertension, tuberculosis, and opiate dependence, in which is needing to use several drugs that may be both substrate and selected inducers or inhibitors of CYP3A4. (Josephson, 2010)

In general, the clinical relevance of a pharmacodynamic DI can often be evaluated, predicted, and monitored easily, because the process is supported by knowledge of the drugs mechanism of action and pharmacological effects (therapeutic and adverse), complemented with the definition and monitoring of parameters related to the drug clinical effects (clinical effects and toxicity profile), if possible in a quantitative way. Whereas, the pharmacokinetic DIs (**alterations in drug plasma concentration associated to changes in the release, dissolution, absorption, distribution, metabolism, or excretion of drug**) are more complex and may not be as easily evaluated, predicted, and monitored as the pharmacodynamic DIs; thus, the process requires both knowledge of pharmacology, pharmacotherapy, and clinical expertise. Thus, it is important to present a development proposal, which have been adjusted with goal to evaluate and predict the clinical relevance of pharmacokinetic DIs in HIV-infected patients receiving ARV therapy. (Amariles et al., 2007b; Giraldo et al., 2010)

2.2.1 Identifying and assessing if one of the medication that the patient is using (or that the patient will be use) is considered as a drug with narrow therapeutic indices

The therapeutic index of a drug is the ratio of the dose that produces toxicity (**drug plasma concentration that elicits the toxic effect in 50 percent of treated individuals -TD_{50}-**), and the dose that produces a clinically desired or effective response in a population of individuals (**drug plasma concentration that elicits the therapeutic effect in 50 percent of the treated individuals -ED_{50}-**) as shown in equation 1 (Katzung, 2009)

Equation 1. Index therapeutic = TD_{50}/ED_{50}

Both TD_{50} and ED_{50} are calculated from dose response curves, which represent the frequency with which each drug plasma concentration elicits the therapeutic effect or the toxic effect in the population (figure 2).

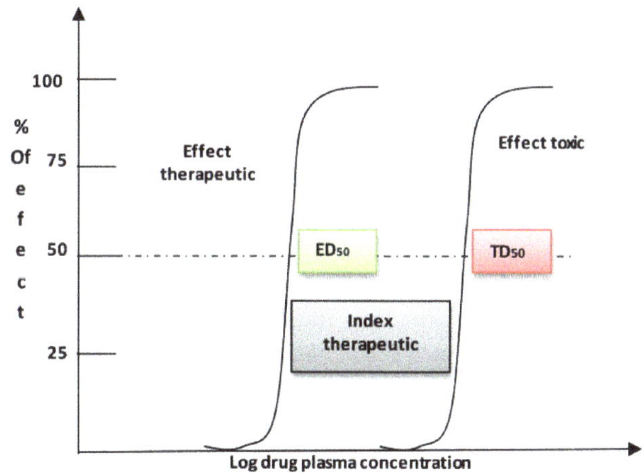

Fig. 2. Dose-responsive curves and Therapeutic Index

From a clinical perspective, drug therapeutic range corresponds at drug plasma concentrations associate to likelihood of achieving, in the most patients, the maximum therapeutic effect with the minimum toxic effect. The probability that a pharmacotherapy process will be effective and safe increases if both the maximum drug plasma concentration and the minimum drug plasma concentration of the steady state **associate to a specific dosing schedule in a patient** are included within the **therapeutic range (population)** or **therapeutic index (individual)** of the drug (**minimum effective level and minimum toxic level, which are theoretical**). If the concentrations achieved at steady state are outside of the therapeutic range or index (excluded), it is increases the probability of drug failure or ineffective (if the concentration is lesser than the minimum effective level) or of adverse or toxic effects (if the concentration is higher than the minimum toxic level). Therefore, drug therapy should obtain that the **achieved drug plasma concentrations** at steady state are included within the therapeutic range or index (**theoretical**) is a specific patient, as shown in figure 3.

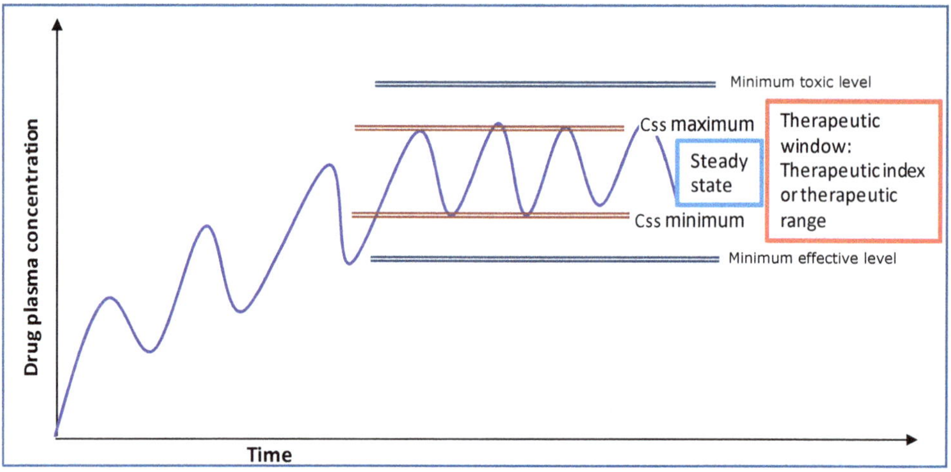

Fig. 3. Relationship between drug plasma concentrations achieved in steady state and the theoretical therapeutic window (therapeutic index or therapeutic margin)

The probability that a pharmacokinetic DI causes that the drug **achieved drug plasma concentrations** at steady state are outside of the therapeutic range or index is inversely proportional to the difference between **minimum effective level and minimum toxic level** that are defined in the therapeutic index or range of the drug. The probability is higher (increased) for drugs with small difference between the minimum effective concentrations and the minimum toxic concentrations (drugs with a narrow therapeutic range or index).

It could be practice to consider a narrow therapeutic range or index drug if the drug: (FDA, 2005) (1) Require pharmacokinetics (therapeutic drug concentration) or pharmacodynamic (measuring clinical effects) monitoring, thus the effective and safe use of the drug require careful dosage titration and patient monitoring; (2) have less than a 2-fold difference in median lethal dose (LD_{50}) and median effective dose (ED_{50}) values; or (3) have less than a 2-fold difference in the minimum toxic plasma concentrations and the minimum effective plasma concentrations

From a clinical practical perspective, there are lists of narrow therapeutic index drugs, including their minimum effective concentrations and the minimum toxic concentrations, which include drug as digoxin, lithium, vancomycin, aminoglycosides, and anticonvulsants. Although it is knowing that some drugs has narrow therapeutic index, for instance oral anticoagulants and insulin, they may not be included in this kind of lists, mainly due to: (1) Absence of population data of minimum toxic concentrations and minimum effective concentrations; (2) presence of a large interindividual pharmacodynamic variability (in some patient a similar drug plasma concentration may cause different magnitude or duration of the clinical effects); and (3) there are not a reasonable relationship between drug plasma concentrations and clinical effects. For that reason, although data for dose-response curves is obtained from several individuals, the therapeutic index is assumed more as an individual perspective whereas therapeutic range is assumed more as a population perspective.

In drug therapy process using drugs with a narrow therapeutic range or index, pharmacokinetic DIs may cause an **increase in blood/serum concentrations and thus could lead to drug toxic effects**, or may cause a **decrease in blood/serum concentrations and thus could lead to drug failure or ineffectiveness**. Therefore, in the process of evaluate and predict the clinical relevance of a DI, **the first stage is to establish whether any drugs that patient is using (or that will use) is considered as a narrow therapeutic range or index drug**. In general, if the drugs used have a broad therapeutic index or margin, the probability of a pharmacokinetic DI makes that the drug be unsafe or ineffective is low, because the probability of a change leads to achieved drug plasma concentrations are excluded at the therapeutic range or index (below of the minimum effective concentrations or above of the minimum toxic concentrations) is minimum. In general, if **pharmacokinetic DIs (as well as pharmacodynamic DIs) involves drug products that are not considered as narrow therapeutic range or index drugs they will be clinical irrelevant**; therefore in these cases the evaluating and predicting of DI may not be needed.

ARV drugs as Narrow Therapeutic or Range Index Drugs. Due to their pharmacological and clinical features, ARV drugs may be considered as narrow therapeutic or range index drugs. (FDA, 2005) For instance, although there are some controversies due to broad intra- and inter-individual pharmacokinetic variability of ARV drugs, (Nettles et al., 2006) PIs and NNRTIs have defined drug plasma concentrations related to maximum efficacy and safety (therapeutic range) and, therefore ARV drugs are susceptible to therapeutic drug monitoring (assessing and monitoring drug concentration) (Justesen, 2006; Wertheimer et al., 2006), as shown in table 1. As consequence, it is possible to establish, that **patients that are receiving PI/NNRT have a high susceptibility to present clinically relevant DIs**. Additionally, some medications used in HIV-infected patients for treatment or prevention of some chronic co-morbidities and opportunistic infections may be considered as narrow therapeutic range or index drugs, for instance rifampin, rifabutin and other antibiotics, anticonvulsants, statins, antidepressants, antihypertensives, and opioids (DHHS, 2011).

2.2.2 Identifying and predicting consequences of drug interaction on the pharmacokinetics, plasma concentrations, and affected drug clinical effects (step more complex)

The consequences of a pharmacokinetic DI on the main pharmacokinetic process, on the drug plasma concentrations, and thus on the affected drug clinical effects, depends among other aspects, of: (1) the magnitude that the respective pharmacokinetic process affects

Drug	Therapeutic range or index (ng/mL)
Saquinavir	250 – 600
Ritonavir (solo)	150 - 2.100
Indinavir	100 - 1.000
Nelfinavir	800 - 3.000
Amprenavir	400 - 2.200
Lopinavir/ritonavir	1.000 - 9.000
Atazanavir	150 - 1.000
Tipranavir	6.500 - 50.000
Nevirapine Cmin	3.500
Efavirenz	1.000 - 4.000
Delavirdine	Limited information

[a]Assessment as its active metabolite (m8). Cmin: minimum concentration

Table 1. Drug plasma concentrations related to effective minimum level and toxic minimum level that defined the therapeutic index or range of ARV drugs. (Justesen, 2006; Nettles et al., 2006; Wertheimer et al., 2006)

achieved drug plasma concentrations with the dosing-schedule used in the patient; and (2) the magnitude of change that the DI causes on altered pharmacokinetic process. These two aspects determine the influence of a DI both on the magnitude of change on drug plasma concentrations and on the probability of achieved drug plasma concentrations at steady state are excluded from the therapeutic range or index. Relate to this issue, the average steady-state concentration (Cpss) is an excellent estimator of achieved drug plasma concentrations, which is determined by the ratio between the drug delivery rate (input rate, which depends directly on the dose –D-, and the bioavailability –F-, and inversely on the dosing interval -τ-), and the clearance rate –CL- (output rate), as shown in equation 2.

Equation 2. $$Cpss = \frac{D \times F}{\tau \times CL}$$

Bioavailability (F). Although, bioavailability of drug is classically defined as the rate and extent to which the active ingredient (drug substance) is absorbed from the dosage form (upon oral administration), from a clinical perspective, this pharmacokinetic parameter may be assumed as the **amount of active ingredient** (drug substance) from the dosage form (drug product, upon oral administration) **that reaches the systemic circulation unchanged.** Therefore, the bioavailability of drug is influenced by: (1) the disintegration of the dosage form, the release of drug from a drug product, and the dissolution of drug in the absorption site; (2) the presystemic metabolism both in the gut lumen (extra-hepatic) and in the liver by CYP450, especially CYP3A4; and (3) the contribution of intestinal transporters, which may decrease the bioavailability, by efflux effect of intestinal P-glycoprotein (P-gp) in drug absorbed from apical to basolateral), or may increase the bioavailability, by effect of the anionic organic polypeptide (TAOP), especially the type B. (Ho & Kim, 2005)

Systemic or total clearance (CL) is defined as the volume of plasma in the vascular compartment cleared of drug per unit of time [volume/time], mainly by hepatic metabolism (hepatic clearance) or by renal excretion (renal clearance) but also by other ways, such as biliary excretion. CL is a measure of the efficiency of human organism to remove irreversibly a drug from the systemic circulation or bloodstream by all routes of elimination, mainly by biotransformation (or drug metabolism) and excretion.

Drugs are metabolized (changed) usually by enzymes found mainly in the liver but also in small intestine, lung, kidney, and skin to a metabolites by process known as drug metabolism or biotransformation. Biotransformation often changes no-polar or lipophilic drugs into metabolites more polar or hydrophilic, which tend to be excreted in the urine (renal excretion) or in the stool (biliary excretion) as glucuronate, sulphate or acetate conjugates. While, polar or hydrophilic drugs may be excreted without drug metabolism through renal excretion.

A renal pharmacokinetic DI may be clinically relevant if: (1) there is a competitive inhibition of tubular secretion of the drug and (2) the **renal clearance contributes more than 30% and drug systemic clearance**. (Bonate et al., 1998; Launay et al., 2006) Additionally, certain drugs, for instance ritonavir may inhibit the renal secretion of certain drugs, which may be critical for drugs that are mainly eliminated by this via. For example, when digoxin is used concomitant with ritonavir, the PI may lead to an increase in the levels and pharmacological effects of digoxin. (Ding et al., 2004)

Concepts provide above, particularly the equation 2, lead to understand why clinically relevant pharmacokinetic DIs are mainly explained by changes in **systemic clearance and bioavailability.** Thus, almost 80% of pharmacokinetic DIs are related to changes in systemic clearance, mainly associated to the systemic inhibition or induction of the metabolic activity of the CYP450 isoenzymes, and approximately 15% related to changes in bioavailability (changes in gastrointestinal pH, presystemic clearance [by hepatic or intestinal CYP3A4 isoenzyme]) or by in P-gp activity). (Amariles et al., 2007b; Giraldo et al., 2010)

The process of evaluating and predicting of the clinical relevance of a pharmacokinetic DI continues with the **identification if the main route of drug elimination is hepatic o renal, and thus if the drug is** remove irreversibly from the systemic circulation or bloodstream by excretion renal or by hepatic metabolism. **Generally, if the drug is eliminating by hepatic metabolism, the probability that a pharmacokinetic DI will be clinical relevant is elevated.** In these cases, subsequent to identify whether the systemic elimination of any drugs that patient is using (or drugs that patient will use) occurs primarily by hepatic metabolism, **the process must continue with the evaluation of the effect that may cause one possible hepatic metabolism inhibition or induction on drug plasma concentrations.**

Because a near to 80% of clinically relevant pharmacokinetic DIs are related to hepatic metabolism, both systemic and presystemic, during the process of developing new drugs it is important to characterize and to predict DIs related to hepatic metabolism. With this goal, both cell cultures are used to establishing the ability of the new drug to modify the activity of major CYP450 isoenzymes, and the assessment of the susceptibility of the drug metabolism to be affected by drugs recognized as enzyme inhibitors and inducers. (Tucker, 2001; Obach et al., 2005, 2006)

The major route of elimination of PIs and NNRTIs is by hepatic metabolism and thus the pharmacokinetic DIs may be clinical relevant. Not at all, for nucleoside or nucleotide analogue reverse transcriptase inhibitors (NRTIs), due to they are eliminated primarily by renal excretion, clinically relevant pharmacokinetic DIs are less frequent. However, among NRTIs, abacavir is metabolized by alcohol dehydrogenase and zidovudine by gucoronil-transferase, which may cause that these two drugs to have interactions associated to changes in the activity of the respective enzymes. Additionally, there is evidence that tenofovir may modify the atazanavir metabolism and thus drug plasma concentrations and clinical effects of this PI; similarly, atazanavir and lopinavir/ritonavir may alter the drug plasma concentrations and clinical effects of tenofovir (see below). In addition, the systemic elimination of some drugs, considered as narrow therapeutic index or margin drugs, and commonly used in patients with HIV/AIDS (such as rifamycins, anticonvulsants, statins, and antidepressants) occurs by hepatic metabolism and, therefore, clinically relevant pharmacokinetic DIs are likely to arise.

2.2.2.1 Evaluation of the effect that may cause one possible hepatic metabolism inhibition or induction on the plasma concentrations of the potentially affected drug

The process of evaluation of a DI associated to hepatic metabolism needs: (1) identify the CYP450 enzyme which is responsible for the biotransformation of the drug whose metabolism can be altered, and (2) identifying agents that alter (induce or inhibit) the metabolic capacity of the CYP450 enzyme. The proper observance of this stage implies following three steps.

a. Identification of the CYP450 enzyme which is responsible for the biotransformation of the drug that may be altered. A detailed and updated list of major CYP450 isoenzymes, together with their most common substrates, inhibitors, and inducers can be found on the following web sites:

- http://medicine.iupui.edu/clinpharm/DDIs/ and
- http://medicine.iupui.edu/clinpharm/DDIs/ClinicalTable.asp

In the case of PIs and NNRTIs, their systemic metabolism occurs primarily by CYP3A4. Additionally, there are other drugs commonly administered to HIV/AIDS patients which are metabolized by CYP3 or CYP2 families.

b. Identifying drugs that may modify (inducing or inhibiting) the metabolic capacity of CYP2 and CYP3 families. For instance, rifampin, rifabutin, carbamazepine, phenobarbital, phenytoin, and Saint-John's-wort may induce the activity of CYP2 and CYP3 families, whereas azole antifungals, macrolides, calcium antagonists, immunosuppressants, and grapefruit juice may inhibit CYP3 family. Most the drugs ARV used in the treatment of HIV are metabolized by the CYP450 enzymes and they have the capacity to modify the activity of CYP3 family and, to a lesser extent, the activity of CYP2 family. Among the NNRTIs, efavirenz and nevirapine mainly induce CYP3A4 and CYP2B6, while delavirdine is primarily an enzymatic inhibitor of the CYP3A4, and etravirine inhibits CYP2C9 and CYP2C19 while inducing CYP3A4. However, efavirenz may inhibit the activity of CYP3A4, CYP2C9, and CYP2C19 isoenzymes. In vitro studies show most of the PIs are inhibitors of activity of CYP3A4 isoenzyme (atazanavir, darunavir/ritonavir, lopinavir/ritonavir, saquinavir, tipranavir/ritonavir) or strong CYP3A4 inhibitors (ritonavir, indinavir, nelfinavir). Some PIs both inhibit and induce CYP3A4 (amprenavir, fosamprenavir). Ritonavir also inhibits CYP2D6. **The NRTIs, the fusion inhibitor enfuvirtide, and the integrase inhibitor raltegravir are not metabolized by the CYP450 system.**

In clinical practice, inhibition of hepatic CYP enzymes or metabolic inhibition is one of the most common DI mechanisms and it is usually reversible and competitive. Most pharmacokinetic DIs occur when a drug increases or decreases metabolism of other drugs in the liver (CYP enzymes or glucuronidation). When a drug or substance causes a decrease in the systemic hepatic metabolism and clearance of a drug, this substance generates an increase in plasma concentrations and may lead to emerge of adverse drug events or toxicities. Thus, the process of evaluating and predicting the effects of this kind of DI needs to identify the drugs that are strong or moderate inhibitors of activity of different CYP450 isozymes known also as "enzyme inhibitors for excellence".

c. Determining if the pharmacokinetic DI related to hepatic metabolism might be either one-way or two-way direction (bidirectional) and if it might affect the levels and effects of the two drugs involved; situation that is likely to occur, because the need to use simultaneously either inhibitor drugs (e.g., macrolides and antifungal azoles) or inducer drugs (for instance rifampicin and carbamazepine) together with PIs and/or NNRTIs is common.

2.2.2.2 Evaluation of changes in the bioavailability of drugs orally administered

Changes in presystemic metabolism (due to inhibition or induction of extra-hepatic or hepatic CYP3A subfamily), in the activity of P-gp, or in the gastrointestinal pH may affect both the amount absorbed and the effects of some ARV drugs. In turn, antiretroviral drugs, particularly PIs, may modify the bioavailability and effects of some drugs, mainly through inhibition of presystemic metabolism and, to a lesser extent, of the activity of P-gp. Didanosine, especially in its dosage form as buffer solution, can change gastrointestinal pH and the amount absorbed by some drugs.

For drugs with kinetics elimination of first order or linear (most drugs used at therapeutic doses, phenytoin is one important exception), as it may be deduced from the equation 2, the increase or decreases of average steady-state concentration (Cpss) is inversely related to the decrease or increase of CL (Cpss≅1/CL). Generally, for narrow range or index drugs, a pharmacokinetic DI may be clinically relevant, if the DI causes a change in the achieved Cpss of +/-20% (FDA, 1999). As Cpss ≅ 1/CL, a decrease (associate to a reduction of hepatic metabolism) in the CL of 10%, 15%, 20%, 30%, 50%, and 75% may produce an increase in the Cpss of 11%, 18%, 25%, 43%, 100%, and 400%, respectively. The expected increasing of Cpss is calculated from the ratio of 100 divided by 100 less the percentage that CL is decreasing [100/ (100 less % of decrease of CL)]. Thus, if CL decreases in 10%, the increase of 11% is obtained from the ratio of 100 divided by 100 less 10 (100/90), which result is 111% and it is showing that Cpss increases in 11%. Similarly, 43% is obtained from the ratio of 100 divided by 100 less 30 (100/70) which result is 143% and it is showing that Cpss increases in 43%; and so similarly for other values. (Amariles, 2002) In the situations of increases of hepatic metabolism (induction enzymatic), it is requiring a minimal increase of 25% in CL, which may be caused a decrease of 20% in the achieved Cpss.

The drug plasma concentration before of the pharmacokinetic DI is another factor that contributes significantly to the magnitude of change in the clinical effect. For example, if diltiazem may decreased CL of quinidine (therapeutic range: 1-4 μg/mL) in 35% (Laganiere et al., 1996), thus it may cause an increase of 54% in the achieved Cpss of quinidine. Thus, if the quinidine Cpss on time interaction was of 2.5 μg/mL, it would increase to 3.85 μg/mL, whereas if the quinidine Cpss was of 3.5 μg mL, it would increase to 5.39 μg/mL. As consequence, the probability of toxicity at 5.39 μg/mL (outside the therapeutic range) is higher than at 3.85 μg/mL (within the therapeutic range). (Amariles, 2002)

2.3 Determining and predicting of the clinical relevance level (Amariles et al., 2007a)

A relevance analysis of a DI should result in determining and predicting the clinical relevance level based on the gravity and probability of occurrence of the DI. The **probability of the DI is set to 3 categories: defined, probable, and possible**, whereas the **gravity of the DI is grouped into 3 categories: grave, moderate, and mild**. Based on the possible combinations of gravity and probability of occurrence, interactions can be grouped into 4 categories:

- **Level 1 (Very high risk)** resulting from the combination of: defined and grave or probable and grave. The simultaneous use of drugs is considered absolutely contraindicated.
- **Level 2 (High Risk)** resulting from the combinations of: possible and severe, defined and moderate, or probable and moderate. The simultaneous use of drugs is considered contraindicated: combined administration should be avoided or, if it is need, the dosage regimen of affected drug may be adjusted and to assess signs and symptoms associated to treatment effectiveness and safety, ideally in a quantitative form.
- **Level 3 (Medium risk)** resulting from the combination of: possible and moderate, defined and mild, or probable and mild. The simultaneous use of drugs requires assessing signs and symptoms associated to treatment effectiveness and safety, ideally in a quantitative form.
- **Level 4 (Low risk)** resulting from the combination can be mild. The interaction is of little clinical relevance.

From a clinical perspective, predicting of the clinical relevance of a DI should be improvement by clinical experience and knowledge obtained from situations similar; thus, the clinical interpretation of the information, including drug history and the patient's clinical condition is critical. Therefore, the presence of concomitant diseases and the need to use other drugs, the condition of renal and hepatic function, as the age and nutritional condition are factors that influence the clinical relevance of a determine DI.

3. Clinical relevance of pharmacokinetic drug interactions in HIV-infected patients receiving antiretroviral therapy

In this apart, using the previously described proposal, the evaluating and predicting the clinical relevance of pharmacokinetic DIs in HIV-infected patients receiving antiretroviral therapy is presented. (Amariles et al., 2007b; Giraldo et al., 2010)

3.1 Drug interactions due to enzyme inhibition mediated by PIs or NNRTIs

The process of evaluating and predicting the effects of this kind of DI needs to identify the drugs that are strong or moderate inhibitors of activity of different CYP450 isozymes known also as "enzyme inhibitors for excellence".

In general, PIs (ritonavir > indinavir ≈ nelfinavir ≈ lopinavir ≈ atazanavir ≈ amprenavir - fosamprenavir- ≈ darunavir ≈ tipranavir > saquinavir) (Boffito et al., 2006), delavirdine (Tran et al., 2001) and, in some cases, efavirenz, (DeSilva et al., 2001) can inhibit the systemic metabolism

Drug group or drugs affected	Clinical relevance: level	Comments and suggestions
Antiarrhythmic drugs [a] • Flecainide • Disopyramide • Amiodarone	2: high risk	Increased likelihood of security problems, especially gastrointestinal, muscular and cardiac conduction problems. Recommendation: dose adjustment and monitoring plasma levels
Antihistamines anti-H1 [a] • Terfenadine	2: high risk	More likelihood of increasing QTc interval on the electrocardiogram and occurrence of cardiac arrhythmias, as well as dizziness Recommendation: avoid co-administration
• Astemizole	1: very high risk	
Ergot alkaloids [a] • Ergotamine • Dihydroergotamine • Ergonovine • Methylergonovine	2: high risk	Increased likelihood of ergotism: hypertension, nervousness, hallucinations, seizures, gastrointestinal, and muscle disorders. Recommendation: dose adjustment and monitoring
Benzodiazepines [a] • Midazolam • Triazolam • Alprazolam	2: high risk	Increased likelihood of respiratory depression, sedation and muscle weakness. Oxazepam, lorazepam or temazepam are an alternative, because they are eliminated by conjugation with glucuronic acid and are hardly affected by the simultaneous use of PIs. Recommendation: dose adjustment and monitoring
Statins [a] (Aberg et al., 2006; Bays, 2006; Benesic et al., 2004; Cooper et al., 2003; Fichtenbaum et al., 2002; Fichtenbaum & Gerber, 2002; Hare et al., 2002; Jacobson, 2004; Sax, 2006; Sudano et al., 2006). • Lovastatin • Simvastatin • Atorvastatin	2: high risk	Increased risk of myopathy, rhabdomyolysis, and even death. Avoid the use of lovastatin or simvastatin in patients using ritonavir, atazanavir and saquinavir. Recommendation: to use the lowest possible dose (for atorvastatin) and to monitor signs and symptoms of muscle toxicity, or use statins involving lower risk for this type of interaction, such as pravastatin, fluvastatin, or rosuvastatin
• Rosuvastatin • Fluvastatin • Pravastatin	3: medium risk	
Calcium antagonists no-dihydro-pyridines [a] • Verapamil • Diltiazem	2: high risk	Increased risk of hypotension and reduced cardiac conduction. It is recommended to reduce the dose of these two drugs by half
Phosphodiesterase type V [a] • Sildenafil • Tadalafil • Vardenafil	2: high risk	Increased risk of hypotension, priapism, headache, and visual disturbances. Doses should be adjusted: sildenafil to 25 mg/48 hours, tadalafil to 10 mg/72 hours, and vardenafil to 2.5 mg/72 hours
Cisapride [a]	2: high risk	Increased likelihood of increasing the QTc interval on the electrocardiogram and cardiac

		arrhythmias, as well as gastrointestinal disturbances and dizziness. Recommendation: Dose adjustment and monitoring
Pimozide [a]	2: high risk	Increased likelihood of involuntary movements (tics), agitation, confusion, behavioral disturbances, and tachycardia. Recommendation: Dose adjustment and monitoring
Warfarina (acenocumarol)	2: high risk	The risk of bleeding may increase, when this combination is used. Recommendation: dose adjustment and monitoring international normalized ratio (INR)
Fluticasone [a] (Arrington-Sanders et al., 2006)	2: high risk	PIs, especially ritonavir alone or with other PIs, tipranavir, and indinavir may increase fluticasone levels, and even lead to the development of Cushing syndrome, especially with the use of ritonavir in children. Recommendation: Dose adjustment and monitoring
Opioid analgesics (Armstrong & Cozza, 2003a, *2003b)* Oxycodone • Oxycodone • Buprenorphine	2: high risk	Protease inhibitors may inhibit CYP2D6 and CYP3A4 and thus the metabolism of oxycodone and buprenorphine, increasing their plasma concentrations as well as the likelihood of toxic effects (sedation and respiratory depression)
• Dihydrocodeine • Hydrocodone	2: high risk	Dihydrocodeine, hydrocodone, and codeine are pro-drugs and require activation by CYP2D6 or glucuronyltransferase. Therefore, protease inhibitors can inhibit the metabolism and the formation of the active compound and, therefore, the pharmacological effect of these drugs. However, codeine is considered a suitable option for pain control in HIV-infected patients receiving antiretroviral therapy
• Codeine	3: medium risk	
Tricyclic and tetracyclic antidepressants (Cvetkovic et al., 2003; de Maat et al., 2003; Oldfield & Plosker, 2006; Von et al., 1998) • Amitriptyline • Desipramine • Nortriptyline • Mirtazapine • Trazodone • Nefazodone	2: high risk	Ritonavir alone or with another PI can inhibit CYP2D6, and thus, the metabolism of these drugs, which can generate toxicity problems, particularly decreased conduction and cardiac arrest, as well as increased anticholinergic effects (constipation, dry mouth, urinary retention) and cardiac abnormalities. It is recommended to reduce the dose by half (or use the lowest dose possible) of these two drugs, with adjustments based on their effectiveness and safety
Antidepressants reuptake inhibitors (SSRI) (Aberg,	2: high risk	Ritonavir alone or with another PI can inhibit CYP2D6, and thus, the metabolism of these

2008; Acosta, 2002; Caballero & Nahata 2005; Currier et al., 2004; de Maat et al., 2003; Isbister & Buckley, 2005; Tseng & Foisy, 1999) • Fluoxetine • Fluvoxamine • Venlafaxine • Paroxetine • Sertraline		drugs, which can lead to increased levels and toxicity of SSRIs (serotonin syndrome). It is recommended using half or the lowest dose possible of either drug, setting the dose in terms of their effectiveness and safety. Citalopram and possibly escitalopram and sertraline, due to their low metabolism and effect on CYP activity, are considered the most suitable option in HIV-infected patients receiving antiretroviral therapy
Integrase inhibitors *Maraviroc* (Aberg, 2008)	2: high risk	PIs increase plasma levels of maraviroc. Recommendation: reduce the dose of maraviroc up to 50% and monitoring

With specific PIs

Drug group or drugs affected	PIs	Clinical relevance: level	Comments and suggestions
Simvastatin (Schmidt et al., 2007)	*Atazanavir*	2: high risk	Inhibition of CYP3A4 by ATV, the increase in the levels and toxicity simvastatin increases the risk of rhabdomyolysis and acute renal failure. Recommendation: dose adjustment and monitoring
• Efavirenz • Paclitaxel • Losartan • Diclofenac • Phenytoin • Amitriptyline • Omeprazole • Fluoxetine • Warfarin • Iibuprofen • Glibenclamide (Dixit et al, 2007)	*Ritonavir, nelfinavir*	3: medium risk	Increased metabolism of drugs metabolized by CYP2B6, CYP2C8, CYP2C9, CYP2C19. Recommendation: monitoring
Tenofovir (Tong et al., 2007)	*ATV, PV, DRV, SQV, FPV*	2: high risk	The coadministration of TDF with ATV, LPV, DRV and SQV increased Cp of tenofovir, while decreases Cp of FPV. Recommendation: dose adjustment and monitoring
Warfarin (Hughes et al., 2007)	*LPV/r*	3: medium risk	LPV/r may increase the metabolism of S enantiomer of warfarin by stimulation of CYP2C9, as well as the R enantiomer by stimulation of

			CYP1A2. Recommendation: INR monitoring
Minociline (DiCenzo et al., 2008)	*ATV*	3: medium risk	Decreased levels and effect of ATV, possibly due to enterohepatic cycle interference associated to alterations of the intestinal bacterial flora. Recommendation: monitoring
Etravirine (Aberg, 2008)	*ATV/r*	1: very high risk	ATV Cp is decreased by 38%. Avoid co-administration.
	Tipranavir	1: very high risk	Etravirine Cp was reduced by 75%. Avoid co-administration
	FPV/r	1: very high risk	FPV Cp is decreased by 77%. Avoid co-administration
	LPV/r	2: high risk	Etravirine Cp may be increased by 85%. Recommendation: dose adjustment and monitoring
	DRV/r	3: medium risk	Etravirine Cp may be decreased by 50%. Recommendation: monitoring
	NFV	2: high risk	Concomitant use increase plasma concentrations of nelfinavir, due to the inhibitory effect of etravirine on CYP3A4. Recommendation: dose adjustment and monitoring (Schöller et al., 2006a; Sekar et al., 2006a)
Raltegravir (Aberg, 2008)	*Tipranavir*	2: high risk	Plasma concentrations of raltegravir are reduced when it is used with tipranavir. Recommendation: dose adjustment and monitoring
	ATV	2: high risk	Plasma concentrations of raltegravir are increased when it is used with ATV. Recommendation: dose adjustment and monitoring
Darunavir	*SQV*(Sekar et al., 2006a)	2: high risk	Plasma concentrations and effects of these PIs may be increased, due to the inhibitory effect of darunavir. Recommendation: dose adjustment and monitoring
	LPV (Sekar et al., 2006b)	2: high risk	
	IDV	3: medium risk	
	NVP	3: medium risk	
• Pravastatin • Sildenafil • Vardenafil • Tadalafil	*DRV* (Sekar et al., 2008)	2: high risk	Plasma concentrations and effects of these medications may be increased, due to the inhibitory effect of darunavir. Recommendation: dose adjustment and/or monitoring
• Budesonide • Quinine	*RTV and LPV/r* (Daveluy et al,	2: high risk	Plasma concentrations and effects of these medications may be increased,

• Docetaxel • Fluticasone • Oxycodone • Alprazolam • Sirolimus • Quetiapine	2009; Gray et al., 2010; Gruber & McCance-Katz, 2010)		due to the inhibitory effect of ritonavir. Recommendation: dose adjustment and monitoring
Cannabinoids (Abrams et al., 2003)	*IDV* *NFV* *RTV*	2: high risk	Plasma concentrations and effects of cannabinoids and marihuana derivates may be increased, due to the inhibitory effect of PIs. Recommendation: dose adjustment and monitoring, or avoid use of cannabinoids
Methadone	*LPV/r* (McCance-Katz et al., 2003)	2: high risk	Plasma concentrations and effects of methadone may be increased, due to inhibitory effect of PIs on CYP3A4. Recommendation: dose adjustment of methadone and/or monitoring adverse effects of methadone
	NFV (McCance-Katz et al., 2004)	2: high risk	
	ATV (Friedland et al, 2005)	3: medium risk	
	FPV (Cao et al., 2008)	3: medium risk	
	IDV	3: medium risk	
Quetiapine (Hantson et al., 2010)	*ATV*	2: high risk	Plasma concentrations and effects of quetiapine are increased, due to inhibitory effect of atazanavir. Recommendation: dose adjustment of quetiapine and monitoring
Antineoplasics (Levêque et al., 2009; Makinson et al., 2010) • Irinotecan • Vinblastine • Vincristine	*LPV/r*	3: medium risk	Plasma concentrations and effects of these antineoplastics may be increased, due to inhibitory effect of LPV/r on CYP3A5. Recommendation: monitoring

[a] Protease inhibitors (ritonavir → indinavir ≈ nelfinavir ≈ atazanavir≈ amprenavir- fosamprenavir- ≈ tipranavir → saquinavir), mainly through inhibition of CYP3A4, may decrease the metabolism of these drugs, which can cause increased plasma concentrations and toxicity.

Table 2. General interactions due to enzyme inhibition by protease inhibitors (Boffito et al., 2006; Busti et al., 2004; DeSilva et al., 2001; DHHS, 2011; Krikorian & Rudorf, 2005; Piscitelli & Gallicano, 2001; Kashuba, 2005a; Robertson et al., 2005a; Tran et al., 2001; Winston & Boffito, 2005; Wire et al., 2006)

of several drugs, increase their plasma levels, and may cause adverse drug reactions, which could cause grave health problems in patients. Thus, according to their clinical relevance, most could be classified in level 1 or 2. Table 2 lists the interactions mediated by enzyme inhibition caused by PIs. Table 3 contains the interactions mediated by delavirdine and efavirenz.

Drug group or drugs affected	Clinical relevance: level		Comments and suggestions
	Delavirdine	Efavirenz	
Anti-H1 antihistamines [a] • Terfenadine	2: high risk	2: high risk	More likely to increase QTc interval on the electrocardiogram and cardiac arrhythmias, as well as dizziness. Recommendation: avoid co-administration
• Astemizole	1: very high risk	1: very high risk	
Ergot alkaloids [a] • Ergotamine • Dihydroergotamine • Ergonovine • Methylergonovine	2: high risk	2: high risk	Increased likelihood of ergotism: hypertension, nervousness, hallucinations, seizures, gastrointestinal and muscle disorders. Recommendation: dose adjustment and monitoring
Benzodiazepines [a] • Midazolam • Triazolam • Alprazolam	2: high risk	2: high risk	Increased likelihood of respiratory depression, sedation and muscle weakness. Oxazepam, lorazepam or temazepam are an alternative, because they are eliminated by conjugation with glucuronic acid and are hardly affected by the simultaneous use of PI
Statins (Bays, 2006; Cooper et al., 2003; Fichtenbaum & Gerber, 2002; Jacobson, 2004; Sax, 2006; Sudano et al., 2006.) • Lovastatin • Simvastatin • Atorvastatin	2: high risk	Efavirenz acts as an inducer of statins metabolism (see interactions induction)	Increased risk of myopathy, rhabdomyolysis, and even death. It should be avoided in patients using delavirdine (see text: 3.1.1 statins with PIs or delavirdine)
• Rosuvastatin • Fluvastatin • Pravastatin	3: medium risk		
Calcium antagonists not dihydro-pyridine [a] • Verapamil	2: high risk	Information not available	Especially with delavirdine, it increases the risk of hypotension and reduced cardiac conduction. Consider to use the half dosing schedule of these two drugs
• Diltiazem	3: medium risk		
Phosphodiesterase Type V inhibitors [a] • Sildenafil • Tadalafil • Vardenafil	2: high risk	2: high risk	It increases the risk of hypotension, priapism, headache, and visual disturbances. Doses should be adjusted: sildenafil to 25 mg/48 hours, tadalafil to 10 mg/72 hours, and vardenafil to 2.5 mg/72 hours

Opioid analgesics (Armstrong & Cozza, 2003a, 2003b) • Oxycodone • Buprenorphine	2: high risk	No information available on clinically relevant interactions	Inhibition of CYP3A4 and metabolism of oxycodone and buprenorphine, increasing plasma concentrations and the likelihood of toxic effects (sedation and respiratory depression)
• Dihydrocodeine • Hydrocodone • Codeine	3: medium risk		Dihydrocodeine, hydrocodone, and codeine are pro-drugs and require activation by CYP2D6 or glucuronyl-transferase. Therefore, delavirdine may inhibit the metabolism and the formation of the active compound and, consequently, the pharmacological effect of these drugs
Antidepressants reuptake inhibitors (SSRI) (Caballero & Nahata, 2005; Currier et al., 2004; DeSilva et al., 2001; Isbister & Buckley, 2005; Tseng & Foisy, 1999) • Fluoxetine • Fluvoxamine • Venlafaxine • Paroxetine • Sertraline	No information available on clinically relevant interactions with delavirdine	2: high risk	Efavirenz, in cases of deficiency of CYP2D6, may inhibit CYP2C9 and CYP2C19, which can lead to increased levels and toxicity of SSRIs (serotonin syndrome). We recommend using half or the lowest dose possible of these two drugs, adjusting the dose in terms of their effectiveness and safety
Warfarin[a] *(acenocumarol)*	2: high risk	Efavirenz induces warfarin metabolism	With delavirdine it increases the risk of bleeding. It is recommended dose adjustment and monitoring of INR
Cisapride [a]	2: high risk	2: high risk	More likelihood of increasing QTc interval on the electrocardiogram and cardiac arrhythmias, as well as gastrointestinal disturbances and dizziness
Raltegravir (Aberg, 2008)	No information available	2: high risk	The Cp of raltegravir is reduced when is co-administered with efavirenz

[a] Delavirdine, primarily through inhibition of CYP3A4, and efavirenz through inhibition of CYP3A4 and CYP2D6, may decrease the metabolism of these drugs, which can cause increased plasma concentrations and toxicity.

Table 3. General interactions due to enzyme inhibition by inhibitors of non-nucleoside transcriptase (DeMaat et al., 2003; DHHS, 2011; Krikorian & Rudorf, 2005; Piscitelli & Gallicano, 2001; Tran et al., 2001)

From a practical perspective and specifying the type of PI, it is generally recommended to avoid the following combinations (level 1 or level 2: very high risk or high risk): (DHHS, 2011)

- Indinavir with: atazanavir, simvastatin or lovastatin, amiodarone, cisapride, pimozide, astemizole or terfenadine, midazolam or triazolam, ergotamine, ergonovine, or methyl ergonovine.
- Ritonavir (alone or with another PI) with: voriconazole (with a ritonavir dose higher than 400 mg/12 hours), fluticasone, simvastatin or lovastatin, amiodarone, flecainide, propafenone, or quinidine, cisapride, pimozide or clozapine, trazodone or nefazodone , astemizole or terfenadine, midazolam or triazolam, ergotamine, ergonovine or methylergonovine.
- Saquinavir with: simvastatin or lovastatin, cisapride, pimozide, astemizole or terfenadine, midazolam or triazolam, ergotamine, ergonovine, or methyl ergonovine.
- Lopinavir/ritonavir with: fluticasone, simvastatin or lovastatin, flecainide or propafenone, cisapride, pimozide, astemizole or terfenadine, midazolam or triazolam, ergotamine, ergonovine, or methyl ergonovine.
- Nelfinavir with indinavir, irinotecan, simvastatin or lovastatin, cisapride, pimozide, astemizole or terfenadine, midazolam or triazolam, ergotamine, ergonovine or methylergonovine.
- Atazanavir with: simvastatin or lovastatin, cisapride, pimozide, astemizole or terfenadine, midazolam or triazolam, ergotamine, ergonovine, or methyl ergonovine.
- Amprenavir (same for the fosamprenavir) with: simvastatin or lovastatin, cisapride, pimozide, astemizole or terfenadine, midazolam or triazolam, ergotamine, ergonovine, or methyl-ergonovina. (Wire et al., 2006)
- Tipranavir with: fluticasone, simvastatin or lovastatin, amiodarone, flecainide, propafenone, or quinidine, cisapride, pimozide, astemizole or terfenadine, midazolam or triazolam, ergotamine, ergonovine, or methyl-ergonovina.(Boffito et al., 2006)

From a practical perspective and specifying the type of NNRTIs, it is generally recommended to avoid the following combinations (level 1 or level 2: very high risk or high risk): (DHHS, 2011)

- Delavirdine with: amprenavir or fosamprenavir, simvastatin or lovastatin, cisapride, astemizole or terfenadine, alprazolam, midazolam or triazolam, ergotamine, ergonovine or methyl ergonovine.
- Efavirenz with: voriconazole, cisapride, astemizole or terfenadine, midazolam or triazolam, ergotamine, ergonovine or methyl ergonovine.

Related to PIs and NNRTIs Di, it is important to note that for delavirdine, its combination with amprenavir or fosamprenavir can cause a decrease in the levels and effects of delavirdine. (Tran et al., 2001; Wire et al., 2006) Additionally, some studies have shown a possible interaction between fosamprenavir with lopinavir/ritonavir, in fact mediated by a two-way increase in CYP3A4 and/or P-glycoprotein (P-gp) metabolic activity by fosamprenavir and lopinavir. (Huang et al., 2001; Taburet et al., 2004; Tranet al., 2002) This interaction is associated to a 50-60% decrease in lopinavir plasma concentration, and a 60-70% decrease in amprenavir levels (ritonavir levels do not change significantly). Consequently, combining these 3 PIs may be inappropriate, due to a high probability of generating a virologic failure (Kashuba et al., 2005) (level 2: high risk). The negative effect of this interaction is not neutralized by increasing ritonavir dose from 100 to 200 mg/12 hours; while this strategy is associated with increased gastric problems associated to the use of ritonavir. (Mauss et al., 2004)

On the other hand, it seems that the combination atazanavir with lopinavir/ritonavir does not generate this problem (although decreased levels of lopinavir by the action of atazanavir may occur (Colombo et al., 2006), which is considered a double pharmacokinetic extension (boosted) with PI, useful in a certain group of patients. (Ribera et al., 2006) Contrary to this effect (of atazanavir on lopinavir levels), when using a saquinavir/ritonavir and atazanavir (1.600/100 and 200 mg) an increase in saquinavir plasma and cellular levels is observed (without effect on ritonavir). Therefore, it is believed that adding atazanavir 200 mg/day to saquinavir/ritonavir 1.600/100 mg/day may be a good strategy for patients in who the Cpss are under the minimum effective one. (Ford et al., 2006)

Due to it is common used of this group of drugs in HIV infected patients receiving antiretroviral therapy; it is important focus following drugs therapeutic class:

Statins. The simultaneous use of PI or delavirdine with statins (lovastatin≈ simvastatin > atorvastatin > rosuvastatin ≈ fluvastatin ≈ pravastatin) increases the risk of myopathy, rhabdomyolysis, and even death. (Hare et al., 2002) Thus, for atorvastatin the lowest possible doses are recommended. Also, it is suggested to monitor muscle toxicity signs and symptoms or to use statins less likely to have this type of interaction, such as pravastatin, fluvastatin or rosuvastatin from. (Benesic et al., 2004; DHHS, 2011; Fichtenbaum et al., 2002; Fichtenbaum & Gerber, 2002; Jacobson, 2004; Sax, 2006) In this regard, statins (simvastatin, lovastatin, and atorvastatin, except pravastatin, fluvastatin, and rosuvastatin) are metabolized by CYP3A4 and, therefore, their use should be avoided in patients using PIs, especially ritonavir, atazanavir and saquinavir. Both metabolism and levels of pravastatin, as well as, most likely, fluvastatin and rosuvastatin are slightly affected by the combined use of ritonavir, indinavir, atazanavir, saquinavir, and nelfinavir and therefore they could be combined in patients receiving cART or HAART. (Aberg et al., 2006; Bays, 2006; Benesic et al., 2004; Cooper et al., 2003; Jacobson, 2004; Sudano et al., 2006). However, in some cases it may be necessary to increase the dose of pravastatin, as appears likely in the case of nelfinavir. (Aberg et al., 2006)

Selective serotonin reuptake inhibitors (SSRI). The use of ritonavir (alone or in combination with another PI) by inhibiting CYP2D6 and efavirenz by inhibiting CYP2C9 and CYP2C19, when a deficit of CYP2D6 exists, may lead to increased levels and toxic effects of SSRIs (fluoxetine, fluvoxamine, venlafaxine, paroxetine and, sertraline). Particularly, it may lead to the development of serotonin syndrome (DeSilva et al., 2001). Therefore, it is advisable to use half the dose or the lowest dose possible of these drugs, setting the dose in terms of their effectiveness and safety. (DHHS, 2011) Additionally, citalopram, and possibly escitalopram and sertraline, due to their pharmacological properties (low metabolism and minimal effect on CYP activity), are considered the most suitable option in patients receiving cART or HAART. (Caballero & Nahata, 2005; Currier et al., 2004; DHHS, 2011; Kashuba, 2005)

Generally, serotonin syndrome is a disorder caused by an increase in serotonin levels, resulting in **cognitive disorders** (lethargy, confusion, coma, agitation, hallucinations, and seizures); **neuromuscular activity disorders** (myoclonus, tremor, hyperreflexia, rigidity, hyperactivity); **autonomic nervous system disorders** (hypotension or hypertension, tachycardia, chills, hyperthermia, diaphoresis, diarrhea, salivation, abdominal pain, tachypnea) (Isbister & Buckley, 2005). In a patient under treatment with a SSRI (or other drugs with serotonergic activity in the central nervous system), such change can occur due to pharmacodynamic interactions (simultaneous treatment with other drugs that increase serotonin activity or agonist) or to pharmacokinetic interactions (treatment with an CYP2D6 inhibitor or because of a situation leading to an increase in serotonin levels and effects). (DeSilva et al., 2001; Tseng & Foisy, 1999)

3.2 Drug interactions mediated mainly by enzymatic inhibition of PIs and NNRTIs with other known enzyme inhibitors (for some drugs metabolism inhibition may occur while for others may occur metabolism induction)

Since PIs and NNRTIs are metabolized by CYP3A, strong inhibitors of CYP3A isoenzyme may inhibit its metabolism, increase plasma levels and therefore the risk of developing adverse drug reactions or toxicities. In these cases, generally, inhibition is bidirectional (the strong inhibitors may increase the PIs and NNRTIs levels and toxicity as well as PIs and NNRTIs may increase the inhibitors plasma concentrations and toxicity). However, in some cases the interaction can be in one direction, while in others both NNRTI metabolism inhibition (by the known inhibitor) and known inhibitor metabolism induction (by the NNRTIs) may occur, especially with efavirenz and nevirapine. In table 4 (for PIs) and table 5 (for NNRTIs) the most relevant interactions of this type are included.

Due to it is important some examples of the **one-way drug interactions mediated mainly by enzymatic inhibition of PIs and NNRTIs are detailed:**

Azoles antifungals

- Azoles antifungals (ketoconazole, itraconazole, fluconazole, voriconazole) with amprenavir. Antifungal may inhibit amprenavir hepatic metabolism (and probably fosamprenavir metabolism), which can lead to an increase in their levels, although such increase does not seem to be clinically relevant (level 3: medium risk). (Vourvahis & Kashuba, 2007)
- Fluconazole with tipranavir/ritonavir. Fluconazole causes an increase in the area under the curve. In any case, similar to what happens when PIs are used with azoles antifungals; it is advisable to monitor the hepatic function and not to exceed a dose of 200 mg/daily fluconazole. (DHHS, 2011)
- Ketoconazole with delavirdine. Ketoconazole may increase delavirdine levels (Level 3: medium risk), (DHHS, 2011) but ketoconazole levels do not change significantly.

Macrolides and immunosuppressants

- Clarithromycin with amprenavir (and probably fosamprenavir). Clarithromycin produces an 18% an increase in the area under the curve of amprenavir, while the effect of PI on macrolide levels is lowest. (Brophy et al., 2000)
- Immunosuppressants with efavirenz or nevirapine. Cyclosporine and tacrolimus may increase the levels and toxicity of these two NNRTIs. It is thus recommended to monitor toxicity signs and symptoms of these drugs and, if required, to adjust its dose (Level 3: medium risk). (Jain et al., 2002; Vogel et al., 2004)

3.3 Drug interactions due to enzyme induction of NNRTIS (Back et al., 2003; Bergshoeff et al., 2005; DHHS, 2011; Kashuba, 2005; Krikorian & Rudorf, 2005; Mildvan et al., 2002; (Pérez et al., 2009; Piscitelli & Gallicano, 2001; Saraga et al., 2006; Young, 2005)

Efavirenz and nevirapine due to their ability to increase the hepatic metabolism may cause a decrease in PIs levels and consequently therapeutic failure. Therefore, in general, using a single PI with efavirenz (in particular) or nevirapine is considered contraindicated (level 2 interaction: high risk). For example, efavirenz can cause a 39% reduction in the minimum

Group drugs or drugs affected	Clinical relevance of the bidirectional inhibition: level	Comments and suggestions
Azole antifungals [a] (Polk et al., 1999; Vourvahis & Kashuba, 2007) • Ketoconazole • Itraconazole • Fluconazole	2: high risk	Except for amprenavir and fosamprenavir, there is a bidirectional increase in the levels of antifungal and PIs, which can lead to toxicity problems. It is recommended using up to 200 mg/day of ketoconazole or 200-400 mg/day of itraconazole. In the case of fluconazole combination with tipranavir / ritonavir an increase in levels of tipranavir, without significant changes in fluconazole is observed. (Vourvahis & Kashuba, 2007)
• Voriconazole	3: medium risk	The coadministration of darunavir and ketoconazole increase the plasma concentrations of both drugs, creating the same toxic effects (Sekar et al., 2008)
Macrolides [a] • Erythromycin • Clarithromycin	2: high risk	Except for amprenavir and fosamprenavir, a bidirectional increase in the levels of macrolides and PIs is generated, which can lead to toxicity problems. Macrolides may increase QTc interval on the electrocardiogram. It is recommended to use maximum 1 g / day of these antibiotics (for clarithromycin it is suggested to reduce 50-75% in the level, if the patient has a creatinine clearance <60 ml / minute). In general, it is considered that using erythromycin with a strong inhibitors of CYP3A4 should be avoided (Ray et al., 2004)
Immuno-suppressants [a] (Jain et al., 2002; Vogel et al., 2004) • Cyclosporine • Tacrolimus	2: high risk	Increased levels and toxicity of immunosuppressants can be generated, so it is recommended to monitor plasma levels and to adjust the treatment regime. In the case of nelfinavir/tacrolimus combination it is recommended to reduce by 50% the dose of the immunosuppressant (Jain et al., 2002). In the case of cyclosporine with lopinavir / ritonavir, a 5% initial reduction is recommended in cyclosporine dose (a reduction of up to 20%) may be necessary. (Vogel et al., 2004) Cyclosporine and tacrolimus may increase the levels and toxicity of PIs and therefore it is recommended to monitor signs and symptoms of toxicity, and if required, to adjust the dose

[a] PIs can inhibit CYP3A4 and may decrease the metabolism of these drugs, which can cause increased plasma concentrations and toxicity. In turn, these drugs, also due to CYP3A4 inhibition, may decrease the metabolism of PIs and increase plasma concentrations and toxicity.

Table 4. Clinical relevant bidirectional drug interactions mediated by PIs enzyme inhibition with other known drugs (Brophy et al., 2000; DHHS, 2011; Kashuba, 2005a, 2005b; Krikorian & Rudorf, 2005; Robertson et al., 2005b; Young, 2005)

Drug group or drugs affected	Clinical relevance: level			Comments and suggestions
	Delavirdine	Efavirenz	Nevirapine	
Azole antifungals [a] • Ketoconazole	3: medium risk	No information available	3: medium risk	With Delavirdine: Delavirdine levels increased with no change in ketoconazole levels. With nevirapine: increased levels of nevirapine and decreased ketoconazole levels
• Itraconazole	3: medium risk	No information available	No information available	In general, slight clinical relevance
• Fluconazole	No significant changes	No information available	2: high risk	With nevirapine: increased levels and potential liver toxicity of nevirapine and no changes on fluconazole
• Voriconazole	3: medium risk	2: high risk	3: medium risk	With delavirdine: increased levels of both drugs. The toxic effects of both drugs should be monitored. Efavirenz and nevirapine: NNRTI levels increased and decreased levels voriconazole
Macrolides [a] • Erythromycin • Clarithromycin	2: high risk	2: high risk	No information available	A bidirectional increase in the levels of macrolides and delavirdine and efavirenz, which may lead to problems of toxicity of macrolides and NNRTIs
Immunosuppressants • Cyclosporine • Tacrolimus	3: medium risk	3: medium risk	3: medium risk	Immunosuppressants inhibit the metabolism of efavirenz and nevirapine. In addition, there are reports of decreased levels of cyclosporine by

				efavirenz, so it is recommended to monitor the levels of immunosuppressants (Tseng et al., 2002)
Pimozide (DHHS, 2011)	No information available	2: high risk	No information available	Efavirenz with drugs primarily metabolized by CYP3A4 may increase plasma concentrations of drugs, due to a weak inhibitory effect on this enzyme. Recommendation: There may be potential for serious or life-threatening reactions such as cardiac arrhythmias with pimozide, so it is not recommended for use concomitantly

[a] NNRTIs may inhibit CYP3A4 and may decrease the metabolism of these drugs, which can cause increased plasma concentrations and toxicity. In turn, these drugs, also due to CYP3A4 inhibition, may decrease the metabolism of NNRTIs and increase plasma concentrations and toxicity.

Table 5. Clinical relevant bidirectional drug interactions mediated by enzyme inhibition (induction in some cases) of NNRTIs with other known enzyme inhibitors (Brophy et al., 2000; Jain et al., 2002; Krikorian & Rudorf, 2005; Piscitelli & Gallicano, 2001; Polk et al., 1999; Ray et al., 2004; Robertson et al., 2005b; Sekar et al., 2008; Vogel et al., 2004; Vourvahis & Kashuba, 2007; Young, 2005)

lopinavir steady state concentration. (Dailly et al., 2005; Solas et al., 2004) The use of another low-dose PI as a pharmacokinetic extension agent (boosted), for instance ritonavir, is a strategy to counter this problem. (Acosta, 2002; Rathbun & Rossi, 2002; Zeldin & Petruschke, 2004) When using atazanavir with efavirenz it is recommended to add 100 mg of ritonavir to the usual dose (300 mg/24 hours). For lopinavir/ritonavir and efavirenz, lopinavir/ritonavir should be increased from 400/100 mg/12 hours (3 capsules) to 533/133 mg/12 hours (4 capsules) without change in the efavirenz dose. (DHHS, 2011; Solas et al., 2004; Dailly et al., 2005). For pediatric patients, in order to compensate the induction of efavirenz hepatic metabolism, it is suggested to increase the lopinavir/ritonavir dose to 300/75 mg/m^2 twice daily. (Dailly et al., 2006) Related to this topic, some studies have shown that cimetidine may be useful as a pharmacokinetic extension agent (effect similar to ritonavir) when combined with saquinavir. (Boffito et al., 2002)

Besides the effect of efavirenz and nevirapine on PIs levels, these ITINNs, (DeJesus et al., 2006) efavirenz (mainly) and nevirapine may increase metabolism, lower levels and cause therapeutic failure with various medications, such as statins (Gerber et al., 2005) and warfarin. In table 6 the most relevant interactions due to enzyme induction mediated by these two NNRTIs are included.

Drug group or drugs affected	Clinical relevance: level			Comments and suggestions
	Delavirdine	Efavirenz	Etravirine	
Protease inhibitors (PI) [a] • Indinavir (IDV) (Harris et al., 2006b) • Nelfinavir (NFV) • Ritonavir (RTV) • Amprenavir (APV) • Tipranavir (TPV) • Lopinavir/Ritonavir (LPV/r) (Bergshoeff et al., 2005; Dailly et al., 2005; Solas et al., 2004)	2: high risk	2: high risk	2: high risk	In general, the use of a single PI with efavirenz (specially) or nevirapine should be avoided. Efavirenz may decrease by 39% the minimum concentration of lopinavir. The dose should be increased to 533/133 mg/12 hours
Saquinavir (SAQ) (Boffito et al., 2002)	4: low risk (Fletcher et al., 2000)	3: medium risk (Baker, 1998)	2: high risk	Concomitant use of etravirine with saquinavir causes a decrease of the saquinavir plasma concentrations, due to etravirine induction effect on CYP3A4. (Etravirine, 2006; Harris et al., 2006b)
Atazanavir (ATZ) (Mullin et al., 2004)	2: high risk	2: high risk	1: Very high risk	It is recommended to add 100 mg of ritonavir. The plasma concentration of atazanavir is reduced by 38% if it is administered concomitantly with etravirine. Recommendation: Concomitant use of etravirine with atazanavir/ritonavir. (Aber, 2008)
Fosamprenavir (f-APV) (Back et al, 2003)	2: high risk	2: high risk	1: Very high risk	Nevirapine may decrease plasma concentrations between 25 and 35% Fosamprenavir plasma concentration is decreased by 77% if it is administered concomitantly with etravirine. Recommendation: avoiding concomitant administration of

				etravirine with fosamprenavir. (Holdich et al., 2007)
Darunavir	No information available	2: high risk	No information available	Efavirenz may decrease plasma concentrations of darunavir (Schöller et al., 2007)
Statins [a](Gerber et al., 2005; Sekar et al., 2007a) • Simvastatin • Atorvastatin • Pravastatin • Lovastatin • Rosuvastatin	3: medium risk	3: medium risk	3: medium risk	Possible reduction effect of these hypolipidemic. Pharmacological response should be traced and dose adjusted, where necessary is recommended to monitor parameters the effectiveness of lovastatin (lipid profile) and if necessary make an adjustment in medication dosage
Methadone (Altice et al., 1999; Bruce et al., 2006; Clarke et al., 2001; Stocker et al., 2004)	2: high risk	2: high risk	No information available	See text: methadone and efavirenz (nevirapine)
Warfarina [a]	3: medium risk	3: medium risk	No information available	Monitoring INR
Ethinyl estradiol [a] (oral contraceptives) (Mildvan et al, 2002)	2: high risk	2: high risk	No information available	Additional contraceptive method should be used (barrier method, for example)
Valproic acid (Saraga et al., 2006)	2: high risk	No information available	No information available	Efavirenz may decrease valproate concentrations by induction of glucoronosil diphosphate transferase
Macrolides • Clarithromycin (Schöller et al., 2006b) • Erythromycin	No information available	No information available	2: high risk	Etravirine may decrease the drugs plasma concentrations, because it exerts on enzyme induction of CYP3A4
Maraviroc	No information available	2: high risk	3: medium risk	Efavirenz is an inducer of CYP3A4 metabolism which can lead to reduced plasma concentrations of maraviroc. Recommendation: In the presence of enzyme inducers such as efavirenz, maraviroc may be increased to 600 mg

				twice daily (Abel et al., 2008) Simultaneous administration of etravirine and maraviroc causes a decrease in plasma concentrations of maraviroc (Cmin decreased 29%, Cmax by 60% and AUC by 53%). Recommendation: dose adjustment (Davis et al., 2007)
NNRTI • Efavirenz • Nevirapine	No information available	No information available	2: high risk	Concomitant use of etravirine with nevirapine and efavirenz can cause a decrease in plasma concentrations of etravirine and its therapeutic effect (Kakuda et al., 2006)
Raltegravir	No information available	2: high risk	2: high risk	Concomitant administration of etravirine and raltegravir with efavirenz can cause a decrease in plasma concentration of raltegravir. Cmin is reduced by 34% and AUC by 10%. (Anderson et al., 2008; Menard et al., 2009; Wittkop et al., 2009)
Sildenafil	No information available	No information available	3: medium risk	Coadministration of etravirine with sildenafil can cause a decrease in sildenafil concentrations by 57%. Recommendation: dose adjustment of sildenafil Pérez et al., 2009)
Buprenorphine	No information available	No information available	2: high risk	Coadministration of efavirenz with buprenorphine may decrease plasma concentrations of its active metabolite, norbuprenorphine, due to the inductive effect exerted by the efavirenz on CYP3A4 (McCance-Katz et al., 2006)

[a] Efavirenz, in particular, and nevirapine can primarily induce CYP3A4 and increase the metabolism of these drugs, which can cause a decrease plasma concentrations and therapeutic effects.

Table 6. Clinical relevant drug interactions due to enzyme induction mediated by NNRTIs (DeJesus et al., 2006; DHHS, 2011; Krikorian & Rudorf, 2005; Young, 2005)

Methadone and efavirenz (nevirapine). Efavirenz and nevirapine may reduce methadone area under curve (AUC) by 57% and 46%, respectively. (Altice et al., 1999) Therefore, when it is necessary to use methadone in patients that are using these NNRTIs, it is advisable to gradually increase the opiate dose from 10 to 10 mg, (Stocker et al., 2004) adjusting it based on effectiveness and safety parameters. Particular attention must be paid to withdrawal clinical manifestations. Withdrawal manifestations usually appear 7-10 days after initiating treatment with NNRTI and must not be confused with neurological toxicity symptoms associated with efavirenz (dizziness, headache, insomnia, concentration difficulty, nightmares, and agitation) that may occur within 1-2 days of starting treatment with efavirenz and which may be present during 14-28 days. (Bruce et al., 2006) Additionally, at sites with a suitable infrastructure, plasma levels of methadone can be monitored, aiming to reach a concentration of 400 and 250 micrograms/mL for (R, S)-methadone and (R) - methadone, respectively. (Bruce et al., 2006; Clarke et al., 2001; DHHS, 2011; Stocker et al., 2004)

Ritonavir as enzymatic inductor. Ritonavir, alone or in combination with other PIs, due to its ability to induce mainly glucuronyl-transferase and, to a lesser extent CYP2B6, which may produce ineffectiveness of some drugs:

- Ethinyl estradiol (oral contraceptive component). The contraceptive effect may be diminished when used simultaneously with ritonavir. (Ouellet et al., 1998) It is therefore advisable to inform the patient of the need to use a barrier method as a complementary birth control method (DHHS, 2011) (level 2: high risk).
- Thyroid hormones. It may cause metabolic inactivation of thyroid hormones and treatment failure (level 2: high risk). It is therefore recommended to monitor and adjust the levels of thyroid hormones in patients under treatment with ritonavir. (Touzot et al., 2006)
- Lamotrigine. It produces a decrease in anticonvulsant plasma levels, which can lead to ineffective treatment (level 2: high risk). It may be necessary to double lamotrigine dose in order to achieve therapeutic levels. (Van der Lee et al., 2006)
- Bupropion. It causes a decrease both in bupropion levels and its metabolite (hydroxy-bupropion), which could lead to ineffective treatment (Level 3: medium risk) and the need to double bupropión dose. (Hogeland et al., 2007) However, in theory, ritonavir can also act as an inhibitor of this isoenzyme and, therefore, increase concentrations of bupropion, so caution is advised until more data are available.

3.4 Drug interactions mediated by known enzyme inducers and consequences on PIs and NNRTIs efficacy (Benator et al., 2007; DHHS, 2011; Hamzeh et al., 2003; Kraft et al., 2004; Krikorian & Rudorf, 2005; Lim et al., 2004; Mullin et al., 2004; Romanelli & Pomeroy, 2003; Young, 2005)

The pharmacological effect of PIs and NNRTIs may be diminished and thus may appear therapeutic failure, associated with the emergence of resistance, when these ARV are combined or used simultaneously with known enzyme inducers (rifampicin, rifabutin, phenobarbital, primidone, carbamazepine, phenytoin), including St. John's wort. Rifabutin, a drug in the same family as rifampicin (rifamycins), is also characterized by inducing the metabolism of certain drugs, although to a lesser degree than rifampicin. (Finch et al., 2002)

3.4.1 Interactions of rifamycins with protease inhibitors (PIs) or with non-nucleoside reverse transcriptase inhibitors (NNRTIs)

Rifampicin and PIs. (Blumberg et al., 2003; Finch et al., 2002; Sekar et al., 2010; Spradling et al., 2002) In general, the use of rifampicin (rifabutin is preferred due to their lesser inductive effect than rifabutin) with a single PI, including the most recent, such as amprenavir and atazanavir, is considered contraindicated (level 1: very high risk), because in most cases, rifampicin produces non-efficacy PIs concentrations. Besides, most treatment guidelines for HIV/AIDS patients extend this contraindication even to PIs combined with ritonavir used as a pharmacokinetic extension agent (enhancer). (DHHS, 2011) However, for saquinavir, (Rolla et al., 2006) atazanavir, (Burger et al., 2006) and lopinavir, (La Porte et al., 2004) some studies show that adding ritonavir may counteract such effect in to some extent. In these cases, both saquinavir/ritonavir dose must be adjusted to 400/400 mg twice daily, (Aaron et al., 2004; de Jong et al., 2004; Rolla et al., 2006;) and lopinavir/ritonavir to 400/400 mg/12 hours or to 800/200 mg/12 hours. (Aaron et al., 2004; de Jong et al., 2004; La Porte et al., 2004)

Regarding the concomitant administration of saquinavir/ritonavir (1000/100 mg once daily) with rifampicin, because of some reports of liver toxicity, it is recommended to avoid such a combination. (Kashuba, 2005) Additionally, some studies show that in order to achieve saquinavir adequate levels, when saquinavir is used in combination with ritonavir, it is advisable to use doses higher than 1.600/200 mg/day of this combination; (Ribera et al., 2007) however this situation could further increase the likelihood of liver toxicity problems. With respect to the advisable rifampicin dose (despite the possible inhibitory effect of PI), changes are not recommended, but liver functioning must be monitored. (La Porte et al., 2004; de Jong et al., 2004; Aaron et al., 2004) For amprenavir (Polk et al., 2001) even with low-dose ritonavir (100 or 200 mg/day), their use in combination with rifampicin is contraindicated (level 1: very high risk). (DHSS, 2011)

Rifampicin and NNRTI. (Finch et al., 2002; de Jong et al., 2004; Ribera et al., 2001; Ramachandran et al., 2006; Weiner et al., 2005) In general, the use of rifampicin together with delavirdine is considered contraindicated (Borin et al., 1997) (level 1: very high risk). When it needs to use simultaneously rifampin with efavirenz, it is recommended to increase the NNRTI dose from 600 to 800 mg/day. (DHHS, 2011; Matteelli et al., 2007) However, some studies conducted with patients weighing 50 kg in Thailand and infected with HIV and tuberculosis, treated with rifampicin and HAART, indicate that the use of the standard efavirenz dose (600 mg/day) may be enough to reach the desired levels and effects with NNRTI at 24 and 48 weeks. (Manosuthi et al., 2005, 2006) Similarly, results achieved in African patients support the use of efavirenz 600 mg/day. (Friedland et al., 2006) Additionally, there are some reports of toxicity with efavirenz at doses of 800 mg/day. (Brennan et al., 2005) Therefore, it is believed that with black patients weighing less than 55 kg, as well as with Hispanic or Asian patients who show evidence of susceptibility to efivarenz toxic effects, it is recommended to use a 600 mg/day dose of this NNRTI. (Matteelli et al., 2007) Thus, when it is indicate to use rifampicin with efavirenz no adjustments are recommended in the dose of rifampicin.

Consequently, in general: a) for patients receiving HAART, rifabutin should preferred to the use of for rifampicin, due to its significantly lower enzyme-inducing effect, b) the use of single PIs with rifampicin should be avoided; c) some studies show that rifampicin could be used with saquinavir, atazanavir, and lopinavir enhanced with ritonavir, but it is needing more evidence on the effectiveness and safety of such combinations, d) the use of delavirdine in conjunction with rifampicin or rifabutin is considered absolutely contraindicated, and e) in most cases where rifabutin or rifampicin is combined with PIs, dosage must be adjusted and potential toxicity must be monitored, particularly liver toxicity due to rifamycins.

Hypericum (St. John's wort) as enzyme inducer and ARV drugs. In general, the combination of this herbal antidepressant with PIs or with NNRTIs, due to high probability of generating therapeutic failure, is considered contraindicated (level 1: very high risk). Thus, there are several reports of therapeutic failure of ritonavir and nevirapine, associated with the use of this herbal product. (Izzo, 2004; Winston & Boffito, 2005; Zhou et al., 2004) This substance may induce both the systemic metabolism by CYP3A4, and the presystemic metabolism by intestinal or hepatic CYP3A4; additionally it may induce P-gp activity (bioavailability related interactions). (Lee et al., 2006)
Table 7 contains details of interactions produced by rifamycins (rifampin and rifabutin), and table 8 contains detailed information on interactions mediated by traditional anticonvulsants.

3.5 Drug interactions related to bioavailability

3.5.1 Drug interactions related to changes in gastrointestinal pH

In general, an increased gastrointestinal pH may affect the amount absorbed of delavirdine, indinavir, fosamprenavir, tipranavir, (Vourvahis & Kashuba, 2007) and atazanavir. (DeSilva et al., 2001; DHHS, 2011; Tomilo et al., 2006) However, it is basic to clarify some aspects:

- Concomitant administration of atazanavir with proton-pump inhibitors (omeprazole, lansoprazole, pantoprazole) (Tomilo et al., 2006) is not recommended (Level 2: high risk). The use of delavirdine with H_2 antihistamines (cimetidine, ranitidine, famotidine, and nizatidine) and with proton-pump inhibitors (level 2: high risk) is also not recommended, due to a decrease near to 90% of the amount absorbed and, consequently, to a reduction in antiretroviral plasma concentrations, which can lead to treatment failure. (DHHS, 2011) In the case of atazanavir, famotidine can be used as an alternative to omeprazole, spacing its administration about 10 hours. A similar result can be achieved by adding low-dose ritonavir (100 mg) at 300 mg/day atazanavir, or by increasing the dose to 400 mg/day of atazanavir. (Kashuba, 2005)

Combined administration of antacids does not seem to significantly affect the amount absorbed of fosamprenavir, (Ford et al., 2005) or raltegravir; however it is recommended to separate the taking of the two drugs when they are used in pharmacological therapy. (Kiser et al., 2010)

Drug group or drugs affected	Clinical relevance: level		Comments and suggestions (see text: rifampicin and PI and rifampicin and NNRTI)
	Rifampicin	Rifabutin	
PIs [a] (Aaron et al., 2004; Benator et al., 2007; Blumberg et al., 2003; Burger et al., 2006; DeJong et al. 2004; Finch et al., 2002; Hamzeh et al., 2003; Kraft et al., 2004; La Porte et al., 2004; Polk et al., 2001; Ribera et al., 2007; Rolla et al., 2006; Spradling et al., 2002) Ritonavir (Aaron et al., 2004; Blumberg et al., 2003; DeJong et al. 2004; Finch et al., 2002; Spradling et al., 2002)	1: very high risk	2: high risk	Adjust rifabutin dose 150 mg/48 hours, with no change in ritonavir

Indinavir (Hamzeh et al., 2003, Kraft et al., 2004)	1: very high risk	2: high risk	Adjust the dose of rifabutin 150 mg/24 hours and indinavir at 1,000 mg/8 hours
Saquinavir (Aaron et al., 2004; Blumberg et al., 2003; DeJong et al. 2004; Finch et al., 2002; Ribera et al., 2007; Rolla et al., 2006; Spradling et al., 2002)	1: very high risk	2: high risk	Use usual dose of rifabutin (300 mg/day), with no change in saquinavir
Nelfinavir (Aaron et al., 2004; Benator et al., 2007; Blumberg et al., 2003; DeJong et al. 2004; Finch et al., 2002; Spradling et al., 2002)	1: very high risk	2: high risk	Adjust rifabutin dose 150 mg/24 hours and nelfinavir to 1,000 mg/8 hours
Atazanavir (Burger et al., 2006)	1: very high risk	2: high risk	Adjust rifabutin dose 150 mg/48hours, with no change in atazanavir
Amprenavir (Polk et al., 2001)	1: very high risk	2: high risk	Adjust rifabutin dose 150 mg/24 hours, with no change in amprenavir
Fosamprenavir (Aaron et al., 2004; DeJong et al. 2004)	1: very high risk	2: high risk	Adjust rifabutin dose 150 mg/24 hours, with no changes in fosamprenavir dose
Tipranavir (Vourvahis & Kashuba, 2007)	1: very high risk	2: high risk	Adjust rifabutin dose 150 mg/48hours, with no changes in tipranavir dose
Lopinavir/ritonavir (Aaron et al., 2004; La Porte et al., 2004; Spradling et al., 2002)	1: very high risk	2: high risk	Adjust rifabutin dose 150 mg/24 hours, with no changes in lopinavir/ritonavir dose
Darunavir	2: high risk	2: high risk	The predominant metabolite of rifabutin (RFB) is 25-O-desacetylrifabutin (desRFB), darunavir by inhibition of CYP3A4 may increase plasma concentrations of RFB, as well as its side effects (Sekar et al., 2010) Rifampin may significantly decrease the plasma concentrations of darunavir (Tibotec, 2008)
Non-nucleosid transcriptase inhibitors (NNRTI)[a] (DeJong et al. 2004; Finch et al., 2002; Friedland et al., 2006; Manosuthi et al., 2005, 2006;	1: very high risk	1: very high risk	This combination is considered absolutely contraindicated

McCance-Katz et al., 2006; Matteelli et al., 2007a; Ramachandran et al., 2006; Ribera et al., 2001) Delavirdine (Borin et al., 1997; DeJong et al. 2004; McCance-Katz et al., 2006; Spradling et al., 2002)			
Nevirapine (Benator et al., 2007; Blumberg et al., 2003; Borin et al., 1997; Burger et al., 2006; Hamzeh et al., 2003; Kraft et al., 2004; La Porte et al., 2004; Polk et al., 2001; Ramachandran et al., 2006; Ribera et al., 2001, 2007; Rolla et al., 2006)	2: high risk	3: medium risk	In general terms, no dosage adjustment is recommended with rifabutin. With rifampicin it may be necessary to increase the dose from 200 mg/12 hours to 300 mg/12 hours, and to monitor liver function
Efavirenz (Brennan et al., 2005; DeJong et al. 2004, Friedland et al., 2006; Manosuthi et al., 2005, 2006; Matteelli et al., 2007a, 2007b; Weiner et al., 2005)	2: high risk	2: high risk	It is recommended to increase rifabutin dose to 450-600 mg/day and to use the usual dose of efavirenz (600 mg/day) (Matteelli et al., 2007b)
Etravirine (Abel et al., 2008)	2: high risk	3: medium risk	Co-administration of etravirine with rifampicin causes a significant decrease in plasma concentrations of etravirine, due to inductor effect on CYP3A4 of rifampicin Co-administration of etravirine with rifabutin causes a decrease by 37% of plasma concentrations of etravirine
Entry inhibitor: Maraviroc (Ogbuokiri, 2009)	2: high risk	3: medium risk	These drugs can reduce the maraviroc plasma concentrations by 66%. Recommendation: dose adjustment of maraviroc to 600 mg

[a] Rifampicin → rifabutin can induce CYP3A4 and increase the metabolism of these drugs, which can cause a decrease in plasma concentrations and virological response. In turn, some PIs or NNRTIs may modify the metabolism and concentrations or rifamycins, particularly by inhibition of CYP3A4, which can decrease their metabolism and increase plasma and concentrations and toxic effects of rifampicin and rifabutin, particularly liver and blood effects.

Table 7. Clinical relevant drug interactions mediated by rifampicin and rifabutin (DHHS, 2011; Tran et al., 2001)

Drug group or drugs affected	Clinical relevance: level			Comments and suggestions
	Phenobarbital and primidone	*Phenytoin*	*Carbamazepine*	
Protease Inhibitors (PI) [a] (Lim et al, 2004; Mullin et al., 2004; Romanelli & Pomeroy, 2003)				
• Ritonavir	2: high risk	2: high risk	2: high risk	Traditional anticonvulsants (except valproic acid) can cause ineffectiveness of PI (including their combination with low dose ritonavir). (Ogbuokiri, 2009) It is recommended the use of second-generation anticonvulsants (gabapentine, lamotrigine, vigabatrin and topiramate). Gabapentine, due to its pharmacological properties (it is not metabolized, it does not affect CYP activity), is considered the best option (Mullin et al., 2004; Romanelli & Pomeroy, 2003)
• Indinavir	2: high risk	2: high risk	2: high risk	
• Saquinavir	2: high risk	2: high risk	2: high risk	
• Nelfinavir	2:high risk	2:high risk	2:high risk	
• Atazanavir	2:high risk	2:high risk	2:high risk	
• Amprenavir	2:high risk	2:high risk	2:high risk	
• Fosamprenavir	2:high risk	2:high risk	2:high risk	
• Tipranavir	2:high risk	2:high risk	2:high risk	
• Lopinavir/ ritonavir	2:high risk	2:high risk	2:high risk	Lopinavir / ritonavir may decrease the plasma concentrations of phenytoin, due to the induction of CYP2C9
Non-nucleoside transcriptase inhibitors (NNRTI) [a] *(Mullin et al., 2004; Romanelli & Pomeroy, 2003; Tran et al., 2001; Tseng & Foisy, 1999)*				
• Delavirdine	1: very high risk	No information available	1:very high risk	Delavirdine with any of the traditional anticonvulsants (except valproic acid) is considered contraindicated. Traditional anticonvulsants (except valproic acid) can cause NNRTI ineffectiveness (Acosta, 2002)
• Nevirapine	2: high risk	No information available	2:high risk	
• Efavirenz	2:high risk	No information available	2: high risk	
Entry inhibitor				
• Maraviroc (Ogbuokiri, 2009)	3: medium risk	3: medium risk	3: medium risk	Traditional anticonvulsants (except valproic acid) can cause ineffectiveness of maraviroc

Table 8. Clinical relevant drug interactions mediated by traditional anticonvulsants (DHHS, 2011; Tran et al., 2001)

- Etravirine-Ranitidine. The concurrently use of etravirine and ranitidine for a period of eight days may cause a reduction in absorption of etravirine due to decrease of gastric (Schöller-Gyüre et al., 2008) acidity (level 3: medium risk).
- Darunavir-Omeprazole/Ranitidine. Due to the absorption of some PIs is pH dependent gastric acid, antacids may inhibit absorption of PIs. However, some studies show that there are not clinically significant DIs between darunavir and omeprazole/ranitidine, thus no dose adjustment is required to concomitant administration. (Sekar et al., 2007b)
- Absorption of delavirdine is noticeably decreased at pH values below 3. Therefore, its administration with antacids may cause a decrease on levels and effects (level 3: medium risk), and it is recommended to space its administration, at least an hour. (Tran et al., 2001)

Broadly, didanosine in buffered tablets may decrease absorption, levels and efficacy of delavirdine and indinavir (as well of other drugs that requiring an acidic environment for absorption), due to didanosine excipients maintain gastric pH above 3. However, the addition of didanosine in a new dosage form (enteric-coated granules within capsules) minimizes this effect, as evidenced by the results of studies on drugs whose bioavailability may be decreased by interactions with antacids such as indinavir, ketoconazole, and ciprofloxacin. (Damle et al., 2002b) Furthermore, the buffered tablet effect cannot be generalized for drugs requiring an acidic pH for absorption, such as itraconazole or fluconazole, whose bioavailability is not altered when administered simultaneously with didanosine, regardless of dosage form used. (Damle et al., 2002a)

Related to this type of mechanism, in general, food (drug-food interactions) can decrease the amount absorbed and effects of several ARV drugs. For example, in the case of didanosine (buffered tablet and enteric-coated granules within capsules), it is recommended to take it on an empty stomach (2 hours before or two hours after meals), (la Porte et al., 2005) because a decrease (between 18 and 55%) in the amount absorbed can be produced (level 3: risk medium). (Damle et al., 2002c; Kearney et al., 2005) Such effect may be minimized if didanosine is administered in combination with indinavir/ritonavir or with tenofovir (La Porte et al., 2005; Kearney et al., 2005) (see didanosine- tenofovir Interaction below).

3.5.2 Interactions related to presystemic metabolism and/or P-glycoprotein activity

P-gp (ABCB1) is one of the most extensively studied transporters regarding DIs. P-gp is expressed in multiple key organs in drug disposition such as small intestine, blood-brain barrier, kidney, and liver. Therefore, P-gp mediated DIs can occur at various organs and tissues. Thus, the induction or inhibition of P-gp can lead to drug-drug interactions. For instance, induction of the intestinal P-glycoprotein activity can cause reduced bioavailability of orally administered drugs and cause therapeutic failure. In contrast, the inhibition of the intestinal P-gp activity can lead to increased bioavailability, concentrations and adverse drug effects. (Josephson, 2010)

Broadly, PIs, particularly ritonavir, are mechanism-based intestinal P-gp efflux activity inhibition, which partially explains the effect on the levels and clinical results of some drugs, (de Maat et al., 2003) such as cyclosporine (Izzedine et al. 2004) and digoxin. (Penzak et al., 2004) Ritonavir can also inhibit renal P-gp activity, which may lead to a decrease in renal clearance of digoxin, associated with an increase in the levels and effects of this drug. (Ding et al., 2004)

Simultaneous administration of saquinavir 500 mg (low dose ritonavir) with omeprazole is associated with an increase of 82% in AUC of saquinavir. Although the mechanism is unclear, it is believed that this effect is due to the fact that omeprazole can inhibit P-gp activity and other membrane transporters activity. (Winston et al., 2006) Similarly, saquinavir bioavailability increases significantly when administered with cimetidine, (Boffito et al., 2002) ranitidine or food, an effect independent of pH increase. (Kakuda & Falcon, 2006) These findings could lead to believe that food is likely to increase solubility and to decrease the hepatic first pass effect, while the effect of cimetidine, ranitidine, and omeprazole, similar to what has been observed with other known inhibitors of intestinal and hepatic CYP3A4, may be associated to decreased presystemic metabolism and, to a lesser extent, to decreased P-gp intestinal activity. (Amariles, 2007)

4. Clinically relevant pharmacodynamic drug interactions in HIV-infected patients receiving antiretroviral therapy

Due to it is important some examples related to pharmacodynamic DIs in HIV-infected patients are detailed:

- Lamivudine and emtricitabine: this combination is considered inadequate, since these drugs show a minimum additive effect, as well as a similar profile of resistance (DHHS, 2011) (level 2: high risk).
- Stavudine and zidovudine: this combination is considered inadequate, because their chemical similarity can lead to competition for intracellular phosphorylation zidovudine inhibits phosphorylation and effects of stavudine (Ray, 2005) which might cause therapeutic failure (Level 2: high risk). Concerning this interaction, it is important to note that prior exposure to zidovudine (2 to 45 months) does not influence the ability of HIV-infected patients to phosphorylate stavudine. (Hoggard et al., 2001) Due to similar mechanism, the lamivudine and zalcitabine combination is considered inadequate, since lamivudine may inhibit the phosphorylation of zalcitabine, which may lead to therapeutic failure (Becher et al., 2004; DHHS, 2011; Havlir et al., 2000) (level 2: high risk).
- Abacavir, tenofovir, and lamivudine (or emtricitabine) as a triple NRTI therapy: This combination is considered contraindicated due to the rapid onset of virologic failure, when used as initial therapy (level 2: high risk). (DHHS, 2011) A similar consideration has been established for combination of tenofovir, didanosine, and lamivudine (emtricitabine). (DHHS, 2011)
- Amprenavir and fosamprenavir: This combination is not recommended, because fosamprenavir is a prodrug of amprenavir, thus their combined use increases the risk of adverse drug reactions without additional benefits (level 2: high risk).(DHHS, 2011)
- Stavudine and aminopterin: This combination is not recommended, because the combination causes an inhibition of hepatic mitochondrial DNA and hepatic toxicity (Setzer et al., 2008) (level 1: very high risk).
- Tenofovir and cisplatin or pemetrexed: The use of tenofovir in patients receiving cisplatin or pemetrexed may increase the risk of renal toxicity (3: medium risk). (Makinson et al., 2010)
- Tenofovir/emtricitabine, disulfiram and nifedipine: The use of nifedipine in HIV-infected patients receiving tenofovir/emtricitabine and disulfiram may cause lactic acidosis (level 2: high risk). (Moling et al., 2009)

- Zidovudine, cisplatin or pemetrexed: The use of zidovudine in patients receiving cisplatin or pemetrexed may increase the risk of hematological toxicity (Makinson et al., 2010) (level 3: medium risk).
- Broadly, the use of drugs with a similar unsafe profile leads to an increased probability and severity of adverse effects, for instance:
  - Stavudine and didanosine: This combination is considered absolutely contraindicated (level 1: very high risk), due to increased likelihood of significant synergism of adverse drug problems associated with mitochondrial toxicity, which may manifest, especially as peripheral neuropathy, pancreatitis, and lactic acidosis. (Boubaker et al., 2001; Catanzaro et al., 2004; Coghlan et al., 2001; DHHS, 2011) Similarly, didanosine/zalcitabine and stavudine/zalcitabine combinations are considered contraindicated because of a greater likelihood and severity of peripheral neuropathy (Dalakas et al., 2001; Simpson & Tagliati, 1995) (level 1: very high risk). In general, NRTIs (lower risk with abacavir and lamivudine) may inhibit competitively the mitochondrial DNA polymerase gamma, an enzyme responsible for repairing mitochondrial DNA associated with oxidative alterations. (Dagan et al., 2002) Therefore, the use of NRTI may lead to depletion of DNA and uncoupling of mitochondrial respiratory chain and thus, to the accumulation of radicals and free fatty acids, as well as dicarboxylic acids, responsible for mitochondrial toxicity associated with this group of drugs. (Petit et al, 2005)
  - Zidovudine and ganciclovir: This combination increases the likelihood of developing bone marrow suppression, a condition associated with the occurrence of severe hematologic toxicity and life threatening infections, including the progression of cytomegalovirus infection (Hochster et al., 1990) (level 1 : very high risk). Related to this type of interaction, another combination with additive hematologic toxicity combination is zidovudine with ribavirin, associated with an increased risk of anemia (DHHS, 2011) (level 2: high risk).
  - Didanosine and ribavirin. This combination increases the likelihood of mitochondrial toxicity, which can lead to lactic acidosis and pancreatitis (Fleischer et al., 2004; Perronne et al. 2006) (level 2: high risk). Similarly, the didanosine-adefovir combination increases the risk of pancreatitis (Perronne et al. 2006) (level 2: high risk).
  - Atazanavir and indinavir: This combination increases the likelihood of developing hyperbilirubinemia (DHHS, 2011) (level 2: high risk).
  - Drugs with additive hepatic toxicity: In general, concomitant use of hepatotoxic drugs enhances the probability of hepatic alterations, for instance, when rifampicin is used with isoniazid (Steele et al., 1991) or with pyrazinamide (Yee et al., 2003) for treatment of tuberculosis; or when acetaminophen is used with zidovudine (Shriner & Goetz, 1992) (Level 2 or 3: high or middle risk).
  - Drugs with additive renal toxicity: Simultaneous use of renal toxic drugs increases the likelihood of problems in this organ, for instance the simultaneously use of adefovir, acyclovir (intravenously), cidofovir, foscarnet, indinavir, ritonavir, tenofovir, pentamidine, aminoglycosides, and amphotericin B (Fisher et al., 1989) (level 2 or 3: high risk or middle).

5. Clinically relevant drug-disease interactions in HIV-infected patients receiving antiretroviral treatment

Due to it is important some examples related to clinically relevant drug-disease interactions in HIV-infected patients are detailed:

- **Pregnancy**
  - Amprenavir oral solution, due to the high content of propylene glycol, as an excipient, can cause toxicity problems (DHHS, 2011) (level 2: high risk).
  - Efavirenz, especially during the first 3 months, because it represents a potential teratogenic risk, it is included in the D category of FDA classification of drugs for teratogenic risk (AIDS Patient Care, 2005; DHHS, 2011) (level 2: high risk).
  - Didanosine and stavudine, because there are reports of severe and even fatal lactic acidosis in pregnant women receiving stavudine and didanosine (DHHS, 2011) (level 2: high risk).
- **Moderate (Child Pugh score: 7-9 points) or severe (Child Pugh: over 9 points) liver failure**
  - NNRTI and PI. In general this class of drugs should be administered with caution or avoided altogether in patients with moderate or severe liver failure (DHHS, 2011) (level 3: medium risk).
  - Amprenavir, fosamprenavir. Avoid their use in the presence of severe liver failure (Amariles et al., 2007c; DHHS, 2011) (level 3: medium risk).
  - Amprenavir/ritonavir, tipranavir / ritonavir. Their use is contraindicated in severe liver failure (Amariles et al., 2007c; DHHS, 2011) (level 2: high risk).
- **Children under 4 years.** Amprenavir oral solution. Due to the high content of propylene glycol, as an excipient, it can cause toxicity problems (DHHS, 2011) (level 2: high risk).
- **Women with CD4 lymphocyte counts> 250 cells/mm^3 or men with CD4 lymphocyte counts > 400 cells/mm^3.** For these groups of patients there are reports of serious, sometimes fatal, liver impairments attributed to nevirapine (DHHS, 2011) (level 2: high risk).
- **Cirrhosis.** The combination of didanosine and ribavirin can lead to liver decompensation. Therefore, this combination is considered no-adequate for patients with advanced liver fibrosis (Perronne, et al. 2006) (level 2: high risk).
- **HIV**. The use of rifapentine (rifamycin) is considered inadequate, due to fewer efficacies in preventing the onset of tuberculosis in this group of patients. For this reason this could be considered as a possible drug-disease interaction (DHHS, 2011) (level 2: high risk).

6. Other clinically relevant drug interactions in HIV-infected patients attributed to different or unclear mechanisms

Other examples of clinically relevant DIs in HIV-infected patients attributed to different or unclear mechanisms are:

- **Zidovudine and enzyme inducers.** Zidovudine is metabolized and inactivated by glucuronyl transferase. Thus, inducers or inhibitors of this enzyme can affect its levels and effects (Kiang et al, 2005). For example, rifampicin may increase zidovudine metabolism and decrease its levels and effects. (Gallicano et al., 1999)
- **Tenofovir and didanosine.** Tenofovir increases didanosine levels and toxicity (particularly, pancreatitis), (Martinez et al., 2004) apparently due to inhibition of its metabolism by purine nucleoside phosphorylase. (Ray et al., 2004) It is thus recommended to reduce the dose from 400 mg to 250 mg/24 hours in patients weighing

less than 60 kg. (Kearney et al., 2005; Martinez et al., 2004; Antoniou et al., 2003) Additionally, even using reduced dose, didanosine toxicity signs and symptoms should be monitored (significant increase in serum amylase or lipase, neuropathy, paresthesia, nausea, vomiting, and abdominal pain). (DHHS, 2011) There are reports of didanosine toxicity (deadly lactic acidosis and acute hepatic failure), (Guo & Fung, 2004; Masía et al., 2005) at doses of 200 mg/day, especially in women weighing 60 or less kg. A similar effect could be observed when administering didanosine with other purine nucleoside phosphorylase inhibitory drugs, such as allopurinol, ganciclovir (Moling et al., 2009) and valganciclovir. (Tseng & Salit, 2007) Additionally, the use of didanosine-tenofovir combination may lead to decrease in the CD4 lymphocyte levels, thus this combination should be avoided (Anderson & Kakuda, 2006; Barreiro & Soriano, 2006) (level 1 or 2: Very high risk" or higher). Similarly, the **didanosine and ganciclovir** combination has also been associated with decreased CD4 cell levels (Tseng & Salit, 2007) (level 2: high risk).

- **Amprenavir oral solution (propylene glycol) and oral ritonavir (ethanol excipient).** Because propylene glycol and ethanol are metabolized by the same enzyme, accumulation and toxicity may occur. (DHHS, 2011) Also, related to the presence of excipients, the use of lopinavir/ritonavir oral solution (4.2% in ethanol) combined with metronidazole or disulfiram, substances that may inhibit the alcohol dehydrogenase, may lead to the development of disulfiram effect. (Cvetkovic & Goa, 2003; de Maat et al., 2003)
- **Atazanavir and tenofovir.** Tenofovir reduces atazanavir levels through a mechanism still to be established, so it is recommend using atazanavir (300 mg) together with low dose ritonavir (100 mg) as an enhancing agent. (Taburet et al., 2004) In addition, lopinavir/ritonavir and atazanavir may increase levels and toxic renal effects of tenofovir. (Perronne et al., 2006) It is important to illustrate that the inductive effects of tenofovir on the metabolism of atazanavir have not been documented to others PIs (Boffito et al., 2005)
- **Saquinavir and adefovir.** Adefovir (antiviral used in the treatment of hepatitis B) lowers saquinavir levels and effects. (Perronne et al. 2006)
- **Tenofovir and enzyme inducers.** NRTIs with inducing capacity (efavirenz and nevirapine) (Droste et al., 2006) and probably rifampicin, (Droste et al., 2005) do not cause variation in tenofovir levels and effects. Therefore, it is not recommended to adjust the dose of either drug, when it is necessary to use such combinations.
- **Amprenavir capsules, vitamin E, and warfarin levels.** Amprenavir capsules contain an amount of vitamin E that exceeds recommended daily dose, so in patients treated with amprenavir in this dosage form, vitamin E supplementation should be avoided. In patients under treatment with warfarin, high levels of vitamin E (associated with intakes higher than 400 IU per day) increase the risk of bleeding. (Amsay et al, 2005, Heck et al., 2000)
- **Strong or moderate inhibitors and PIs.** Some known enzyme inhibitors such as ketoconazole may decrease the extra-intestinal P-gp efflux activity and increasing PIs levels and effects in certain body areas, such as the cerebrospinal fluid, which have been evidenced for ritonavir and saquinavir. (Cvetkovic & Goa, 2003; Oldfield & Plosker, 2006; Lin & Yamazaki, 2003; Lin, 2003; Khaliq et al., 2000)
- **Rosiglitazone and nevirapine.** Rosiglitazone, apparently due to increased CYP3A4 or P-gp activity, may decrease nevirapine levels. This effect does not occur when using

lopinavir/ritonavir with nevirapine. (Oette et al., 2005) Thus, it is recommended to monitor nevirapine levels and effects, when this drug is used in combination with rosiglitazone (level 2: high risk).

- **Maraviroc and raltegravir.** The concomitantly administration of these drugs can reduce peak concentrations of both drugs due to changes in pre-systemic elimination associated to changes in absorption and/or first pass metabolism; however, the exact mechanism of interaction has not been determined (Andrews et al., 2010) (3: medium risk).

7. Software for evaluating and predicting clinical relevance of drug interactions in HIV-infected patients receiving antiretroviral therapy

The identification, systematization, evaluation, and prediction of DIs may be easier by using computer applications. Additionally, these kinds of informatics tools may contribute to reduce the risk to arise of clinical relevant DIs, and thus, the negative effect in goals of HAAR or cART in patients with HIV/SIDA. Thus, the design software that facilitates the identification and prediction the clinical relevance of drug interactions may be an important contribution to get the possible outcomes best in HIV-infected patients receiving HAART or cART. (Amariles et al., 2008) In this way, the following tasks have been done:

a. **Structured and systematic review of publications on Pubmed/Medline and other electronic databases, supplemented by other primary and secondary information sources to identify DIs in HIV-infected patients receiving ART therapy.** Thus, published articles of DIs in HIV-infected patients were identified by a comprehensive literature search using electronic databases of information sources (Medline/Pubmed, SIETES, Medscape, and Tripdatabase) to identify all full text or abstracts published in English and Spanish from January 1996 to February 2011. Additionally, a search was done in some specify journals: New England Journal of Medicine, British Medical Journal, and other recognized information sources: the electronic sheet drug interactions: www.drug-interactions.com; Philip D. Hansten, John R. Horn. Managing Clinically Important Drug Interactions, facts and comparison, 2003; Stockley IH. Drug Interactions. First edition. Pharma Editores. Spain, 2004, and Drug Interaction Facts, Micromedex (Drug-REAX) computer program.

b. **Classification of the clinical relevance of pairs of the identified DIs.** The accessing and predicting the clinical relevance of pairs of the identified DIs were based on the severity and probability of occurrence of the DIs. Based on the possible combinations of severity and probability of occurrence, DIs were grouped into 4 categories: Level 1 (very high risk), level 2 (high risk), level 3 (medium risk), an level 4 (low risk) as it was mentioned in numeral 2.3 (Determining and predicting of the clinical relevance level) (Amariles et al., 2007a)

c. **Software design.** The results of the review and evaluation of clinical relevance of the DIs were used to design a platform with alert generator, report generator, constant evolution support systems data integrity, network management intranet and Internet Web and Windows platforms. The developed software facilitates the identification, evaluation, and prediction of clinical relevant of 1,082 drug pairs of potential DIs, near to 80% of them due to pharmacokinetic mechanism (changes in plasma concentration), mainly associated to enzyme inhibition. The scaling of these 1,082 drug pairs of the recognized DIs according to different dosage forms and strengths of identified drugs, generates a total of 6,087 pairs of DIs, which, according their clinical relevance, 4,158

(68.3%) are clinical relevant (Levels 1 and 2) in HIV-infected patients receiving ARV therapy. Thus, the software meets the requirements defined for this type of programs. (Gaikwad et al., 2007; Rodríguez et al., 2009)

d. **Software implementation.** The program, posterior to entering drug treatment of a specific patient, generate the list of possible interactions with clinical relevance, accompanied by the suggestion of the most appropriate process to be followed by the healthcare professional user of the program. In Colombia, the program have been implemented in 24 health institutions, in addition the access is free and it is available on the website http:www.udea.edu.co/pypfarmaceutica. However, further investigation to evaluate in more detail information regarding to positive predictive and negative predictive values of alert generates by program is required.

8. Conclusions

Due to ARV therapy is one of the most dynamic in terms of launching new products in the market, it is necessary to carry out structured and systematic review of publications on Pubmed/Medline and other electronic databases to identify new DIs in HIV-infected patients, receiving ART therapy, which must be complemented with evaluating the scientific evidence and classifying their clinical relevance.

In HIV-infected patients receiving antiretroviral therapy, closer to 80% of relevant clinical pharmacokinetic DIs are associated to induction or inhibition of the systemic hepatic metabolism, which is associated to systemic clearance for a significant number drugs. While closer to 20% of relevant clinical pharmacokinetic DIs are associated to changes in bioavailability related interactions, including changes in gastrointestinal pH, presystemic metabolism and/or P-gp transport activity. Therefore, in HIV-infected patients receiving HAART of cART, the assessing and predicting clinical relevance of a given pharmacokinetic DI need to understand and use of concepts related to induction and, particularly with enzyme inhibition (mainly in CYP3 and CYP2 subfamilies) and, to a lesser extent, to bioavailability (especially with changes in a drug presystemic metabolism and/or P-gp transport activity).

It is becoming more evident that ARV drugs are metabolized via common pathways by CYP450 enzymatic complex, which leads to an increased probability of new clinical relevant pharmacokinetic DIs due to the inhibition or stimulation of CYP isoforms (mainly in CYP3 and CYP2 subfamilies).

In general, for a patient using more than one drug with differential capacity to modify CYP3A4 and/or P-gp enzymatic activity (some induce while some others inhibit), it is difficult to predict the net effect on the levels and effects of a drug whose metabolism is affected. (Spradling et al., 2002) Therefore, it is necessary, from a theoretical perspective, to avoid the use of such schemes, which is difficult in patients with HIV/AIDS. In this context, some studies conducted to establish the influence of several antiretroviral drugs on CYP3A activity show that ritonavir/nelfinavir inhibitory effect is maintained and it counteracts efavirenz/nevirapine inducing effect, when they are administered in combination. Additionally, it has been found that chronic administration of ritonavir (200 mg/day) or nelfinavir (2.5 g/12 hours) does not increase CYP3A activity. (Fellay et al., 2005; Mouly et al., 2006)

Similar to other groups of patients, it is important to systematize, distribute, and use guidelines and recommendations based on the findings of studies indicating which

combinations of a specified drug, of some specify therapeutic class, are the most appropriate for patients receiving cART or HAART. Such appropriate combinations should be chosen considering the lowest probability of the DIs, which should lead to a decrease in the use of less adequate combinations, as evidenced by studies in other countries. (Hulgan et al., 2005) The developing software based both on the severity of the effect, and on the probability of occurrence of a specify DI, including quality and quantity of literature that supports the interaction (evidence) in order to establish its clinical relevance, could be a notable contribution to the management of DIs in VIH-infected patients receiving ARV therapy.
Since proprietary databases and clinician assessment of severe DIs do not agree, developing a knowledge base for a DI alert system likely requires proprietary database information in conjunction with clinical opinion. (Smithburger et al., 2010) Thus, evaluation and prediction of relevant clinical DIs involves not only using DI alert system, but also the clinical interpretation of the alert and information, including drug history and the patient's clinical condition. In this task, a computer program that facilitates the evaluation, prediction, and decision on the clinical relevance of the DIs in HIV-infected patients receiving ART therapy have been designed, however its clinical utility requires be assessed in a study designed for this goal.

9. References

Aaron, L.; Saadoun, D.; Calatroni, I.; Launay, O.; Memain, N.; Vincent, V.; et al. (2004). Tuberculosis in HIV-infected patients: A comprehensive review. *Clin Microbiol Infect*, Vol. 10, pp. 388-398, ISSN 1469-0691.

Abel, S.; Jenkins, T.; Whitlock, L.; Ridgway, C. & Muirhead, G. (2008). Effects of CYP3A4 inducers with and without CYP3A4 inhibitors on the pharmacokinetics of maraviroc in healthy volunteers. *Br. J. Clin. Pharmacol*, Vol. 65, No. 1, pp. 38–46, 1365-2125.

Aberg, J. (2008). Drug-drug interactions with newer antiretroviral agents. *Top HIV Med*, Vol.16, pp. 146–150, ISSN 15428826.

Aberg, J.; Rosenkranz, S.; Fichtenbaum, C.; Alston, B.; Brobst, S.; Segal, Y.; et al. (2006). Pharmacokinetic interaction between nelfinavir and pravastatin in HIV-seronegative volunteers: ACTG Study A5108. *AIDS*, Vol. 20, pp. 725-729, ISSN 1473-5571.

Abrams, D.; Hilton, J. & Leiser, R. (2003). Short-term effects of cannabinoids in patients with HIV-1 infection: A randomized, placebo-controlled clinical trial. *Ann Intern Med*, Vol. 139, pp. 258–266, ISSN 1539-3704.

Acosta, E. (2002). Pharmacokinetic enhancement of protease inhibitors. *J Acquir Immune Defic Syndr*, Vol. 29, No. 1, pp. 11-18, ISSN 1525-4135.

AIDS Patient Care. (2005). Antiviral briefs: Pregnancy category change for efavirenz. *AIDS Patient Care STDS* Vol. 19, pp. 413, ISSN 1557-7449.

Altice, F.; Friedland, G. & Cooney, E. (1999). Nevirapine induced opiate withdrawal among injection drug users with HIV infection receiving methadone. *AIDS*, Vol. 13, pp. 957-962, ISSN 1473-5571.

Amariles, P. (2002). Interacciones medicamentosas. En: Amariles P, editor. El medicamento. Compendio básico para su utilización correcta. Medellín: *Impresos LTDA*, pp. 155-246.

Amariles, P. (2007). Food consumption, cytochrome P450 3A4 (CYP3A4) presystemic inhibitors, and bioavailability of saquinavir. *Farm Hosp*, Vol. 31, pp. 68-70, ISSN 1130-6343.

Amariles, P.; Giraldo, N. & Faus, M. (2007a) Clinical relevance of drug interactions. *Med Clin (Barc)*, Vol. 129, pp. 27-35, ISSN 1578-8989.

Amariles, P.; Giraldo, N. & Faus, M. (2007b). Interacciones medicamentosas en pacientes infectados con el VIH: aproximación para establecer y evaluar su relevancia clínica. *Farm Hosp*. Vol. 31, pp. 283-302, ISSN 1130-6343.

Amariles, P.; Giraldo, N.; Faus, M. & Gutiérrez, F. (2008). Proposal of a software for analysis of clinical relevance of antiretroviral drug interactions. *Pharm World Sci*. Vol. 30, pp. 711, ISSN 2210-7711.

Amariles, P.; Lacampa, P. & Sáez-Benito, L. (2007c). Dosage adjustments for hepatic dysfunction *Am J Health Syst Pharm*, Vol. 64, No. 24, pp. 2536-2538, ISSN 1535-2900, December.

Amsay, N.; Kenny, M.; Davies, G. & Patel, J. (2005). Complimentary and alternative medicine use among patients starting warfarin. *Br J Haematol*, Vol. 130, pp. 777-780, ISSN 1365-2141.

Anderson, P. & Kakuda, T. (2006). Comment on: Suboptimal CD4 gains in HIV-infected patients receiving didanosine plus tenofovir. *J Antimicrob Chemother*, Vol. 58, pp. 220-221, ISSN 1460-2091.

Armstrong, S. & Cozza, K. (2003). Pharmacokinetic drug interactions of morphine, codeine, and their derivatives: Theory and clinical reality, Part II. *Psychosomatics*, Vol .44, pp. 515-520, ISSN 1545-7206.

Arrington-Sanders, R.; Hutton, N.; & Siberry, G. (2006). Ritonavir-fluticasone interaction causing Cushing syndrome in HIV-infected children and adolescents. *Pediatr Infect Dis J*, Vol . 25, pp. 1044-1048, ISSN 0891-3668.

Andrews, E.; Glue, P.; Fang, J.; Crownover, P.; Tressler, R. & Damle, B. (2010). Assessment of the pharmacokinetics of co-administered maraviroc and raltegravir. *Br J Clin Pharmacol*, Vol. 69, No. 1, pp. 51-57, ISSN 1365-2125, January.

Antoniou, T.; Park-Wyllie, L. & Tseng, A. (2003). Tenofovir: A nucleotide analog for the management of human immunodeficiency virus infection. *Pharmacotherapy*, Vol. 23, pp. 29-43, ISSN 0277-0008.

Back, D.; Gibbons, S. & Khoo, S. (2003). Pharmacokinetic drug interactions with nevirapine. *J Acquir Immune Defic Syndr*, Vol. 34, No. 1, pp. 8-14, ISSN 1077-9450.

Baker, R. (1998). Efavirenz and Fortovase. *BETA*. Jul:9.

Barreiro, P. & Soriano, V. (2006). Suboptimal CD4 gains in HIV-infected patients receiving didanosine plus tenofovir. *J Antimicrob Chemother*, Vol. 57, pp. 806-809, ISSN 1460-2091.

Bays, H. (2006). Statin safety: An overview and assessment of the data-2005. *Am J Cardiol*, Vol. 97, No. 1, pp. 6-26, ISSN 0029149.

Becher, F.; Landman, R.; Mboup, S.; Kane, C.; Canestri, A.; Liegeois, F.; et al. (2004). Monitoring of didanosine and stavudine intracellular trisphosphorylated anabolite concentrations in HIV-infected patients. *AIDS*, Vol. 18, pp. 181-187, ISSN 1473-5571.

Benator, D.; Weiner, M.; Burman, W.; Vernon, A.; Zhao, Z.; Khan, A. et al. (2007). Clinical evaluation of the nelfinavir-rifabutin interaction in patients with tuberculosis and human immunodeficiency virus infection. *Pharmacotherapy*, Vol. 27, pp. 793-800, ISSN 0277-0008.

Benesic, A.; Zilly, M.; Kluge, F.; Weissbrich, B.; Winzer, R.; Klinker, H.; et al. (2004). Lipid lowering therapy with fluvastatin and pravastatin in patients with HIV infection and antiretroviral therapy: Comparison of efficacy and interaction with indinavir. *Infection*, Vol . 32, pp. 229-233, ISSN 0153-4453.

Bergshoeff, A.; Fraaij, P. & Ndagijimana, J. (2005). Increased dose of lopinavir/ritonavir compensates for efavirenz-induced drug-drug interaction in HIV-1-infected children. *J Acquir Immune Defic Syndr*, Vol. 39, pp. 63-68, ISSN 1077-9450.

Blumberg, H.; Burman, W.; Chaisson, R.; Daley, C.; Etkind, S.; Friedman, L.; et al. (2003). American Thoracic Society/Centers for Disease Control and Prevention/Infectious Diseases Society of America: Treatment of tuberculosis. *Am J Respir Crit CareMed*, Vol. 167, pp. 603-662, ISSN 0003-0805.

Boffito, M.; Carriero, P. & Trentini, L. (2002). Pharmacokinetics of saquinavir co-administered with cimetidine. *J Antimicrob Chemother*, Vol. 50, pp. 1081-1084, ISSN 1460-2091.

Boffito, M.; Maitland, D. & Pozniak, A. (2006). Practical perspectives on the use of tipranavir in combination with other medications: Lessons learned from pharmacokinetic studies. *J Clin Pharmacol*, Vol. 46, pp. 130-139, ISSN 0091-2700.

Boffito, M.; Pozniak, A.; Kearney, B.; Higgs, C.; Mathias, A.; Zhong, L.; et al. (2005). Lack of pharmacokinetic drug interaction between tenofovir disoproxil fumarate and nelfinavir mesylate. *Antimicrob Agents Chemother*, Vol. 49, pp. 4386-4389, ISSN 1098-6569.

Bonate, P.; Reith, K. & Weir, S. (1998). Drug interactions at the renal level. Implications for drug development. *Clin Pharmacokinet*, Vol. 34, pp. 375-404, ISSN 1179-1926.

Borin, M.; Chambers, J.; Carel, B.; Gagnon, S. & Freimuth, W. (1997). Pharmacokinetic study of the interaction between rifampin and delavirdine mesylate. *Clin Pharmacol Ther*, Vol. 61, pp. 544-553, ISSN 1532-6535.

Boubaker, K.; Flepp, M.; Sudre, P.; Furrer, H.; Haensel, A.; Hirschel, B.; et al. (2001). Hyperlactatemia and antiretroviral therapy: The Swiss HIV Cohort Study. *Clin Infect Dis* Vol. 33, pp. 1931-1937, ISSN 1537-6591.

Brennan, P.; Lyus, R.; Harrison, T.; Pakianathan, M. & Macallan, D. (2005). Pharmacokinetic interactions between efavirenz and rifampicin in the treatment of HIV and tuberculosis: One size does not fit all. *AIDS*, Vol. 19, pp. 1541-1543. ISSN 1473-5571.

Brophy, D.; Israel, D.; Pastor, A.; Gillotin, C.; Chittick, G.; Symonds, W.; et al. (2000). Pharmacokinetic interaction between amprenavir and clarithromycin in healthy male volunteers. *Antimicrob Agents Chemother*, Vol. 44, pp. 978-984, ISSN 1098-6596.

Bruce, R.; Altice, F.; Gourevitch, M. & Friedland, G. (2006). Pharmacokinetic drug interactions between opioid agonist therapy and antiretroviral medications: Implications and management for clinical practice. *J Acquir Immune Defic Syndr*, Vol. 41, pp. 563-572, ISSN 1077-9450.

Burger, D.; Agarwala, S.; Child, M; Been-Tiktak, A.; Wang, Y. & Bertz, R. (2006). Effect of rifampicin on steady-state pharmacokinetics of atazanavir with ritonavir in healthy volunteers. *Antimicrob Agents Chemother*, Vol. 50, pp. 3336-3342, ISSN 1098-6596.

Caballero, J. & Nahata, M. (2005). Use of selective serotonin-reuptake inhibitors in the treatment of depression in adults with HIV. *Ann Pharmacother*, Vol. 39, pp. 141-145, ISSN 0012-6667.

Cao, Y.; Smith, P. & Wire, M. (2008). Pharmacokinetics and pharmacodynamics of methadone enantiomers after coadministration with fosamprenavir-ritonavir in opioid-dependent subjects. *Pharmacotherapy*, Vol. 28, pp. 863–874, ISSN 0277-0008.

Catanzaro, L.; Slish, J.; DiCenzo, R. & Morse, G. (2004). Drug interactions with antiretrovirals. *Curr Infect Dis Rep* Vol. 1, pp. 89-96.

Chan, L. (2002). Drug-nutrient interaction in clinical nutrition. *Curr Opin Clin Nutr Metab Care*. Vol. 5, pp. 327-332, ISSN 1473-6519.

Clarke, S.; Mulcahy, F.; Tjia, J.; Reynolds, H.; Gibbons, S.; Barry, M.; et al. (2001). The pharmacokinetics of methadone in HIV-positive patients receiving the non-nucleoside reverse transcriptase inhibitor efavirenz. *Br J Clin Pharmacol*, Vol. 51, pp. 213-217, ISSN 1365-2125.

Coghlan, M.; Sommadossi, J.; Jhala, N.; Many, W.; Saag, M. & Johnson, V. (2001). Symptomatic lactic acidosis in hospitalized antiretroviral treated patients with human immunodeficiency virus infection: A report of 12 cases. *Clin Infect Dis*, Vol. 33, pp. 1914-1921, ISSN 1537-6591.

Colombo, S.; Buclin, T.; Franc, C.; Guignard, N.; Khonkarly, M.; Tarr, P.; et al. (2006). Ritonavir-boosted atazanavir-lopinavir combination: A pharmacokinetic interaction study of total, unbound plasma and cellular exposures. *Antivir Ther* Vol. 11, pp. 53-62, ISSN 2040-2058.

Cooper, K.; Martin, P.; Dane, A.; Warwick, M.; Schneck, D. & Cantarini, M. (2003). Effect of itraconazole on the pharmacokinetics of rosuvastatin. *Clin Pharmacol Ther*, Vol. 73, pp. 322-329, ISSN 0009-9236.

Currier, M.; Molina, G. & Kato, M. (2004). Citalopram treatment of major depressive disorder in Hispanic HIV and *AIDS* patients: A prospective study. Psychosomatics, Vol. 45, pp. 210-216, ISSN 1545-7206.

Cvetkovic, R. & Goa, K. (2003). Lopinavir/ritonavir: A review of its use in the management of HIV infection. *Drugs*, Vol. 63, pp. 769-802, ISSN 0012-6667.

Dagan, T.; Sable, C.; Bray, J. & Gerschenson, M. (2002). Mitochondrial dysfunction and antiretroviral nucleoside analogue toxicities: What is the evidence? *Mitochondrion* Vol. 1, pp. 397-412, ISSN 1567-7249.

Dailly, E.; Allavena, C.; Raffi, F. & Jolliet, P. (2005). Pharmacokinetic evidence for the induction of lopinavir metabolism by efavirenz. *Br J Clin Pharmacol*, Vol. 60, pp. 32-34, ISSN 1365-2125.

Dailly, E.; Tribut, O.; Tattevin, P.; Arvieux, C.; Perré, P.; Raffi, F.; et al. (2006). Influence of tenofovir, nevirapine and efavirenz on ritonavir-boosted atazanavir pharmacokinetics in HIV-infected patients. Eur *J Clin Pharmacol*, Vol. 62, pp. 523-526, ISSN 1432-1041.

Dalakas, M.; Semino-Mora, C. & Leon-Monzon, M. (2001). Mitochondrial alterations with mitochondrial DNA depletion in the nerves of *AIDS* patients with peripheral neuropathy induced by 2′3′dideoxycytidine (ddC). *Lab Invest*, Vol. 81, pp. 1537-1544, ISSN 1530-0307.

Damle, B.; Hess, H.; Kaul, S. & Knupp, C. (2002a). Absence of clinically relevant drug interactions following simultaneous administration of didanosine-encapsulated, enteric-coated bead formulation with either itraconazole or fluconazole. *Biopharm Drug Dispos*, Vol. 23, pp. 59-66, ISSN 0142-2782.

Damle, B.; Mummaneni, V.; Kaul, S. & Knupp, C. (2002b). Lack of effect of simultaneously administered didanosine encapsulated enteric bead formulation (Videx EC) on oral absorption of indinavir, ketoconazole, or ciprofloxacin. *Antimicrob Agents Chemother*, Vol. 46, pp. 385-391, ISSN 1098-6569.

Damle, B.; Yan, J.; Behr, D.; O'Mara, E.; Nichola, P.; Kaul, S.; et al. (2002c). Effect of food on the oral bioavailability of didanosine from encapsulated enteric-coated beads. *J Clin Pharmacol*, Vol. 42, pp. 419-427, ISSN 0091-2700.

Daveluy, A.; Raignoux, C.; Miremont-Salamé, G.; Girodet, P.; Moore, N.; Haramburu, F.; et al. (2009). Drug interactions between inhaled corticosteroids and enzymatic inhibitors. Eur *J Clin Pharmacol*, Vol.65, No. 7, pp. 743-745, ISSN 1432-1041. July

Davis, J.; Schöller-Gyre, M.; Kakuda, T.; Ridgway, C.; Tweedy, S.; Ndongo, N.; et al. (2007). An open, randomized, two period, crossover study in 2 cohorts to investigate the effect of steady state TMC125 and the combination of TMC/darunavir/ritonavir on the steady state pharmacokinetics of oral maraviroc in healthy subjects. 11th European *AIDS* Conference. Madrid, Spain. Oct 24-27. Abstract P4.3/02.

De Jong, B.; Israelski, D.; Corbett, E. & Small, P. (2004). Clinical management of tuberculosis in the context of HIV infection. *Annu Rev Med*, Vol. 55, pp. 283-301, ISSN 0066-4219.

De Maat, M.; Ekhart, G.; Huitema, A.; Koks, C.; Mulder, J. & Beijnen J. (2003). Drug interactions between antiretroviral *Drugs* and comedicated agents. *Clin Pharmacokinet*, Vol. 42; pp. 223-282, ISSN 0312-5963.

DeJesus, E.; Piliero, P.; Summers, K.; Wire, M.; Stein, D.; Masterman, A.; et al. (2006). Interaction between fosamprenavir, with and without ritonavir, and nevirapine in human immunodeficiency virus-infected subjects. *Antimicrob Agents Chemother*, Vol. 50, pp. 3157-3159, ISSN 1098-6569.

DeSilva, K.; Le Flore, D.; Marston, B. & Rimland, D. (2001). Serotonin syndrome in HIV-infected individuals receiving antiretroviral therapy and fluoxetine. *AIDS*, Vol .15, pp. 1281-1285, ISSN 1473-5571.

DHHS. (2005). Panel on Antiretroviral Guidelines for Adult and Adolescents. Guidelines for the use of antiretroviral agents in HIV-infected adults and adolescents. Department of Health and Human Services. In: *AIDS* INFO, 10.01.2011; Available from: http://www.*AIDS*info.nih.gov/contentfiles/AdultandAdolescentGL.pdf. ISBN 1588-080048

DiCenzo, R.; Peterson, D.; Cruttenden, K.; Mariuz, P.; Rezk, N.; Hochreiter, J.; et al. (2008). Effects of minocycline and valproic acid coadministration on atazanavir plasma concentrations in human immunodeficiency virus-infected adults receiving atazanavir-ritonavir. *Antimicrob Agents Chemother*, Vol. 52, pp. 3035–3059, ISSN 0066-4804.

Ding, R.; Tayrouz, Y.; Riedel, K.; Burhenne, J.; Weiss, J.; Mikus, G.; et al. (2004). Substantial pharmacokinetic interaction between digoxin and ritonavir in healthy volunteers. *Clin Pharmacol Ther*, Vol. 76, pp. 73-84, ISSN 1532-6535.

Dixit, V.; Hariparsad, N.; Li, F.; Desai, P.; Thummel, K. & Unadkat J. (2007). Cytochrome P450 enzymes and transporters induced by antihuman immunodeficiency virus protease inhibitors in human hepatocytes: Implications for predicting clinical drug interactions. Drug Metab Dispos, Vol. 35, pp.1853–1859, ISSN 0090-9556.

Droste, J.; Kearney, B.; Hekster, Y. & Burger, D. (2006). Assessment of drug-drug interactions between tenofovir disoproxil fumarate and the nonnucleoside reverse transcriptase inhibitors nevirapine and efavirenz in HIV-infected patients. *J Acquir Immune Defic Syndr*, Vol. 41, pp. 37-43, ISSN 1077-9450.

Droste, J.; Verweij-van, C.; Kearney, B.; Buffels, R.; Vanhorssen, P.; Hekster, Y.; et al. (2005). Pharmacokinetic study of tenofovir disoproxil fumarate combined with rifampin in healthy volunteers. *Antimicrob Agents Chemother*, Vol. 49, pp. 680-684, ISSN 1098-6569.

Etravirine: R165335, TMC 125, TMC-125, TMC125. *Drugs* R & D 2006;7(6):367–73.

FDA. (1999). US Food and Drug Administration. Guidance for Industry: In vivo Drug Metabolism/Drug Interaction Studies - Study Design, Data Analysis, and Recommendations for Dosing and Labeling. Center for Drug Evaluation and Research (CDER), Center for Biologics Evaluation and Research (CBER), Rockville, MD, November 1999.

FDA. (2005). Food and Drug Administration. Title 21, Volume 5: CFR 320.33. Code of Federal Regulations. Available from: http://www.accessdata.fda.gov/scripts/cdrh/cfdocs/cfcfr/CFRSearch.cfm?fr=320.24.

Fellay, J.; Marzolini, C.; Decosterd, L.; Golay, K.; Baumann, P.; Buclin, T.; et al. (2005). Variations of CYP3A activity induced by antiretroviral treatment in HIV-1 infected patients. Eur *J Clin Pharmacol*, Vol. 60, pp 865-873, ISSN 1432-1041.

Fichtenbaum, C. & Gerber J. (2002). Interactions between antiretroviral *Drugs* and *Drugs* used for the therapy of the metabolic complications encountered during HIV infection. *Clin Pharmacokinet*, Vol . 41, pp. 1195-1211, ISSN 84-7666-135-5.

Fichtenbaum, C.; Gerber, J.; Rosenkranz, S.; Segal, Y.; Aberg, J.; Blaschke, T.; et al. (2002). Pharmacokinetic interactions between protease inhibitors and statins in HIV seronegative volunteers: ACTG Study A5047. *AIDS*, Vol . 16, pp. 569-577, ISSN 1473-5571.

Finch, C.; Chrisman, C.; Baciewicz, A. & Self, T. (2002). Rifampin and rifabutin drug interactions: An update. *Arch Intern Med*, Vol. 162, pp. 985-989, ISSN 1538-3679.

Fisher, M.; Talbot, G.; Maislin, G.; McKeon, B.; Tynan, K. & Strom, B. (1989). Risk factors for amphotericin B-associated nephrotoxicity. *Am J Med*, Vol. 87, pp. 547-552.

Fleischer, R.; Boxwell, D. & Sherman, K. (2004). Nucleoside analogues and mitochondrial toxicity. *Clin Infect Dis*, Vol. 38, pp. 79-80, ISSN 1537-6591.

Fletcher, C.; Acosta, E.; Cheng, H.; Haubrich, R.; Fischl, M.; Raasch, R.; et al. (2000). Competing drug-drug interactions among multidrug antiretroviral regimens used in the treatment of HIV- infected subjects: ACTG 884. *AIDS*, Vol. 14, No. 16, pp. 2495-2501, ISSN 1473-5571.

Ford, S.; Wire, M.; Lou, Y.; Baker, K. & Stein DS. (2005). Effect of antacids and ranitidine on the single-dose pharmacokinetics of fosamprenavir. *Antimicrob Agents Chemother*, Vol. 49, pp. 467-469, ISSN 1098-6569.

Ford, J.; Boffito, M.; Maitland, D.; Hill, A.; Back, D.; Khoo, S.; et al. (2006). Influence of atazanavir 200 mg on the intracellular and plasma pharmacokinetics of saquinavir and ritonavir 1600/100 mg administered once daily in HIV-infected patients. *J Antimicrob Chemother*, Vol. 58, pp. 1009-1016, ISSN 1460-2091.

Friedland, G.; Andews, L. & Schreibman, T. (2005). Lack of an effect of atazanavir on steady-state pharmacokinetics of methadone in patients chronically treated for opiate addiction. *AIDS*, Vol. 19, pp. 1635–1641, ISSN 1473-5571.

Friedland, G.; Khoo, S.; Jack, C. & Lalloo, U. (2006). Administration of efavirenz (600 mg/day) with rifampicin results in highly variable levels but excellent clinical outcomes in patients treated for tuberculosis and HIV. *J Antimicrob Chemother*, Vol. 58, pp. 1299-1302. ISSN 1460-2091.

Gaikwad, R.; Sketris, I.; Shepherd, M. & Duffy, J. (2007). Evaluation of accuracy of drug interaction alerts triggered by two electronic medical record systems in primary healthcare. *Health Informatics J*, Vol. 13, pp. 163-177, ISSN 1741-2811.

Gallicano, K.; Sahai, J.; Shukla, V.; Seguin, I.; Pakuts, A.; Kwok, D.; et al. (1999). Induction of zidovudine glucuronidation and amination pathways by rifampicin in HIV-infected patients. *Br J Clin Pharmacol*, Vol. 48, pp. 168-179, ISSN 1365-2125.

Gerber, J.; Rosenkranz, S.; Fichtenbaum, C.; Vega, J.; Yang, A.; Alston, B.; et al. (2005). Effect of efavirenz on the pharmacokinetics of simvastatin, atorvastatin, and pravastatin: Results of AIDS Clinical Trials Group 5108 Study. *J Acquir Immune Defic Syndr*, Vol. 39, pp. 307-312, ISSN 1077-9450.

Giraldo, N.; Amariles, P.; Gutiérrez, F.; Monsalve, M. & Faus, M. (2010). Aproximación para establecer y evaluar la relevancia clínica de las interacciones medicamentosas en pacientes infectados con virus de la inmunodeficiencia humana: actualización 2009. *Farm Hosp*, Vol. 34, pp. 90-93, ISSN 1130-6343.

Gray, D.; Roux, P.; Carrihill, M. & Klein, M. (2010). Adrenal suppression and Cushing's syndrome secondary to ritonavir and budesonide. S Afr Med J, Vol. 100, No. 5, pp. 296-297, ISSN 2078-5131.

Grimes, R.; Lal, L. & Lewis, S. (2002). Frequency of medical history items, drug interactions, and lifestyle characteristics that may interfere with antiretroviral medications. *HIV Clin Trials*, Vol. 3, pp. 161-167, ISSN 1528-4336.

Gruber, V. & McCance-Katz, E. (2010). Methadone, buprenorphine, and street drug interactions with antiretroviral medications. *Curr HIV/AIDS Rep*, Vol. 7, No. 3, pp. 152-160, ISSSN 1548-3576.

Guo, Y. & Fung, H. (2004). Fatal lactic acidosis associated with coadministration of didanosine and tenofovir disoproxil fumarate. *Pharmacotherapy*, Vol. 24, pp. 1089-1094, ISSN 0277-0008.

Hamzeh, F.; Benson, C.; Gerber, J.; Currier, J.; McCrea, J.; Deutsch, P.; et al. (2003). Steady-state pharmacokinetic interaction of modified-dose indinavir and rifabutin. *Clin Pharmacol Ther* Vol. 73, pp. 159-69, ISSN 1532-6535.

Hantson, P.; Di Fazio, V. & Wallemacq, P. (2010). Toxicokinetic interaction between quetiapine and antiretroviral therapy following quetiapine overdose. *Drug Metab Lett*, Vol.4, No. 1, pp.7-8, ISSN 1872-3128.

Hare, C.; Vu, M.; Grunfeld, C. & Lampiris, H. (2002). Simvastatin-nelfinavir interaction implicated in rhabdomyolysis and death. *Clin Infect Dis*, Vol . 35, pp. 111-112, ISSN 1058-4838.

Harris, M.; Zala, C.; Ramírez, S.; Woodfall, B.; Peeters, M.; Scholler, M.; et al. (2006). Pharmacokinetics and safety of adding TMC125 to stable regimens of saquinavir, lopinavir and ritonavir in HIV+adults. 13th Conference on Retroviruses and Opportunistic Infections.Denver (CO). 5-8 Feb. Abstract 575.

Havlir, D.; Tierney, C.; Friedland, G.; Pollard, R.; Smeaton, L.; Sommadossi, J.; et al. (2000). In vivo antagonism with zidovudine plus stavudine combination therapy. *J Infect Dis*, Vol. 182, pp. 321-325, ISSN 1537-6613.

Heck, A.; DeWitt, B. & Lukes, A. (2000). Potential interactions between alternative therapies and warfarin. *Am J Health Syst Pharm*, Vol. 57, pp. 1221-1227, ISSN 1535-2900.

Ho, R. & Kim, R. (2005). Transporters and drug therapy: implications for drug disposition and disease. *Clin Pharmacol Ther*, Vol. 78, pp. 260-277, ISSN 1532-6535.

Hochster, H.; Dieterich, D.; Bozzette, S.; Reichman, R.; Connor, J.; Liebes, L.; et al. (1990). Toxicity of combined ganciclovir and zidovudine for cytomegalovirus disease associated with *AIDS*. An *AIDS* Clinical Trials Group Study. *Ann Intern Med*, Vol. 113, pp. 111-117, ISSN 1539-3704.

Hogeland, G.; Swindells, S.; McNabb, J.; Kashuba, A.; Yee, G. & Lindley, C. (2007). Lopinavir/ritonavir reduces bupropion plasma concentrations in healthy subjects. *Clin Pharmacol Ther* Vol. 81, pp. 69-75, ISSN 1532-6535.

Hoggard, P.; Sales, S.; Phiboonbanakit, D.; Lloyd, J.; Maher, B.; Khoo, S.; et al. (2001). Influence of prior exposure to zidovudine on stavudine phosphorylation in vivo and ex vivo. *Antimicrob Agents Chemother*, Vol. 45, pp. 577-582, ISSN 1098-6569.

Holdich, T.; Shiveley, L. & Sawyer, J. (2007). Effect of Lamivudine on the plasma and intracellular pharmacokinetics of apricitabine, a novel nucleoside reverse transcriptase inhibitor, in healthy volunteers. *Antimicrob Agents Chemother*, Vol. 51. No. 8, pp. 2943-2947, ISNN 1098-6569.

Huang, L.; Wring, S.; Woolley, J.; Brouwer, K.; Serabjit-Singh, C. & Polli, J. (2001). Induction of P-glycoprotein and cytochrome P450 3A by HIV protease inhibitors. *Drug Metab Dispos* Vol. 29, pp. 754-760, ISSN 0090-9556.

Hulgan, T.; Sterling, T.; Daugherty, J.; Arbogast, P.; Raffanti, S. & Ray, W. (2005). Prescribing of contraindicated protease inhibitor and statin combinations among HIV-infected persons. *J Acquir Immune Defic Syndr*, Vol. 38, pp. 277-282, ISSN 1077-9450.

Hughes, C.; Freitas, A. & Miedzinski LJ. (2007). Interaction between lopinavir / ritonavir and warfarin. *CMAJ*, Vol. 177, pp. 357–359, ISSN 1488-2329.

Isbister, G. & Buckley, N. (2005). The pathophysiology of serotonin toxicity in animals and humans. *Clin Neuropharmacol*, Vol. 28, pp. 205-214, ISSN 0362-5664.

Izzedine, H.; Launay-Vacher, V.; Baumelou, A. & Deray, G. (2004). Antiretroviral and immunosuppressive drug-drug interactions: An update. *Kidney Int*, Vol. 66, pp. 532-541, ISSN 1523-1755.

Izzo, A. (2004). Drug interactions with St. John's Wort (Hypericum perforatum): A review of the clinical evidence. Int J *Clin Pharmacol Ther*, Vol. 42, pp. 139-148, ISSN 0174-4879.

Jacobson, T. (2004). Comparative pharmacokinetic interaction profiles of pravastatin, simvastatin, and atorvastatin when coadministered with cytochrome P450 inhibitors. Am J Cardiol, Vol . 94, pp. 1140-1146, ISSN 0029149.

Jain, A.; Venkataramanan, R.; Shapiro, R.; Scantlebury, V.; Potdar, S.; Bonham, C.; et al. (2002). The interaction between antiretroviral agents and tacrolimus in liver and kidney transplant patients. *Liver Transpl*. Vol. 8, pp. 841-845, ISSN 1527-6473.

Josephson, F. (2010). Drug-drug interactions in the treatment of HIV infection: focus on pharmacokinetic enhancement through CYP3A inhibition. *J Intern Med*, Vol. 268, No. 6, pp. 530-539, ISSN 1365-2796, December.

Justesen, U. (2006). Therapeutic drug monitoring and human immunodeficiency virus (HIV) antiretroviral therapy. *Basic Clin Pharmacol Toxicol*, Vol. 98, pp. 20-31, ISSN 1742-7843.

Kakuda, T. & Falcon, R. (2006). Effect of food and ranitidine on saquinavir pharmacokinetics and gastric pH in healthy volunteers. *Pharmacotherapy* Vol. 26, pp. 1060-1068, ISSN 0277-0008.

Kakuda, T.; Schöller-Gyüre, M.; Woodfall, B.; De Smedt, G.; Peeters, M.; Vandermeulen, K.; et al. (2006). TMC125 in combination with other medications: summary of drug-drug interaction studies. 8th International Congress on Drug Therapy in HIV Infection. Glasgow. 12-16 November. Oral presentation PL5.2.

Kashuba, A.; Tierney, C.; Downey, G.; Acosta, E.; Vergis, E.; Klingman, K.; et al. (2005). Combining fosamprenavir with lopinavir/ritonavir substantiallyreduces amprenavir and lopinavir exposure: ACTG protocol A5143 results. *AIDS*, Vol. 19, pp. 145-152, ISSN 1473-5571.

Kashuba, A. (2005). Drug-drug interactions and the *Pharmacotherapy* of HIV infection. Top HIV Med, Vol. 13, pp. 64-69, ISSN 1542-8826.

Katzung, B. (2009). Basic and Clinical Pharmacology. 11th ed. McGraw Hill Medical, ISBN 0071604057.

Kearney, B.; Sayre, J.; Flaherty, J.; Chen, S.; Kaul, S. & Cheng, A. (2005). Drug-drug and drug-food interactions between tenofovir disoproxil fumarate and didanosine. *J Clin Pharmacol*, Vol. 45, pp. 1360-1367, ISSN 0091-2700.

Khaliq, Y.; Gallicano, K., Venance, S.; Kravcik, S. & Cameron, D. (2000). Effect of ketoconazole on ritonavir and saquinavir concentrations in plasma and cerebrospinal fluid from patients infected with human immunodeficiency virus. *Clin Pharmacol Ther*, Vol. 68, pp. 637-646, ISSN 1532-6535.

Kiang, T.; Ensom, M. & Chang, T. (2005). UDP-glucuronosyltransferases and clinical drug-drug interactions. *Pharmacol Ther*, Vol. 106, pp. 97-132, ISSN 0163-7258.

Kiser, J.; Bumpass, J.; Meditz, A.; Anderson, P.; Bushman, L.; Ray, M.; et al. (2010). Effect of antacids on the pharmacokinetics of raltegravir in human immunodeficiency virus-seronegative volunteers. *Antimicrob Agents Chemother*, Vol. 54, No. 12, pp. 4999-5003, ISSN 1098-6569.

Kraft, W.; McCrea, J.; Winchell, G.; Carides, A.; Lowry, R.; Woolf, E.; et al. (2004). Indinavir and rifabutin drug interactions in healthy volunteers. *J Clin Pharmacol*, Vol. 44, pp. 305-313, ISSN 1552-4604.

Krikorian, S. & Rudorf, D. (2005). Drug-drug interactions and HIV therapy: What should pharmacists know? *J Pharm Pract*, Vol. 18, pp. 278-294, ISSN 0897-1900.

La Porte, C.; Colbers, E.; Bertz, R.; Voncken, D.; Wikstrom, K.; Boeree, M.; et al. (2004). Pharmacokinetics of adjusted-dose lopinavir-ritonavir combined with rifampin in healthy volunteers. *Antimicrob Agents Chemother*, Vol. 48, pp. 1553-1560, ISSN 1098-6596.

La Porte, C.; Verweij-van, C.; van Ewijk, N.; Aarnoutse, R.; Koopmans, P.; Reiss, P.; et al. (2005). Pharmacokinetic interaction study of indinavir/ritonavir and the enteric-coated capsule formulation of didanosine in healthy volunteers. *J Clin Pharmacol*, Vol. 45, pp. 211-218, ISSN 0091-2700.

Laganiere, S.; Davies, R.; Carignan, G.; Foris, K.; Goernert, L.; Carrier, K.; et al. (1996). Pharmacokinetic and pharmacodynamic interactions between diltiazem and quinidine. *Clin Pharmacol Ther*, Vol. 60, pp. 255-264, ISSN 1532-6535.

Launay, V.; Izzedine, H.; Karie, S.; Hulot, J.; Baumelou, A. & Deray, G. (2006). Renal tubular drug transporters. *Nephron Physiol*, Vol. 103, pp. 97-106, ISSN 1660-2137.

Lee, L.; Andrade, A. & Flexner, C. (2006). Interactions between natural health products and antiretroviral *Drugs*: Pharmacokinetic and pharmacodynamic effects. *Clin Infect Dis* Vol. 43, pp. 1052-1059, ISSN 1537-6591.

Levêque, D.; Santucci, R.; Pavillet, J.; Herbrecht, R. & Bergerat J. (2009). Paralytic ileus possibly associated with interaction between ritonavir/lopinavir and vincristine. *Pharm World Sci*, Vol. 31, No. 6, pp. 619-621, ISSN 2210-7711.

Lim, M.; Min, S.; Eron, J.; Bertz, R.; Robinson, M.; Gaedigk, A.; et al. (2004). Coadministration of lopinavir/ritonavir and phenytoin results in twoway drug interaction through cytochrome P-450 induction. *J Acquir Immune Defic Syndr*. Vol. 36, pp. 1034-40, ISSN 1077-9450.

Lin, J. & Yamazaki, M. (2003). Role of P-glycoprotein in pharmacokinetics: Clinical implications. *Clin Pharmacokinet*, Vol. 42, pp. 59-98, ISSN 0312-5963.

Lin, J. (2003). Drug-drug interaction mediated by inhibition and induction of P-glycoprotein. *Adv Drug Deliv Rev*, vol. 55, pp. 53-81, ISSN 0169-4092.

Maddox, R.; Groves, W. & Ensom, R. (1980). Automated pharmaceutical assistance systems. I. Clinical pharmacokinetics. II. Drug interference with laboratory tests results. *J Med Syst*, Vol. 4, pp. 151-168, ISSN 0148-5598.

Makinson, A.; Pujol, J.; Le Moing, V.; Peyriere, H. & Reynes J. (2010). Interactions between cytotoxic chemotherapy and antiretroviral treatment in human immunodeficiency virus-infected patients with lung cancer. *J Thorac Oncol*, Vol. 5, No. 4, pp. 562-571, ISSN 1556-1380.

Manosuthi, W.; Sungkanuparph, S.; Thakkinstian, A.; Vibhagool, A.; Kiertiburanakul, S.; Rattanasiri, S.; et al. (2005). Efavirenz levels and 24- week efficacy in HIV-infected patients with tuberculosis receiving highly active antiretroviral therapy and rifampicin. *AIDS*, Vol. 19, pp. 1481-1486, ISSN 1473-5571.

Manosuthi, W.; Kiertiburanakul, S.; Sungkanuparph, S.; Ruxrungtham, K.; Vibhagool, A.: Rattanasiri, S.; et al. (2006). Efavirenz 600 mg/day versus efavirenz 800 mg/day in HIV-infected patients with tuberculosis receiving rifampicin: 48 weeks results. *AIDS* , Vol. 20, pp. 131-132, ISSN 1473-5571.

Markowitz, J. & DeVane, C. (2001). The emerging recognition of herb-drug interactions with a focus on St. John's wort (Hypericum perforatum). *Psychopharmacol Bull*. Vol. 35, pp. 53-64.

Martinez, E.; Milinkovic, A.; de Lazzari, E.; Ravasi, G.; Blanco, J.; Larrousse, M:; et al. (2004). Pancreatic toxic effects associated with co-administration of didanosine and tenofovir in HIV-infected adults. *Lancet*, Vol. 364, pp. 65-67, ISSN 0140-6736.

Masía, M.; Gutiérrez, F.; Padilla, S.; Ramos, J. & Pascual, J. (2005). Severe toxicity associated with the combination of tenofovir and didanosine: Case report and review. *Int J STD AIDS* Vol. 16, pp. 646-648, ISSN 0956-4624.

Matteelli, A.; Regazzi, M.; Villani, P.; De Iaco, G.; Cusato, M.; Carvalho, A.; et al. (2007). Multiple-dose pharmacokinetics of efavirenz with and without the use of rifampicin in HIV-positive patients. *Curr HIV Res*, Vol. 5, pp. 349-353, ISSN 1570-1621.

Mauss, S.; Scholten, S.; Wolf, E.; Berger, F.; Schmutz, G.; Jaeger, H.; et al. (2004). A prospective, controlled study assessing the effect of lopinavir on amprenavir concentrations boosted by ritonavir. *HIV Med*, Vol. 5, pp. 15-17, ISSN ISSN 1542-8826.

McCance-Katz, E.; Moody, D. & Morse, G. (2006). Interactions between buprenorphine and antiretrovirals I: Non-nucleoside reverse transcriptase inhibitors: Efavirenz and delavirdine. *Clin Infect Dis*, Vol. 43, pp. S224–S234, ISSN 1537-6591.

McCance-Katz, E.; Rainey, P. & Friedland G. (2003). The protease inhibitor lopinavir/ritonavir may produce opiate withdrawal in methadone-maintained patients. *Clin Infect Dis*, Vol. 37, pp. 476–482, ISSN 1537-6591.

McCance-Katz, E.; Rainey, P. & Smith, P. (2004). Drug interactions between opioide and antiretroviral medications: Interaction between methadone, LAAM and nelfinavir. *Am J Addict*, Vol.13, pp.163–180, ISSN 1521-0391.

Menard, A.; Solas, C.; Mokthari, S; Bregigeon, S.; Drogoul, M.; Tamalet, C.; et al. (2009). Etravirine- raltegravir, a marked interaction in HIV-1 infected patients: about four cases. *AIDS*, Vol. 23, pp. 869-871, ISSN 1473-5571.

Mildvan, D.; Yarrish, R.; Marshak, A.; Hutman, H.; McDonough, M.; Lamson, M.; et al. (2002). Pharmacokinetic interaction between nevirapine and ethinyl estradiol/norethindrone when administered concurrently to HIV-infected women. *J Acquir Immune Defic Syndr*, Vol. 29, pp. 471-477, ISNN 1077-9450.

Miller, C.; El-Kholi, R-; Faragon, J. & Lodise, T. (2007). Prevalence and risk factors for clinically significant drug interactions with antiretroviral therapy. *Pharmacotherapy*, Vol. 27, No. 10, pp. 1379-1386, ISSN 0277-0008.

Moling, O.; Rimenti, G.; Pristerà, R.; Vedovelli, C.; Pagani, L.; Spoladore, G.; et al. (2009). Fatal lactic acidosis precipitated by nifedipine in a patient treated with disulfiram and antiretrovirals. *Drug Metab Lett*. Vol. 3, No. 3, pp. 176-180, ISSN 1872-3128.

Mouly, S.; Rizzo-Padoin, N.; Simoneau, G.; Verstuyft, C.; Aymard, G.; Salvat, C.; et al. (2006). Effect of widely used combinations of antiretroviral therapy on liver CYP3A4 activity in HIV-infected patients. *Br J Clin Pharmacol*, Vol. 62, pp. 200-209, ISSN 1365-2125.

Mullin, P.; Green, G. & Bakshi, R. (2004). Special populations: The management of seizures in HIV-positive patients. *Curr Neurol Neurosci Rep*, Vol.4, pp.308-14, ISSN: 1534-6293.

Nettles, R.; Kieffer, T.; Parsons, T.; Johnson, J.; Cofrancesco, J.; Gallant, J.; et al. (2006). Marked intraindividual variability in antiretroviral concentrations may limit the utility of therapeutic drug monitoring. *Clin Infect Dis*, Vol. 42, pp. 1189-1196, ISSN 1537-6591.

Obach, R.; Walsky, R.; Venkatakrishnan, K.; Gaman, E.; Houston, J. & Tremaine, L. (2006). The utility of in vitro cytochrome P450 inhibition data in the prediction of drug-drug interactions. *Pharmacol Exp Ther*, Vol. 316, pp. 336-348, ISSN 1521-0103.

Obach, R.; Walsky, R.; Venkatakrishnan, K.; Houston, J. & Tremaine, L. (2005) In vitro cytochrome P450 inhibition data and the prediction of drug-drug interactions:

qualitative relationships, quantitative predictions, and the rank-order approach. *Clin Pharmacol Ther*, Vol. 78, pp. 582-592, ISSN 1532-6535.

Oette, M.; Kurowski, M.; Feldt, T.; Kroidl, A.; Sagir, A.; Vogt, C.; et al. (2005). Impact of rosiglitazone treatment on the bioavailability of antiretroviral compounds in HIV-positive patients. *J Antimicrob Chemother*, Vol. 56, pp. 416-419, ISSN 1460-2091.

Ogbuokiri, J. (2009). Optimizing care for patients on maraviroc salvage therapy. *HIV Clin Summer*, Vol. 21, No. 3, pp. 11-15, ISSN 1551-8850

Oldfield, V. & Plosker, G. (2006). Lopinavir/ritonavir: A review of its use in the management of HIV infection. *Drugs*, Vol. 66, pp. 1275-1299, ISSN 0012-6667.

Ouellet, D.; Hsu, A.; Qian, J.; Locke, C.; Eason, C.; Cavanaugh, J.; et al. (1998). Effect of ritonavir on the pharmacokinetics of ethinyl estradiol in healthy female volunteers. *Br J Clin Pharmacol*, Vol. 46, pp. 111-116, ISSN 1365-2125.

Pau, A. & Boyd, S. (2010). Recognition and management of significant drug interactions in HIV patients: challenges in using available data to guide therapy. *Clin Pharmacol Ther*, Vol. 88, No. 5, pp. 712-719, ISSN 1532-6535.

Penzak, S.; Shen, J.; Alfaro, R.; Remaley, A.; Natarajan, V. & Falloon J. (2004). Ritonavir decreases the nonrenal clearance of digoxin in healthy volunteers with known MDR1 genotypes. *Ther Drug Monit*, Vol. 26, pp. 322-330, ISSN 1536-3694.

Pérez, V.; Sánchez, P. & Villar, S. (2009). Etravirine drug interactions. *Enferm Infecc Microbiol Clin*, Vol. 27, No. 2, pp. 27-31, ISSN 1578-1852.

Perronne, C. (2006). Antiviral hepatitis and antiretroviral drug interactions. *J Hepatol*, Vol. 44, No. 1, pp. 119-125.

Petit, F.; Fromenty, B.; Owen, A. & Estaquier, J. (2005). Mitochondria are sensors for HIV Drugs. *Trends Pharmacol Sci*, Vol. 26, pp. 258-264, ISSN 0165-6147.

Piscitelli, S & Gallicano, K. (2001). Interactions among *Drugs* for HIV and opportunistic infections. *N Engl Med*, Vol . 344, pp. 984-996, ISSN 0028-4793.

Polk, R.; Brophy, D.; Israel, D.; Patron, R.; Sadler, B.; Chittick; G.; et al. (2001). Pharmacokinetic interaction between amprenavir and rifabutin or rifampin in healthy males. *Antimicrob Agents Chemother*, Vol. 45, pp. 502-508, ISSN 1098-6596.

Polk, R.; Crouch, M.; Israel, D.; Pastor, A.; Sadler, B.; Chittick, G.; et al. (1999). Pharmacokinetic interaction between ketoconazole and amprenavir after single doses in healthy men. *Pharmacotherapy*, Vol.19, pp. 1378-1384, ISSN 0277-0008.

Ramachandran, G.; Hemanthkumar, A.; Rajasekaran, S.; Padmapriyadarsini, C.; Narendran, G.; Sukumar, B.; et al. (2006). Increasing nevirapine dose can overcome reduced bioavailability due to rifampicin coadministration. *J Acquir Immune Defic Syndr*, Vol. 42, pp. 36-41. ISSN 1077-9450.

Rathbun, R. & Rossi, D. (2002). Low-dose ritonavir for protease inhibitor pharmacokinetic enhancement. *Ann Pharmacother* Vol. 36, pp. 702-706, ISSN 0012-6667.

Ray, A.; Olson, L. & Fridland, A. (2004). Role of purine nucleoside phosphorylase in interactions between 2′,3′-dideoxyinosine and allopurinol, ganciclovir, or tenofovir. *Antimicrob Agents Chemother* Vol. 48, pp. 1089-1095, ISSN 1098-6569.

Ray, A. (2005). Intracellular interactions between nucleos(t)ide inhibitors of HIV reverse transcriptase. *AIDS* Rev, Vol. 7, pp. 113-125.

Ray, W.; Murray, K.; Meredith, S.; Narasimhulu, S.; Hall, K. & Stein, C. (2004). Oral erythromycin and the risk of sudden death from cardiac causes. *N Engl J Med*, Vol. 351, pp. 1089-1096, ISSN 1533-4406.

Ribera, E.; Azuaje, C.; López, R.; Díaz, M.; Feijoo, M.; Pou, L.; et al. (2006). Atazanavir and lopinavir/ritonavir: Pharmacokinetics, safety and efficacy of a promising double-boosted protease inhibitor regimen. *AIDS*, Vol. 20, pp. 1131-1139, ISSN 1473-5571.

Ribera, E.; Azuaje, C.; López, R.; Domingo, P.; Curran, A.; Feijoo, M.; et al. (2007). Pharmacokinetic interaction between rifampicin and the once-daily combination of saquinavir and low-dose ritonavir in HIV-infected patients with tuberculosis. *J Antimicrob Chemother*, Vol. 59, pp. 690-697, ISSN 1460-2091.

Ribera, E.; Pou, L.; López, R.; Crespo, M.; Falco, V.; Ocaña, I.; et al. (2001). Pharmacokinetic interaction between nevirapine and rifampicin in HIVinfected patients with tuberculosis. *J Acquir Immune Defic Syndr*, Vol. 28, pp. 450-453, ISSN 1077-9450.

Robertson, S.; Penzak, S. & Pau, A. (2005). Drug interactions in the management of HIV infection. *Expert Opin Pharmacother*, Vol. 6, pp. 233-253, ISSN 1744-7666.

Rodríguez, A.; Caraballo, M.; Palma, D.; Santos, B.; Molina, T.; Desongles, T.; et al. (2009). Quality of interaction database management systems. *Farm Hosp*, Vol. 33, pp. 134-146, ISSN 1130-6343.

Rolla, V.; da Silva Vieira, M.; Pereira, P.; Lourenço, M.; de Jesus, C.; Gonçalves, M.; et al. (2006). Safety, efficacy and pharmacokinetics of ritonavir 400 mg/saquinavir 400 mg twice daily plus rifampicin combined therapy in HIV patients with tuberculosis. *Clin Drug Investig*, Vol. 26, pp. 469-479, ISSN 1179-1918.

Romanelli, F. & Pomeroy, C. (2003). Concurrent use of antiretrovirals and anticonvulsants in human immunodeficiency virus (HIV) seropositive patients. *Curr Pharm Des*, Vol.9, pp. 1433-1439, ISSN 1381-6128.

Santos, C. & Boullata, J. (2005). An approach to evaluating drug-nutrient interactions. *Pharmacotherapy*. Vol. 25, pp. 1789-1800, ISSN 0277-0008.

Saraga, M.; Preisig, M. & Zullino, D. (2006). Reduced valproate plasma levels possible after introduction of efavirenz in a bipolar patient. Bipolar Disord, Vol. 8, pp. 415-417, ISSN 1399-5618.

Sax, P. (2006). Strategies for management and treatment of dyslipidemia in HIV/AIDS. *AIDS* Care, Vol . 18, pp. 149-157, ISSN 0954-0121.

Schmidt, G.; Hoehns, J.; Purcell, J.; Friedman, R. & Elhawi, Y. (2007). Severe rhabdomyolysis and acute renal failure secondary to concomitant use of simvastatin, amiodarone, and atazanavir. *J Am Board Fam Med*, Vol. 20, pp. 411–416, ISSN 1558-7118.

Schöller, M.; Woodffall, B.; De Marez, T.; De Smedt, G.; Peeters, M.; Vandermeulen, K.; et al. (2006). Pharmacokinetics of TMC125 with atazanavir and atazanavir/ritonavir. 8th Internacional Congress on Drug Therapy in HIV Infection. Glasgow. Nov 12-16, Abstract P278.

Schöller-Gyüre, M.; Kakuda, T.; De Smedt, G.; Vanaken, H.; Bouche, M.; Peeters, M.; et al. (2008). A pharmacokinetic study of etravirine (TMC125) co-administered with ranitidine and omeprazole in HIV–negative volunteers. *Br J Pharmacol*, Vol. 66, pp. 508-516, ISSN 1476-5381.

Schöller-Gyüre, M.; Kakuda, T.; De Smedt, G.; Woodfall, B.; Bollen, S.; Peeters, M.; et al. (2007). Pharmacokinetic interaction between the non-nucleoside reverse transcriptase inhibitor TMC125 and atorvastatin in HIV-negative volunteers. 4th

International *AIDS* Society Conference on HIV Pathogenesis, Treatment and Prevention. Sydney. 22-25 Jul. Abstract WEPEA 106.

Schöller-Gyüre, M.; Woodfall, B.; Debroye, C.; De Marez, T.; Peeters, M.; Vandermeulen, K.; et al. (2006). Pharmacokinetic interaction between TMC125 and rifabutin. 44th Annual Meeting of the Infectious Diseases Society of America. Toronto. 12-15 Oct. Abstract 963

Sekar, V.; De Pauw, M. & Mariën, K. (2007a). Pharmacokinetic interaction between TMC114/r and efavirenz in healthy volunteers. *Antivir Ther,* Vol. 12, No. 4, pp. 509–514, ISSN 2040-2058.

Sekar, V.; Lefebvre, E. & Boogaerts, G. (2006a). Pharmacokinetic interaction between the protease inhibitors TMC114 and lopinavir/ritonavir. 46th Interscience Conference on Antimicrobial Agents and Chemotherapy, Sep 27-30, San Francisco (CA), abstract no. A-367.

Sekar, V.; Lefebvre, E.; De Marez, T.; De Pauw, M.; De Paepe, E.; Vangeneugden, T.; et al. (2008). Effect of repeated doses of darunavir plus low-dose ritonavir on the pharmacokinetics of sildenafil in healthy male subjects: phase I randomized, open-label, two-way crossover study. *Clin Drug Investig,* Vol. 28, No. 84, pp. 79-85, ISSN 1179-1918.

Sekar, V.; Lefebvre, E. & De Paepe, E.; et al. (2007b). Pharmacokinetic interaction between darunavir boosted with ritonavir and omeprazole or ranitidine in human immunodeficiency virus-negative healthy volunteers. *Antimicrob Agents Chemother,* Vol. 51, No. 3, pp. 958–961, ISSN 1098-6569, March.

Sekar, V.; Lefebvre, E. & Mariën, K. (2006b). Pharmacokinetic interaction between the HIV protease inhibitors TMC114 and saquinavir, in the presence of low-dose ritonavir. 44th Annual Meeting of the Infectious Disease Society of America, Oct 12-15; Toronto (ON). abstract no. 959.

Sekar, V.; Lavreys, L; Van de Casteele, T; Berckmans, C.; Guzman, S.; Vangeneugden, T.; et al. (2010). Pharmacokinetics of darunavir/ritonavir and rifabutin coadministered in HIV-negative healthy volunteers. *Antimicrob Agents Chemother,* Vol. 54, No. 10, pp. 4440-4445, ISSN 1098-6569.

Setzer, B.; Lebrecht, D. & Walker, U. (2008). Pyrimidine nucleoside depletion sensitizes to the mitochondrial hepatotoxicity of the reverse transcriptase inhibitor stavudine. *Am J Pathol.* Vol. 172, No. 3, pp. 681-690.

Shriner, K. & Goetz, M. (1992). Severe hepatotoxicity in a patient receiving both acetaminophen and zidovudine. *Am J Med,* Vol. 93, pp. 94-96.

Simpson, D. & Tagliati, M. (1995). Nucleoside analogue associated peripheral neuropathy in human immunodeficiency virus infection. *J Acquir Immune Defic Syndr Hum Retrovirol,* Vol. 9, pp. 153-161.

Smithburger, P.; Kane-Gill, S.; Benedict, N.; Falcione, B. & Seybert, A. (2010). Grading the severity of drug-drug interactions in the intensive care unit: a comparison between clinician assessment and proprietary database severity rankings. *Ann Pharmacother.* Vol. 44, No. 11, pp. 1718-1724, ISSN 0012-6667.

Solas, C.; Poizot-Martin, I.; Drogoul, M.; Ravaux, I.; Dhiver, C.; Lafeuillade, A.; et al. (2004). Therapeutic drug monitoring of lopinavir/ritonavir given alone or with a non-nucleoside reverse transcriptase inhibitor. *Br J Clin Pharmacol,* Vol. 57, pp. 436-440, ISSN 1365-2125.

Spradling, P.; Drociuk, D.; McLaughlin, S.; Lee, L.; Peloquin, C.; Gallicano, K.; et al. (2002). Drug-drug interactions in inmates treated for human immunodeficiency virus and Mycobacterium tuberculosis infection or disease: An institutional tuberculosis outbreak. *Clin Infect Dis*, Vol. 35, pp. 1106-1112, ISSN 1537-6591.

Steele, M.; Burk, R. & DesPrez, R. (1991). Toxic hepatitis with isoniazide and rifampin: A meta-analysis. *Chest*, Vol. 99, pp. 465-71, ISSN 1931-3543.

Stocker, H.; Kruse, G. & Kreckel, P. (2004). Nevirapine significantly reduces the levels of racemic methadone and (R)-methadone in human immunodeficiency virus-infected patients. *Antimicrob Agents Chemother*, Vol. 48, pp. 4148-4153, ISSN 1098-6569.

Sudano, I.; Spieker, L.; Noll, G.; Corti, R.; Weber, R. & Luscher, T. (2006). Cardiovascular disease in HIV infection. *Am Heart J*, Vol . 151, pp. 1147-1155, ISSN 0002-8703.

Taburet, A.; Piketty, C.; Chazallon, C.; Vincent, I.; Gerard, L.; Calvez, V:; et al. (2004). Interactions between atazanavir-ritonavir and tenofovir in heavily pretreated human immunodeficiency virus-infected patients. *Antimicrob Agents Chemother*, Vol. 48, pp. 2091-2096, ISSN 1098-6569.

Taburet, A.; Raguin, G.; Le Tiec, C.; Droz, C.; Barrail, A.; Vincent, I.; et al. (2004). Interactions between amprenavir and the lopinavir-ritonavir combination in heavily pretreated patients infected with human immunodeficiency virus. *Clin Pharmacol Ther*, Vol 75, pp. 310-323, ISSN 1532-6535.

Tibotec (2008). Prezista® (darunavir) tablet: US prescribing information. Raritan (NJ), 25.03.2009 Available from:
http://www.prezista.com/prezista/documents/us_package_insert.pdf

Tomilo, D.; Smith, P.; Ogundele, A.; Difrancesco, R.; Berenson, C.; Eberhardt, E.; et al. (2006). Inhibition of atazanavir oral absorption by lansoprazole gastric acid suppression in healthy volunteers. *Pharmacotherapy*, vol. 26, pp. 341-436, ISSN 0277-0008.

Tong, L.; Phan, T.; Robinson, K.; Babusis, D.; Strab, R.; Bhoopathy, S.; et al. (2007). Effects of human immunodeficiency virus protease inhibitors on the intestinal absorption of tenofovir disoproxil fumarate in vitro. *Antimicrob Agents Chemother*, Vol.51, pp. 3498–3504, ISSN 1098-6596.

Touzot, M.; Beller, C.; Touzot, F.; Louet, A. & Piketty, C. (2006). Dramatic interaction between levothyroxine and lopinavir/ritonavir in a HIV-infected patient. *AIDS*, Vol. 20, pp. 1210-1212, ISSN 1473-5571.

Tran, J.; Gerber, J. & Kerr, B. (2001). Delavirdine: Clinical pharmacokinetics and drug interactions. *Clin Pharmacokinet*, Vol. 40, pp. 207-226, ISSN 0312-5963.

Tran, J.; Petersen, C.; Garrett, M.; Hee, B. & Kerr, B. (2002). Pharmacokinetic interaction between amprenavir and delavirdine: Evidence of induced clearance by amprenavir. *Clin Pharmacol Ther*, Vol. 72, pp. 615-626, ISSN 1532-6535.

Tseng, A.; Nguyen, M.; Cardella, C.; Humar, A & Conly, J. (2002). Probable interaction between efavirenz and cyclosporine. *AIDS*, Vol. 16, pp. 505-506, ISSN 1473-5571.

Tseng, A. & Foisy M. (1999). Significant interactions with new antiretrovirals and psychotropic *Drugs. Ann Pharmacother*, Vol. 33, pp. 461-473, ISSN 0012-6667.

Tseng, A. & Salit, I. (2007). CD4+ cell count decline despite HIV suppression: A probable didanosine-valganciclovir interaction. *Ann Pharmacother*, Vol. 41, pp. 512-517, ISSN 0012-6667.

Tucker, G.; Houston, J. & Huang, S. (2001). Optimizing drug development: strategies to assess drug metabolism/transporter interaction potential-toward a consensus. *Clin Pharmacol Ther*, Vol. 70, pp. 103-114, ISSN 1532-6535.

Van der Lee, M.; Dawood, L.; Hofstede, H.; Graaff-Teulen, M.; Ewijk-Beneken, Caliskan, N.; et al. (2006). Lopinavir/ritonavir reduces lamotrigine plasma concentrations in healthy subjects. *Clin Pharmacol Ther*, Vol. 80, pp. 159-168, ISSN 1532-6535.

Vogel, M.; Voigt, E.; Michaelis, H.; Sudhop, T.; Wolff, M.; Turler, A.; et al. (2004). Management of drug-to-drug interactions between cyclosporine A and the protease-inhibitor lopinavir/ritonavir in liver-transplanted HIV-infected patients. *Liver Transpl*, Vol 10, pp. 939-944, ISSN 1524-6473.

Von, L.; Greenblatt, D.; Duan, S.; Daily, J.; Harmatz, J. & Shader, R. (1998). Inhibition of desipramine hydroxylation (Cytochrome P450-2D6) in vitro by quinidine and by viral protease inhibitors: Relation to drug interactions in vivo. *J Pharm Sci*, Vol. 87, pp. 1184-1189, ISSN 1520-6017.

Vourvahis, M. & Kashuba, A. (2007). Mechanisms of pharmacokinetic and pharmacodynamic drug interactions associated with ritonavirenhanced tipranavir. *Pharmacotherapy*, Vol. 27, pp.888-909, ISSN 0277-0008.

Weiner, M.; Benator, D.; Peloquin, C.; Burman, W.; Vernon, A.; Engle, M.; et al. (2005). Evaluation of the drug interaction between rifabutin and efavirenz in patients with HIV infection and tuberculosis. *Clin Infect Dis*,Vol.41, pp. 1343-1349. ISSN 1537-6591.

Wertheimer, B.; Freedberg, K.; Walensky, R.; Yazdanapah, Y. & Losina, E. (2006). Therapeutic drug monitoring in HIV treatment: A literature review. *HIV Clin Trials*, Vol. 7, pp. 59-69, ISSN 1528-4336.

Winston, A.; Back, D.; Fletcher, C.; Robinson, L.; Unsworth, J.; Tolowinska, I.; et al. (2006). Effect of omeprazole on the pharmacokinetics of saquinavir-500 mg formulation with ritonavir in healthy male and female volunteers. *AIDS*, Vol. 20, pp. 1401-1406, ISSN 1473-5571.

Winston, A. & Boffito, M. (2005). The management of HIV-1 protease inhibitor pharmacokinetic interactions. *J Antimicrob Chemother*, Vol . 56, pp. 1- 5, ISSN 0305-7453.

Wire, M.; Shelton, M. & Studenberg S. (2006). Fosamprenavir: Clinical pharmacokinetics and drug interactions of the amprenavir prodrug. *Clin Pharmacokinet*, Vol . 45, pp. 137-168, ISSN 0312-5963.

Wittkop, L.; Breilh, D.; DaSilva, D.; Duffau, P.; Mercié, P.; Raymond, I.; et al. (2009). Virological and immunological response in HIV-1-infected patients with multiple treatment failures receiving raltegravir and optimized background therapy, ANRS CO3 Aquitaine Cohort. *J Antimicrob Chemother*, Vol. 63, 1251-1255, ISSN 1460-2091.

Yee, D.; Valiquette, C.; Pelletier, M.; Parisien, I.; Rocher, I. & Menzies, D. (2003). Incidence of serious side effects from first-line antituberculosis *Drugs* among patients treated for active tuberculosis. *Am J Respir Crit Care Med*, Vol. 167, pp. 1472-1477.

Young, B. (2005). Review: Mixing new cocktails: Drug interactions in antiretroviral regimens. *AIDS Patient Care STDS*, Vol. 19, pp. 286-297, ISSN 1557-7449.

Zeldin, R. & Petruschke, R. (2004). Pharmacological and therapeutic properties of ritonavir-boosted protease inhibitor therapy in HIV-infected patients. *J Antimicrob Chemother*, Vol. 53, pp. 4-9, ISSN 1460-2091.

Zhou, S.; Chan, E.; Pan, S.; Huang, M. & Lee, E. (2004). Pharmacokinetic interactions of *Drugs* with St John's wort. *J Psychopharmacol*, Vol. 18, pp. 262-276, ISSN 1461-7285.

15

Exploring the Nanotechnology-Based Drug Delivery Systems for AIDS Treatment

Flávia Chiva Carvalho[1], Rubiana Mara Mainardes[2] and Maria Palmira Daflon Gremião[1]
[1]*School of Pharmaceutical Sciences, State University of São Paulo, UNESP, Araraquara,*
[2]*State University of West-Center, UNICENTRO, Guarapuava,*
Brazil

1. Introduction

The Acquired Immunodeficiency Syndrome (AIDS) and Human Immunodeficiency Virus (HIV) infection are a worldwide public health challenge. The emergence of antiretroviral therapy agents has significantly increased the life expectancy and the patient´s quality of life. In the 1990's, there was a great improvement in the knowledge of the disease, enlargement of therapeutic resources, a rise in life expectancy and the epidemiologic profile. Since the mid-1990's, the advancement of pharmacology studies and the arrival of protease inhibitor antiretroviral have given rise to a new era of anti-HIV agents, known as Highly Active Antiretroviral Therapy (HAART) (Geocze et al., 2010, Richman et al., 2009). The HAART's adhesion improved the clinical results, the control of the advancement of the disease and decreased the mortality rate, which resulted in an improvement of the patient's life quality. Despite the successful administration of HAART, latently infected cells can escape the viral immune response and persist for long periods of time (Alexaki et al., 2008). In addition, the HAART presents several collateral effects, such as fatigue, nausea, sickness, diarrhea and lipodystrophy. These symptoms contribute to a lack of treatment adhesion in the patient, resulting in a rise in the blood viral load and a decline in CD4+ T cells count, as well as an increased tolerance of anti-HIV drugs, treatment failure, increased opportunistic infections and in wasted investments (Geocze et al., 2010). Moreover, many antiretroviral drugs undergo extensive pre-systemic metabolism and instability in the gastrointestinal environment, resulting in inadequate and erratic oral absorption as well as low bioavailability. The half-life for most anti-HIV drugs is short, and thus, it requires frequent dosage administrations, leading to a decrease in patient compliance. Also, some antiretroviral classes present poor solubility, low absorption and limited bioavailability. Another limitation of the current HAART is the inefficiency of the regimens to eradicate HIV from various anatomical reservoirs (e.g., central nervous system (CNS) and gastrointestinal tract) and intracellular sites (e.g., macrophages, hepatocytes, dendritic cells and Langerhans cells) (Ojewole et al., 2008, Saksena & Haddad, 2003). Large concentrations are essential for eliminating HIV from these reservoirs to achieve the desired therapeutic effect, but these large doses contribute to severe side effects associated with anti-HIV therapy (Ojewole et al., 2008). Because drug development in the HIV field has slowed

(Hawkins, 2010), strategies currently being investigated to overcome these limitations include the design and development of novel drug delivery systems that can improve the efficacy of both existing and novel antiretroviral drugs (Ojewole et al., 2008). With the aim to reduce dosing frequency and to improve the compliance of the existing pharmacotherapy with patients, drug delivery system design is becoming complementary to new drug discovery (Sosnik et al., 2009). In the past decade, there has been an explosion of interest in the development of anti-HIV delivery systems (Ojewole et al., 2008). Evidence of this new interest is the emergence of several revision papers that have focused attention to the development of anti-HIV delivery systems, which have been published in the last two years (Geocze et al., 2010; Gupta & Jain, 2010; Hawkins, 2010; Neves et al., 2010; Sosnik et al., 2009, Wong et al., 2010, Khalil et al., 2011).

There is a special trend in research concerning the development of anti-HIV drug delivery systems, which apply nanotechnology to improve AIDS treatment. The basic concept behind the use of nanotechnology-based systems for antiretroviral drug delivery is the ability of these systems to compartmentalize as well as modify the properties and behavior of drugs in the biological medium. Through drug association with nanostructured systems, the properties that govern drug release are determined by the physicochemical properties of the nanosystems and not by the drug properties (Neves et al., 2010). These properties can include the protection of incorporated drugs from the metabolism, an increase of drug residence time in the human body and the possibility of targeting drugs to specific cells or organs. In addition, these properties can allow a dosage reduction, more appropriate dosage regimens, fewer adverse effects and increased patient compliance. Moreover, there is the possibility of incorporating different anti-HIV drugs in the same delivery system, which can also contribute to a simplification of drug administration schedules (Neves et al., 2010).

Despite the improvement of the nanotechnology-based studies, many of them are still in the pre-formulation or pre-clinical phases. However, the potential of nanotechnology-based drug delivery systems to improve AIDS treatment is evident. Thus, the goal of the current chapter is to organize a systematic review about this area of study. Particular emphasis was placed on surfactant and nanoparticulated systems. The surfactant systems are formed by amphiphilic compounds and include several types of arrangements; these systems self-organize with different physicochemical properties, which can be used to design new drug delivery systems. The most popular surfactant system that incorporates antiretroviral drugs are the liposomes (Zidan et al., 2010; Clayton et al., 2009; Kaur et al., 2008); however, anti-HIV drugs were also found to be associated with microemulsions (Vyas et al., 2008), polymeric micelles (Chiappetta et al. 2010; Kaparissides et al., 2006), self-assembled drug delivery systems (Jin et al., 2010) and liquid crystals (Carvalho et al., 2010a). In addition to surfactant systems, polymeric nanoparticles have been extensively studied as nanometric carriers, and these carriers presenting different morphologies, including nanospheres or nanocapsules. In this document, these are referred to as polymeric nanoparticles (Mainardes et al., 2010; Sharma & Garg, 2010, Schäfer et al., 1992, Shah & Amiji, 2006, Destache et al., 2009, Mahajan et al., 2009) and solid lipid nanoparticles (Aji Alex et al., 2010; Kuo & Chen, 2009; Shegokara et al., 2010). The advantages and limitations of each system are discussed, thus, this work can be used as a start point for researchers focusing on nanotechnology-based drug delivery systems for the treatment of AIDS.

2. Surfactant systems

Surfactants are extensively used as excipients in drug delivery and the understanding of the physicochemical properties and behavior of these amphiphilic compounds has undergone significant development. One reason for this development is that surface chemistry is a relatively young scientific discipline, and many studies have recognized its importance for the design and controlled use of drug delivery formulations (Malmsten, 2002). The surfactant systems comprise several types of arrangements, and they self-organize with different physicochemical properties that can be used to design new drug delivery systems that are able to solubilize both water-soluble and oil-soluble compounds. Depending on the composition and molecules of the component, surfactant systems can infinitely dilute or form highly stiff matrices, both in physiological conditions. Due the capacity of surfactant systems, which can form viscous and gel-like structures with different rheological characteristics, these systems are extremely versatile and can be delineated to be applied for different routes of administration, e.g., transdermal or mucosal administration, such as vaginal, nasal, rectal and sublingual. However, almost all studies aim oral administration, where anti-HIV drugs are associated in microemulsions, polymeric micelles, self-assembled drug delivery systems, liquid crystals and liposomes. Liposomes, contrary to the other surfactant organizations, have been widely explored for orally administered anti-HIV drugs. Although the oral route is still the primary mode of delivery for antiretroviral surfactant systems, they were found to be a suitable vehicle for anti-HIV intravenous and mucosal administration (described below).

2.1 Microemulsions

Microemulsions are systems consisting of water, oil, and surfactant(s), which constitute a single optically isotropic and thermodynamically stable liquid dispersion. Such systems are useful for drug delivery due to their excellent stability, ease of preparation, optical clarity, as well as their capacity to dissolve hydrophilic and lipophilic drugs, frequently in high amounts. Microemulsions differ from emulsions and nanoemulsions because of their thermodynamic stability; these systems form spontaneously, exhibit reduced droplets sizes (typically 10–100 nm) (Malmsten, 2002), higher surface areas and free energy without the inherent creaming, flocculation, coalescence and sedimentation associated with emulsions (Gupta & Jain, 2010). Thus, microemulsions are considered to be an interesting possibility for anti-HIV drug delivery systems (Gupta & Jain, 2010). Carvalho et al. (2009) developed and characterized PPG-5-CETETH-20/oleic acid/water zidovudine-loaded microemulsions; the in vitro drug release assay showed that the drug release followed the Fickian diffusion through a disordered matrix, and the mechanism was identified by the use of Weibull mathematical model. Vyas et al. (2008), investigated the oral bioavailability of saquinavir incorporated in oil-in-water microemulsions in the study of enhanced brain disposition, a potential sanctuary site for HIV. Pharmacokinetics parameters were found to be higher in the brain, suggesting an enhanced rate and extended saquinavir absorption following oral administration of microemulsions. Thus, microemulsions may be very promising for HIV/AIDS therapy, in particular, for reducing the viral load in important anatomical reservoir sites (Vyas et al., 2008).

2.2 Polymeric micelles

Polymeric micelles are nanostructures that have been utilized for improving aqueous solubility, mucosal permeability and disease-site targeting of several drug molecules.

Compared to the conventional surfactant based micelles, polymeric micelles are composed of block copolymers. Although the structural "core-shell" arrangement is similar to surfactant-based micelles, polymer micelles self associate at much lower concentrations. Consequently, the thermodynamic and in vivo stability of polymeric micelles is relatively high (Sharma & Garg, 2010). A study by Chiappeta et al. (2010) showed that the solubility of efavirenz, a lipophilic first-line antiretroviral drug, could be improved. Micellar systems composed of N-methylated and N-alkylated poloxamines (X-shaped poly(ethylene oxide)-poly(propylene oxide, PEO-PPO) diblocks connected to a central ethylenediamine group), were investigated to optimize the oral pharmacotherapy effects of efavirenz. The in vitro release was sustained for at least 24 h. The authors suggested that the polymeric micelles could be promising nanocarriers for oral or parenteral drug delivery. The aqueous solubility of the drug was increased from 0.004 mg/mL to approximately 30 mg/mL, representing the best solubilization performance in an aqueous medium of any nanocarrier described thus far (Chiappetta et al. 2010). Other characteristics of polymeric micelles present the possibility for substitution of the block copolymer micelles with specific ligands, which is a very promising strategy for a broader range of sites of activity with a considerably higher selectivity (Kaparissides et al., 2006). Micelles can be tailored by attaching hydrophilic blocks to antibodies or other ligands specific for the type of receptors present within the disease site. Lectin receptors are present on HIV reservoirs, such as T lymphocytes, dendritic cells and macrophages; therefore, this can be a promising approach for viral reservoir targeting (Sharma & Garg, 2010).

2.3 Self-assembled drug delivery systems of antiretroviral prodrugs

A novel technology involving antiretroviral prodrugs with amphiphilic properties have been developed by Jin and co-workers (Jin et al., 2008, 2009, 2010). The molecular self-assembly properties of those prodrugs in aqueous media permit the formation of nanostructures with amphiphilic characteristics, allowing them to cross biomembranes and deliver themselves in vivo without carriers (Jin et al., 2008). Recently, a series of cholesteryl derivatives of antiviral nucleoside analogues were synthesized by this group, which involved acyclovir, zidovudine and didanosine. The morphologies and the morphological transformation of cholesterylsuccinyl didanosine was investigated as a prodrug with representative self-assembly behavior in aqueous media. Results showed that the resulted nanoparticulate system had a narrow size distribution, which allowed heat sterilization and showed a site-specific distribution for the anti-HIV therapy after IV administration (Jin et al., 2008). Another example of this technology was the synthesis of the amphiphilic prodrug anti-HIV zidovudine, cholesteryl-phosphonyl zidovudine. This system degraded quickly in biological environments and showed high anti-HIV activity; in addition, the system targeted the mononuclear phagocyte system (MPS) and was followed by degradation at the targeted organs (Jin et al., 2009). Furthermore, a study was recently published on the synthesis of an amphiphilic prodrug containing dual zidovudine (Jin et al., 2010). The stable and concentrated vesicular self-assemblies were prepared through injecting the prodrug solution into water followed by adding stabilizers and removing solvents. Properties, such as their nanoscale size, stability, anti-HIV activity and macrophage targeting effects, have demonstrated that the prodrug is a promising self assembled drug delivery system. Moreover, this kind of system containing different drugs would benefit a combination therapy for AIDS treatment (Jin et al., 2010).

2.4 Liquid cristal

Liquid crystals combine the properties of both liquid and solid states. They can be made to form a range of different nanostructures, including rods, lamellae, and bicontinuously interconnected structures, with alternative polar and non-polar layers, where aqueous drug solutions can be included. (Kaparissides et al., 2006; Malmsten, 2001). The spontaneous self-assembly of some lipids used to form liquid crystalline structures can offer a potentially new class of sustained release matrices. Depending to the liquid crystalline materials, they can be highly stable to dilution, which means they can persist as a reservoir for slow drug release in excess fluids, such as the gastrointestinal tract or subcutaneous regions. Drug release rates are directly related to the nanostructure of the matrix. The particular geometry into which the lipids assemble can be manipulated through either the use of additives to modify the assembly process or through modifying conditions, such as temperature (Boyd, 2010). The structure-forming lipids can absorb a certain amount of water and then spontaneously form gel-like phases with unique internal structures into which drugs can be incorporated. Moreover, non-toxic, biodegradable and bioadhesive properties also contribute to their applications towards drug delivery (Guo et al., 2010). Liquid crystal phases have been found to be mucoadhesive, with a range of mucosal surfaces; and the mechanism of mucoadhesion probably involves the rheological properties of the system, which are similar to the in situ gelling vehicles. These liquid crystal systems can be arranged in a very strong and viscous matrix that favors the mucosal retention, impeding the immediate removal of the formulation by the mucociliary clearance (Carvalho et al., 2010b). This property was used by Carvalho et al. (2010a) to develop a mucoadhesive surfactant system for the nasal administration of zidovudine. The nasal route has been explored to avoid the extensive, first-pass metabolism and poor oral bioavailability of drugs that suffer hepatic metabolism or gastric degradation when administered by the oral route. Thus, the nasal route is an option for enhancing the therapeutic efficacy of drugs and to reduce the extent of their first-pass effect because this route is highly vascular and has a great superficial area of absorption. However, there are some mechanisms that limit the intranasal absorption, such as the mucociliary clearance, which rapidly removes the formulation from the nasal cavity. Systems composed of PPG-5-CETETH-20 as surfactant, oleic acid and water have shown to display phase transition to the lamellar phase when put in contact with the aqueous nasal-simulated mucus (SM). The phase transition was accompanied by an increase in the system's elasticity, in addition to the presentation of suitable mucoadhesive force. Thus, a viscous and mucoadhesive liquid crystalline matrix can be formed when the formulations are in contact with the SM, which may prolong the residence time of zidovudine in the nasal cavity. These findings indicate a potentially useful system for the nasal administration of zidovudine (Carvalho et al., 2010a).

2.5 Liposomes

Liposomes can be defined as associations of colloidal amphipathic lipids that spontaneously arrange themselves in closed structures, such as spherical shells containing aqueous cores. The unique aspect of the liposomes is that the hydrophilic drugs can be encapsulated in the aqueous layer, while the hydrophobic drugs can be incorporated into the phospholipid bilayer. They can range in size from 25 nm up to several microns, and liposomes are prepared from natural or synthetic phospholipids and cholesterol; in addition, they may include other substances, such as lipids and proteins (Sharma & Sharma, 1997). Conventional liposomes (without surface modification) are naturally taken up by cells of the

MPS, an important HIV reservoir. Additionally, the liposome surface can be modified to improve its properties. Ligands that promote active targeting of liposomes to HIV-infected cells and organs are interesting alternatives. Liposomes represent a convenient approach to improve the delivery of anti-HIV agents into infected cells, thereby improving the efficacy of drugs and reducing their adverse side effects (Desormeaux et al., 1998).

Monocytes/macrophages (M/Ms) are widely recognized as the secondary cellular target of HIV-1 and a crucial virus reservoir. HIV-1-infected M/Ms cells are widely distributed in all tissues and organs, including the CNS, and the HIV-1 replication in these cells is a crucial pathogenic event during the progression of viral infection. Also, M/Ms are resistant to the cytopathic effect of HIV-1 and produce viruses over a prolonged period, consisting of a long-term viral reservoir (Gartner et al., 1986; Garaci et al., 1999).

The primary research studies involving the application of liposomes in AIDS treatment are based in in vitro and in vivo (animals) experiments that consider the ability of liposomes to increase the intracellular delivery of antiretroviral drugs. The most popular drugs studied are zalcitabine, zidovudine, didanosine, stavudine and indinavir. One of the first studies that introduced the application of liposomes as carriers for anti-HIV drugs was realized by Szebeni and co-workers (1990). The group suggested that the capability of liposomes for targeting drugs in vivo to macrophages could potentially be exploited to improve the therapeutic index of dideoxynucleoside drugs. They also demonstrated the antiviral effects of 2',3'-dideoxycytidine-5'-triphosphate-loaded liposomes in cultured human M/Ms infected with HIV-1 and the higher drug stability in presence of liposome. Another study involving 2',3'-dideoxycytidine (zalcitabine) showed that the anionic character of the liposome seemed to be an important factor to obtain a high intracellular uptake. The lipid component can interfere in interactions between the cell and the liposome (Makabi-Panzu et al., 1998).

After the discovery of the zidovudine associated hematotoxicity (Ganser et al., 1989), the effect of liposome encapsulation on the bone marrow toxicity and antiviral activity of zidovudine in mice was determined by the Phillips group (1991, 1992). The results showed that zidovudine encapsulated in liposomes exhibited no bone marrow toxicity at doses that were cytotoxic with zidovudine solution; in addition, erythrocyte and leukocyte levels remained normal. Also, zidovudine loaded liposomes presented a better and prolonged antiretroviral response compared to the zidovudine solution. A more recent study showed that galactosylated liposomes reduced hematopoietic toxicity, enhanced cellular uptake and altered pharmacokinetics of zidovudine (Gard & Jain, 2006). Studies performed by the Jain group (2006, 2008) reported on the application of zidovudine loaded liposomes via transdermal route. The results showed that zidovudine permeation was higher from liposomal formulations, and it was able to target the drug to MPS organs more effectively than the free drug. In 2008, Kaur and co-workers demonstrated that mannosylated-liposomes were able to target zidovudine to the spleen and lymph nodes after subcutaneous administration. The mannose receptors in the spleen explain the role of mannose on the liposome surface and the highest drug localization in this organ.

The Désormeaux group (1994) was one of the first to study liposomal formulations for didanosine. They found that the liposomes modified the drug tissue distribution and plasma pharmacokinetics, resulting in a marked improvement of drug biodistribution, especially into the MPS. Furthermore, they reported that didanosine was efficiently targeted to lymph nodes and macrophage-rich tissue when it was loaded in liposomes. The group showed that the liposomes were able to increase the plasma half-life of the drug, and also the sterically stabilized liposomes remain concentrated in the spleen (Harvie et al., 1995, 1996). In a recent study, a prodrug of didanosine in a liposomal formulation displayed antiviral activity and showed a promising enhancement of the drug activity against HIV-1 in in vitro infected cell cultures (Lalanne et al., 2007).

The effect of the liposome composition and cholesterol on the cellular uptake of stavudine by human M/Ms was verified by Katragadda and co-workers (2000). The cells were up-taken more expressively by the negatively charged liposomes (containing phosphatidylserine and dicetyl phosphate) compared to either the neutral or positive liposomes. The authors suggested that the difference in stavudine liposome uptake in the presence of charge might be due in part to the extent of the interaction between the charged bilayer and the cells. Other studies involving stavudine and liposomes were studied by Garg et al. (2006, 2007). Primarily, they observed that the elimination half-life and mean residence time of stavudine were increased when they were encapsulated in the mannosylated and galactosylated liposomes. Stavudine-loaded mannosylated liposomes presented in vitro antiretroviral activity. In addition, the two liposomal formulations resulted in reduced hematological toxicity and enhanced the hepatic cellular uptake of the stavudine. Furthermore, the group demonstrated that the antiretroviral activity of stavudine in galactosylated liposomes is dose-dependent, in a study with infected cell culture (Garg et al., 2008).

Immunoliposomes (liposomes with antibody attached) have also been used to deliver antiretroviral drugs to HIV targets. The Betageri group (1993a, 1993b) attached a mouse antibody in liposomes containing stavudine-triphosphate or zalcitabine-triphosphate and observed a significant increase in uptake by human macrophages compared to the free drug and unmodified liposomes. Gagné and co-workers (2002) showed that immunoliposomes were very efficient in delivering high concentrations of indinavir to lymphoid tissues (126 times higher than the free drug) for at least 15 days, post a single subcutaneous injection in mice. The HLA-DR determinant of major histocompatibility complex class II is highly expressed on macrophages and activated CD4+ T cells. Also, the authors showed that the immunoliposomal indinavir was as efficient as the free drug to inhibit HIV-1 replication in cultured cells. A recent study (Clayton et al., 2009) demonstrated specific targeting and delivery of a novel protease inhibitor encapsulated in PEGylated immunoliposomes (coated with a F105 Fab' fragment). The immunoliposome was shown to enable selective delivery of the drug to HIV-1-infected cells and also demonstrated that the effect of the targeted drug on viral replication was greater than the effect of a comparable concentration of the free drug or non-targeted drug. Therefore, the potential of liposomes and various ligands for the active targeting of antiretroviral drugs loaded on liposomes has on development. These studies have shown potential benefits of liposomes for improving antiretroviral drug therapy.

3. Polymeric nanoparticles

Nanoparticles are solid, colloidal particles consisting of macromolecular substances varying in size from 10 to 1,000 nm. The drug can be dissolved, entrapped, adsorbed, attached or encapsulated into a nanoparticle. Depending on the method of preparation, nanospheres or nanocapsules can be developed with different properties; in addition, different release characteristics for the encapsulated therapeutic agent can also be developed. For nearly three decades, polymeric nanoparticles have been extensively studied due to their unique and valuable physicochemical and biological properties. Nanoparticles can improve drug actuation by the following characteristics: protecting it from degradation (higher physical stability during storage and in biological fluids), enhancing its transport and distribution (possibility through drug targeting by modification of surface charge with inserted ligands, such as antibodies, surfactants, and polymers) and prolonging its release (ability to sustain the drug release over a period of days to weeks). Therefore, nanoparticles may improve the plasma half-life of the entrapped drug (Allémann et al., 1993; Oppenheim, 1981). The drug pharmacokinetics parameters are altered when the drug is loaded in nanoparticles, and the particle surface composition plays an important role in drug bioavailability, which can be greater or lower than the drug solution/powder ratio, depending on the polymer used (Ubrich et al., 2005). Some characteristics of nanoparticles, such as particle size and surface charge, can be modulated by modifying some process parameters of formulation; they can be used in various applications. The research involving the applications of polymeric nanoparticles in AIDS treatment is primarily directed to increasing the intracellular and brain delivery of antiretroviral drugs. Thus, it is clear that M/Ms represent an important target for antiretroviral drugs and for carriers loaded with these drugs. The nanoparticles represent an attractive alternative in AIDS treatment because they consist of a carrier system intended for targeting M/Ms. When administered intravenously, conventional nanoparticles are rapidly cleared from the bloodstream by the MPS, represented by M/Ms. The particle uptake by cells is affected by the particle's physicochemical properties, such as particle size, surface charge, hydrophobicity and presence of a coating (varying in density/conformation) (Stolnik et al., 2005; Owens & Peppas, 2006).

Schäfer and co-workers (1992) were pioneers in studies involving antiretroviral drugs and macrophage targeting using nanoparticles. The authors found that the physicochemical properties, including the composition, surface characteristics and size, of poly(alkylcyanoacrylate) (PACA), poly(metylmethacrylate) (PMMA) and human serum albumin (HSA) nanoparticles containing zidovudine influenced the rate of uptake by macrophages, particularly when these cells were infected by HIV (up to 60% more than for uninfected macrophages). Also, the group demonstrated the effectiveness of poly(hexylcyanoacrylate) (PHCA) and HSA nanoparticles containing zidovudine and didanosine in preventing HIV infection in M/Ms cultures in vitro (Bender et al., 1994). Furthermore, the group prepared PHCA nanoparticles as carriers for saquinavir or zalcitabine and demonstrated that the both nanoparticles formulations led to a dose-dependent reduction of HIV-1 antigen production in vitro in primary human M/Ms cultures (Bender et al., 1996). In a similar study, saquinavir carried in poly(ethyleneoxide)-modified poly(epsilon-caprolactone) (PEO-PCL) nanoparticles was significantly internalized by the THP-1 human M/Ms cell line at a 10-fold higher rate than an aqueous solution of saquinavir (Shah & Amiji, 2006). In another study, Hillaireau et al. (2006) demonstrated that nanocapsules composed of PIBCA and poly(ethyleneimine) increased the intracellular uptake of azidothymidine-triphosphate 10- to 30-fold higher that the free drug, in a mouse macrophages culture. Destache and co-workers (2009) developed poly(lactic-co-glycolic) acid (PLGA) nanoparticles containing ritonavir, lopinavir and efavirenz and the results of the in vitro release of the drugs from the nanoparticles in human peripheral blood mononuclear cells showed an intracellular peak of each drug over a 28-day period, while the free drugs were eliminated in 2 days. The authors also demonstrated that nanoparticles were not significantly cytotoxic over macrophages. These results are important because they demonstrate that the three drugs can be incorporated into a single nanoparticle for drug delivery and because the use of a single antiretroviral in the treatment of HIV-1 only resulted in the development of resistant strains and treatment failures. In another study, the same group showed that these nanoparticles were able to maintain the plasmatic drug concentrations for a prolonged period, after intraperitoneal administration in mice. Also, the drug concentration in the brain was significantly higher with drug-loaded nanoparticles than with the free drug. Additionally, the antiretroviral drug-loaded nanoparticles were able to interact with the M/Ms infected with HIV-1 and inhibit virus replication up to 1000-fold for 10 days compared to the free drugs (Destache et al., 2010). Poly(lactic) acid (PLA) and PLA-polyethylene glycol (PLA-PEG) blended nanoparticles containing zidovudine were developed, and their uptake by polymorphonuclear leucocytes from rats was studied in vitro. The results showed that the PLA nanoparticles were more efficiently phagocytosed than PLA-PEG blends and were able to activate a larger number of cells than the blended PLA-PEG nanoparticles (Mainardes et al., 2009). Furthermore, the group evaluated the pharmacokinetic profile of these nanoparticles in rats after a single intranasal administration. Blended PLA-PEG nanoparticles exhibited a sustained release of the drug over 24 h, while PLA nanoparticles were sustained up to 10 h. The half-life of zidovudine also varied among the formulations. The slow elimination rate (Ke) resulted in significantly prolonged $t_{1/2}$ values for zidovudine from the PLA and blended PLA-PEG nanoparticles compared to the zidovudine solution. Because of the slow release of zidovudine from the nanoparticles, its metabolic breakdown was also slower, increasing the mean half-life. The significant increase ($p< 0.05$) in the value of the area under curve (AUC) for the zidovudine-loaded PLA-PEG nanoparticles, compared to the PLA nanoparticles and zidovudine aqueous solution, distinctly indicated the improved intranasal bioavailability of the blended system (Mainardes et al., 2010). Thus, the results of this study corroborated those of the first study, indicating that the physicochemical characteristics of nanoparticles intended for controlled drug release is very important because these characteristics can govern the application of the formulation and can be used to predict its behavior in the biological medium. The size and surface charge are also important parameters in a nanostructured system because these characteristics interfere directly in biological processes, such as the transport across biological membranes and the recognition by M/Ms and biodistribution.

Another important factor that must be taken into account in the design strategies used to improve AIDS treatment is the brain delivery system of antiretroviral drugs. Because of the restricted entry of anti-HIV drugs, the brain is thought to form a viral sanctuary, and the treatment and control of HIV within this reservoir must be primordial. Nanoparticles can enhance the brain-drug delivery by three major pathways, which include the following: i) increasing the local drug gradient at the Blood Brain Barrier (BBB) by passive targeting, ii) allowing drug-trafficking by non-specific or receptor-mediated endocytosis and iii) blocking drug efflux transporters at the BBB (Wong et al., 2010). Consequently, the use of nanocarriers should help to achieve higher concentrations of encapsulated drugs and also allow their prolonged residence in the CNS.

One of the most used polymers for the development of nanoparticles intended for brain delivery is poly-(butylcyanoacrylate) (PBCA) (Koziara et al., 2006). Studies have shown that the surface modification of PBCA nanoparticles using other polymers or surfactant agents, such as polysorbate 80, could increase the transport of particles through the BBB. Polysorbate 80 has been found to increase the translocation of nanoparticles by increasing the particle interaction with the low density lipoprotein (LDL) receptor-mediated endocytic pathway in brain endothelial cells and by inhibition the efflux function of P-gp (Goppert & Muller, 2005).

Kuo and Chen (2006) showed that methylmethacrylate-sulfopropylmethacrylate (MMSPM) nanoparticles were able to significantly increase the BBB permeability of zidovudine and lamivudine by 100%, using blood-brain-microvascular endothelial cells model. In the same study, PBCA nanoparticles increased the BBB permeability of zidovudine 8- to 20-fold and lamivudine 10- to 18-fold. The authors also demonstrated that the drug permeability increased with the decrease in particle size of the two polymeric carriers. Furthermore, these authors observed an increase in the BBB permeability (in vitro) of stavudine-, delaviridine- and saquinavir-loaded PBCA and MMSPM nanoparticles coated with polysorbate 80 and solid lipid nanoparticles; in addition, a higher drug permeability was obtained with smaller particles (Kuo & Fu, 2007).

The transferrin receptors present in the luminal membrane of brain endothelial cells have been used as preferential targets for enhanced antiretroviral drug delivery to the CNS by means of nanoparticulate systems (Kreuter, 2001). PEGylated albumin nanoparticles encapsulating zidovudine were prepared, and its surface was modified by anchoring transferrin as a ligand for brain targeting. A significant enhancement of brain localization of zidovudine was observed when it was delivered by transferrin-anchored PEGylated albumin nanoparticles compared to unmodified nanoparticles (Mishra et al., 2006).

Recently, the properties of cell-penetrating peptides have been explored to further enhance the cellular permeability of drug carrier systems. In this approach, certain proteins or peptides can be tethered to the hydrophilic drug of interest, and together, the construct possesses the ability to translocate across the plasma membrane and to deliver the payload intracellularly (Jeang et al., 1999). The Tat peptide, the most frequently used cell-penetrating peptide, is derived from the transcriptional activator protein encoded by HIV-1 (Torchilin, 2008). Thus, nanoparticles containing Tat are promising systems for transport across the BBB and entry into the brain. Therefore, Rao and co-workers (2008) hypothesized that anti-HIV drugs loaded in nanoparticles could bypass the efflux action of P-gp and that Tat conjugation would enhance their transport across the BBB, thereby enhancing the CNS bioavailability of anti-HIV drugs. In their study, ritonavir-loaded PLA nanoparticles conjugated with the Tat peptide were developed, and it was demonstrated to enhance and sustained brain delivery of the system without influencing the integrity of the BBB; these data suggested that the transport occurred through transcytosis across the endothelium of the brain vasculature. At two weeks post administration, the brain ritonavir level after administration of the conjugated nanoparticles was 800-fold higher than that with the drug delivered in solution. It was concluded that Tat-conjugated nanoparticles enhanced the ritonavir CNS bioavailability and maintained therapeutic drug levels in the brain for an effectively sustained period for reducing the viral load in the CNS, which acts as a reservoir for the replicating HIV-1 virus.

4. Solid Lipid Nanoparticles (SLN)

In the last decade of the last century, SLN have gained considerable interest as novel particulate drug delivery systems. SLN are solid, particulate carriers that are nano-sized and composed of biodegradable/biocompatible lipids, suitable for the incorporation of lipophilic and hydrophilic drugs in the lipid matrix in high concentrations. SLNs can be prepared from fatty acids and the stabilization of dispersions with emulsifiers and co-emulsifiers, such as polysorbates, poloxamers, fatty acid co-esters, lecithin and bile salts (Gupta & Jain, 2010). Although few reports about the anti-HIV drug SLN have been published, some studies have proved the suitability of this system to dissolve lipophilic anti-HIV drugs and sustain the drug release; in addition, these studies have shown the feasibility of scaling up SLN production. Cationic SLN were found to be beneficial to the entrapment efficiency of saquinavir. SLN were fabricated via a microemulsion method and stabilized by polysorbate 80; in addition, the lipid phase contained cationic stearylamine, dioctadecyldimethyl ammonium bromide, non-ionic Compritol 888 ATO and cacao butter. The in vitro drug release assay suggested that the carriers could sustain drug delivery without an apparent initial burst (Kuo & Chen, 2009). Aji Alex et al. (2010) investigated the use of SLNs to target intestinal lymphatic vessels. Lopinavir, a poor orally available anti-HIV, was successfully encapsulated in glyceryl behenate-based SLNs produced via a hot homogenization process followed by ultrasonication. In vitro release studies showed that SLNs presented a low release profile; the intestinal lymphatic transport study showed an increase in the cumulative percentage dose of lopinavir secreted into the lymph. These results significantly enhanced the percentage of lopinavir bioavailability. SLNs have been obtained using large-scale production methods, and the study of Shegokara et al. 2010 showed promising results, in which the scaling up of the stavudine production for intravenous injection was possible. The SLNs were produced by the high-pressure homogenization of the stavudine lipid melt, dispersed in a hot surfactant solution (pre-emulsion). For the investigated formulation, the homogenization system seemed to be rather robust, producing very similar SLN sizes.

5. Challenges involving clinical trials of antiretroviral drug delivery systems

Despite the current increase of published original studies on nanotechnology-based antiretroviral drug delivery systems with promising strategies and pre-clinical results, these studies generally have not extended to the clinical studies and, consequently, patients have not received the benefits. Clinical trials are the best way to confirm the efficacy of new medicines; however, this type of study also utilizes placebos, which present serious ethical challenges. The placebo-group has been disapproved in cases of AIDS research because the patient that does not receive the effective regimen can suffer serious consequences in the absence of AIDS therapy. Studies using placebos have been considered unethical in the case where an efficient treatment is known (Scheffer, 2000). Since the Declaration of Helsinki (World Medical Association, 2008), a document with guidelines of ethical principles for the medical community about human experimentation, researchers worldwide must protect the life, health, privacy, and dignity of the human subject, although those principles may contradict many economic and political interests. Thus, a discussion about human experimentation and the investigation of new in vitro models in cells and animals are also extremely important to circumvent the problems with clinical trials of new antiretroviral drug delivery systems.

6. Conclusion

The development of systems for drug delivery will not only benefit the therapy of AIDS and other viral diseases but also accelerate the development of systems for bacterial diseases, fungi and mycobacteria. For this, new challenges for the future of drug delivery systems are the feasibility of scaling-up processes to bring to the market quickly innovative therapeutic and the possibility of obtaining multifunctional systems that will be able to fulfill the different biological and therapeutic requirements.

7. Acknowledgment

The authors would like to thank the FAPESP (Fundo de Apoio a Pesquisa do Estado de São Paulo) and the CNPQ (Conselho Nacional de Desenvolvimento Científico e Tecnológico) from Brazil for financial support.

8. References

Aji Alex M.R., Chacko A. J., Jose S., Souto E. B. (2011). Lopinavir loaded solid lipid nanoparticles (SLN) for intestinal lymphatic targeting. European Journal of Pharmaceutical Sciences, Vol. 18, n. 42, 11-18. DOI:10.1016/j.ejps.2010.10.002

Alexaki A., Liu Y, Wigdahl B. (2008). Cellular reservoirs of HIV-1 and their role in viral persistence. Current HIV Research, Vol. 6, pp. 388-400. DOI:10.2174/157016208785861195

Allémann E., Gurny R., Doelker E. (1993). Drug loaded nanoparticles preparation methods and drug targeting issues. European Journal of Pharmaceutics and Biopharmaceutics, Vol. 39, pp. 173-91.

Bender A.R., Schäfer V., Steffan A.M., Royer C., Kreuter J., Rübsamen-Waigmann H., Von Briesen H. (1994). Inhibition of HIV in vitro by antiviral drug-targeting using nanoparticles. Research Virology, Vol. 145, pp. 215–20. DOI: 10.1016/S0923-2516(07)80025-2

Bender A.R., von Briesen H., Kreuter J., Duncan B., Rübsamen-Waigmann H. (1996). Efficiency of nanoparticles as a carrier system for antiviral agents in human immunodeficiency virus-infected human monocytes/macrophages in vitro. Antimicrobial Agents and Chemotherapy, Vol. 40, pp. 1467–1471.

Betageri G.V., Black S.D., Szebeni J., Wahl L.M., Weinstein J.N. (1993a). Fc-receptor-mediated targeting of antibody-bearing liposomes containing dideoxycytidine triphosphate to human monocyte/macrophages. Journal of Pharmacy and Pharmacology, Vol. 45, pp. 48–53.

Betageri G.V., Jenkins S.A., Ravis W.R. (1993b). Drug delivery using antibody-liposome conjugates. Drug Development and Industrial Pharmacy, Vol. 19, pp. 2109–2116. DOI:10.3109/03639049309069345

Boyd B., (2010) Liquid crystals as drug delivery systems, http://www.pharm.monash.edu.au/research/mips/d4/liquidcrystals.html

Carvalho F. C., Barbi M. S., Sarmento V. H. V., Chiavacci L. A., Netto F. M., Gremião M. P. D. (2010a) Surfactant systems for nasal zidovudine delivery: structural, rheological and mucoadhesive properties. Journal of Pharmacy and Pharmacology, Vol. 62, pp. 430–439. DOI: 10.1211/jpp/62.04.0004

Carvalho F. C., Bruschi M. L., Evangelista R. C., Gremião M. P. D. (2010b) Mucoadhesive drug delivery systems. Brazilian Journal of Pharmaceutical Sciences, Vol. 46, pp. 1-17. DOI: 10.1590/S1984-82502010000100002

Carvalho F. C., Sarmento V. H. V., Chiavacci L. A., Barbi M. S., Gremião M. P. D. (2009). Development and in vitro evaluation of surfactant systems for controlled release of zidovudine. Journal of Pharmaceutical Sciences, Vol. 99, pp. 2367-74. DOI:10.1002/jps

Chiappetta D.A., Alvarez-Lorenzo C., Rey-Rico A., Taboada P, Concheiro A., Sosnik A. (2010) N-alkylation of poloxamines modulates micellar assembly and encapsulation and release of the antiretroviral efavirenz. European Journal of Pharmaceutics and Biopharmaceutics, Vol. 76, pp. 24–37, DOI:10.1016/j.ejpb.2010.05.007

Clayton R., Ohagen A., Nicol F., Del Vecchio A.M., Jonckers T.H., Goethals O., Van Loock M., Michiels L., Grigsby J., Xu Z., Zhang Y.P., Gutshall L.L., Cunningham M., Jiang H., Bola S., Sarisky R.T., Hertogs K. (2009). Sustained and specific in vitro inhibition of HIV-1 replication by a protease inhibitor encapsulated in gp120-targeted liposomes. Antiviral Research, Vol. 84, pp. 142-149. DOI:10.1016/j.antiviral.2009.08.003

Desormeaux A., Bergeron M.G. (1998). Liposomes as drug delivery system: a strategic approach for the treatment of HIV infection. Journal of Drug Targeting, Vol. 6, pp. 1–15. DOI:10.3109/10611869808997877

Désormeaux A., Harvie P., Perron S., Makabi-Panzu B., Beauchamp D., Tremblay M., Poulin L., Bergeron M.G. (1994). Antiviral efficacy, intracellular uptake and pharmacokinetics of free and liposome-encapsulated 2', 3'-dideoxyinosine. AIDS, Vol. 8, pp. 1545-1153.

Destache C.J., Belgum T, Goede M, Shibata A., Belshan M.A. (2010). Antiretroviral release from poly(DL-lactide-co-glycolide) nanoparticles in mice. Journal of Antimicrobial Chemotherapy, Vol. 65, pp. 2183-7. DOI: 10.1093/jac/dkq318

Destache C.J., Belgum T., Christensen K., Shibata A., Sharma A., Dash A. (2009). Combination antiretroviral drugs in PLGA nanoparticle for HIV-1. BMC Infectious Diseases, Vol. 9, pp.198-206. DOI: 10.1186/1471-2334-9-198

Gagné J.F., Désormeaux A., Perron S., Tremblay W.J., Bergeron M.G. (2002). Targeted delivery of indinavir to HIV-1 primary reservoirs with immunoliposomes. Biochimica et Biophysica Acta - Biomembranes, Vol. 1558, pp. 198-210. DOI: 10.1016/S0005-2736(01)00432-1

Ganser A., Greher. J, Völkers B., Staszewski S., Hoelzer D. (1989). Inhibitory effect of azidothymidine, 2'-3'-dideoxyadenosine, and 2'-3'-dideoxycytidine on in vitro growth of hematopoietic progenitor cells from normal persons and from patients with AIDS. Expert Hematology, Vol. 17, pp. 321-5.

Garg M., Asthana A., Agashe H.B., Agrawal G.P., Jain N.K. (2006). Stavudine-loaded mannosylated liposomes: in-vitro anti-HIV-I activity, tissue distribution and pharmacokinetics. Journal of Pharmacy and Pharmacology, Vol. 58, pp. 605–616. DOI: 10.1211/jpp.58.5.0005

Garg M., Dutta T., Jain N.K. (2007). Reduced hepatic toxicity, enhanced cellular uptake and altered pharmacokinetics of stavudine loaded galactosylated liposomes. European Journal of Pharmaceutics and Biopharmaceutics, Vol. 67, pp. 76–85. DOI:10.1016/j.ejpb.2006.12.019

Geocze L., Mucci S., Marco M. A. D., Nogueira-Martins L. A., Citero V. A. (2010). Qualidade de vida e adesão ao tratamento anti-retroviral de pacientes portadores de HIV. Rev. Saúde Pública, Vol. 44, pp. 743-9, DOI: 10.1590/S0034-89102010000400019

Goppert T.M., Muller R.H. (2005). Polysorbate-stabilized solid lipid nanoparticles as colloidal carriers for intravenous targeting of drugs to the brain: comparison of plasma protein adsorption patterns. Journal of Drug Targeting, Vol.13, pp. 179–87. DOI: 10.1080/10611860500071292

Gupta U., Jain N. K. (2010) Non-polymeric nano-carriers in HIV/AIDS drug delivery and targeting. Advanced Drug Delivery Reviews, Vol. 62, pp. 478–490, DOI: 10.1016/j.addr.2009.11.018

Harvie P., Desormeaux A., Bergeron M.C., Tremblay M., Beauchamp D., Poulin L., Bergeron M.G. (1996). Comparative pharmacokinetics, distributions in tissue and interactions with blood proteins of conventional and sterically stabilized liposomes containing 2, 3-dideoxyinosine. Antimicrobial Agents and Chemotherapy, Vol.40, pp. 225–229.

Harvie P., Desormeaux A., Gagne N., Tremblay M., Poulin L., Beauchamp D., Bergeron M.G. (1995). Lymphoid tissues targeting of liposome-encapsulated 2, 3-dideoxyinosine. AIDS, Vol.9, pp. 701–707.

Hawkins T. (2010). Understanding and managing the adverse effects of antiretroviral therapy. Antiviral Research, Vol. 85, pp. 201–209, DOI:10.1016/j.antiviral.2009.10.016

Hillaireau H., Le Doan T., Appel M., Couvreur P. (2006). Hybrid polymer nanocapsules enhance in vitro delivery of azidothymidine-triphosphate to macrophages. Journal of Controlled Release, Vol. 116, pp. 346–52. DOI:10.1016/j.jconrel.2006.09.016

Jain S., Tiwary A.K, Jain N.K. (2006). Sustained and targeted delivery of an anti-HIV agent using elastic liposomal formulation: mechanism of action. Current Drug Delivery, Vol.3, pp. 157–166. DOI: 10.1016/j.antiviral.2009.08.003

Jain S., Tiwary A.K., Jain N.K. (2008) PEGylated elastic liposomal formulation for lymphatic targeting of zidovudine. Current Drug Delivery, Vol. 5, pp. 275–281. DOI:10.2174/156720108785915078

Jeang K.T., Xiao H., Rich E.A. (1999). Multifaceted activities of the HIV-1 transactivator of transcription, Tat. The Journal of Biological Chemistry, Vol. 274, pp. 28837–40. DOI: 10.1074/jbc.274.41.28837

Jin Y., Qia N., Tong L., Chen D. (2010). Self-assembled drug delivery systems. Part 5: Self-assemblies of a bolaamphiphilic prodrug containing dual zidovudine. International Journal of Pharmaceutics, Vol. 386, pp. 268–274, DOI:10.1016/j.ijpharm.2009.11.018

Jin Y., Ai P., Xina R., Chen D. (2008) Morphological transformation of self-assembled nanostructures prepared from cholesteryl acyl didanosine and the optimal formulation of nanoparticulate systems: Effects of solvents, acyl chain length and poloxamer 188. Journal of Colloid and Interface Science, Vol. 326, pp. 275-282. DOI:10.1016/j.jcis.2008.07.014

Jin Y., Xinga L., Tian Y., Li M., Gao C., Du L., Dong J., Chen H. (2009) Self-assembled drug delivery systems. Part 4. In vitro/in vivo studies of the self-assemblies of cholesteryl-phosphonyl zidovudine. International Journal of Pharmaceutics, Vol. 381, pp. 40–48.
DOI:10.1016/j.ijpharm.2009.07.024

Kaparissides C., Alexandridou S., Kotti K., Chaitidou S. (2006). Recent advances in novel drug delivery systems, In: Journal of nanotechnology online, November 25th, 2010, Available from <http://www.azonano.com/Details.asp?ArticleID=1538>
DOI: 10.2240/azojono0111

Katragadda A., Bridgman R., Betageri G. (2000). Effect of liposome composition and cholesterol on the cellular uptake of stavudine by human monocyte/macrophages. Cellular Molecular Biology Letters, Vol. 5, pp. 483–493.

Kaur C.D., Nahar M., Jain N.K. (2008). Lymphatic targeting of zidovudine using surfaceengineered liposomes. Journal of Drug Targeting, Vol. 16, pp. 798–805.
DOI: 10.1080/10611860802475688

Khalil N.M., Carraro E., Cótica L.F., Mainardes R.M. (2011). Potential of polymeric nanoparticles in AIDS treatment and prevention. Expert Opinion on Drug Delivery, Vol. 8, pp. 95-112.
DOI: 10.1517/17425247.2011.543673

Koziara J.M., Lockman P.R., Allen D.D., Mumper R.J. (2006). The blood-brain barrier and brain drug delivery. Journal of Nanoscience and Nanotechnology, Vol. 6, p. 2712-35.
DOI: 10.1166/jnn.2006.441

Kreuter J. (2001). Nanoparticulate systems for brain delivery of drugs. Advanced Drug Delivery Reviews, Vol. 47, pp. 65–81.
DOI: 10.1016/S0169-409X(00)00122-8

Kuo Y. C. Chen H. H. (2009). Entrapment and release of saquinavir using novel cationic solid lipid nanoparticles. International Journal of Pharmaceutics, Vol. 365, pp. 206–213,
DOI: 10.1016/j.ijpharm.2008.08.050

Kuo Y.C. Chen H.H. (2006). Effect of nanoparticulate polybutylcyanoacrylate and methylmethacrylate-sulfopropylmethacrylate on the permeability of zidovudine and lamivudine across the in vitro blood-brain barrier. International Journal of Pharmaceutics, Vol. 327, pp. 160–69.
DOI: 10.1016/j.ijpharm.2006.07.044

Kuo Y.C. Su FL. (2007). Transport of stavudine, delavirdine, and saquinavir across the blood-brain barrier by polybutylcyanoacrylate, methylmethacrylatesulfopropylmethacrylate, and solid lipid nanoparticles. International Journal of Pharmaceutics, Vol. 340, pp. 143–152.

DOI: 10.1517/17425247.2011.543673

Lalanne M., Paci A., Andrieux K., Dereuddre-Bosquet N., Clayette P., Deroussent A., Ré M., Vassal G., Couvreur P., Desmaële D. (2007). Synthesis and biological evaluation of two glycerolipidic prodrugs of didanosine for direct lymphatic delivery against HIV. Bioorganic Medicinal Chemistry Letters, Vol. 17, pp. 2237–2240.

Mainardes R.M., Gremião M.P.D., Brunetti I.L., da Fonseca, A.M., Khalil, N.M. (2009). Zidovudine-loaded PLA and PLA-PEG blend nanoparticles: influence of polymer type on phagocytic uptake by polymorphonuclear cells. Journal of Pharmaceutical Sciences, Vol. 98, pp. 257-67.
DOI: 10.1002/jps.21406

Mainardes, R.M.; Khalil, N.M.; Gremião, M.P.D. (2010) Intranasal delivery of zidovudine by PLA and PLA-PEG blend nanoparticles. International Journal of Pharmaceutics, Vol. 16, pp. 266-271,
DOI: 10.1016/j.ijpharm.2010.05.020.

Makabi-Panzu B., Gourde P., Desormeaux A., Bergeron M.G. (1998). Intracellular and serum stability of liposomal 2', 3'-dideoxycytidine. Effect of lipid composition. Cellular Molecular Biology, Vol. 44, pp. 277–284.

Malmsten, M. (2002). Surfactants and polymers in drug delivery. Marcel Dekker, ISBN 978-0-8247-0804-7, New York.

Mishra V., Mahor S., Rawat A., Gupta P.N., Dubey P., Khatri K., Vyas S.P. (2006). Targeted brain delivery of AZT via transferrin anchored pegylated albumin nanoparticles. Journal of Drug Targeting, Vol. 14, pp. 45–53.
DOI: 10.1080/10611860600612953

Neves J., Amiji M. M., Bahia M. F., Sarmento B. (2010). Nanotechnology-based systems for the treatment and prevention of HIV/AIDS, Advanced Drug Delivery Reviews, Vol. 62, pp. 458–477,
DOI: 10.1016/j.addr.2009.11.017

Ojewole E., Mackraj I., Naidooa P., Govender, T. (2008) Exploring the use of novel drug delivery systems for antiretroviral drugs. European Journal of Pharmaceutics and Biopharmaceutics, Vol. 70, pp. 697-710.
DOI 10.1016/j.ejpb.2008.06.020

Oppenheim R.C. (1981). Solid colloidal drug delivery systems: nanoparticles. International Journal of Pharmaceutics, Vol.8, pp. 217-34.
DOI: 10.1016/0378-5173(81)90100-9

Owens D.E., Peppas N.A. (2006). Opsonization, biodistribution, and pharmacokinetics of polymeric nanoparticles. International Journal of Pharmaceutics, Vol. 307, pp. 93-102.
DOI: 10.1016/0169-409X(95)00025-3

Phillips N.C., Skamene E., Tsoukas C. (1991). Liposomal encapsulation of 3`-azido-3`-deoxythymidine (AZT) results in decreased bone marrow toxicity and enhanced activity against murine AIDS-induced immunosuppression. Journal of Acquired Immune Deficiency Syndrome, Vol. 4, pp. 959–966.

Phillips N.C., Tsoukas C. (1992). Liposomal encapsulation of azidothymidine results in decreased hematopoietic toxicity and enhanced activity against murine acquired immunodeficiency syndrome. Blood, Vol. 79, pp. 1137–1143.

Rao K.S., Ghorpade A., Labhasetwar V. (2009). Targeting anti-HIV drugs to the CNS. Expert Opinion on Drug Delivery, Vol. 6, pp. 771-84. DOI:10.1517/17425240903081705

Richman D.D., Margolis D.M., Delaney M., Greene W.C., Hazuda D, Pomerantz R.J. (2009). The challenge of finding a cure for HIV infection. Science, Vol. 323, pp. 1304–07. DOI: 10.1126/science.1165706

Saksena N.K., Haddad D.N. (2003). Viral reservoirs an impediment to HAART: new strategies to eliminate HIV-1. Current Drug Targets Infection Disorders, Vol. 3, pp. 179–206. DOI: 10.2174/1568005033481187

Schäfer V., von Briesen H., Andreesen R., Steffan, A.M., Royer, C., Tröster, S., Kreuter, J., Rübsamen-Waigmann, H. (1992). Phagocytosis of nanoparticles by human immunodeficiency virus (HIV)-infected macrophages: a possibility for antiviral drug targeting. Pharmaceutical Research, Vol. 9, pp. 541–46. DOI: 10.1023/A:1015852732512

Scheffer M. (2000) Tecnologia, AIDS e ética em pesquisa. Interface - Comunicação, Saúde, Educação, Vol. 6, pp. 173-176.

Shah L.K., Amiji M.M. (2006). Intracellular delivery of saquinavir in biodegradable polymeric nanoparticles for HIV/AIDS. Pharmaceutical Research, Vol. 23, p. 2638-45. DOI: 10.1007/s11095-006-9101-7

Sharma A., Sharma U.S. (1997). Liposomes in drug delivery: progress and limitations. International Journal Pharmaceutics, Vol. 154, pp. 123–140. DOI:10.1016/S0378-5173(97)00135-X

Sharma P., Garg S. (2010). Pure drug and polymer based nanotechnologies for the improved solubility, stability, bioavailability and targeting of anti-HIV drugs. Advanced Drug Delivery Reviews, Vol. 62, pp. 491–502. DOI: 10.1016/j.addr.2009.11.019

Shegokara R., Singha K. K., Müller R. H. (2010). Production & stability of stavudine solid lipid nanoparticles — From lab to industrial scale, International Journal of Pharmaceutics, In press, DOI: 10.1016/j.ijpharm.2010.08.014

Sosnik A., Chiappetta D. A., Carcaboso A. M. (2009). Drug delivery systems in HIV pharmacotherapy: What has been done and the challenges standing ahead. Journal of Controlled Release, Vol. 138, pp. 2–15, DOI: 10.1016/j.jconrel.2009.05.007

Stolnik S., Illum L., Davis S.S. (1995). Long circulating microparticulate drug carriers. Advanced Drug Delivery Reviews, Vol. 16, pp. 195–214. DOI: 10.1016/0169-409X(95)00025-3

Szebeni J., Wahl S.M., Betageri G.V., Wahl L.M., Gartner S, Popovic, M, Parker R.J., Black C.D., Weinstein J.N. (1990). Inhibition of HIV-1 in monocyte/ macrophage cultures

by 2′, 3′-dideoxycytidine-5′-triphosphate, free and in liposomes. AIDS Research and Humum Retroviruses, Vol. 6, pp. 691–702.
DOI: 10.1089/aid.1990.6.691

Torchilin V.P. (2008). Tat peptide-mediated intracellular delivery of pharmaceutical nanocarriers. Advanced Drug Delivery Reviews, Vol. 60, pp. 548-58.
DOI: 10.1016/j.addr.2007.10.008

Ubrich N., Schmidt C., Bodmeier R., Hoffman M., Maincent, P. (2005). Oral evaluation in rabbits of cyclosporine-loaded Eudragit RS or RL nanoparticles. International Journal of Pharmaceutics, Vol. 288, p. 169-75.
DOI:10.1016/j.ijpharm.2004.09.019

Vyas T. K., Shahiwala A., Amiji M. M. (2008). Improved oral bioavailability and brain transport of saquinavir upon administration in novel nanoemulsion formulations. International Journal of Pharmaceutics, Vol. 347, pp. 93–101,
DOIi:10.1016/j.ijpharm.2007.06.016

Wong H. L., Chattopadhyay N., Wu X. Y., Bendayan R. (2010). Nanotechnology applications for improved delivery of antiretroviral drugs to the brain. Advanced Drug Delivery Reviews, Vol. 62, pp. 503–517,
DOI:10.1016/j.addr.2009.11.020

World Medical Association (2008) Declaration of Helsinki - Ethical Principles for Medical Research Involving Human Subjects.
http://www.wma.net/en/30publications/10policies/b3/index.html.

Zidan A.S., Spink C., Fortunak J., Habib M., Khan M.A. (2010). Near-infrared investigations of novel anti-HIV tenofovir liposmes. The AAPS Journal, Vol. 12, pp. 202-214.
DOI: 10.1208/s12248-010-9177-1

16

Acute Kidney Injury in Hospitalized HIV-Infected Patients in the HAART Era: An Epidemiological View

José António Lopes and Sofia Jorge
Department of Nephrology and Renal Transplantation,
Hospital de Santa Maria,
Centro Hospitalar Lisboa Norte,
Lisboa,
Portugal

1. Introduction

Actually, more than 30 million people are affected with human immunodeficiency virus (HIV) infection worldwide [1]. Since the introduction of the highly active antiretroviral therapy (HAART) at the end of 1995, overall mortality of patients with HIV infection decreased dramatically as well as mortality caused by HIV infection or by an Acquired Immunodeficiency Syndrome (AIDS)-defining disease. Conversely, mortality due to kidney disease, liver disease, heart disease, and non-AIDS-defining cancers has proportionally increased [2,3,4].

Renal disorders in HIV-infected patients can present as an acute or chronic condition and they are associated with increased morbidity and mortality in this population [5,6,7,8,9]. Acute kidney injury is a common complication in ambulatory HIV-infected patients treated with HAART and has been associated with prior renal impairment, lower CD4 levels, AIDS, hepatitis C virus (HCV) co-infection, and liver disease [10,11]. HIV-infected patients are also at increased risk for AKI development within hospitalization, related to volume depletion, sepsis, and the acute administration of nephrotoxic medications or radiocontrast. Before the advent of HAART, studies addressing AKI on HIV-infected patients typically included only severe cases of AKI which were identified through hospital records or biopsy databases [12,13,14]. The epidemiology of AKI in hospitalized HIV-infected patients in the HAART era has also not been extensively analyzed. In fact, few studies have focused on the clinical characteristics of AKI in hospitalized HIV-infected patients in the HAART era [15,16,17,18]. In this chapter, we provide a critical and contemporary review of AKI in hospitalized HIV-infected patients in the HAART era, focusing on the incidence, risk factors, and outcome.

2. Incidence of AKI in hospitalized HIV-infected patients

Three recent studies [15,16,17] have addressed specifically the incidence of AKI in hospitalized HIV-infected patients (Table 1). Wyatt et al [15] compared the incidence of AKI in HIV-infected patients before and after the introduction of HAART. For this purpose, all adult patients who were discharged from acute care hospitals in New York State during 1995 (pre-HAART era) and during 2003 (post-HAART era) were evaluated. The presence of AKI was determined by a diagnosis code 584 of the International Classification of Diseases, 9th Revision (ICD-9), which identified AKI based on the clinical judgement of the treating physician. There were 52.580 patients with documented HIV infection discharged from hospital in 1995, and 25.114 in 2003. Acute kidney injury was reported significantly more often during hospitalizations for HIV-infected patients than for uninfected patients in both 2003 (6% versus 2.7%) and 1995 (2.9% versus 1.0%). After adjusting for other covariates, HIV infection remained associated with an increased risk of AKI both in 2003 [adjusted odds ratio (OR) 2.82, 95% confidence interval (CI) 2.66-2.99) and in 1995 (adjusted OR 4.62, 95% CI 4.3-4.95). Lopes et al [16] conducted a cohort study including 489 HIV-infected patients hospitalized in a tertiary and teaching Portuguese Hospital between 2005 and 2007 to characterize AKI in this population. Acute kidney injury was defined and categorized according to "Risk Injury Failure Loss of kidney function End-stage kidney disease" (RIFLE) classification [19], and it was considered if there was an increase of baseline serum creatinine × 1.5 or in patients with baseline serum creatinine > 4 mg/dl if there was an acute rise in serum creatinine of at least 0.5 mg/dl. They found that 18% of patients had AKI within the hospitalization which was much higher than the incidence previously reported (6%) in hospitalized HIV-infected patients in HAART era [15]. It should be remembered that in the study of Wyatt et al [15] the diagnosis of AKI was determined by a diagnosis code 584 of the ICD-9 based on the clinical judgement and documentation of the treating physician, and laboratory values were not reported. Administrative databases may be a powerful tool for the study of AKI, although the low sensitivity of the AKI codes still remains an important caveat [20]. Therefore, in the study of Wyatt et al [15] the utilization of diagnostic code to identify AKI could not have captured an important number of cases.

In a previous report, Lopes et al [17] have also studied AKI in a small cohort of critically ill HIV-infected patients hospitalized in a tertiary and teaching Portuguese Hospital between 2002 and 2006. In this retrospective study, 47% of patients had AKI (defined by the RIFLE criteria) during the intensive care unit (ICU) stay.

3. Risk factors of AKI in hospitalized HIV-infected patients

In the HAART era, clinical conditions commonly associated with increased risk of AKI in the general population such as older age, Male, Black race, diabetes, prior hypertension, liver disease and pre-existing chronic kidney disease have also been reported as independent risk factors of AKI in hospitalized HIV-infected patients [15,16,17] (Table 1). Accordingly, renal function should be closely monitored during the hospitalization, and an adequate control of glycemia and blood pressure as well as the appropriate management of patients with acute or chronic liver insufficiency and/or chronic kidney disease could prevent the occurrence of AKI.

	N	Design	Setting	Year of hospitalization	Definition of AKI	Incidence of AKI	Risk factors of AKI	Mortality (AKI versus non-AKI)
Wyatt et al [15]	25.114	Retrospective, multicenter	Hospitalized	2003	Code 584 of the ICD-9	6%	Age (per year above mean) (adjusted OR 1.03, 95% CI, 1.02-1.04), Male (adjusted OR 1.16, 95% CI 1.04-1.30), diabetes mellitus (adjusted OR 1.27, 95% CI 1.08-1.49), chronic kidney disease (adjusted OR 5.48, 95% CI 4.58-6.56), liver disease (adjusted OR 1.59, 95% CI 1.40-1.79)	In-hospital mortality [27% versus 4.5% (adjusted OR 5.83; 95% CI, 5.11-6.65, $P<0.0001$)]
Lopes et al [16]	489	Retrospective, single-center	Hospitalized	2005-2007	↑> 1.5X SCr or ↑ SCr $\geq$0.5mg (if baseline SCr >4mg/dl)	18%	Pre-existing hypertension (adjusted OR 2.4, 95% CI 1.04-5.6, P=0.04), AIDS (adjusted OR 2.7, 95% CI 1.2-6, P=0.02), sepsis (adjusted OR 23, 95% CI 11-45.3, $P<0.001$), and nephrotoxic drugs administration (adjusted OR 2.8, 95% CI 1.4-5.8, P=0.004)	In-hospital mortality [27.3% versus 8% (adjusted OR 2.7, 95% CI 1.3-5.6, P=0.008)]
Lopes et al [17]	97	Retrospective, single-center	Intensive care unit	2002-2006	↑> 1.5X SCr or ↑ SCr $\geq$0.5mg (if baseline SCr >4mg/dl)	47%	Age >60 years (adjusted OR 5.32, 95% CI 1.23-23, P=0.025), HCV co-infection (adjusted OR 3.42, 95% CI 1.08-10.85, P=0.037), SAPS II >50 (adjusted OR 2.35, 95% CI 1.2-5.9, P=0.008)	60-day mortality (65% versus 24%, $P<0.0001$)

Table 1. Studies reporting the incidence, risk factors and mortality of acute kidney injury in the highly active antiretroviral therapy era. AKI- acute kidney injury. ICD-9- International Classification of Diseases, 9th Revision. OR- odds ratio. CI- confidence interval. HCV- hepatitis C virus. SCr- serum creatinine. AIDS- Acquired Immunodeficiency Syndrome. SAPS II- Simplified Acute Pathophysiology Score version II.

Hepatitis C virus co-infection has also been associated with increased risk for AKI (Table 1). Hepatitis C virus co-infection is an increasingly important cause of morbidity and mortality in patients with HIV [2], and affects approximately 30% of HIV-infected individuals [21]. Studies have demonstrated that co-infection with HIV and HCV translates into higher morbidity and mortality related to end-stage liver disease [22]. A recent meta-analysis of 27 studies including data of more than 18.000 HIV-infected patients has also demonstrated that HCV co-infection was associated with an increased risk of AKI by 64% [23]. Therefore, the association between HCV co-infection and risk for acute and chronic kidney disease supports existing guidelines for the diagnosis and management of kidney disease in patients with HIV [5].

Only two studies have specifically analyzed the etiology of AKI in hospitalized HIV-infected patients [16,17]. In the study of Lopes et al [16], the etiology of AKI was multifactorial in 48.9% of patients. The most common etiologies of AKI in this cohort were sepsis (59%), nephrotoxic drugs administration (i.e. aminoglycosides, amphotericine B, vancomycin, acyclovir, gancyclovir and foscarnet) (37.5%), volume depletion (21.6%), and use of radiocontrast (20.5%). Other less common causes of AKI were tumour lysis syndrome, hemorrhage, acute urinary tract obstruction and thrombotic microangiopathy. In the ICU setting, Lopes et al [17] have also identified sepsis as the most common cause of AKI (86%) in HIV-infected patients. Therefore, prompt recognition and aggressive treatment of sepsis, adequate hydration, avoidance and serum monitoring of nephrotoxic drugs, and prophylaxis of contrast induced nephropathy could be important in diminishing the occurrence of AKI in this population [24,25].

The influence of HIV-related variables namely type of HIV, HAART, CD4 lymphocyte count, viral load and AIDS diagnosis in the development of AKI in hospitalized HIV-infected patients still remains to be established. In fact, only one study has attempted to study the impact of those variables on renal function in hospitalized HIV-infected patients [16]. In this study, only AIDS-defining conditions were independently associated with AKI and none association was found with type of HIV, HAART, CD4 lymphocyte count and viral load. However, the limited number of studied patients did not allow the authors to conclude definitively about the influence of those variables in the development of AKI. Therefore, prospective and randomized studies with a large number of patients are still warranted to better determine the precise impact of those HIV-related variables on renal function among HIV-infected patients who are hospitalized.

4. Impact on outcome of AKI in hospitalized HIV-infected patients

Acute kidney injury is a risk factor for short- and long-term mortality, and there is a graded relationship between severity of AKI and increased mortality [26,27,28,29,30,31,32]. The mechanism by which AKI contributes to increased mortality is not completely understood. Volume overload, coagulation abnormalities, an increased incidence of sepsis with multi-organ failure, and cytokine or immunemediated major organ dysfunction are other possible explanations for poor survival among AKI patients. The permanent injury to other vital organs caused by AKI, although the potential reversible nature of clinical AKI, in which serum creatinine can return to baseline after the acute episode, could account for decreased long-term survival of patients who developed AKI [33,34,35]. Moreover, CKD disease with subsequent hypertension, proteinuria and increased cardiovascular disease has been appointed as a possible cause of poor long-term outcome among AKI patients [36].

The development of AKI during the hospitalization also portends an ominous outcome among HIV-infected patients (Table 1). In the study of Wyatt et al [15], hospitalizations of HIV-infected patients that were complicated by AKI were also complicated by much higher in-hospital mortality that seen in admissions of HIV-infected patients without AKI and, furthermore, AKI independently increased in-hospital mortality of those patients. In the study of Lopes et al [16], the development of AKI was associated with lengthened time of hospitalization and increased in-hospital mortality. In fact, patients who developed AKI within the hospitalization had higher in-hospital mortality than those patients who did not develop AKI. After adjusting for other covariates, AKI still remained associated with increased in-hospital mortality. Furthermore, there was a relationship between more severe AKI and increased in-hospital mortality. In critically ill HIV-infected patients [17], AKI has also been associated with increased mortality, and there was a graded relationship between AKI severity and mortality.

The detrimental impact of AKI on patient outcome seems to persist after hospital discharge even in those patients who exhibit renal function recovery. Recently, Choi et al [17] conducted an observational cohort study in a national sample of 17.325 HIV-infected persons receiving care in the Veterans Health Administration who survived at least 90 days after discharge from their first hospitalization to examine the association between AKI experienced during their first hospitalization with the development of heart failure, atherosclerotic cardiovascular events, end-stage renal disease (ESRD), and death over a period of 2 decades. They found a graded and independent association between severity of AKI with heart failure, cardiovascular disease, ESRD, and death.

5. Conclusions

Acute kidney injury is a common complication in hospitalized HIV-infected patients in the HAART era. Older patients, Male, Black race patients, diabetic and /or hypertensive patients and patients with pre-existing chronic kidney disease, HCV co-infection and/or liver disease are at increased risk for AKI within the hospitalization and, therefore, renal function should be closely monitored in those patients. Sepsis is the most common etiology of AKI in this setting and should be promptly diagnosed and treated. The occurrence of AKI is associated with both increased short- and long-term mortality. Therefore, prevention of AKI should be an important task to accomplish in order to improve morbidity and mortality in this specific population.

6. References

[1] UNAIDS. UNAIDS/WHO AIDS Epidemic Update: December 2009, 2009

[2] Selik RM, Byers RH Jr, Dworkin MS. Trends in diseases reported on U.S. death certificates that mentioned HIV infection, 1987-1999. *J Acquir Immune Defic Syndr.* 2002;29:378-387

[3] Krentz HB, Kliewer G, Gill MJ. Changing mortality rates and causes of death for HIV-infected individuals living in Southern Alberta, Canada from 1984 to 2003. *HIV Med.* 2005;6:99-106

[4] Palella FJ Jr, Baker RK, Moorman AC, et al. Mortality in the highly active antiretroviral therapy era: changing causes of death and disease in the HIV outpatient study. *J Acquir Immune Defic Syndr.* 2006;43:27-34

[5] Gupta SK, Eustace JA, Winston JA, et al. Guidelines for the management of chronic kidney disease in HIV-infected patients: recommendations of the HIV Medicine Association of the Infectious Diseases Society of America. *Clin Infect Dis.* 2005;40:1559-1585

[6] Szczech LA, Hoover DR, Feldman JG, et al. Association between renal disease and outcomes among HIV-infected women receiving or not receiving antiretroviral therapy. *Clin Infect Dis.* 2004;39:1199-1206

[7] Fine DM, Atta MG. Kidney disease in the HIV-infected patient. *AIDS Patient Care STDS.* 2007;21:813-824

[8] Wyatt CM, Winston JA, Malvestutto CD, et al. Chronic kidney disease in HIV infection: an urban epidemic. *AIDS.* 2007;21:2101-2103

[9] Fine DM, Perazella MA, Lucas GM, et al. Renal disease in patients with HIV infection: epidemiology, pathogenesis and management. *Drugs.* 2008;68:963-980

[10] Franceschini N, Napravnik S, Eron JJ Jr, et al. Incidence and etiology of acute renal failure among ambulatory HIV-infected patients. *Kidney Int.* 2005;67:1526-1531

[11] Ibrahim F, Claire Naftalin C, Cheserem E, et al. Immunodeficiency and renal impairment are risk factors for HIV-associated acute renal failure. *AIDS.* 2010,24:2239-2244

[12] Valeri A, Neusy AJ. Acute and chronic renal disease in hospitalized AIDS patients. *Clin Nephrol.* 1991;35:110-118

[13] Rao TK, Friedman EA. Outcome of severe acute renal failure in patients with acquired immunodeficiency syndrome. *Am J Kidney Dis.* 1995;25:390-398

[14] Peraldi MN, Maslo C, Akposso K, et al. Acute renal failure in the course of HIV infection: a single institution retrospective study of ninety-two patients and sixty renal biopsies. *Nephrol Dial Transplant.* 1999;14:1578-158

[15] Wyatt CM, Arons RR, Klotman PE, et al. Acute renal failure in hospitalized patients with HIV: risk factors and impact on in-hospital mortality. *AIDS.* 2006;20:561-565

[16] Lopes JA, Fernandes J, Jorge S, et al. Acute renal failure in critically ill HIV-infected patients. *Crit Care.* 2007;11:404

[17] Choi AI, Li Y, Parikh C, et al. Long-term clinical consequences of acute kidney injury in the HIV-infected. *Kidney Int.* 2010;78:478-485

[18] Lopes JA, Melo MJ, Viegas A, et al. Acute kidney injury in hospitalized HIV-infected patients: a cohort analysis. *Nephrol Dial Transplant.* 2011 May 4. [Epub ahead of print]

[19] Bellomo R, Ronco C, Kellum JA, et al. Acute renal failure - definition, outcome measures, animal models, fluid therapy and information technology needs: the Second International Consensus Conference of the Acute Dialysis Quality Initiative (ADQI) Group. *Crit Care*. 2004;8:R204

[20] Waikar SS, Wald R, Chertow GM, et al. Validity of International Classification of Diseases, Ninth Revision, Clinical Modification Codes for Acute Renal Failure. *J Am Soc Nephrol*. 2006;17:1688-1694

[21] Alter MJ. Epidemiology of viral hepatitis and HIV co-infection. *J Hepatol*. 2006;44:S6-S9

[22] Graham CS, Baden LR, Yu E, et al. Influence of human immunodeficiency virus infection on the course of hepatitis C virus infection: a meta-analysis. *Clin Infect Dis*. 2001;33:562-569

[23] Wyatt CM, Malvestutto C, Coca SG, et al. The impact of hepatitis C virus coinfection on HIV-related kidney disease: a systematic review and meta-analysis. *AIDS*. 2008;22:1799-807

[24] Dellinger RP, Levy MM, Carlet JM, et al. Surviving Sepsis Campaign international guidelines for management of severe sepsis and septic shock: 2008. *Crit Care Med*. 2008;36:296-327

[25] Venkataraman R. Can we prevent acute kidney injury? *Crit Care Med*. 2008;36 (4 Suppl):S166-S171

[26] Hoste EA, Clermont G, Kersten A, et al. RIFLE criteria for acute kidney injury are associated with hospital mortality in critically ill patients: a cohort analysis. *Crit Care*. 2006;10:R73

[27] Bagshaw SM, Laupland KB, Doig CJ, et al. Prognosis for long-term survival and renal recovery in critically ill patients with severe acute renal failure: a population-based study. *Crit Care*. 2005;9:R700-709

[28] Lopes JA, Jorge S, Resina C, et al. Acute kidney injury in patients with sepsis: a contemporary analysis. *Int J Infect Dis*. 2009;13:176-181

[29] Lopes JA, Fernandes P, Jorge S, et al. Long-term risk of mortality after acute kidney injury in patients with sepsis: a contemporary analysis. *BMC Nephrol*. 2010;11:9

[30] Parikh CR, Coca SG, Wang Y, et al. Long-term prognosis of acute kidney injury after acute myocardial infarction. *Arch Intern Med*. 2008;168:987-995

[31] Covic A, Schiller A, Mardare NG, et al. The impact of acute kidney injury on short-term survival in an Eastern European population with stroke. *Nephrol Dial Transplant*. 2008;23:2228-2234

[32] Tsagalis G, Akrivos T, Alevizaki M, et al. Long-term prognosis of acute kidney injury after first acute stroke. *Clin J Am Soc Nephrol*. 2009;4:616-622

[33] Kelly KJ. Distant effects of experimental renal ischemia/reperfusion injury. *J Am Soc Nephrol*. 2003;14:1549-1558

[34] Hassoun HT, Lie ML, Grigoryev DN, et al. Kidney ischemia-reperfusion injury induces caspase-dependent pulmonary fibrosis. *Am J Physiol Renal Physiol*. 2009;1:F125-137

[35] Li X, Hassoun HT, Santora R, et al. Organ crosstalk: the role of the kidney. *Curr Opin Crit Care*. 2009;15:481-487

[36] Tonelli M, Wiebe N, Culleton B, et al. Chronic kidney disease and mortality risk: a systematic review. *J Am Soc Nephrol*. 2006;17:2034-2047

Permissions

The contributors of this book come from diverse backgrounds, making this book a truly international effort. This book will bring forth new frontiers with its revolutionizing research information and detailed analysis of the nascent developments around the world.

We would like to thank Fyson H. Kasenga, MPH, PhD, for lending his expertise to make the book truly unique. He has played a crucial role in the development of this book. Without his invaluable contribution this book wouldn't have been possible. He has made vital efforts to compile up to date information on the varied aspects of this subject to make this book a valuable addition to the collection of many professionals and students.

This book was conceptualized with the vision of imparting up-to-date information and advanced data in this field. To ensure the same, a matchless editorial board was set up. Every individual on the board went through rigorous rounds of assessment to prove their worth. After which they invested a large part of their time researching and compiling the most relevant data for our readers. Conferences and sessions were held from time to time between the editorial board and the contributing authors to present the data in the most comprehensible form. The editorial team has worked tirelessly to provide valuable and valid information to help people across the globe.

Every chapter published in this book has been scrutinized by our experts. Their significance has been extensively debated. The topics covered herein carry significant findings which will fuel the growth of the discipline. They may even be implemented as practical applications or may be referred to as a beginning point for another development. Chapters in this book were first published by InTech; hereby published with permission under the Creative Commons Attribution License or equivalent.

The editorial board has been involved in producing this book since its inception. They have spent rigorous hours researching and exploring the diverse topics which have resulted in the successful publishing of this book. They have passed on their knowledge of decades through this book. To expedite this challenging task, the publisher supported the team at every step. A small team of assistant editors was also appointed to further simplify the editing procedure and attain best results for the readers.

Our editorial team has been hand-picked from every corner of the world. Their multi-ethnicity adds dynamic inputs to the discussions which result in innovative outcomes. These outcomes are then further discussed with the researchers and contributors who give their valuable feedback and opinion regarding the same. The feedback is then collaborated with the researches and they are edited in a comprehensive manner to aid the understanding of the subject.

Apart from the editorial board, the designing team has also invested a significant amount of their time in understanding the subject and creating the most relevant covers. They scrutinized every image to scout for the most suitable representation of the subject and create an appropriate cover for the book.

The publishing team has been involved in this book since its early stages. They were actively engaged in every process, be it collecting the data, connecting with the contributors or procuring relevant information. The team has been an ardent support to the editorial, designing and production team. Their endless efforts to recruit the best for this project, has resulted in the accomplishment of this book. They are a veteran in the field of academics and their pool of knowledge is as vast as their experience in printing. Their expertise and guidance has proved useful at every step. Their uncompromising quality standards have made this book an exceptional effort. Their encouragement from time to time has been an inspiration for everyone.

The publisher and the editorial board hope that this book will prove to be a valuable piece of knowledge for researchers, students, practitioners and scholars across the globe.

List of Contributors

Ali Mirzazadeh
Regional Knowledge Hub for HIV/AIDS Surveillance, Kerman University of Medical Sciences, Kerman, Iran
HIV/AIDS & Communicable Disease Unit, WHO Representative Office, Tehran, Iran

Saharnaz Nedjat
School of Public Health, Knowledge Utilization Research Center, Tehran University of Medical Science, Iran

Rupali Kotwal Doshi, Carlos del Rio and Vincent C. Marconi
Emory University School of Medicine and Rollins School of Public Health, United States

Dominique Berger
PAEDI, EA 4281, Claude Bernard University - Lyon 1 – IUFM, France

Zitha Mokomane and Mokhantšo Makoae
Human Sciences Research Council of South Africa, South Africa

Ali A. Al-Jabri
1Head of Immunology Division, Department of Microbiology and Immunology, College of Medicine and Health Sciences, Sultan Qaboos University, Muscat, Oman

Abdullah A. Balkhair
Head of Infectious Diseases Unit, Department of Medicine, Sultan Qaboos University Hospital,Muscat, Oman

Mohammed S. Al-Balosh and Sidgi S. Hasson
Department of Microbiology and Immunology, College of Medicine and Health Sciences, Sultan Qaboos University, Muscat, Oman

Fabio Buelli and Francesco Castelli
Institute for Infectious and Tropical Diseases, University of Brescia, Brescia, Italy

Fabio Buelli, Virginio Pietra, Richard Fabian Schumacher, Salvatore Pignatelli and Francesco Castelli
Medicus Mundi Italy, Brescia, Italy

Virginio Pietra, Jacques Simpore and Salvatore Pignatelli
St. Camille Medical Center, Ouagadougou, Burkina Faso

Richard Fabian Schumacher
University Children's Hospital, Brescia, Italy

Fabio Buelli
Ph.D. in Appropriate Methods and Technologies for International Development Co-operation, University of Brescia (A. Archetti Fund), Italy

Elvira Ivanova and Nadezhda Shmagel
Perm Regional AIDS Center, Russian Federation

Natalia Vorobeva
Vagner Perm State Academy of Medicine, Russian Federation

Subra Caroline, Burelout Chantal, Proulx Sophie, Simard Sébastien and Gilbert Caroline
Centre de Recherche en Rhumatologie et Immunologie (CRRI), Département de Médecine, Faculté de Médecine, Université Laval, Québec, Canada

Fiona T. van den Berg and Marc S. Weinberg
Antiviral Gene Therapy Research Unit (AGTRU), University of the Witwatersrand, South Africa

Georgy A. Nevinsky
Institute of Chemical Biology and Fundamental Medicine of SD of RAS, Russia

E. Castellanos-Velasco
Facultad de Ciencias, Electrónica, Universidad Autónoma de San Luis Potosí, San Luis Potosí, S.L.P., Mexico

J. Sants-Feorreira
Centro Universitário do Leste de Minas Gerais, Campus Coronel Fabriciano-M.G., Programa de Mestrado em Engenharia Industrial, Minas Gerais, Brasil

Norah L. Katende-Kyenda
Walter Sisulu University, Department of Pharmacology, P Bag X 1, Mthatha, South Africa

Donald R. Branch
Department of Medicine, University of Toronto, Canada

Clifford A. Lingwood and Donald R. Branch
Department of Laboratory Medicine and Pathobiology, University of Toronto, Canada

Clifford A. Lingwood
Department of Biochemistry, University of Toronto, Canada
Research Institute, Hospital for Sick Children, Toronto, Ontario, Canada

Donald R. Branch
Division of Cell and Molecular Biology, Toronto General Research Institute, Canada
Research and Development, Canadian Blood Services, Toronto, Ontario, Canada

Pedro Amariles and Newar Giraldo Alzate
University of Antioquia, Medellin, Colombia

Maria Jose Faus
University of Granada, Granada, Spain

Flávia Chiva Carvalho and Maria Palmira Daflon Gremião
School of Pharmaceutical Sciences, State University of São Paulo, UNESP, Araraquara, Brazil

Rubiana Mara Mainardes
State University of West-Center, UNICENTRO, Guarapuava, Brazil

José António Lopes and Sofia Jorge
Department of Nephrology and Renal Transplantation, Hospital de Santa Maria, Centro Hospitalar Lisboa Norte, Lisboa, Portugal

The ESTHER-Brescia Study Group

www.ingramcontent.com/pod-product-compliance
Ingram Content Group UK Ltd.
Pitfield, Milton Keynes, MK11 3LW, UK
UKHW022206051026
15624UKWH00001B/20

9 781632 412553